Bob Lyon
USD
1978

DAN LENNEN

ABOUT THE COVER

Man and one aspect of his besieged environment are shown in color thermo-grams—"thermal images" or "heat maps"—in which the different colors portray different surface temperatures. The full range, from coldest to hottest, is black, blue, green, yellow, orange, and red.

Thermography is useful in detecting and diagnosing various medical conditions, including strokes and other vascular damage, breast cancer, and arthritis. For although a thermogram shows only skin surface temperatures, these reflect blood circulation and other cellular activity beneath the skin. In the center thermogram, for example, the hand on the left is cooler than the one on the right because of its poorer circulation.

The top and bottom pictures are parts of a thermogram of a section of the Con-necticut River at the site of a large industrial plant. Heated waste water from the plant is discharged into the river and appears here in the "warm" colors. Ecologists are concerned about the effects of such industrial "thermal pollution" on the life processes of fishes and on the ecological balance of all aquatic life. (Thermograms courtesy Barnes Engineering Company, Stamford, Connecticut.)

Health:
man in a changing environment

ABOUT THE AUTHOR

Benjamin A. Kogan received his M.D. from Wayne State University College of Medicine and his M.S.P.H. and Dr.P.H. from the University of Michigan. He is Director of the Bureau of Medical Services of the County of Los Angeles Health Department. An experienced classroom teacher, Dr. Kogan holds the following appointments: Associate Clinical Professor of Community Medicine and Public Health, University of Southern California School of Medicine; Lecturer in Health Science, San Fernando Valley State College; Lecturer in Public Health, University of California at Los Angeles; Lecturer in Public Health, California State College at Los Angeles; Lecturer in Preventive Medicine, University of California at Irvine, College of Medicine. Dr. Kogan has made frequent television appearances and has written a number of articles on public health.

BENJAMIN A. KOGAN, M.D., Dr. P.H.

HEALTH

man in a changing environment

HARCOURT, BRACE & WORLD, INC.

New York   Chicago   San Francisco   Atlanta

The following anatomical drawings are by Zena Bernstein: Chapter 4 (Figure 5, left), Chapter 7 (Figures 7, 9, 10b, 11, 16, 20, 21), Chapter 8 (Figures 2, 3, 8, 10, 11, 15), Chapter 9 (Figures 6, 7), Chapter 12 (Figure 9), Chapter 13 (Figures 4, 6, 7, 9, 10, 11).

ISBN: 0-15-535580-5

Library of Congress Catalog Card Number: 78-113709

Printed in the United States of America

ACKNOWLEDGMENTS AND COPYRIGHTS
The author wishes to thank the companies and persons listed below for permission to use material in this book.

TEXTUAL MATERIAL AND TABLES
American Cancer Society, Inc., for Table 7-1, "Cancer: The Casualty Figures, Warning Signals, and Safeguards," from the American Cancer Society, *1970 Cancer Facts and Figures.* Reprinted by permission of the American Cancer Society.

E. W. R. Best, for Table 12-5, "Causes of Death of Current Male Cigarette Smokers," adapted from E. W. R. Best et al., "Summary of a Canadian Study of Smoking and Health," *Canadian Medical Association Journal,* Vol. 96 (April 15, 1967), p. 1104.

Acknowledgments and copyrights for further textual material and tables and for illustrations continue on page 619.

This book is for my parents
as well as for Barbara and Ellen

Preface

Man is in trouble. He is trapped in the web of his own technological triumphs. Never before has he known so much of both his inner mechanisms and his outer world. Yet never before has he been so oppressed by the imbalances between them. Since ecological balance is essential to human health, people need to know what is causing ecological imbalance. They must seek and find ways of achieving harmony between their slowly changing inner environment and their rapidly changing outer environment. This is the central and recurring theme of this book.

And so, the study of man's inner and outer ecosystems has been the guiding principle in the very structure of this health book. The first two chapters explore the meanings of health and relate them to ecology. But ecology includes more than human interrelationships with other living communities, whether plant or animal. Human ecology also encompasses the kaleidoscopic facets of human culture. The next two chapters (Chapters 3 and 4) describe some of the imbalances between man's internal and external environments. Whether it is noise pollution disturbing the cilia of the hair cells of the inner ear, or air pollution interfering with the cilia of the respiratory tract, the threat of the accumulating poisons of this plundered planet is presented to the student as his urgent business. Chapter 5 traces the historical course of disease (particularly plague), and the impact of individual illness (particularly Napoleon's) on history. Disease has twisted human destiny, and the past provides lessons for the future. The survey of communicable diseases in Chapter 6 is designed to continue this sense of the past with a view of the future. However, the major microscopic threats in the present ecosystem, as well as practical ways of meeting them, are covered.

This same concern with a relevant view of health and illness underlies Chapters 7 and 8, which are concerned with body structure and function and chronic impairments to them. Heart disease and cancer receive particular attention, although other major chronic ailments such as asthma, arthritis, and diabetes are not neglected. Still again, whether the problem is the stress contributing to heart disease or viruses involved in cancers, the approach is ecological. Here, as elsewhere, the facts of anatomy and physiology are described not in isolation but in the context of the meaningful problems and challenges today. Nourishment (Chapter 9) is also seen as both a process and a practical problem to be solved. Chapters 10 and 11 explore man's personality development and the range of his anxieties as they relate to his environment. The range is wide, yet the components are intertwined. Whether the subject is the working mother or campus unrest, health aspects are present and are examined.

In the long chapter on drugs, Chapter 12, a special effort has been made to provide up-to-date scientific information about an ill-understood area. Inconclusive data is so labeled. For example, as 1969 drew to a close, two separate issues of a national medical journal published the results of some drug research. One careful investigation, conducted at the National Institutes of Health, reported on the effects of LSD on human chromosomes. The results showed no effect. The other paper detailed twelve clinical cases of marihuana-induced psychoses diagnosed among U.S. soldiers in Vietnam. Both findings are in this book. They are included, however, with the caution that the final decision about the effect of LSD on human chromosomes has yet to be made, and that marihuana-induced psychoses are rarely reported in this country. The known hazards associated with the use of these and other drugs are explicitly detailed; but opinionated comment is not needed and unsubstantiated statements are avoided.

Chapter 13 is concerned with overpopulation problems and reproduction. These two are hardly more separable than are overpopulation and pollution. Chapter 14 explores the significance of courtship and premarital sex. The marriage chapter (Chapter 15) includes a discussion of the physiology of sexuality; it has, however, purposefully been preceded by a consideration of the meaning and arts of mutuality and love. Recent progress is presenting humankind with previously unimaginable opportunities and dilemmas. The genetic ecosystem is considered in Chapter 16, along with the development of the human embryo. The hazards of the intrauterine environment are explained, as are modern methods of decreasing them. The final chapter emphasizes a paradox: modern health miracles occur daily but in the midst of the enduring misery of millions for whom miracles have no reality. Here the role of the individual, organized with other individuals in the pursuit of health for all, is examined. The book opens with a question: "What is health?" It ends with a question: "Health—whose responsibility?" Answers are, it is hoped, provided.

A basic feature of this book is the great number of sources upon which it draws. This is inevitable. The subject matter of health is broad, sometimes controversial, and always subject to change as new discoveries are made. Only by consulting the vast literature of the biological and medical sciences can one hope to present an accurate account of what is and is not known. Moreover, the extensive footnotes provide the student with a bibliography for further study. But the book also draws heavily on the humanities and social sciences. Education, no less than health or life itself, must have unity. The student of health is simultaneously a student of economics, religion, ancient and modern literature and history, political science, anthropology, and other disciplines. If health is part of the rich fabric of life, it follows that it is part of the fabric of all aspects of education.

Space permits mention of only a few of those who helped with this book. Gerald A. Heidbreder, M.D., the Health Officer of the County of

Los Angeles, and a teacher, was a constant source of encouragement. The support of members of his staff, particularly that of Maxwell Rosenblatt, M.D., and Mr. Charles A. Norris, cannot be overestimated. Nor could this book have been written without Mrs. Ruby Pearson's enduring secretarial help. Dr. Helen Nakagawa, Assistant Professor of Nursing at the University of Washington School of Nursing, and Bernard Portnoy, M.D., Associate Professor of Pediatrics, Community Medicine, and Public Health at the University of Southern California School of Medicine, critically read the entire manuscript, as did Dr. John T. Fodor and L. H. Glass, Dr. P. H., Professors of Health Science at San Fernando Valley State College, Los Angeles. The support of the Chairman of Health Science of that college, Dr. Claude T. Cook, is deeply appreciated. John M. Leedom, M.D., Associate Professor of Medicine at the University of Southern California School of Medicine, was helpful with various aspects of the manuscript, particularly with those chapters dealing with chronic diseases, nourishment, and heredity. S. Douglas Frasier, M.D., Associate Professor of Pediatrics and Physiology at the University of Southern California School of Medicine, was of assistance with some of the material relating to the endocrine glands. Others who read sections of the manuscript are Dr. Deryck Calderwood, Consultant in Family Life and Sex Education; Marie A. Hinrichs, M.D., Medical Consultant, Department of Health Education, American Medical Association; Dr. Wayne H. Jepson, Director of the Office of Health-Related Programs, Illinois State University; Dr. Cyrus Mayshark, Associate Dean and Professor of Health Education, University of Tennessee College of Education; Dr. Ann E. Nolte, Associate Director, School Health Education Study; Dr. Oscar H. Paris, Associate Professor of Zoology, University of California at Berkeley; Dr. James G. Paulat, Professor and Director of Teacher Education, Sacramento State College; Mr. D. Allen Rude, Assistant Professor of Health Education, Foothill College; and Dr. Esther D. Schulz.

However, it is the author who must accept total responsibility for errors; corrections would be most gratefully appreciated.

BENJAMIN A. KOGAN

Contents

Health:
man in a changing environment

1

Health:
a fabric
richly woven

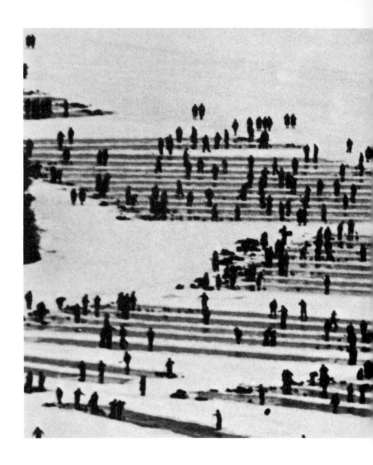

The scale of health

What is health? Is it visible? Is it seen as a gleaming smile, for example? Not to those Asians who chew betel nuts to blacken their teeth for beauty. Or is health felt? Many people feel well yet harbor infectious illness. Perhaps a formula, something short and magical, like $E = mc^2$, could define health. But formulae such as Einstein's equation apply best not to men but to things. Since there is no human equation, there is no health equation. Health is as complex as man, as variable as life. An attempt to define health within strict limits is as idle as to seek the mind in the dissecting laboratory. This is its encompassing problem, its endless fascination.

Among the many existing definitions of health, there is this famous one devised by the World Health Organization: health is "a state of complete physical, mental and social well-being and not merely the absence of disease or infirmity." In its positive approach this definition has virtue: it is uncompromising. The mere absence of disease or infirmity is indeed

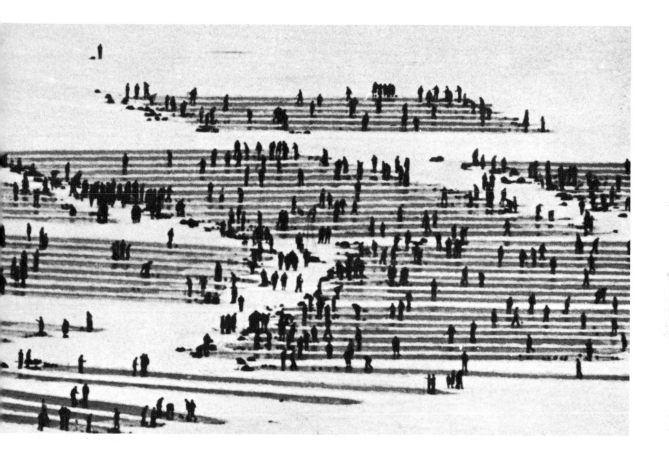

not enough for health. The statement is also inclusive: man is not healthy unto himself; man and health are both of culture and society and are reciprocally influenced by the mind.

But has the World Health Organization provided a realistic definition or an idealistic policy? Even though they labor for a Valhalla of health, WHO's most devoted workers (and they are legion) hardly expect to attain "complete physical, mental and social well-being" for everyone. They have given much, but they have not given a usable definition of health.

Any concept of health must be viewed as much with imagination as with words. Imagine, then, a scale or a ruler, of as yet unmeasured length. At one end of the scale is zero health (death); at the other end is perfect health, which as yet remains an unknown optimum. In developing this concept, Marston Bates points out that health is a "polar word" and "its meaning is relative only to some standard or scale."[1] Between the poles

[1] Marston Bates, "The Ecology of Health," in Iago Galdston, ed., *Medicine and Anthropology* (New York, 1959), p. 59.

of death and perfect health are the many gradations of health—the scale is a continuum along which living things constantly move and shift directions.

Stand back and watch someone living on the scale of health. His life is a series of constantly changing happenings. So long as he breathes, so long as his heart beats, so long as his cells multiply, so long does he constantly move on the health scale. His health, then, is a dynamic attribute of his life. From one moment to the next, it is never the same. Sometimes illness strikes. He moves toward the death end of the scale. Should he recover, he moves away from death—toward, but probably never reaching, perfect health.

An example? At about 6 A.M. one Sunday morning, a man who had been feeling below par develops a sudden shaking chill. At 10 A.M. the doctor is called. Within the hour he arrives. By that time the man has chilled violently half a dozen times. A sharp pain knifes his right chest. His slight cough produces a rusty-colored sputum. His breathing is labored. His oral temperature: 104°F. After examining the patient, the physician promptly hospitalizes him. X-ray and other studies quickly confirm the diagnosis: pneumonia. The man is perilously ill. He has been rapidly moving toward the death pole of the health scale. Apprehension fills his eyes.

Treatment is prompt. The patient is placed in an oxygen tent. Fluids are dripped into his veins. Antibiotics are administered. His doctor visits him several times every day. Nurses hover at his bedside. Efficiently they carry out the physician's directives. Slowly, the patient improves. He moves away from death toward a safer, healthier level on the scale. He regains his strength. Hopefully, brushing elbows with death has given him wisdom about living. He develops a good health regimen. He moves along the scale of health, approaching perfect health.

Things are never dull on the health scale. Something is always happening to every individual. It is affecting him and he is reacting to it individually. That is because each person is unique. Does this statement seem obvious? Actually it is neither understood nor accepted by everyone.

Health and the individual

All men are not created equal —in health "We hold these truths to be self-evident, that all men are created equal." These words are revered by the people of this nation and well they might be. Written in a passion for liberty, they still give the nation purpose in time of trial. There is only one thing wrong with them: they are not true. All men are not created equal. On the scale of health each human being is born to a particular place and pace. No two people occupy the same place. All have individual speeds. When one considers the infinite genetic variations that exist in the more than three billion inhabitants of the earth, the concept of equal birth becomes ludicrous. One infant, born a symphony of nerve and muscle, is destined to run the hundred-yard dash in nine seconds. Another, cruelly palsied, will find five feet an agony. One human being may be born a congenital idiot, the other a congenital genius.[2] Differences may be much more subtle than this, and the variations may be hardly noticeable. It is good that man is not created equal, for only duplicates are equal. Men want freedom for themselves, not duplicates of themselves. (What the founding fathers meant was that all men are equal in the eyes of a divine personality. So it followed that opportunity should be made equal for all. With equal opportunity, men could attain the high responsibilities of freedom.)

If man is born biologically unequal, then it follows that he is biologically individual. True, as a member of a species each man shares countless characteristics with other men. He is erect. His gut enables him to digest a variety of foods unheard of among other creatures. These characteristics, combined with his thumb and clever brain, empower him to rule all else that lives. Yet man also shares basic qualities with other animals, particularly the higher species. Kendeigh notes that "primitive man has few if any characteristics not also found in animals."[3] Like men, birds walk on two legs. A bird will care for its young in a fashion that in some respects is as highly developed as that of a human. A squirrel uses its hands to manipulate a nut or a banana. When they are at play, some animals laugh. The Galapagos finch uses a stick as a tool "to pry insect larvae out of holes of dead wood." These are but a few examples Kendeigh cites of human and animal activities that are similar.

There are others. On the little Japanese island of Koshima, for example, lives the fastidious macaque monkey (Figure 1-1). Dipping a sand-covered potato in the sea, he will busily scrub it with his paw. Not until he has carefully peeled the potato with his teeth will he eat it. Nor does he tolerate sand on his wheat. By putting sandy wheat grains into water he separates them. Wheat, he has learned, floats. It can be picked out clean from the water for eating. Man is distinguished from animals by culture, and culture is what man has learned. But at this point, the difference between man and macaque becomes slender indeed.

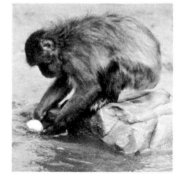

1-1 A fastidious and creative monkey.

Despite the broad scope of attributes shared by man and animals, there is room for the individual characteristics of each single varying creature. So it is that each man, as a biological individual, has health problems that must be considered individually.

This individuality explains why tissue transplants from one human to another are so difficult. For a transplant to succeed, profound changes, created and maintained in the recipient, are necessary. With few exceptions (such as transplants of the cornea of the eye), successful tissue transplants were, until recently, exceedingly rare. As yet, not even a

---

[2] It should not be inferred that either an innate difference or an innate equality in all people's intellectual capacity has been proved.

[3] Charles S. Kendeigh, "The Ecology of Man, the Animal," *Bioscience*, Vol. 15, No. 8 (August 1965), p. 521.

mother may donate skin to her burned child. But transplantation of skin from one part of a person's body to another part is successful.

Lower on the biological scale, tissue transplants are less difficult. Among mammals, the golden hamster is unique in that its cheek pouch will accept grafts not only from other hamsters but from many other creatures, including the frog. Skin from one frog may also be successfully grafted to any member of the same species. On a still lower level, different parts of certain worms may be grafted together as long as all the segments point in the same direction.[4] Two complete earthworms have even been successfully grafted together.

Viruses, which contain only materials for self-propagation, are at the bottom of the scale of "living things." Indeed, many experts place them in an intermediate position—between living creatures and nonliving things. They are composed of large molecules. Recently, scientists at the California Institute of Technology performed a remarkable experiment. They placed various parts of a number of viruses of the same type into a test tube. All of these viruses were genetically defective in some way. Some lacked genes to make heads, others had no genes for tails, still others had no "collar" genes, and so on. Mixing these incomplete viruses together in a test tube, the researchers were able to assemble a complete virus.[5] Compare this singular lack of individuality to the infinitely complex human being whose mother's skin will not stay grafted to him.

On the basis of individuality human beings occupy the top position on the biological scale. Variety is possible not only in such obvious external features as height, eye color, and bone structure but in internal organs as well. Studies[6] of the human stomach show its numerous normal variations in size and shape. The liver too varies greatly, yet normally, in size and shape. But what about the heart? Surely any deviation from a single heart structure would be fatal. Nonsense. Hearts vary so much in normal people that careful training and experience are needed to tell sick hearts from normal variations. No organ of any person is exactly like that of another person. It follows that the chemical functions of these organs differ from person to person. Human patterns of excretion, of glandular activity, of enzyme activity, and the very composition of the hair, skin, bone, stomach juices, saliva, and blood—all these vary from individual to individual.[7]

In sexual appetite enormous differences also exist. These are at least partly due to variations in such organs as the pituitary, sex, and adrenal glands. As one writer sees it:

According to one important measure, normal men—those who had been able to pass for normal—varied in their sex appetites by as

[4] Roger J. Williams, *Free and Unequal* (Austin, Tex., 1953), p. 15.
[5] *Science News*, Vol. 91, No. 15 (April 1967), p. 356.
[6] Roger J. Williams, *Biochemical Individuality* (New York, 1956), pp. 21–30.
[7] *Ibid.*, Chapter IV.

much as forty thousand fold. If "abnormals" were included, how great would the variation be? . . . when two men brought up in the same society differ in their sex activities by ten, one thousand, or ten thousand fold, there is bound to be something back of the variation besides what their mammas, or some naughty boy, told them.[8]

Realizing the normally wide variations of people should make one cautious about making hasty comparisons. The pointless comparisons that parents sometimes make between children is illustrated by the following series of events.

Recently a worried mother brought her seventeen-month-old baby daughter to their family physician. A sturdy child, she had not yet walked.

"She sits in the sun all day long," the mother fretted. "And everybody hits her."

The doctor bent to examine the child. "Everybody?" he asked slowly.

"That boy next door—the thin one . . . You delivered him too. Ten months ago."

The doctor gave the child a tongue blade to play with and cautiously looked into her ear. He nodded. "He's not thin."

"Well," the woman went on, "he's not weak, that's for sure. He's been walking for ten days. His mother says it's three weeks, but it's really ten days. And yesterday, he just loped up to my baby and stuck his finger in her eye."

The doctor straightened. "Her eyes are all right. What did she do?"

"What did she do? What could she do? She just sat there and screamed. When will she walk? She can't just sit there."

"Why not?" the doctor wanted to know. He was being irritating, and he knew it. "She'll walk when she's ready," he added. "She's perfectly normal. We just all do things differently. In due time, one day she'll get up and walk away in the sun. Just watch her."

Two weeks later the mother telephoned in excitement. The child had begun to walk a few moments before. Holding a toy wooden hammer, she had walked right up to that "kid" from next door. (He had just happened to be in the room.) "They'll be calling you about stitches," she said, and hung up.

Unfortunately, most parents do not fully realize the uniqueness of their child. Were they to do so, much pain for both child and parent could be avoided. Apparently, there is a certain embarrassment in being too different. Most people want to be a trifle different, but never beyond what is acceptable. To put it another way, they want to be acceptably extraordinary. In great measure, the desire to belong to a common group accounts for this.

[8]Roger J. Williams, *Free and Unequal*, p. 22.

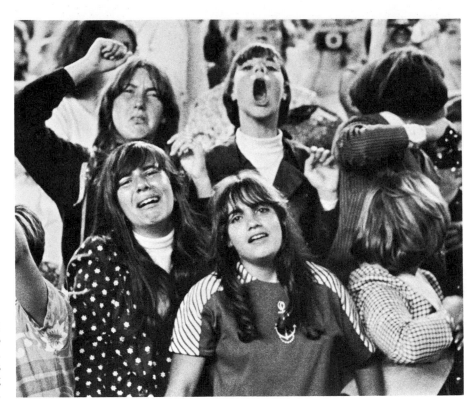

1-2 Each unique person reacts differently to the same stimulus. This group of teen-agers is responding to the Beatles.

But on the health scale there is no common man. Thus one should not attempt to enforce one's personal health ideas on anyone else. Most ideas of health are personal: writers of health rules usually write about themselves. Eight hours sleep may be what some people need. Many people get along beautifully on six. Some need ten. "Drink milk" is good advice for most people, but there are those who are sickened by milk; they may even be allergic to it. "I can't start the day without a good breakfast," one person insists. Another finds the thought of a heavy breakfast nauseating. A singularly predictable trait of man is his unpredictability.

Health rules should be taken with a grain of salt, and only if salt suits the taste. For effective living, health rules must allow for individuality. A hundred years ago Thoreau wrote in *Walden,* "If a man does not keep pace with his companions, perhaps it is because he hears a different drummer. Let him step to the music which he hears, however measured or far away." An old cockney story makes a similar point. Watching her soldier son marching in a company of recruits, a doting mother exclaimed proudly, "All out of step but Bill!" A poignant example both of human individuality and of the rich range within which a life can be lived under adverse health conditions is provided by the life of Mary Lamb, who grew to realize not only her limitations but also her potential. She was the gifted sister of the brilliant English essayist Charles Lamb. All their adult lives they lived together. Lamb wrote of her in his celebrated *Essays of Elia* (in which she appears as Bridget Elia):

> [*She*] *has been my housekeeper for many a long year, I have obligations to Bridget, extending beyond the period of memory. We house together, old bachelor and maid, in a sort of double singleness; with such tolerable comfort, upon the whole, that I, for one, find in myself no sort of disposition . . . to bewail my celibacy.*[9]

Mary Lamb conducted a gracious home for her celebrated brother, skillfully entertaining his literary friends. She wrote with grace, too, collaborating with her brother on the classic *Tales Founded on the Plays of Shakespeare* (1807). She also suffered tragically from insanity.

A careful study[10] has been made of her case. Briefly, it is as follows. Her first mental attack occurred when she was thirty. It lasted a month. Two years later she had her second attack, and during it, killed her beloved mother. Only the intervention of a close friend of the family, an attorney, saved her from prosecution. For the rest of her life, she was placed in the care of her brother.

She died at eighty-two, a respected figure in English literature. Never, in the forty years that he cared for her, did her brother forsake her. (He died at sixty-nine.) A slight irritability would warn them both of an attack of insanity. She would then be placed into the strait jacket they always carried with them or would be immediately taken to a hospital. During the fifty-two years of her illness, she was hospitalized at least thirty-eight times. Between the eighth and ninth hospitalizations (and between her forty-second and forty-fourth birthdays), she collaborated with her brother in writing the *Shakespeare Tales.*

Few facts about man are more enigmatic than his rhythms. In a study of biological rhythms,[11] Richter wrote of a Cambridge team that adjusted its schedule to the accumulation of water in the knee joints of its star player, whose illness occurred regularly every nine days and lasted for two or three days. This is a rather gross example; yet it is by means of his biological rhythms that man adapts to much of his changing environment and becomes synchronized and in harmony with it. Genetic messages may direct these rhythms. Recent research indicates that the basic timing mechanism may lie in the chemical structure of some of the cell's nuclear DNA. This timing mechanism is what is meant by an "inner biological clock." Its rhythm, integrated into every living cell, is part of the biological organization of the organism. Other research indicates the

Health and rhythm

[9]Charles Lamb, "The Last Essays of Elia," quoted from the essay "Mackery End, in Hertfordshire," in H. K. Russell, William Wells, and Donald A. Stauffer, eds., *Literature in English* (New York, 1948), p. 764.
[10]E. C. Ross, *The Ordeal of Bridget Elia, A Chronicle of the Lambs* (Norman, Okla., 1940).
[11]Curt Paul Richter, *Biological Clocks in Medicine and Psychiatry* (Springfield, Ill., 1965), p. 92.

additional presence of a natural time rhythm, an "outer cosmic clock," which is correlated with the relative position of earth, sun, and moon, as well as with other physical factors of the cosmos, such as cosmic radiation and magnetic fields.

Rhythm characterizes all life patterns. Whether rhythm is governed by the inner biological clock or the outer cosmic clock has become a question for avid research. That there is a relationship between the two seems indisputable. Raise a bean plant in darkness. Its leaves will develop no natural daily sleep movement. Expose it to but a flash of light. Natural sleep movement will be induced. Returned to darkness, the leaves then persist in elevating each day at the time of the single exposure. At sunrise the fiddler crab begins to blacken. In this way it is protected from both the sun's glare and its predators. At sunset its dark coat rapidly blanches to a cool silvery gray. Captured and kept in a dark room it maintains this gray color. These examples illustrate how closely all creature life is related to the universe. Man's rhythms are no less marked. There are the obvious rhythms of a beating heart, of walking, sleeping, breathing, loving. And there are the more subtly secret rhythms of body functions. Within a twenty-four-hour cycle, for example, a person's temperature may vary from 1 to 1.5 degrees Fahrenheit. In the late afternoon or early evening, the "normal" temperature (98.6°F. orally) is normally maximal, at 100.1°F. At four or five in the morning, it is normally minimal (97.6°F.). Rhythmical biological cycles that recur at approximately twenty-four-hour intervals are called *circadian*. Most people who travel by jet over several time zones in one day will testify to the fatigue (and even illness) resulting from interference with their timed cycles. A man leaves Chicago at 6 P.M. The flight takes nine hours, but he arrives in London at dawn. The English are having breakfast. For the Chicagoan it is bedtime. He may feel ill. How can he avoid this affront to his body rhythms? He can begin the trip rested. He should allow a day to adjust, or arrange to arrive before nightfall. He should avoid overeating.

Rhythm also characterizes the onset of labor and even birth.[12] For human beings, active during the day and resting at night, the peak frequency of the onset of labor is 1 A.M. and the peak of birth frequency is 3 A.M. to 4 A.M.

Even attacks of illness seem to occur in a rhythmic cycle. Asthmatic and heart attacks are more common at 4 A.M.[13] Epileptic fits have been found to occur on a periodic or rhythmic basis. Studies[14] of thousands of epileptics in England show that many patients tend to have an epileptic seizure at the same time every day. Many patients tend to have seizures between 6 A.M. and 7 A.M. or between 10 P.M. and midnight.

[12] "Biologic Rhythms," *Therapeutic Notes*, Vol. 74 (March–April 1947), p. 35.
[13] *Ibid.*
[14] G. M. Griffiths and J. T. Fox, "Rhythm in Epilepsy," cited in Curt Paul Richter, *Biological Clocks in Medicine and Psychiatry*, p. 60.

Were Mary Lamb's attacks rhythmic? Richter has written: "The attacks occurred with regularity over some periods, and with little regularity in others—possibly owing in part to failure of the records to show all the attacks."[15]

Periodicity has been observed among some patients with nervous diseases. For years Richter recorded a twenty-four-hour cycle in a hospitalized young female with Parkinson's disease[16] (also called "shaking palsy"). During the day, although her mind was clear, she suffered the symptoms of the illness. She was unable to walk, speak clearly, or write legibly. She endured severe rigidity and tremors of her legs and arms. This was her condition all day. Every evening, at 9 P.M., she suddenly became quite well. She could walk, eat, drink, write, and talk. For two or three hours she was thus remarkably improved. Then she would lapse into her state of symptoms to remain helpless until 9 P.M. the following evening.

Some mentally ill patients have been noted to be very abnormal for twenty-four hours, then, within a few minutes, to become normal for twenty-four hours, and then, again within a brief few moments, to revert to abnormalcy. Richter observed this kind of cycle in one patient for thirty years.[17] Such abnormal-normal transitions have occurred in certain patients in cycles ranging from a few days to as long as ten years.

Whether manifested normally or abnormally, creature rhythms remain utterly individual. The billions of cells in the human body function in a harmony (or disharmony) that is unique for each person. True, all men develop daytime and nighttime (and countless other) patterns. Nevertheless, those patterns vary endlessly from person to person. Each inner biological clock is set differently. The external cosmic clock, however, is the same for all people in the same locale. The established cosmic time patterns in Tokyo, for example, determine the external cosmic clock of all the residents of Tokyo. But people do not stay in one place. And, even when they do, their reactions to local time intervals are individual. At a certain time one person may feel rushed. This may cause his body temperature to rise. His heart rate may increase. Under the same circumstances another person may respond differently. Even in deep sleep, responses differ.

Every man maintains his own loom of life. Every man has his own patterned fabric of good health and disease. Yet these billions of different looms manufacture infinitely varying fabrics that must fit together into a functional harmony called mankind. And the same unified system of life exists not only between men but between him and all other life. Everything that lives has a rhythm that is synchronized with the individual rhythms of all that relates to it.

---

[15] Curt Paul Richter, *Biological Clocks in Medicine and Psychiatry*, pp. 60–61.
[16] *Ibid.*, p. 61.
[17] *Ibid.*

The complex rhythmic individuality of human beings should caution against total reliance on average health measurements. In proper perspective, averages are indispensable. Health workers use average measurements—such as height and weight, blood sugar content, and white cell counts—in a host of ways. However, many people do not fit into averages, nor may they be forced into them. For the average population, smog tolerance levels are valuable indices of whether the smog level is safe or not. But for those with severe chronic bronchitis the same level may be dangerous. They may become ill and even die before the average tolerance to smog is reached. Those who set legal tolerances for allowable smog levels must, then, set them low enough to protect the sick.

Sometimes nonaverage reactions are misleading. For example, most people undergoing a prolonged period of emotional deprivation soon show evidences of trauma. This has been commonly observed among those suffering intensive bombing or cruel imprisonment. The conscience of men is etched with the tragedies of the Spanish revolution, with the bombings of Hiroshima and Nagasaki, with Auschwitz. Yet, in the midst of such suffering, there have also been those, few it is true, who endured the suffering best. Their apparent fortitude lent strength to their brethren. However, closer observation often revealed that what was thought to be nobility in these people was really indifference. What served as a source of strength was in reality a sick inability to form and experience human attachments. Under normal conditions such cold alienation would have been considered mental illness. Here again one sees the treachery of applying averages to all men.

Man is individual, but neither man nor any other living creature moves along the scale of health alone. Life, health, sickness, recovery, and death are dynamically related episodes, shared by all that lives. But this sharing goes on in an all-inclusive environment. The environment molds, and, in turn, is molded, by all within it. To understand health one must be concerned with how man relates to his environment.

Ecology: a system of environmental checks and balances

Consider a community of giant redwoods in northern California. The trees are cathedral. Away from the choking freeways, a man can observe a hurrying ant and not feel like one. The quiet is so palpable that he does not think that much is happening there.

Yet, amidst the seeming serenity of the forest as much is happening as on the freeways. From its roots each tree must slake its thirst and feed its outermost bud. At the tree's top each leaf must find light or die. With silent ferocity, each tree competes with every other for life. In living together, however, trees better resist wind and water erosion. A dense grove of trees prevents fallen leaves from being blown away, thus helping to maintain soil moisture and nutrients. About the tree, on it, and in it are numberless forms of life similarly striving for existence, competing with and adapting to one another. "The community, as well as the individual organism, is 'something happening,'"[18] Clarke has written.

So it is with man within his community. He is not rooted to one place, of course, but, like the tree, he competes with the rest of life for his place in the sun. Swarming inside of him and outside of him are countless other organisms all competing, all adapting.

Marston Bates has distinguished these events quite simply as "skin-in" and "skin-out" biology.[19] This convenient distinction by no means implies that they are separable. What goes on outside the body influences what occurs inside. For example, the number of red cells in human blood will normally increase at high altitudes. The Aymara Indians, therefore, living in the Andes Mountains of Peru and Ecuador, have a normal red cell count of about eight million per cubic millimeter.[20] At sea level, the normal red cell count is four-and-a-half to five million. At that level, therefore, a red cell count of eight million would be distinctly abnormal. The barrel chests of the Aymaras, and other changes in their respiratory systems, help them to adapt to the thin mountain air. The sea level dweller, however, accustomed to a higher oxygen tension in the air, is grossly uncomfortable in the mountains. His work capacity is markedly reduced, as is his lung efficiency. There is some evidence of temporarily reduced fertility and a diminished ability to carry a fetus to term. Sixteenth-century Spaniards reported that in the high South American mining areas, the production of a live child by Spanish parents was almost unknown. So profoundly does Bates's "skin-out" environment influence what is "skin-in."

In discussing the environment, one is automatically involved in a major field of science—*ecology*. This word is derived from the Greek, *oikos* meaning "home" or "household," and *logos* meaning "discourse." It is the mutual interaction between living things and their environmental household that is of interest to the ecologist. A key word in his vocabulary is *ecosystem*, a term so new that it did not even appear in *Webster's Unabridged Dictionary* published just two decades ago. *Ecosystem* refers to the systematic, orderly combination or arrangement of living organisms mutually interacting with a shared environment. One may sharply define the area of an ecosystem even to the simplest unit of ecology. A single-celled bacterium thriving in the human gut has its own ecosystem. But the concept of an ecosystem may be wider. There are complex interrelationships between the bacterium and millions of other bacterial ecosystems within the gut. Nor could anyone deny a relationship between the bacterial ecosystems and those of their human hosts. So, innumerable ecosystems interrelated with one another can be distinguished. One may speak of the ecosystem of the Atlantic Ocean or of a man swimming in

---

[18] George L. Clarke, *Elements of Ecology* (New York, 1966), p. 16.
[19] Marston Bates, *The Forest and the Sea* (New York, 1960), p. 12.
[20] Jacques M. May, *The Ecology of Human Disease* (New York, 1958), p. 1.

it, or of a bacterium swimming in him. Ecosystems cannot be separated from one another. They are interdependent, and all within them is interdependent too. This concept of interdependence within the universe was movingly described more than half a century ago by the English poet Francis Thompson:

> All things by immortal power,
> Near or far,
> Hiddenly
> To each other linked are,
> That thou canst not stir a flower,
> Without troubling of a star.[21]

As the modern ecologist Frederick Sargent has written: "All living things are related to one another in societies and communities, and each organism is inexorably bound to its habitat. This interdependence is an essential characteristic of the ecosystem."[22] The ecosystem, then, is structured like a spider's web. In the coordination of the whole, each strand depends on its intimate connection with every other strand.

Nonhuman ecology: balance within two dimensions

Within any intact ecosystem, there is a constant pattern of cause (stimulus) and effect. Only *physical-biological* stimuli and effects operate within plant and animal ecosystems. At the root of all life is the green plant. Endlessly powered by the sun's physical energy, photosynthesis occurs within the leaves. The plant grows. Upon being eaten, it begins to decompose. With digestion and evacuation, it breaks down into simpler forms. The final products of plant decomposition contribute chemicals to the ecological cycle of food production. Should any stimulus disturb this interdependent balance between the physical and the biological aspects of the ecological cycle, changes would occur within the ecosystem in an attempt to achieve a new balance between these two dimensions. For an example of this process, consider a garden.

There are many ways to regard a garden. One may admire the delicate turn of a petal or an armored ladybug resting upon it. One patient Englishman looked even closer. While studying his own modest garden, he counted hundreds of different living species. In their harmonious garden environment they lived in ecological balance with one another. This does not mean they all survived their entire life span. Many, perhaps most, did not. However, in that orderly English garden community, no single species completely overran another. But were that garden to be permanently deprived of most of its sun, a profound ecological imbalance would

---

[21] Francis Thompson, "The Mistress of Vision," from *Complete Poetical Works of Francis Thompson,* Vol. XXII, (New York, 1900), p. 184.
[22] Frederick Sargent, "Weather Modifications and the Biosphere," *Technology Review,* Vol. 71, No. 5 (March 1969), p. 44.

result. Much life of the garden would die or leave. Yet, some plants and animals would prevail. Eventually, species needing less sun would begin to develop. Counterbalancing changes would be set in motion. In a now dimmer garden, a new ecological balance would be achieved. A new and shady ecosystem would have replaced the former sunny garden. But the principle of interrelatedness would remain unchanged.[23]

A question arises here. Does counterbalance always succeed in rectifying ecological imbalance? As a result of overwhelming ecological change, is there no possible cataclysm? In terms of life, ecological changes can indeed be cataclysmic. Ecosystems would still exist but the changes within them could exclude life. As will be seen, this is the core of man's environmental health problem. He must maintain his garden in an ecological balance that averts the threat of cataclysm and assures him the opportunities of the good life.

All life is imprisoned within the shared, weblike ecosystem. This creates for its inhabitants a life of paradox—of competition and dependency. Recall the pneumonia patient referred to previously. For the man's life to be saved, bacteria had to be killed. For life, life was sacrificed. Thus life and health for one species may spell disease and death for another. All living organisms are susceptible to parasitic invasion, and sometimes this invasion kills the host. This is all a part of the natural order. For the parasite (the bacterium that caused the pneumonia), human health was not only unnatural, it was fatal. Another bacterial victim is shown in Figure 1-3.

Clarke's reference to a distinguished study by Petrunkevitch unforgettably illustrates such a life and death relationship:

The biotic drama within the ecosystem

> *When the female of the giant wasp* Pepsis marginata *is ready for egg laying, she somehow locates a tarantula* Cryptopholis portoricia, *and explores it with her antennae to make sure that it is the correct species. The larvae of each species of wasp can be nourished by only one species of tarantula. Although the tarantula could easily kill the wasp, it does not do so, and makes little attempt to escape. After the wasp has dug a grave for its intended victim, she stings it, drags it into the grave, and lays a single egg, which she attaches to the abdomen of the paralyzed monster. At hatching the wasp larva is only a tiny fraction of the bulk of the tarantula, but, by the time it is ready for metamorphosis and independent life, it has consumed all the soft tissue of the giant spider.[24]*

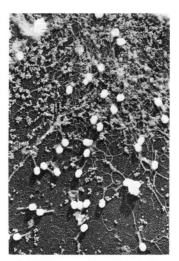

1-3 Debris of a bacterial cell victimized by the T2 virus. The viruses (the large round white objects) multiplied inside the host cell, dissolved its walls, and spilled out. (×23,850)

---

[23] In the case of the individual cell, the nature of this interrelationship is different. For the cell to survive, there must be a physical and chemical *imbalance* between the inner cell and its outer environment, causing nutrients to enter the cell and wastes to leave it. Nevertheless, this very imbalance makes possible ecological balance within and between cells.

[24] George L. Clarke, *Elements of Ecology*, p. 387.

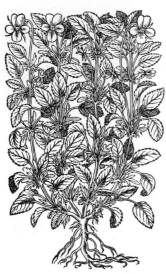

1-4 Heartsease.

There is still more to this biotic drama. The permanent paralysis, induced by the wasp sting, does not promptly kill the tarantula. Initially, it is a living but helpless recipient of the wasp's egg. Only later does it become a source of food for the larva. Instinct serves the wasp well but the tarantula poorly.

Still another example of the competitive interdependence of living creatures in the environment was provided by Darwin. He showed that the heartsease (Figure 1-4), a lovely wild pansy, could not be fertilized without the humblebee.[25] The humblebee was constantly threatened by field mice. The number of field mice depended on the number of available cats. The number of available cats, in turn, was dependent (this last association was not Darwin's) upon the number of cat lovers who kept cats. So, theoretically, the future of a pretty flower, such as the heartsease, depends on the inclination of some people to keep a cat!

But is ecological existence pure exploitation? By no means. The foraging Pederson shrimp (*Periclimenes pedersoni*) of the Bahamas, in taking food from a host fish, provides its host with a health-giving cleaning. Limbaugh writes:

> *When a fish approaches, the shrimp will whip its long antennae and sway its body back and forth. If the fish is interested, it will swim directly to the shrimp and stop an inch or two away. The fish usually presents its head or a gill cover for cleaning, but if it is bothered by something out of the ordinary such as an injury near its tail, it presents itself tail first. The shrimp swims or crawls forward, climbs aboard and walks rapidly over the fish, checking irregularities, tugging at parasites with its claws and cleaning injured areas. The fish remains almost motionless during this inspection and allows the shrimp to make minor incisions in order to get at subcutaneous parasites. As the shrimp approaches the gill covers, the fish opens each one in turn and allows the shrimp to enter and forage among the gills. The shrimp is even permitted to enter and leave the fish's mouth cavity. Local fishes quickly learn the location of these shrimp. They line up or crowd around for their turn and often wait to be cleaned when the shrimp has retired into the hole.*[26]

Symbiosis is the general term given to such close association of two dissimilar organisms. The results of this phenomenon range from mutual benefit to mutual destruction. There are occasions when symbiosis is essential for health. A mouse raised in a germ-free environment develops profound structural abnormalities of the digestive tract (Figure 1-5). If the mouse is brought into contact with proper bacteria, its anatomic abnormalities are quickly corrected.

[25]The heartsease has also been known as the wallflower; the derivation is, however, obscure.
[26]Conrad Limbaugh, "Cleaning Symbiosis," *Scientific American*, Vol. 205, No. 2 (August 1961), p. 42.

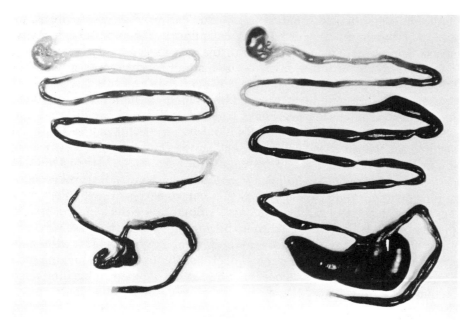

1-5 Symbiosis: microbe and mouse may need each other— normal (*left*) and germ-free (*right*) digestive tracts of mice.

As the giant wasp lives at the expense of the tarantula, as the heartsease needs the humblebee, as the Pederson shrimp relieves a fish of its parasites, as the mouse needs some germs to maintain health, so does man grow healthy and live in cooperation with or at the expense of a wide variety of living creatures. He consumes endless quantities of meat. Within his digestive tract are countless bacteria helping to maintain his health. Other bacteria he destroys with drugs. Both mammals and microbes may pay with their lives for man's ingenuous will to live. Or they may cooperate with man in a joint struggle for survival. With this in mind, still another aspect can be added to the bipolar health scale. All life on the scale is interrelated; the life of one species may depend either on the life or death of another. Frequently, the relationship is parasitic and exploitive; frequently, it is not. In this world man is not isolated. He peoples the "web of life" in plenty of company. Yet in one major respect man's ecosystem is unique. For all other life the ecosystem is comprised of two interrelated dimensions—physical and biological. Man's ecosystem, his web, is complicated and enriched by a third dimension—*culture.*

Unique to man, culture is the sum of what he has learned. It is the substance of that sum that differentiates him from all other life, giving him singular adaptive powers. Like all other living things, man is subject to physical and biological stimuli. But his culture permits their planned alteration and, therefore, changes their effects. Man's cultural processes may also operate independently of the physical or biological stimuli that instigated them.

To human ecology a third dimension is added: culture

Within the pneumonia patient, discussed earlier, there occurred a biological imbalance between his lung cells and a pneumonia-causing microbe. But it was only to the patient that this biological imbalance was a threat. For the invading microbes the man's sickness was a boon, an opportunity to propagate its species. However, man's culture had provided that patient with penicillin. It turned the ecological tables. With the antibiotic, man created a disastrous ecological imbalance for the microbe. Combining with the patient's natural biological resistance, the antibiotic secured for the afflicted lung cells first, counterbalance, and finally, ecological balance.

Consider this second example. Uranium miners have at least three times the incidence of lung cancer as other men in their age group. This is due to years of breathing radioactive dust. Formed in the decay of radon gas, the dust particles are inhaled during the mining operation. These particles emit alpha rays that physically affect normal lung cells. The cells may change biologically and become cancerous. Exposed to undue amounts of uranium, a miner experiences such biological changes in his lung cells. He develops lung cancer. Helplessly, he moves towards the death end of the health scale. But are not all people subjected to the physical stimulus of some natural radiation? Yes. Some cells are damaged. Some cells die. With most people, however, the total radiation dose at any one time is small. There is time for cellular recovery and replacement, for restoration of the ecological balance.

The uranium miner is less fortunate. For a long time he has suffered an excessive dose of radiation. Adequate counterbalance is impossible. He is overwhelmed. He sickens critically. The biological events within him stimulate cultural changes that are reflected by his own responses and those of his loved ones. He must, for example, "be brave," and his family must attempt to conceal their anguish. Moreover, his society, which embraces him culturally, becomes deeply involved. Crusading newspaper articles anger the public. The miner dies. Coming into play now are cultural processes utterly unrelated to the original stimuli causing the tragedy. The miner is mourned in a certain way. His funeral is in strict accordance with cultural dicta. He is buried according to a rigid set of cultural rules. Bitterly, the miner's union pressures the officials in Washington. Public clamor is now vast, insistent. A cultural imbalance has occurred and must be set aright. To restore the cultural balance laws are passed. The original physical stimulus and biological effect happened deep in a mine. But the actual operation of the legislative process, a cultural event, occurred independently of them.

To what extent is man affected by imbalance in his ecosystems? Are his environmental competitors able to nullify his cultural powers? René Dubos has written:

All living things, from men to the smallest microbe, live in association with other living things . . . an equilibrium is established which permits the different components of biological systems to live at peace together, indeed often to help one another. Whenever the equilibrium is disturbed by any means whatever, either internal or external, one of the components of the system is favored at the expense of the other . . . and then comes about the process of disease.[27]

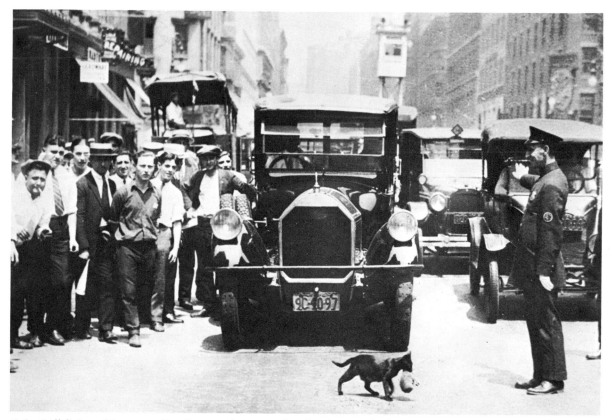

1-6 "All living things . . . live in association with other living things."

Study now some of mankind's challenges for environmental control. Their actions spell ecological imbalance for man. Their weapon is disease.

The *Staphylococcus aureus* is a microorganism carried in the nose and throat by numberless people throughout the world—including those working in hospitals. Most people who carry the germ, however, are unaffected by it. They are in a state of ecological balance with it.

Occasionally, however, the germ overcomes the resistance of its host.

The staphylococcus versus man's penicillin: a world war

[27] René Dubos, "The Germ Theory Revisited," quoted in *Harold G. Wolff's Stress and Disease,* rev. and ed. by Stewart Wolf and Helen Goodell, 2nd ed. (Springfield, Ill., 1968), p. 190.

It then causes conditions such as pimples, boils, or eye infections. At one time, most staphylococci were exquisitely sensitive to penicillin. Small doses of the antibiotic destroyed vast numbers of these staphylococci. Doctors, therefore, saturated the environment of these microorganisms with this antibiotic. Most staphylococci could not live in the penicillin environment but a few could. They were resistant. The original penicillin-resistant staphylococci were not the result of change brought about by the antibiotic. The resistant bacteria were present in the original bacterial population. These resistant germs lived through the penicillin deluge. They multiplied enormously. Today, they are a spectre of infection in every hospital in the world. But staphylococci have developed resistance to more antibiotics than penicillin. There now exist strains of this microorganism also resistant to other valuable antibiotics such as the tetracyclines. Most types of the *Staphylococcus aureus* have thus become resistant to a man-made physical change in their environment.[28]

Organisms of higher species also exhibit this resistance to man's connivance. Consider the louse.

Of lice and men Man struggles to control his environment. His ability to behave according to what he has learned molds his culture. Insects do not learn. Their environmental control is entirely by instinct. They have a society, not a culture. About three-fourths of the insect's brain is eye. He sees much, but learns nothing. Instinct governs him. His sexual instincts, for example, generally depend on his exquisite sensitivity to odor. The scientist can isolate the insect sex chemical and spray it over an area. One can imagine the confusion of the male insect. He is completely surrounded by glamorous females who are not there. One would think the frustration enough to kill him. It is. Man, in this instance at least, has outwitted the insect.

But in his constant war with insects for environmental control, man is hardly the instant winner. Temporarily, at least, the humble body louse can thwart man. On the warm body of a human the louse can find comfort for some time. Left to his own devices, he gets free board, room, and transportation. He finds a transient ecological peace. The compliment goes unreturned. The satisfaction is not mutual. In the first place, infestation by lice will make a person itch. Second, some lice can carry serious, even fatal, epidemic disease (typhus fever). Lice are notorious for their partiality to soldiers and their clothing. However, anybody will do. It was with some relief, therefore, that during the Second World War, DDT was found to be fatal to the body louse. For some time during and immediately after the war, soldiers and affected populations alike were effectively deloused with this agent (see Figure 1-7).

[28]More than a decade ago, at Keio University in Tokyo, Dr. Tsutomu Watanabe identified a *resistance factor* in certain bacteria. It is made up of genes—DNA (Chapter 16). Many bacteria, such as those causing typhoid fever and infant diarrhea, can contain these resistant genes. By simple contact, antibiotic-resistant germs may transmit their resistance factor to germs of a different species. Drug immunity can thus be spread to a whole population of different bacteria. How to meet this potential threat to antibiotic effectivity is a major problem of modern science.

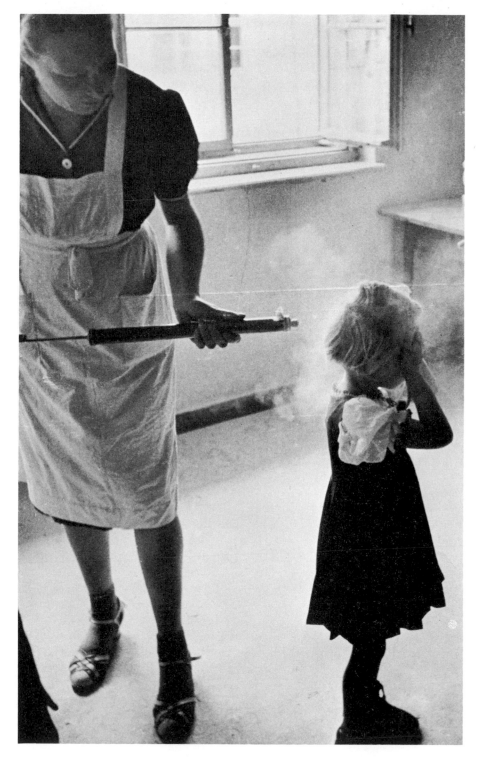

1-7 A European child deloused with DDT. Such spraying was commonplace during and just after the Second World War.

Imagine the consternation that occurred when, during the Korean War, it was found that DDT was useless in killing the body louse. The foot soldier had lost a valuable chemical ally. What had happened? During the Second World War, DDT had been introduced into the louse environment. That environment became more tolerable for humans, but intolerable for many lice. Most of the exposed lice died. Most. Not all. Some lice lived. To understand why, one must remember that great numbers and varieties of lice exist. Enormous numbers of lice, with various genetic combinations, produced astronomic numbers of offspring. These offspring contained even greater numbers of genetic combinations. A few of these genetic combinations resulted in lice that were resistant to DDT. These DDT-resistant lice produced offspring with genetic combinations as resistant to DDT as their predecessors (some were even more resistant). In this way DDT acted as a selector of DDT-resistant lice. Since all the DDT-susceptible lice were killed, in the end only DDT-resistant lice were left. Adaptation to DDT meant survival of the louse.

This is a classic example of a biological (genetic) adaptation by an organism to a man-made change in physical environment. The adaptation by the louse profoundly affects man's culture. To completely defeat the body louse, to protect health, the ecology of lice and men will need to be changed even more.

Rain, potatoes, and tuberculosis

It is more than a hundred years since the Irish potato famine, but the scars of its deep societal wounds are still apparent. The famine was the result of an ecological imbalance. Climate, a physical factor in the Irish ecosystem, had not previously disturbed the biological balance between the potato (their "root of delight") and one of its parasites. Suddenly, climate did upset that subtle relationship. Like a house of cards, the whole ecosystem collapsed.

1-8 A funeral during the Irish potato famine.

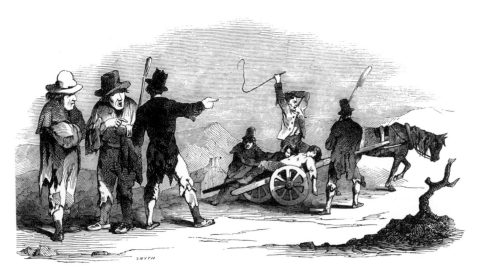

In 1845, a black cloud hung over Ireland. This is what had happened. The parasitic fungus *Phytophthora infestans* had long infested the Irish potato. This potato, originally an inedible tuber growing wild in the Andes, had been brought to Ireland as a new food. The fungus had come along. With careful farming and reasonably good weather, the fungus had been kept at bay. Ireland prospered and her population multiplied.

Then the crop failed. Why? For two basic reasons. First, by growing the best varieties, the Irish had refined the potato for edibility and yield. The tastier potato was now delicate. It could no longer resist a fungus as well as its hardy Andean ancestor could. Second, in 1845 the weather in Ireland was pitiless. Rain and fog upset the now delicate ecological-biological balance between potato and fungus. The potato was overwhelmed by the fungus. It lay soaked, rotting. The crop was ruined, and so was Ireland.

The enormity of the calamity has been recorded in a masterpiece by Salaman.[29] More than a million people died of sheer hunger. Others were plagued by scurvy (from vitamin C deficiency), dysentery, and typhus. Insanity and blindness were rampant. The former was doubtless due to prolonged shock and lack of vitamins. The latter was probably caused by lack of decent nourishment. An Irish famine song of unknown authorship tells the melancholy story:

> *Oh, the praties, they are small*
> *Over here, over here.*
> *Oh, the praties, they are small,*
> *When we dig 'em in the fall.*
> *And we eat 'em coats and all,*
> *Full of fear, full of fear.*[30]

Fearful people of Europe, then as now, looked to the New World. In desperate droves, the rural Irish, starved, disease-ridden, left Ireland for New York, Philadelphia, and Boston. There they met with other miseries. Accustomed to the pace and space of the Irish farm, they were now forced into the congestion and speed of the cities. Their situation could not have been more conducive to the spread of tuberculosis. As Dubos points out, "The sudden and dramatic increase of tuberculosis mortality in the Philadelphia, New York and Boston areas around 1850 can be traced in large part to the Irish immigrants who settled in these cities at that time."[31]

So, because it rained in Ireland in 1845, tuberculosis increased in Boston

---

[29] N. Redcliffe Salaman, *The History and Social Influence of the Potato* (Cambridge, Eng., 1949).

[30] A Kansas version of the Irish Famine Song, similarly of unknown authorship:
> *Oh, potatoes, they grow small in Kansas,*
> *Oh, potatoes, they grow small.*
> *For they plant them in the fall,*
> *And they eat 'em skins and all,*
> *In Kansas.*

[31] René Dubos, *Mirage of Health* (Garden City, N.Y., 1961), p. 90.

and New York and Philadelphia in 1850. The arm of ecology is long and the results of ecological imbalance are extensive. The physical change in the climate, resulting in a change in the biological balance between the potato and its fungal parasite, brought about vast physical, biological, and cultural imbalances affecting the health of human beings thousands of miles away.

And note this: in the succession of imbalances, there were counterbalances. The ecological scales were but temporarily tipped against man. In the end, he survived. And with his help, so did the Irish potato. Why? Because man is able to think.

Of unwelcome guests, their unprepared hosts, and imbalanced ecosystems

Much has been written of the friendly Indian reception given early European invaders of the New World. Perhaps there were isolated instances of such behavior. On the whole, however, the Europeans were met with bitter hostility. Had it not been for a powerful ally, the Indians might have successfully, albeit temporarily, driven the invaders from the New World. That ally was disease. To the Indians, the Europeans brought grievous ecological imbalance.

Cortez brought smallpox to the Indians. Most of the Conquistadores were probably immune to the virus causing the illness. The Indians, however, had been bred in an environment completely free of it. They were hopelessly susceptible. Resistance was impossible. The disease decimated them. It was not so much the bravery of the Spaniards that broke down the resistance of the Indians. Sick and frightened, the Indians had little choice but to flee or seek peace. Interestingly, sickness, the friend of the Spaniard and the enemy of the Indian, confused the more devout Europeans. The Indians who converted to Christianity seemed to be rewarded with disease and death.

With the arrival of the English, early in the seventeenth century, the North American Indians met a similar fate. The Indians resisted, trying to free their lands of the ruthless invaders. They failed. Their greatest enemy was the smallpox brought them from Europe. Modern celebrants of Thanksgiving Day portray the Puritan relationship with the Indian as pious and benevolent. Dubos tells a different story:

> Europeans soon became aware of the fact that smallpox was one of their most effective weapons against Indians, and they did not hesitate to spread the infection intentionally by means of contaminated blankets, always on the pretext that it helped destroy the enemies of the faith. God is always on the side of the strong battalions, even when they are made up of microbes.[32]

It has been estimated that of the twelve million seventeenth-century American Indians six million died of smallpox.

[32] *Ibid.,* p. 189.

In 1887, Tha Combau, the native Chief of the Fiji Islands, returned with his retinue from a visit to Sydney, Australia. At the time, he had a slight cough. Thus he generously shared his microbes with other members of his delegation. He was developing measles. Within four months, twenty thousand Fijians died of the disease. The introduction of the measles virus into a population that had no previous experience with it was catastrophic. The people, without previous immunity, could not achieve an ecological balance with the microorganism. The cost in life was devastating.

Similar incidents have been recorded involving the effects of tuberculosis, venereal disease, scarlet fever, and polio on populations newly exposed to them. At various times both Polynesians and Africans have been cruelly decimated by these afflictions. But one need not seek out exotic countries to provide excellent examples of biological imbalance caused by the occurrence of a new infectious agent in a community.

In February and March 1966, type A2 influenza sent half a million Los Angeles school children to bed. They complained of headaches, sore throats, and coughing. Some had muscle pains. Oral temperatures rose as high as 104°F. Not many vomited or had diarrhea. Gastrointestinal symptoms are not usually part of the true influenza picture. Their parents, who had been adequately exposed to the virus some five years before, were immune and were hardly affected by the disease. The virus, absent in epidemic amounts from the Los Angeles area for five years, found a receptive host in the child. Why? In his preschool years, the Los Angeles child had no previous opportunity to develop immunity. Almost two years later (in December 1968), a new A2 influenza virus type, originating in Hong Kong, brought sickness to millions. In this Los Angeles epidemic, both adults and children were affected. In this case neither had been previously exposed to the Hong Kong type of influenza A2 virus. The Hong Kong influenza virus had changed genetically from the previous A2 influenza virus. The population had not developed a resistance to this changed virus.

These examples demonstrate biological imbalance resulting from the introduction of a new microbe into a community. It is well to remember that a microorganism can exist in the human body quite harmlessly. However, man's activities, resulting in a changed ecosystem, can transform a harmless relationship into a destructive battle. An example is the yeast-like fungus *Candida albicans*, which usually inhabits the human intestine without harm. It can cause a disease of infants (rarely of adults) called *thrush*. This condition is characterized by whitish spots in the mouth. Oral antibiotics, such as penicillin, have been known to kill certain microorganisms in the intestine that keep the *Candida* in check. *Candidiasis*, an infection that occurs when there is an overgrowth of these fungi, can result in serious liver abscesses.

Sometimes, biological imbalances are purposely instigated by man to his own advantage. The rabbit of Australia is a case in point. Once these animals were a major agricultural pest. In an attempt to control them, ferrets and weasels, the natural enemies of the rabbit, were introduced into Australia. This attempt met little success. A virus was then tried, which caused a rabbit disease called *myxomatosis*. The introduction of the virus into Australia seemed to solve the problem. However, one is reminded of the genetic success achieved by the louse against DDT and the staphylococcus against penicillin. Already strains of rabbits resistant to the virus have appeared. Another method of rabbit control will be needed soon.[33]

Clarke relates an incident in which the purposeful use of biological imbalance boomeranged. Some sheep ranchers, convinced that coyotes were killing their young sheep, destroyed all the coyotes that could be found. The decrease in the predator coyote made life safe for such grass-eating rodents as rabbits and field mice. To meet this second threat, the sheep men stopped killing the coyotes and turned on the rodents. Coyotes from neighboring areas then wandered into and about the area, relatively undisturbed. Finding their natural rodent diet gone, they started doing what they had not done before—eating the sheep![34]

For balance, ecologic challenge alters man

Every creature characteristic, varying from the opening of a flower to the opening of a hand, is determined by both genes and environment (see Chapter 16). Formed and stored many millenia ago, the structured chemical pattern of man's uniquely arranged set of genes changes with the deliberate speed of evolution. The patterned detail of his genetic make-up changes as environmental conditions favor the selective activity of some genes over others. Genes and environment interplay in subtle concert to produce a creature with the best chance of meeting the particular environmental challenge. Thus man, by means of his genetic structure, remains in balance with his environment. As Mindel has written,

> Man, then, is a creature shaped by the distant past, as it has been conserved by evolution and stored in his genes, as well as by the present environment, which favors the development of some stored potentials over others. He changes not only in the course of thousands of years but also in a generation . . . Man becomes human because his genetic potential interacts not only with his natural environment but also with his social and cultural environment.[35]

Can environmental stimulus alone produce rapid change? Yes. Normally, the human genetic pool changes little, if at all, from a single generation to the next. Yet, in the years since the Second World War, one environmental change, diet, helped produce a whole generation of larger Japanese and Israeli children. Another recent environmental change ac-

---

[33] Marston Bates, *Animal Worlds* (New York, 1963), p. 296.
[34] George L. Clarke, *Elements of Ecology*, p. 19.
[35] Joseph Mindel, "The Living Experience," a review of René Dubos' *So Human an Animal, Technology Review*, Vol. 71, No. 4 (February 1969), p. 13.

counts for the earlier sexual maturity of today's Western teen-ager. From his grandparents the teen-ager has inherited an unchanged reproductive system. But the culture within the modern ecosystem, independent of his genes, stimulates early marriage.

That environmental or ecological changes such as diet may have marked effects on future generations is shown by research indicating a close relationship between maternal stature and the death rates of newborns. "The deleterious effects of malnutrition in childhood will not be confined to the skeleton but must affect the development of the whole body, and thus the quality of the response to pregnancy."[36] The mother's reproductive capacity (profoundly influenced by her diet) plus the standards of her care are two basic factors in determining the viability of her newborn.

The environment of the Aymara Indians (discussed earlier in this chapter) negatively influences their stature and reproductive maturity. Deficiency of oxygen and cold are characteristic of the high Peruvian Altiplano. Such stresses are associated with the lessened birth weight, slower growth rate, and diminished adolescent spurt of the children in that area. There, the earliest age at which any woman gives birth to a child is eighteen.[37]

The needs of man's ecosystem exert even more profound changes in his physical characteristics. The fair skin of the Northwest European affords him the maximum benefit of the little ultraviolet radiation that passes through the cloudy skies of his country. Conversely, the dark skin of the Negro, evolved in the distant past, was doubtless protective. It guarded him against overexposure to the ultraviolet rays of the sun while allowing him to get enough of those rays so that synthesis of vitamin D could occur. Without adequate vitamin D rickets results. It is of interest to note that Negro children are somewhat more liable to rickets than white children in the same climate. This is thought to be due to the filtering action of the skin pigment.[38] An analogous situation can be found in some sections of India and Egypt, where the custom of shielding women (purdah) is still commonly practiced. In those areas, girls and women are always shielded from public view by curtains and screens. Thus, chronically deprived of light, these unfortunate females suffer serious vitamin D deficiencies with resultant advanced rickets.[39]

"There is no doubt," Dubos has written,

that, just like other living things, man was molded and chiseled into shape by his physical environment . . . A short, stocky body frame covered with fat helps the Eskimo economize body heat in the arctic climate. In contrast, some tribes of Equatorial Africa

---

[36] Dugald Baird, "Perinatal Mortality," *The Lancet,* Vol. 1, No. 7593 (March 8, 1969), p. 511.

[37] Paul T. Baker, "Human Adaptation to High Altitudes," *Science,* Vol. 163, No. 3872 (March 14, 1969), p. 1156.

[38] Sonia Cole, *Races of Man,* 2nd ed. (London, 1965), p. 21.

[39] Jacques M. May, *The Ecology of Human Disease,* p. 5.

exhibit a tall, lanky, gracile structure which probably helps in dispelling body heat . . . On level lands where it is often helpful to see far and move fast, tall men are at an advantage over short-legged, rotund ones, whereas the situation is different in densely wooded areas. [The work of living in the forest] depends upon the use of a variety of muscles that are less often called into play for locomotion on the plains. As a result, the forest dweller is likely to be short legged, long trunked, barrel chested, and broad handed. A stocky muscular build is as important for his survival as the greyhound body form is of advantage to the plainsman.[40]

Eskimos (Figure 1-9) have short noses. Were their noses as long as those of the average desert dweller, there would surely be an epidemic of frozen noses in the Arctic. The Tongus and Mongoloids of eastern Siberia live in probably the coldest places in the world. They have short noses, narrow nasal passages, and flat faces. Their squat bodies are fat-padded to help keep them warm. In the African heat, a body frame so covered with fat would be a discomfort. To the Eskimo and the Siberian, it is essential for survival.

Diet also influences body structure. Meat eaters are large. Rice eaters are small. The effect of diet on height has already been noted (page 26). Eskimos eat fatty foods because they need twice as many calories as do people living in the tropics. The fat they accumulate also insulates them against the cold, as was noted above. These people have had no instruction in nutrition. Their physical environment has taught them their needs.

René Dubos[41] points to still another example of a physical adaptation resulting from a genetic mechanism—the curious, recently discovered

[40] René Dubos, *Mirage of Health* (New York, 1959), pp. 30–31.
[41] *Ibid.,* p. 43

1-9 *"Man was molded . . . by his physical environment."* Masai elephant trackers (*left*) and a Copper Eskimo (*right*).

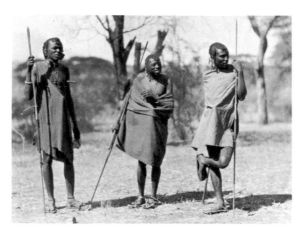
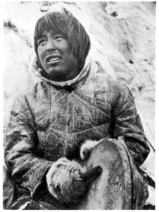

relationship of the sickle-cell trait to resistance to malaria. Sickle-cell anemia is a hereditary (genetically determined) illness, occurring almost exclusively in Negroes. Some people may carry the trait in their genes without having the disease. The symptoms of this illness, characterized by fragility of the red blood cells, include pains in the joints, acute attacks of abdominal pain, and leg ulcerations. The red blood cells of those who have the disease, instead of being circular discs, are crescent-shaped (hence the name "sickle cell," see Figure 1-10). Sickle-cell anemia markedly lessens the chances of survival to reproductive age. Since sickle-celled people would probably not live to produce sickle-celled children, one might reasonably assume that, in time, the proportion of the population who have the sickle-cell trait would decrease. Curiously enough, this has not been the case. Why?

Children with the sickle-cell trait develop resistance to malaria. Their death rate from malaria is lower than that of children without the sickle-cell trait. So, the death rates of children with the sickle-cell trait are offset by the deaths from malaria of children without the sickle-cell trait. As would be expected, when a population with a high incidence of sickle-cell trait moves from a malarial to a nonmalarial area, the proportion of people with the sickle-cell trait to those with normal red blood cells decreases. The "survival advantage" gained by resistance to malaria is lost.

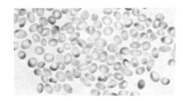
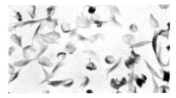

1-10 Red blood cells: normal cells (*top*) and sickle cells (*bottom*).

To meet their needs, creatures modify their ecosystems

A living organism may change the environment to suit itself. The romantic little firefly has a characteristically unique code of flashing light. Seeing the signal of the flying male, the female firefly signals her response, thereby attracting him. In the deep darkness of the sea, some shrimp resist attack by producing a discharge of light that distracts or frightens the attacker. The temperature inside the hive of the honeybee is maintained by the bee at a relatively constant level. In winter time, muscle activity within the cluster in the hive keeps the temperature high enough for survival. In summertime, the beating of wings forces cooling air through the hive. Adult white pelicans protect their young from the hot sun of Salton Sea, California, by wetting their plumage. Their brooding is surely unusual. Instead of keeping her young and eggs warm, the mother keeps them cool! Of all the creatures of this planet, none can modify his ecosystem so much as man. How his very ingenuity has produced an ecosystem that threatens his health is explored in Chapters 3 and 4.

This first chapter, however, has reviewed some ways to regard health. An ever changing biotic adventure of varying individuals, health is a part of the weave of life, coloring it brightly here, subtly shading it there, obvious in one place, obscure—almost lost—in another. In holding the fabric to the light, one sees the infinite variety of health. So singular and so varied a pattern does mankind's all-pervasive culture give his ecosystems that it is the subject of the entire following chapter.

2

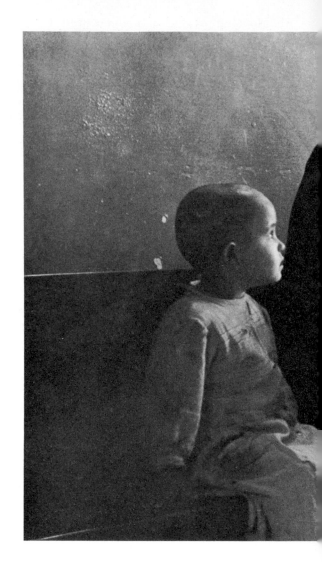

Health and
the community

Culture and health

Up to this point a variety of rhythmic, balanced interrelationships between living things has been considered. The redwood tree struggling silently to survive, the selfless tarantula, the obliging Pederson shrimp, the greedy potato fungus, the stubborn staphylococcus resisting its antibiotic enemy, the devious louse changing genetically to foil man's clever chemicals, and man, himself, changing physically to meet his needs—all these speak of dynamic operations in the environment. They both remind man of the basic environmental threats challenging him and suggest

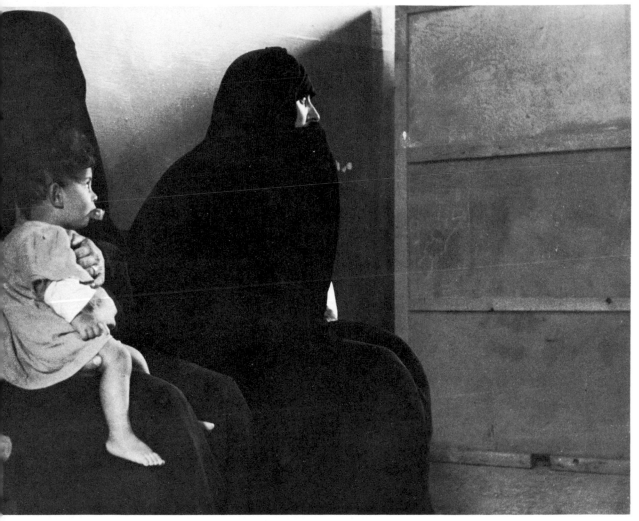

At a Syrian dispensary, children wait to be examined for favus, a scalp infection.

possible ways of coping with these challenges. For example, in Chapter 1 it was noted that a certain species of wasp was able to propagate itself only by sacrificing a tarantula. Mankind's knowledge of such events as this, combined with his cultural achievements, enable him to manipulate ecosystems to his own benefit. For example, large milk supplies in California were recently found to be polluted by a pesticide. How did this happen? Cows eat alfalfa. Competing for their food were voracious alfalfa weevil larvae. Wanting milk, man brought his culture to bear on the side of the cow. To save the cow-food crop, alfalfa growers first used a pesticide. The weevil was eliminated. But the milk was polluted by the pesti-

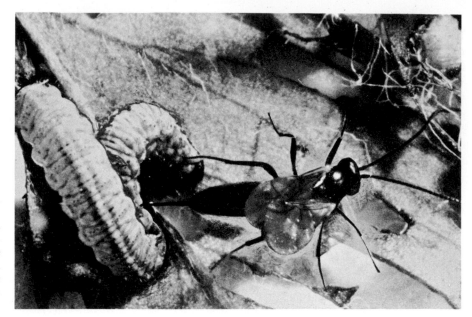

2-1 The wasp and the weevil. A natural enemy of the alfalfa weevil and a friend of the alfalfa grower, the wasp deposits its eggs within the alfalfa weevil larva, as shown here. The eggs hatch within the host. The host dies.

cide. Another method of destroying the weevil had to be found. Within the ecosystem lay the answer. It had been observed that certain wasps deposited their eggs inside the alfalfa weevil (Figure 2-1). Within the host, the eggs hatched and the weevil died. And so, into the weevil's ecosystem great numbers of wasps were deliberately let loose. By this manipulation of the environment, the threat of the alfalfa weevil was removed. No longer was there a need for dangerous pesticides. The milk pollution was eliminated.

Thus man's complex, learned culture enters into the simpler ecological picture of a biological relationship. Scientific skill is wholly learned and taught. But science, as much as any other aspect of culture, can harm as well as help man. His culture has brought him both health and disease. In distinguishing man from all else that lives, it has lent him power over all other life. Yet within his own ecosystem man has become his own worst enemy. To comprehend this ecological threat, man must examine mankind and the consequences of group living. Other creatures live successfully in groups. Why is man so different? To what extent does man's culture, patterned into the web of his ecosystem, control him? How does it create his health problems and yet at the same time offer him solutions? This chapter will seek answers to these questions. But first it might be well to examine the behavior of a species existing in a singularly successful society. "Go to the ant, thou sluggard; consider her ways, and be wise" (Proverbs 6:6). Man need not emulate the ant. It is inefficient, a slaveholder, and a thief. But ant society has so much in common with human society, as well as having so many instructive differences, that it merits a careful examination.

A morsel to tempt the most finicky Mexican bride at her wedding breakfast might well be an insect honeyball. This delicacy is a collection of ants, swollen like tiny barrels, purposely stuffed by worker ants with honeydew. In times of short supply these cask ants provide food for worker ants. Being a living mason jar is but one of the countless ingenuities of the ant. For millions of years, several thousand recorded species of ants, the members of the family *Formicidae,* have scurried about on the face of the earth.

As the example of the cask ant shows, these insects have a caste structure. Ants maintain babysitters, keep cattle, and have an elaborate and regular system of patrols. Soldiers (undeveloped females) defend the nest from outside invasion. Let a stray ant wander into a strange nest and he is attacked, but a prodigal, gone for weeks, is welcomed back. There is even a "doorkeeper" ant, whose head is fashioned into a plug to close nest entrances.[1]

Some ants lay trails, construct cities and freeways, and build elaborate skyscrapers characteristic of, and suitable for, the species. So consistently do Swiss yellow ants build their elongated mounds pointed to the east that mountaineers use them as compasses.[2] Some ants also engage in agriculture. The suava ants industriously collect pieces of leaves cut from various plants. Within the nest, workers (which, like soldiers, are undeveloped females) chew the leaves to a spongy pulp. This pulp is then stored in special chambers and purposely infected with spores of a fungus. The resulting growth is used as food for all members of the ant colony.

One genus of ants uses slave labor. *Polyergus,* the slave-making ant, will raid the nests of the *Formica* ants and carry home the larvae and pupae. After maturation, these become willing captives and, as mature workers, are kept busy feeding their masters and building their nests. Who is slave and who is master? Who is dependent and who is independent? These questions are open to philosophic discussion. For, even in the presence of food, *Polyergus* will starve unless he is fed by the slave.

Army ant warfare has been studied, presumably with profit, by generals. These "Huns and Tartars of the insect world"[3] (which make up a particular subfamily of ants) eat only meat. As temporary guests, they are quite welcome in some tropical houses because they clean the place of vermin. Marching in military columns and carrying their larvae between their legs (nobody stays home), they pillage the countryside, devouring other insects and ripping the flesh from even small animals. Some of the meat is devoured on the spot; the rest is saved for later. Bending their bodies, some soldier ants point their heads upward and eject scalding streams of formic acid at an enemy.

Such coordinated devotion by the individual to the common societal good would be hard to surpass. But, as Dobzhansky states, "Among the

[1]Theodosius Dobzhansky, *Evolution, Genetics, and Man* (New York, 1955), p. 343.
[2]*M.D., Medical Newsmagazine,* Vol. 6, No. 5 (May 1962), p. 168.
[3]W. M. Wheeler, quoted in John Tyler Bonner, *Cells and Societies* (Princeton, N.J., 1955), p. 67.

marvels of ant and termite societies, one thing is conspicuously absent. Nowhere is there a school for the young workers or soldiers!"[4] The ant's behavioral patterns are not learned.

Man and learned culture

This is the crux of the difference between *Hominidae* and *Formicidae*, between human and ant society. For the insect, behavior is instinctual. The ant need not learn. Without training, it becomes expert at particular tasks when it reaches a given stage of development. The human must be trained, and only after prolonged growth and development does he achieve a certain ability. Moreover, what the ant does is suitable for its limited environment. In a new environment its inherited instinctual effort is useless or fatal. The human, however, can adapt to new environments. Paul has written:

> Should all the members of an ant community perish, for example, except one fertilized female, the lone survivor would be capable of rebuilding the entire social edifice in all its original complexity within the span of a few short generations. A society of humans could not similarly recover from catastrophe if all humans suddenly disappeared except one adult couple organically intact but innocent of knowledge and all other social learning ... it would take tedious thousands of generations to rediscover the ways and wisdom needed to run any human society now in existence. This is because humans, unlike insects, order their lives and interpersonal relations largely by means of socially acquired signals.[5]

So human beings rely primarily on learned behavior, or culture, for survival. It is this acquired guidance, this cultural instruction, that enables man to constantly adapt to change. Insect societies do not change; human societies change constantly, and change makes progress possible.

Still another remarkable difference between human beings and life that is lower on the biological scale is the great length of time required for the development of independence. No other creature in nature is forced into so long a dependency as is the human. Usually the insect has a brief period of immaturity followed by a relatively long period of productivity. While the young monkey busily forages in the supermarkets of nature, the human of the same age idly contemplates his fingers. For a man to mature requires almost one-third of his life span. He needs this time to learn the rules of adaptation to his culture. Also, man has an unusually long postreproductive life span. In the length of her life after menopause, the woman is unique among mammals. Nature grants humankind extra years—precious time in which to learn the demands of his culture and even more years in which to make use of his wisdom. But, in his develop-

---

[4] Theodosius Dobzhansky, *Evolution, Genetics, and Man*, p. 343.
[5] Benjamin D. Paul, ed., *Health, Culture, and Community* (New York, 1955), p. 461.

mental years, man picks up problems as well as wisdom. And, in his productive years, he creates even more problems for himself. In growing, he often flaws his health and thus his productive energy.

In *Childhood and Society,* Erikson points to the price of "becoming":

> *One may scan work after work on history, society, and morality and find little reference to the fact that all people start as children and that all peoples begin in their nurseries. It is human to have a long childhood; it is civilized to have an ever longer childhood. Long childhood makes a technical and mental virtuoso out of man, but it also leaves a lifelong residue of emotional immaturity in him. While tribes and nations, in many intuitive ways, use child training to the end of gaining their particular form of mature human identity, their unique version of integrity, they are, and remain, beset by the irrational fears which stem from the very state of childhood which they exploited in their specific way.*[6]

So, although man is unique in his learned behavior (culture), the process of his learning has a price. Too often the cost of some aspect of this culture is his health. The price will depend on his ability to create a balance between himself and his surroundings. The relationship between culture and environment and health is aptly stated by Mead: "In many cultures throughout the world, man is continuous with his environment. Therefore, he is not healthy unless his environment is 'healthy' or conversely, the well-being of his environment depends upon his acts."[7]

Health, then, helps to create culture and culture creates health, for man is not alone. But culture can be tyranny.

The power of culture

All men and their communities share a common denominator of problems. However, various cultures have various solutions to these similar problems.

In the face of sickness, every culture defines what must be done, by whom, with what, when, and so forth.[8] Herb medicines and antibiotic therapy are highly dissimilar treatments, but they are both specific. Even how to behave in the presence of illness is strictly prescribed by culture. In his autobiographical novel *Of Human Bondage* W. Somerset Maugham expresses this through the sensitive thoughts of the hero, Philip Carey. At the time, Philip is a medical student in an English hospital dispensary. This is what passes through his mind:

> *Sometimes you saw an untaught stoicism which was profoundly moving. Once Philip saw a man, rough and illiterate, told his case*

[6]Erik H. Erikson, *Childhood and Society* (New York, 1950), from the Foreword.
[7]Margaret Mead, ed., *Cultural Patterns and Technical Change* (New York, 1955), pp. 217–18.
[8]Ralph Linton, *The Study of Man,* cited in Leo J. Simmons and Harold G. Wolff, *Social Science in Medicine* (New York, 1954), pp. 74–75.

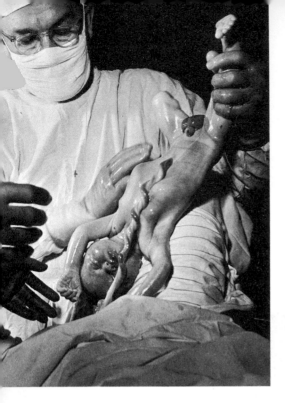

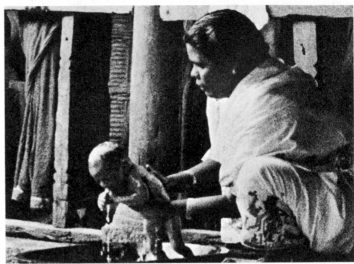

Economics and health: a baby is born. The child pictured at the left is the beneficiary of all that modern science can offer the newborn; the infant shown below, born in an underdeveloped society, is washed off by a midwife.

2-2 Culture and Health

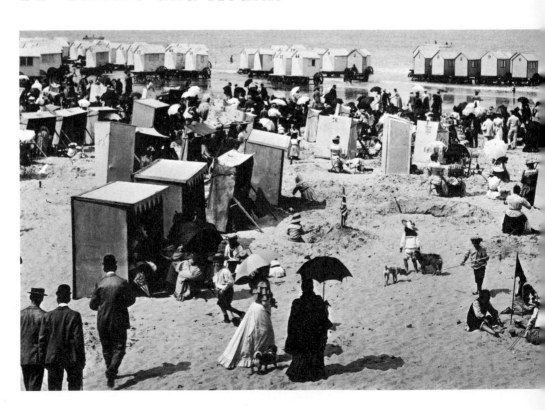

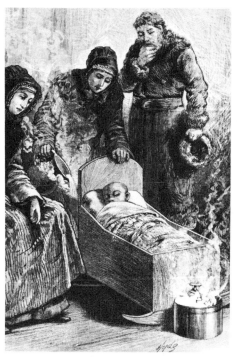

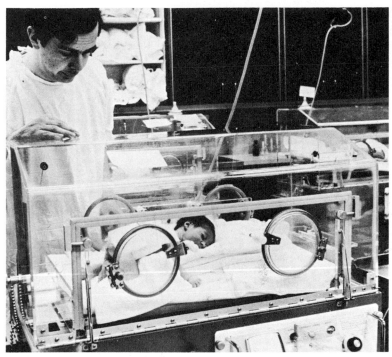

Technology and health: the premature baby. This 19th-century incubator (*left*) was kept warm by hot water poured into a container behind the head of the bed. The hot water flowed into a canal under the mattress and was let out through a spigot at the foot of the bed. Today's incubator (*right*) is designed to give the infant its best chance for life.

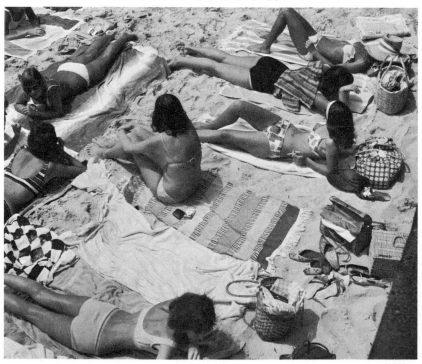

Fashion and health: the ecosystem of human skin. In Ostende, Belgium, in 1898 (*left*), ladies were not to be seen in bathing costumes. They were kept from public view by remaining in little changing cabins or "bathing boxes," which were drawn to the water by ponies. After a dip, the ladies resumed their ruffles while being wheeled back to the dry beach. The contemporary beach, by contrast (*right*), is a study in skin exposure. Modern bathing customs are a peril to some: the sun's ultraviolet light radiation is responsible for most skin cancers.

was hopeless; and, self-controlled himself, he wondered at the splen-
did instinct which forced the fellow to keep a stiff upper-lip before
strangers. But was it possible for him to be brave when he was by
himself, face to face with his soul, or would he then surrender to
despair?[9]

Clearly, this man's "stiff upper lip before strangers" is ordered by his culture. He may tremble within, but to the outside world, his cultural world, he must show a brave face. So does culture at times force man into a cruel paradox. It gives him company and sustenance and yet it enforces loneliness, too. As the man becomes sicker, and even as he approaches death, his culture will still make demands based on set rules, which, so long as he is able, he will obey. Indeed, so it was with the previously mentioned uranium miner who died of lung cancer.

Death is the ultimate unknown. That men have been known to accept death and even to embrace it because their culture so dictates is remarkable. A community that believes in magic can literally condemn a man to death by pointing a bone at him. Malinowski describes bone-pointing in Melanesia:

> *For the sorcerer has, as an essential part of the ritual performance, not merely to point the bone dart at his victim, but with an intense expression of fury and hatred he has to thrust it in the air, turn and twist it as if to bore it in the wound, then pull it back with a sudden jerk. Thus not only is the act of violence, or stabbing, reproduced, but the passion of violence has to be enacted.*[10]

Simmons and Wolff tell of the overwhelming impact of this condemnation on the damned individual.[11] To be read out of the living, already to be considered dead by one's own, means death. Terrified by belief in magic, utterly alone through loss of support from kin, excommunicated in an organized manner by the culture and society that sheltered him, the tragic figure undergoes profound physical changes. Sinking from trembling fear to choking terror to tormented collapse to mute agony and, finally, to utter resignation, the "boned" man awaits death. The members of the community who have forsaken him return, but only to organize his doom. The rules must yet and ever be obeyed. He is prepared for "death and ritual mourning." The condemned man utters no sound, partakes neither of food nor water.

He dies quietly. So overwhelming are the cultural powers of man.

To find "boning" in his own culture, the reader need merely be reminded of the torment of the "witches" of the sixteenth and seventeenth centuries and the activities of Nazi Germany some three decades ago.[12]

[9] W. Somerset Maugham, *Of Human Bondage* (Garden City, N.Y., 1915), pp. 497–98.
[10] Bronislaw Malinowski, *Magic, Science and Religion* (Garden City, N.Y., 1955), p. 71.
[11] Leo J. Simmons and Harold G. Wolff, *Social Science in Medicine*, pp. 92–94.
[12] There are those who separate these actions from the people and attribute them rather to their leaders.
But the British historian Trevor-Roper put this idea to rest in this way: "No ruler has ever carried out

Today, more subtle examples of "boning" are commonplace. And so are its consequences. In the first half of this century, as Wolff has pointed out, stomach ulcers became principally a male disorder.[13] Among the reasons for this phenomenon is increased male stress due to the changed relationship between the sexes. Millions of married women seek careers. A married woman failing in an occupational venture endures no societal approbation; she may honorably retire to caring for her family. In the event of the husband's failure, no such escape is possible. Indeed the reverse is true. Cultural sanctions often endorse the public humiliation (or "boning") of a man failing to provide for his family. "Thus while society's requirements of the male are essentially as stringent as before, the emotional support accorded him in return has become less."[14] Furthermore, those women who remain in the competitive world previously occupied largely by men suffer an increasing rate of "stress diseases," of which the stomach ulcer is but one.

The effect of "boning" on the modern adolescent is no less disturbing. Menninger writes,

> It is logical to suggest that our adolescents' provocative behavior may be their way of saying to us, "I object." They may be telling us how they feel about our systematically segregating them from adult society . . . Nowhere are the starkness and the meagerness of this social isolation more apparent than in the lot of the 15-year old. Except for going to school, virtually nothing that he can do is legal. He can't quit school, he can't work, he can't drink, he can't smoke, he can't drive in most states, he can't marry, he can't vote, he can't enlist, he can't gamble. He cannot, in fact, participate in any of the adult virtues, vices, or activities . . . this infantilizing of the adolescent provokes adventure-seeking, thrill-seeking, serious risk-taking behavior, such as taking drugs.[15]

This "enforced sidelining of the adolescent" ill prepares him for adulthood. Explaining his restrictions to him would be helpful.

Still another consequence of "boning" is to be found in ghetto rioting; this is how two investigators summarized the results of their 1967 survey done in Detroit and Newark:

> One is led to conclude that the continued exclusion of Negroes from American economic and social life is the fundamental cause of riots. This exclusion is the result of arbitrary racial barriers rather

a policy of wholesale expulsion or destruction without the cooperation of society . . . Without general social support, the organs of isolation and expulsion cannot even be created." (H. R. Trevor-Roper, "Witches and Witchcraft," *Encounter*, Vol. 28, No. 5 [May 1967], p. 14.)

[13] *Harold G. Wolff's Stress and Disease*, rev. and ed. by Stewart Wolf and Helen Goodell, 2nd ed. (Springfield, Ill., 1968) pp. 216–17.

[14] *Ibid.*, p. 217.

[15] Roy Menninger, "What Troubles Our Troubled Youth?" *Mental Hygiene*, Vol. 52, No. 3 (July 1968), pp. 324–27.

than a lack of ability, motivation or aspiration on the part of the Negroes who perceive it as arbitrary and unjust.

One important question remains to be answered: "Why do they riot now?" After all, the opportunity structure has been closed for 100 years. Our data suggest that Negroes who riot do so because their conception of their lives and their potential has changed without commensurate improvement in their chances for a better life.[16]

Emotions and ecosystems

For the primitive, belief often means fear. Death from "boning," for example, could not occur without complete belief in magic. But in primitive cultures belief in the community is as strong as belief in magic. Only by community support may one be saved from evil happenings. When someone finds himself utterly forsaken by the community, he is lost.[17] The primitive community, in turn, fearful of inadequate control of its ecosystem, sticks together. Together, ecological threats can be best met by the group. In the primitive community, anxiety is a cohesive force.

Unlike the primitive, however, civilized man has brought the techniques of ecological control to a high state. Never in human history has man ordered his ecosystem about so successfully. This control is a triumph of Western civilization. And yet, both within and without, man is ridden with problems. His very creativity has boomeranged. Too often it has also meant the creation of disease.

Western man is threatened. Not only is he endangered by the results of his own ecological mismanagement (Chapters 3 and 4), but he is also tormented by confusions and doubts. He has created and developed emotional disorders that profoundly affect his adjustment to the physical, biological, and cultural aspects of his ecosystem. For example, a diabetic may, as a result of emotional distress, impair his ability to metabolize sugar. He may develop symptoms that can kill him if they remain uncontrolled. Even with the proper dosage of insulin, the diabetic might, in such circumstances, become listless, weak, and thirsty. He may vomit, experience extreme dizziness, and finally lapse into a coma. (This critical situation is called diabetic crisis.)

Although several factors, such as acute injuries, may be involved, the profound influence of emotional disturbance in precipitating diabetic crisis is undeniable. Conflicts with parents or relatives, a bitter quarrel with a friend, indeed any severe emotional upset, can precipitate a diabetic crisis. Why? Human beings normally respond to any stressful situa-

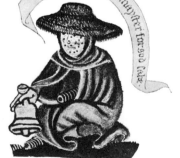

2-3 Woman leper with a warning bell (late 14th or early 15th century).

[16]Nathan S. Caplan and Jeffrey M. Paige, "A Study of Ghetto Rioters," *Scientific American,* Vol. 219, No. 2 (August 1968), p. 21.

[17]No better example of "boning" can be found than in the treatment of the leper in medieval Europe. Clad in a white shroud and with a grave cloth covering his garments, the leper was led to the church, where he kneeled in the place customarily used for putting the bodies of the dead. Then the clergy intoned over him the rites for the dead. The leper was then led to the leper's cemetery, and there he knelt as earth was thrown over him three times. He was then excluded from ordinary communal life and often wore a bell to warn those who approached him. This cruel quarantine is partly responsible for the reduction of the disease in Europe.

tion with an increased sugar metabolism. This response fulfills the body's sudden need for energy, a result of the psychic stress. With normal people, this increase is protective. To the diabetic, it is a hazard. His precarious, delicately attuned metabolism, exquisitely balanced by highly refined medication, cannot handle the rapidly elevated sugar supply. A disturbance in his interpersonal relationships may, therefore, cause him to go into the shock of a diabetic crisis. It may even cost him his life. The balance of his personal ecosystem—the balance between his drug and his sugar metabolism, between his emotions and his motions, between himself and those about him—so carefully engineered by decades of elegant medical research and centuries of cultural training is sacrificed to the costly luxury of human disagreement.

Hinkle suggests another kind of relationship between emotion and environment.[18] Sad, tearful, tired women do not seem to be able to withstand some viral infections as successfully as do those who are happy and rested. In a comparative study of happy and sad women, Hinkle observed that the common cold was both more frequent and more severe in the grieving group. A weepy woman's nasal mucosa often becomes engorged (filled with blood). So, for reasons other than infection, it secretes more profusely. It is during this time that she seems most susceptible to a cold. When she is gloomy, her symptoms are aggravated.

Thus a woman, weeping and restless with unrequited love, either real or imagined, may lose even more than an expected amount of balance with her ecosystem. She may lose some resistance to infection. As she regains her composure, she ostensibly regains resistance to the viruses of her environment, and her ecological balance is restored.

Symptom interpretation is closely related to culture. What would be considered illness in some communities might be considered the natural state in others. Among some people living in the southern United States and among Africans, diarrhea is not considered unusual. Many African mothers become concerned unless their children have six or seven bowel movements daily. Trachoma (a serious viral eye disease associated with severe inflammation and a variety of other symptoms) is considered a way of life among some Greeks.[19] Most observers would consider pinta an unsightly skin disease. Seen in some parts of South America, it is characterized by colored spots on the skin. These may be white, coffee-colored, red, blue, or violet. But among the North Amazonian Indians it is so common that the disfigured are regarded as normal and the normal are considered sick. In that area, Indians without pinta are excluded from marriage.[20] Among the Thonga in Africa, the ever present intestinal

Cultural interpretation of symptoms

[18]Lawrence E. Hinkle, "Studies on Human Ecology in Relation to Health and Behavior," *Bioscience*, Vol. 15, No. 8 (August 1965), pp. 518–19.
[19]Irving Kenneth Zola, "Culture and Symptoms—An Analysis of Patients Presenting Complaints," *American Sociological Review*, Vol. 31, No. 5 (October 1966), p. 617.
[20]Erwin W. Ackerknecht, "The Role of Medical History in Medical Education," cited in Irving Kenneth Zola, "Culture and Symptoms—An Analysis of Patients Presenting Complaints," p. 618.

worms are appreciated—the natives consider them essential for digestion. And, in the nineteenth century, malaria was so ordinary in the Mississippi Valley that the residents did not consider it a disease.

Religion and health For most of the world's religious people, faith has profound emotional connotations. But there is more to religion than emotion. Into its dogma have often been built pragmatic society-saving precepts—precepts that are often involved with health. For example, consider the question of the sacred cow in India. Westerners are prone to despair of India. Newspapers are filled with stories of the starvation in that overpopulated country. In her history, she has endured dozens of famines. One has read of "starving fields" where people go to die. Then one realizes that the Hindu religion prohibits Indians from killing and eating cows. In that hungry country, cows consume ten million tons of human food yearly. To the practical peoples of this nation, such a situation would be intolerable. Resistance to Indian aid is widespread.

But why do so many Indians reject beef? Is the religious concept of the sacred cow a product of stupidity? Foolishness? Ignorance? No. Without the bullock the Indian farm could not exist. In India cows produce the bullocks that pull the plows. Cows, even if old and ailing, produce lavish amounts of manure. For millions of Indians, manure is the only source of fertilizer and fuel. It also provides a usable building material.

What the Indian farmer has developed, ecologically speaking, is a cultural balance. To kill and eat the cows would feed several million Indians for a short while. But the resulting ecological imbalance would cause an agricultural catastrophe of incalculable dimensions. True, technological change will eventually alter the situation. But at this point the destruction of the cow—a major source of agricultural traction, fuel, manure, and building material—would be anti-life, irreligious. And just as Moses forbade pork to the ancient Jews (to protect them, it is thought, from a serious disease, now known as trichinosis), so the Hindu religion forbids the destruction of the cow. To some extent, the Indian's refusal to eat a sacred cow could be compared to the Westerner's reaction to dogmeat. In some societies puppy-hams are a popular food. Some observers have suggested that Western man's reaction to this usually amiable animal borders on worship.

The mainland Chinese present a comparable example of incorporating a societal need into virtual religious belief. Even in 1930 China was the most populous nation on earth. Today the Chinese population problem is enormously compounded. Reasons for this are not hard to find. The Communist government of China has long been interested in the public health. Since it took control in 1949, the Chinese mainland government has generated interest in health by massive propaganda concerning the threat of "bacteriological warfare" by the United States. "There are nonetheless plans to control the diseases that have long plagued the Chinese populace; these have met with some success."[21]

Public health success lowers death rates. With the combination of an uncontrolled birth rate and a decreasing death rate, China can expect nothing but continued population growth. It is extremely important, both to China and to the world, that this increase be controlled. But her population continues to grow. Why? It is Chinese tradition to have sons. Daughters are not too important, but the old rural farmer needs many sons to continue the tilling of his miserable bit of soil. For the aged, a supply of sons plus a carefully developed (religious) respect for parents (and age) combine to provide a social security of sorts. To the Chinese farmer, a program to reduce the number of sons is a threat.

So, among its other functions, religion incorporates practical health rules to meet societal needs. However, most religious experience is also permeated with mysticism. Perhaps it was this element in man's culture to which the German philosopher Goethe referred when he said that "There is in nature what is within reach and what is beyond reach . . . He who is unaware of the distinction may waste himself in lifelong toil trying to get at the inaccessible without ever getting close to truth." The true mystic would disagree. For him divine truths only seem beyond reach. They are, however, accessible through contemplation. To avoid distractions, various asceticisms—such as fasting and poverty—may willingly be endured. In this milieu, suffering becomes a part of religious experience. All the world's great religions have some element of this kind of mysticism. But about two centuries ago a curious, nonreligious offshoot of this philosophy developed. It reached a peak in about the middle of the nineteenth century. The notion gained acceptance that illness per se lent a beautiful intelligence to people. Greatness rose intrinsically from suffering. Sickness became the mark of the poet. He was the sensitive inheritor of the earth. This romantic concept of suffering does not entirely belong to the past. It has modern followers and it merits close examination.

"We are so fond of one another," wrote Jonathan Swift in his *Journal to Stella* (1711), "because we share the same ailments." This practical if unchivalrous observation anticipated a common view of the writers of the late eighteenth and early nineteenth centuries. As always, illness was often shared. But, in those days, even when it went unshared, it had romantic nuances.

This notion of illness found expression as a central theme in much Romantic literature and music. After long centuries of disrepute, after generations of ostracism, suspicion, and indifference, some of the sick

The Romantic age of suffering

[21]Robert M. Worth, "Health Trends in China Since the 'Great Leap Forward,'" *American Journal of Hygiene*, Vol. 78, No. 3 (November 1963), pp. 349, 357.

became not only respected, but envied. This was particularly true of the tuberculous. Blood spitting, night-sweats, loss of weight, pinched fatigue, racking coughs—all these woeful symptoms became emblems of talent, charm, and beauty. To sicken piteously, elegantly flecking a white blouse with blood, became romantic.

René and Jean Dubos note this theme in the words of several famous writers.[22] Lord Byron expressed a courtly desire to die of tuberculosis so the ladies would rhapsodize over "how interesting he looks in dying." The wistful emotions of the ladies of the time were expressed by Marie Bashkirtsev, who wrote in her diary, "I cough continually! But for a wonder, far from making me look ugly, this gives me an air of languor that is very becoming." In his memoirs, Alexander Dumas wrote, "It was the fashion to suffer from the lungs; everybody was consumptive, poets especially; it was good form to spit blood after each emotion that was at all sensational and to die before reaching the age of thirty."

Superior intelligence and tuberculosis became oddly equated. "Is it possible that genius is only scrofula?"[23] Elizabeth Barrett Browning overheard someone ask tremulously of her doctor. John Keats, long afflicted with tuberculosis, wrote to Fanny Brawne, "I must premise that, illness so far as I can judge in so short a time, has relieved my mind of a load of deceptive thoughts and images, and makes me perceive things in a truer light." But his perceptions grew gloomy as his time grew short. Among the last words he read were those from Alfieri's tragedies: "Unhappy me! No solace remains for me but weeping, and weeping is a crime." Living a nightmare of fear that he would suffocate, he died in Rome at twenty-six. Immediately after the funeral the Roman police unromantically "took charge of the apartment at the Piazza di Spagna, burning all the furniture, scraping the walls and floors and even making new doors and windows."[24] "I have been half in love with easeful Death," Keats had written in his "Ode to a Nightingale."

In this century, the writer Katherine Mansfield found in her tuberculosis a link with great writers of the past. Her scrapbooks are full of references to Anton Chekhov and Keats, and she notes that Keats's letters "written during his fatal illness are terrible to one in my situation. It is frightening that he too should have known this mental anguish."[25] She died on January 9, 1923. Her husband, John Middleton Murry, romanticizing her death, wrote:

> I have never seen, nor shall I ever see, any one so beautiful as
> she was on that day; it was as though the exquisite perfection which
> was always hers had taken possession of her completely . . . As

[22]René and Jean Dubos, "Consumption and the Romantic Age," in Berton Roueche, ed., *Curiosities of Medicine* (New York, 1958), pp. 47, 48, 55–56.
[23]Scrofula is tuberculosis of the lymph glands, and sometimes of the surfaces of the bones and joints. In this country it is now very rare.
[24]Aileen Ward, *John Keats: The Making of a Poet* (New York, 1963), p. 388.
[25]John Middleton Murry, ed., *The Scrapbook of Katherine Mansfield* (New York, 1940), p. 195.

she came up the stairs to her room at 10 P.M. she was seized by a fit of coughing which culminated in a violent hæmorrhage. At 10:30 she was dead.[26]

To the well, the sadly sick have always had a certain fascination. The fragility of the ill, the flushed and hollow cheek, the fevered, lustrous eye, the cough-racked body, have been successful themes for all manner of expression, from poetry to television plays. True, the ladies of *Playboy* have apparently replaced "the body rather flat beneath a dress that might have been worn by a slender seraphim."[27] But many moderns still sense something romantic about sickness.

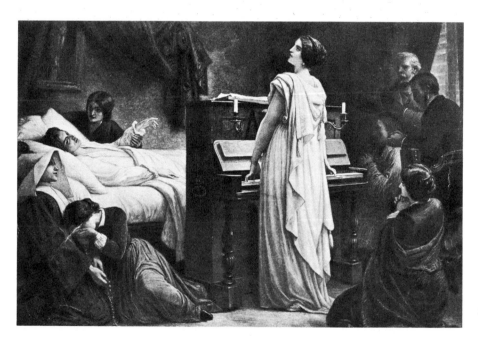

2-4 The death of Chopin: a Romantic view.

People today are often touched by the celebrated nineteenth-century love affair between George Sand and Frederic Chopin. Often she refused him sexual intercourse because she feared it would make him spit blood. This, she wrote, hurt his vanity.[28] There is something romantic about Chopin delicately hemorrhaging on the keyboards of Europe. What cruel boors were those who came to his concerts only to complain that he could not be heard! The truth was that he had barely enough strength to depress the keys.

[26] John Middleton Murry, ed., *The Journal of Katherine Mansfield* (New York, 1940), pp. 255–56.
[27] From the journals of Edmund and Jules de Goncour, quoted in René and Jean Dubos, "Consumption and the Romantic Age," p. 47.
[28] Considerate of his health as she was, she still became somewhat impatient with him, addressing him as "my dear corpse."

And there are those who cannot forget Greta Garbo as Camille. Playing the coughing courtesan with languid passion, she collected her presumably positive sputum (for tuberculosis) in a fluttering, lacy handkerchief. Watching the melancholy scenes with her unhappy lover, who could think of insanitation? Yes, the romantic aspect of sickness has been a valuable tool for the writer, the composer, and the painter. There is even a folk belief to the effect that suffering enriches and deepens character. For some saints this is true. But for most of humanity, suffering is not civilizing, it is demeaning. In *The Moon and Sixpence,* W. Somerset Maugham expressed this clearly: "It is not true that suffering ennobles the character; happiness does that sometimes; but suffering, for the most part, makes men petty and vindictive."[29]

Indifference and resistance to health programs

A view of illness as romantic or ennobling can militate against efforts to curb illness. But in this culture today, health workers confront a more powerful obstacle to their efforts: indifference and active resistance that are decidedly unromantic in origin. What place does health have in life? And why do some people resist health measures?

In its proper place, health is important
"Although health is a common need and the effort to attain it represents a common drive it is actually of secondary rather than of primary importance."[30] If health is not a primary need, then what is? The basic human needs are generally considered to be food, shelter, and sexual expression. Only insofar as health furthers or thwarts the satisfaction of these needs do normal people pay much attention to it. It is to the hypochondriac that health is a continually central thought—an obsession. Indisputably, however, health is a superb adornment to life.

How does man consider death—the end of health—in his scheme of things? Freud called death the goal of all life. The Elizabethan poet John Donne bid "Death, be not proud." After they died, the ancient Roman emperors were customarily deified. It was recorded by the Roman historian Suetonius that the Emperor Vespasian's last words were: "Woe's me. Methinks I'm turning into a god." During the First World War, British soldiers used to sing a song that asked, "O death, where is thy sting-a-ling-a-ling?" A modern wit spoke of death as "nature's way of telling you to slow down." But although such wry references to death are numerous, they merely emphasize mankind's sense of inadequacy in dealing with it. Death is a central event of life, before which all ordinary men stand in awe.

But does death stimulate universally similar reactions? The death of

[29] W. Somerset Maugham, *The Moon and Sixpence* (New York, 1919), p. 94.
[30] John J. Hanlon, *Principles of Public Health Administration* (St. Louis, 1969), p. 55.

a child is instructive in this regard. In an old English churchyard, on the small gravestone of a three-week-old child, is this inscription:

> It is so soon that I am done for,
> I wonder what I was begun for.

These poignant lines reflect the deep and sharp pain caused by the suffering and death of a child. All scriptures—whether Hindu, Buddhist, Zoroastrian, Moslem, Confucianist, Taoist, or Judeo-Christian—cherish the child, and modern civilized societies are geared to nourish and protect the child. However, there have been tragic lapses during which this was not so. Winslow writes:

> Tyler in Primitive Culture relates the Thuringian tale that to make the castle of Liebenstein fast and impregnable, a child was bought for hard money of its mother and walled in. It was eating a cake while the masons were at work and it cried out, "Mother, I see thee still"; then later, "Mother, I see thee a little still"; and as they put in the last stone, "Mother, now I see thee no more."[31]

But one need not go back in history to find people who accept a child's death with equanimity. Hanlon, in discussing the customs of some developing societies, describes the characteristics of the funeral of an infant or young child:

> Often there appears to be surprisingly little mourning; the physical appearance of the funeral procession, if anything, tends to be much brighter and, among some people, even rather cheerful. Songs may be sung, bands may play, and, when the small body is finally removed, there may be a somewhat enthusiastic social event with dining, drinking, dancing and indulgence in all other pleasures of the flesh.[32]

It is, to them, immutable economic logic. The loss of a child cannot be compared to that of a hunter. The unproven child is destined to a prolonged dependence unsuited to the emergencies of tribal life. The child is a consumer, not a contributor. The hunter, however, sustains the group by solving the immediate problem of hunger. And so the death of a great hunter is a signal for the women to wail and for the men to offer sacrifices.

Health, then, is an aspect of life that helps satisfy man's primary needs. As such, it merits serious (though not obsessive) concern. Yet in this culture, those who attempt to improve the public's health are often stymied by a seeming indifference that does not necessarily stem from attitudes

Poverty: the mother of diseases

[31]C.-E. A. Winslow, *The Conquest of Epidemic Disease* (Princeton, N.J., 1943), p. 4.
[32]John J. Hanlon, *Principles of Public Health Administration*, p. 56.

to health and death. This indifference is a mark of social disadvantage. It is an indifference born of poverty and bred by a hopeless sense of helplessness.

Every health worker is witness to this societal tragedy; no complete health survey fails to demonstrate it. A survey recently conducted by a large West Coast health department is illustrative. It had been part of the preplanning activity necessary for a campaign to promote immunization against "regular" measles (rubeola). A safe and effective vaccine was available. The year before a similar effort had seemed to abort an epidemic. For protection against the disease, thousands of parents had brought their children either to their family doctors or to the health department. The new survey revealed that there were still large pockets in the community containing thousands of unvaccinated children. It was statistically certain that a high proportion of them had not had the disease. Lacking immunity by vaccination or by an attack of the illness, they were susceptible not only to the illness but to its serious complications.

The health workers studied a pin-studded map indicating areas of inadequate vaccination levels. They drew circles around a few pockets in the middle-class areas. The survey showed that relatively few children in these sections of the county were still susceptible to measles. The circles surrounding the areas of poverty enclosed the majority of the pins. Although health department workers had provided the vaccinations free of charge, the children of the poor were the least immunized. Here was the old story of the *behavioral* or *performance gap*—the gap between the preventive health services offered and those accepted. That gap between the available benefits of modern preventive care and the indifference to them by a large segment of the poor is hard to bridge.

The great majority of poor people do take advantage of health facilities. Nor do they fail to understand the importance of health. Chancellor Lee of the University of California has pointed out that,

> *A recent Harris poll makes it very clear that poor people understand the relationship between their ill health and poverty. Health is one of their major concerns. Mr. Harris found that 59 percent of the poor blacks and 72 percent of poor whites give health a higher priority than having a good job, compared to 51 percent of Americans as a whole, and he wrote, "Good health to the poor is the lifeline to all else."* [33]

But a large segment of the poor do not take advantage of available preventive health programs. Most of these people are part of what anthropologist Oscar Lewis calls "the culture of poverty." [34] The people in this culture feel deeply alienated from the major institutions of the sur-

[33] Philip R. Lee, "The Problems of the Minorities Rest Not with Them, but with the White Majority," *California's Health*, Vol. 26, No. 11 (May 1969), p. 4.
[34] Oscar Lewis, "The Culture of Poverty,"*Scientific American*, Vol. 215, No. 4 (October 1966), pp. 20–25.

rounding society, generally have little or no effective community organization beyond the family, have a sharply curtailed period of childhood dependency, and often feel helpless and inferior. Lewis distinguishes between poverty and the culture of poverty. Despite their desperate circumstances, many of the poor of Africa, Asia, and South America, for example, have a sense of belonging to and participation with the larger group. Of the estimated 20 to 50 million poor people in the United States, only 20 percent (4 to 10 million) live in the culture of poverty.

In the United States, those in the culture of poverty are mostly blacks, Chicanos (Mexican-Americans), Puerto Ricans, American Indians, and Southern poor whites. And since the culture of poverty perpetuates itself, the children within it are most likely condemned to the behavioral gap too. In this country the largest number of people in the behavioral gap are black. They encounter a double lock on the door to societal opportunities—poverty and prejudice. While the fires of Watts were still burning, a resident of the area summed up the problem of alienation this way: "We have absentee leadership, absentee ministers, absentee landlords and absentee merchants. They provide what services they can during the day, and when the sun goes down in Watts, it's just us and the cops."[35] James Baldwin has been no less direct: "To be a Negro in this country," he has said, "and to be relatively conscious, is to be in a rage almost all of the time."[36] What does the black man want? He wants what the white man wants. Despite the deep sense of alienation within black and other minority communities, the vast majority still seek to advantage themselves of societal opportunities. In this there is hope.

Money alone will solve neither alienation nor the behavioral gap, for these problems are not merely economic. But money is essential to relieving them. High death rates of children and pregnant women, shorter adult life expectancies, malnutrition—these are among the bitter realities of the poor.[37] Health programs are one area where more money must be spent. But is it expenditure or investment? As the following section indicates, a health program can show a financial profit.

Some years ago a physician addressed the regular meeting of the city council of a large Midwestern city. A deliberate man, he developed his theme carefully: to cure a child cost more than to prevent his disease. His audience, largely composed of businessmen, regarded him with curious interest. Unaccustomed to this approach, some of his listeners were not quite sure they liked it. They were more comfortable with sentiment. Not a month before someone had brought a crippled child of seven to the meeting. The child's eyes were brown, enormous, and reproachful. A lot of money had been raised that afternoon for a crippled children's clinic.

Meeting community resistance—health is a bargain

[35] Gladwin Hill, *The New York Times* (August 28, 1965), p. 54.
[36] Quoted in Charles Silberman, *Crisis in Black and White* (New York, 1964), p. 36.
[37] For a discussion of malnutrition and retardation see pages 296–97.

Now the physician told them that contributions were needed to support a psychiatrist for the crippled children's clinic. Treatment was needed for the mental limp. A child, benefited by such treatment, would be less likely to inhabit costly psychiatric wards, would be less prone to populate prisons, would more likely work and pay taxes someday. Such a child would cost now but repay later. Health was an investment. Contributions to it, deductible from personal income tax this year, would lower taxes in the future. They did not need to be told of their obligations to children, the physician told them. But had they realized that health was good business? It was a bargain.

His theme was not new, he admitted. At the turn of the century, summer was the season of death in the New York tenements. Thousands of babies died of summer diarrhea. New York physicians, hurrying to beat the undertaker to the tenement baby, had a slogan: "It costs $25 to save a baby, but $75 to bury it."

"Let us take another example you all know about," the physician continued. "Recently, we vaccinated 100,000 children against measles. At $1.50 per vaccination, the cost was $150,000. This means, however, that 100,000 children won't get the disease. But without the vaccine, just about all the children would have contracted measles. One measles case out of 1,000 develops encephalitis.[38] This is a brain inflammation. Had we not vaccinated the 100,000 children, we would have had 100 cases of measles encephalitis. Of these, 25 children would have died and 40 would have been permanently retarded physically and mentally, or both. We won't talk now about the 25 children that would have been lost. But to care for one retarded child during his lifetime costs $200,000. It is simple arithmetic. Forty children times $200,000 equals $8,000,000. Subtract the $150,000 cost of the vaccination program from the $8,000,000. The net profit— $7,850,000."

The speaker sat down. There was a pause and then a murmur of approval. The chairman asked for comments. One after another the businessmen rose to support the speaker. Saving a child appealed to their emotions; saving a dollar, to their business sense. It was a good way to be good.

The physician's talk had convinced the businessmen of the community that preventive health measures were indeed good business. By unanimous vote, adequate funds for the psychiatrist were made available.

Despite misinformed opposition, health programs can also be good politics. But those who wield political power in the ballot box must make their wishes felt. Otherwise they may be victimized by a misinformed minority.

"Them dogs don't vote"   A short time ago the elected city council of a large western city met in regular session. The council chambers were even more crowded and

[38] Saul Krugman and Robert Ward, *Infectious Diseases of Children*, 4th ed. (St. Louis, 1968), p. 140.

tense than usual. Television lights and cameras had been set up. In the rear a voice could be heard rising in anger.

With difficulty the meeting was called to order. The subject was introduced. It was fluoridation of the municipal water supply for the purpose of preventing dental cavities in children. New York, Philadelphia, Chicago, Detroit—all had long ago provided the benefits of fluorides to their children. When the subject of fluoridation had been brought up in those cities, all major scientific and lay agencies, from the American Dental Association to local PTA's, had testified in its favor. Years of experience had proved beyond a doubt that a safe level of fluoridation in the water supply, costing about ten cents per person per year, would prevent over sixty percent of the children's cavities.

Today, at the council meeting, dental and public health experts presented a quiet case for fluoridation. They remained calm, objective, and accurate. Their opponents were strident, adamant, and even threatening. Hinting about "election time," they exhorted the council to beware of "a Communist plot to poison the water." Some spoke darkly of "secret animal and human experiments that need looking into."

The majority of the council voted against fluoridation. And so millions of children in this city will needlessly become dental cripples. The suffering will begin with those who, of course, could not speak for themselves at the meeting—the children. It will continue throughout their lives in endless pain and expense. And until the council changes its mind, each new bumper crop of children in that western city will be condemned to the same fate. Even more discouraging was the lack of support from some council members representing the poor. Although their constituents could not afford dental care, they voted against fluoridation.

Fluoridation, as a recognized effective method of preventing dental cavities in children, is discussed in Chapter 9. The point here is that a loud minority of the community deprived the suppliant majority of a proven health practice.

Not long ago it was unsafe for a child in that same western city to play in the street, much less walk home from school. Rabid dogs roamed the streets, biting, and possibly infecting, any human being who happened across their path. A safe and effective vaccine to prevent rabies in dogs had long been available. All responsible scientific organizations supported compulsory vaccination of dogs. Yet for many years, a small, militant, seemingly well-financed minority successfully led the fight against rabies vaccinations of dogs. The advice of public health officials, distinguished deans of medical and veterinary schools, and other leading scientific figures in the community went unheeded.

Again, it was usually the child who paid. A child does not easily understand that a sick dog can carry death and must be left alone. And when he does understand this, his compassion usually gains the upper hand over his judgment. In that city children had to be taught to fear dogs—sick dogs in particular. Frequently, both children and adults had to endure the fourteen to twenty-eight painful injections that constitute the dangerous Pasteur treatment. Since human rabies is always fatal, the preventive vaccine was the only treatment. However, it caused paralysis about once every two thousand times it was used.[39] The following true story illustrates the dilemma.

Tommy, a nine-year-old newsboy, was brought to a physician by his mother because he had been bitten by a dog that "was acting funny—he was limping around and had a funny bark." The boy had tried to help the animal, and it had bitten him savagely on the hand. Before coming to the doctor, the mother had reported the dog bite to the health department. The doctor immediately telephoned the health department and asked their veterinarian about the animal. The dog had been caught. It was rabid. The bite in the child's thumb was a deep tear. The doctor washed the wound for a long time. He then sutured it, and started the injections against rabies.

After nine injections into the soft tissue around the umbilicus, the child developed a fever (103°F. orally), a headache, and an "'lectric like" feeling over the right ribs and arm. "See doctor," he said, more curious than concerned, "I can't hold a pencil." The doctor saw only too well. The boy's symptoms heralded a treatment paralysis. He turned to the mother. "We will have to stop his treatments," he said slowly.

"But won't he get rabies?" Her voice rose. She fought to control it.

"He could. But right now, with this reaction from the vaccine, the chances of his getting rabies are not as great as the chances of a permanent treatment paralysis. It's a matter of measuring the risks. And there is a good chance, the best chance, that nothing at all will happen and he will be all right."

"When will we know?"

The doctor paused. He had seen two cases of human rabies. Now, as he regarded the boy, he remembered them. "In about a week or two we should know pretty well. But we can't be absolutely positive, not for some months."

After the distraught woman left with her child, the doctor telephoned a city councilman. He explained the case in detail. "Why don't you vote for rabies vaccination?" he asked. "It's even good for the dogs."

"Listen doc," the politician said bluntly, "when we took up this rabies vaccination thing, the council chambers were swarming with dog lovers. They raised a row. These days two things bring people to a council meeting—taxes and dogs. You know how many people came to talk for vaccination? One was this rundown botany professor whose sleeves are too long for him. The other was the president of the medical society, and nobody likes him because he drives a Cadillac. Where were you? There were twenty dog lovers for every kid lover. Everybody gets what he deserves. As for them sick dogs, well, them dogs don't vote."

---

[39] A much safer vaccine is now available, but there is some doubt as to whether it is equally effective in some instances.

The doctor telephoned the mother. "I just wanted to ask you," he said, "do you remember the council meeting on compulsory rabies vaccination last month? Were you there?"

There was a long pause. "I wasn't there," she said. "I'm getting what I deserve."

The child recovered, but his mother did not rest until, in the next year, compulsory rabies vaccination for dogs was the law in her town.

So it has been since this country began. Public health is sometimes accepted only after years of effort by an informed and a finally aroused citizenry. In Colonial America, Cotton Mather was widely hated for his advocacy of smallpox vaccination. Indeed, in 1791, a hand grenade was thrown into his house. Attached to it was this message: "Cotton Mather, you Dog, Damn you, I'll inoculate you with this, and a Pox to you."

Smallpox vaccination, rabies vaccination, water fluoridation and chlorination, milk pasteurization—these and a host of other health advances have been met with the bitter resistance of the misinformed. Though experience may teach the misinformed, too often the paths of experience are littered with the dead and disabled.

The first chapter of this book placed man on a health scale within a dynamic ecosystem. This second chapter has considered him within his culture. Alone among living creatures, man has added thought to instinct, culture to inherited impulse. Human health is inextricably tied to culture. It is profoundly affected not only by such basic cultural concerns as ethics, religion, money, and freedom but also by the environmental changes that man has continually wrought. Many of these changes he has used productively. As a primitive, the harnessing of fire brought him warmth and cooked food. As a sophisticate, the harnessing of the laser beam enabled him to perform delicate eye surgery. But the environmental changes of mankind are rarely unmixed blessings. DDT has multiplied man's crops, but now it threatens his well-being. The automobile has extended his world, but, too often, it has ended his life. Has man remained in healthful balance with his environment? Or has he, for temporary advantage, been too careless with his ecological future? These questions will be discussed in the next two chapters.

3

Man versus man: waters of affliction and ill winds

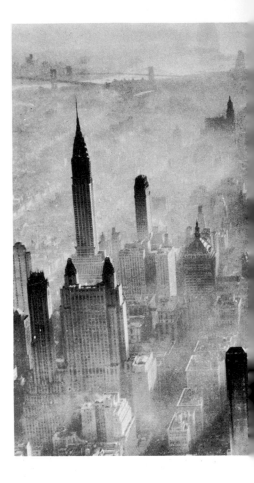

"To insure health, a man's relation to Nature must come very near to a personal one; he must be conscious of a friendliness in her . . . I cannot conceive of any life which deserves the name, unless there is a certain tender relation to Nature."[1]

Samples from the polluted past

To live is to pollute. This condition of existence man shares with all creatures. Even, however, as evolution granted man greater gifts to control environment, so did it enable him to dirty it most. Beginning with the Neanderthal and Cro-Magnon peoples of the Paleolithic period (who have occupied ninety-eight percent of the total human time on earth so far),

[1] Henry David Thoreau, *Journal*, January 23, Saturday, 1858, in Carl Bode, ed., *The Portable Thoreau* (New York, 1947), p. 590.

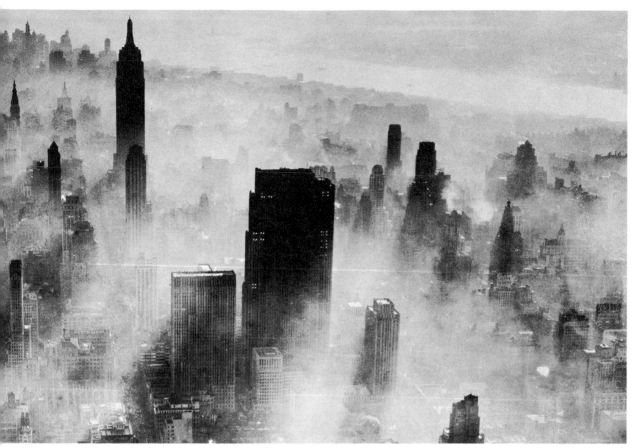

Smog over New York.

man has constantly befouled the planet. It was stated on page 5 that, in adapting and evolving, primitive man had acquired thumbs, a complex brain, an erect posture, an accommodating digestive tract. Slowly, he learned how best to use them. His wants stimulated him. He was dissatisfied with vegetable roots. He wanted meat. Using his thumb, therefore, he grasped a lit torch and thought enough to set woods afire. The flames drove wild game out for the kill, but smoke filled the air. Much of earth was once forest. The trees failed to outlast man. Around the charred stumps, farmers planted their crops. People gathered. Little cities rose. Sharing each other's company, people had to also share each other's residues, and because they came to believe that sickness rose from filth, they sought ways of cleanliness.

"And the Lord God took the man, and put him into the garden of Eden to dress it and to keep it" (Genesis 2:15). Expelled from the storied garden, man presumably took his custodial function with him. But in this stewardship of nature, his performance left much to be desired. Still lacking humility, he considered the world to be his. "We make our greatest mistake when we believe that the world belongs to us. It does not—we belong to it."[2] Not comprehending this, man has polluted his environment ceaselessly, carelessly, and with abandon. Should he persist, he may ultimately find as little room for himself in the world as he found in Eden. Nor has his garbage been limited to earth. Today, the junk from man's space ships orbits the globe. The first human litter has even invaded the moon. Man's pollutions are now literally out of this world. Considering man's sufferings at the hands of nature's pollutions, one would think he would hesitate to indiscriminately add his own.

Lucretius, Pliny the Younger, and the forces of nature

In his most ancient writings man made melancholy reference to nature's threats to his ecosystem. In *On the Nature of Things*, the Roman poet Lucretius wrote eloquently of those who ventured deep into the earth to mine the ore: "What hurtful damps, what noxious vapours rise! / The wretched miner o'er the metal dies."

Lucretius was concerned with the occupational disease of gold miners. In those days only slaves worked the mines. Presumably the ancient Greeks of Herculaneum and Pompeii were not so unfortunate. Indifferent to the shadow of the seething volcano Vesuvius, they had settled in suburban villas on the sunny Bay of Naples. But in A.D. 79, Vesuvius erupted. The air pollution was appalling. "We had scarce considered what was to be done," wrote Pliny the Younger to Tacitus, "when we were surrounded with darkness . . . you might then have heard the shrieks of women, the moans of infants, and outcries of men . . . ashes poured down upon us."[3] In two days Herculaneum lay beneath forty-five feet of hardening volcanic ash and mud, Pompeii under twenty-four.

Medieval smog and the reign of cholera

Centuries passed. New lands were settled. Wars were fought. Early in European history English influence arose and spread. But the English homeland was cold country. The early English burned wood for warmth. Then wood became scarce. Englishmen were forced to seek elsewhere for heat's comfort. Perhaps they had heard that the Chinese had been using coal as a fuel for a thousand years. Tardily, Henry III permitted his shivering subjects to burn coal. This resulted in a formidable thirteenth-century English smog. To pacify the coughing, complaining barons, Henry's son Edward decreed death as punishment for coal burning while Parliament was in session, "lest the health of the Knights of the Shire should suffer during their residence in London."[4] One early Englishman certainly found coal unhealthful. In 1307, he was hanged for burning it.

[2] Phillip Kellerin, quoted in Robert and Leona Train Rienow, *Moment in the Sun* (New York, 1967), p. 33.

[3] John Boyle, Earl of Orrery, *The Letters of Pliny the Younger with Observations on Each Letter*, 2nd ed., Vol. II (London, 1751), p. 54.

[4] Eugene Ayres, "The Age of Fossil Fuels," in William L. Thomas, Jr., ed., *Man's Role in Changing the Face of the Earth* (Chicago, 1956), p. 368.

London smog persisted as a dangerous nuisance, as is shown by these rhymes from a book of collected verse published in about 1663.

> He[5] shewes that 'tis the seacoale smoake
> That allways London doth Inviron,
> Which doth our Lungs and Spiritts choake
> Our hangings spoyle, and rust our Iron.
> Lett none att Fumifuge be scoffing
> Who heare att Church our Sunday's Coughing.[6]

Air pollution was hardly the only environmental problem of early England. In 1290, the good monks of Whitefriars begged the King to attend to the "putrid exhaltations" rising from the Thames. Their complaint: the stench rose above the sweet scent of incense burnt upon the altar. More important, they thought it had caused the death of several brethren.[7] Centuries passed and brought no relief. The October 17, 1710, edition of *The Tatler* carried an especially pungent description of the turgid waters of the Thames. It reads in part:

> Filth of all hues and odours seem to tell
> What street they sail'd from, by their sight and smell . . .
> Sweepings from butcher's stalls, dung, guts, and blood,
> Drown'd puppies, shaking sprats, all drenched in mud,
> Dead cats, and turnip tops, come tumbling down the flood.[8]

The whole area around the Thames became known as the "capital of cholera." It well deserved this name. In those days, this bacterial, water-borne disease was rampant in London.

Meanwhile, what had been going on in the New World?

On a basic use of waste

Some historians are fond of referring to pre-Columbian America as a virgin land. But it had been raped long before the Italian and his crew reached its shores. In ravaging the land, the early Central American Mayan Indians destroyed their civilization. First they burned the trees. Then they planted crops for quick harvest. They did not think to replenish the land with their excreta. This failure to use their own organic wastes cost them their survival as a great people. As soon as the unfed soil of their farms became too exhausted to provide more food, they moved. From place to place they went, from despoiled to unspoiled soil, always taking, never giving. Under ordinary conditions, nature needs three hundred to a thousand years to build one inch of topsoil. The Mayan method of agriculture

---

[5]This verse, among others, was dedicated to John Evelyn (1620–1706), whose work on London smog, *Fumifugium,* had attracted wide attention.
[6]Quoted in Marjorie Hope Nicolson, *Pepys' Diary and the New Science* (Charlottesville, Va., 1965), p. 149.
[7]N. J. Barton, *The Lost Rivers of London* (London, 1962), p. 107.
[8]*Ibid.,* p. 106.

gave nature neither time nor help to rebuild. Eventually exhausted, the soil could yield no more food. Kept on the move, constantly forced to reconstruct anew at each new site, in a thousand years the Mayans were also exhausted. Today, they are a people of monuments and memories. By contrast, the Chinese did not take food from their soil without feeding the soil their wastes. They survived.

The Mayans are an example of what not to do. The Oriental exemplifies what must be done.[9] "The function of all waste organic matter, animal and vegetable, is to maintain the fertility of the soil, and while man's ingenuity may produce wonderful as well as monstrous things, he is incapable of getting round this fundamental fact."[10] In considering waste control, it is well to remember this.

In parts of modern Africa this principle has yet to be applied. Many of the herdsmen are nomads. The migrating animals in their keep do not remain in one area long enough to provide adequate manure for agricultural purposes. Instead, farmers must use poor fertilizer such as ashes and bushes. As soon as the soil is exhausted, whole tribes move on to another area to repeat their agricultural errors. Much of Africa has thus become a vast farming problem.[11]

Life in a new republic
"Why should cities be erected," Noah Webster asked mournfully, "if they are to be only the tombs of men?" Even from his tomb, Webster's contemporary, Doctor Benjamin Franklin, acted to avoid this gloom. On May 10, 1790, the Aldermen and Common Councilmen of Philadelphia gathered to read excerpts from Franklin's last will and testament. He had left Philadelphia a little money, advice on how to increase it, and still more advice on how to spend it.

> Whence the water of wells must gradually grow worse, and in time be unfit for use, as I find has happened in all old cities . . . I recommend . . . the corporation of the city Employ a part of the hundred thousand pounds in bringing by pipes, the water of Wissahickon Creek into town, so as to supply the inhabitants, which I apprehend may be done without great difficulty, the level of that creek being much above that of the city and may be made higher by a dam.[12]

The wise old man had not been unduly concerned. According to the May 3, 1799, issue of the *Aurora,* Philadelphians of the day were often "saluted with a great variety of fetid and disgusting smells . . . exhaled

[9]The modern Japanese, too, provide a lesson in frugality. During the Second World War, they carefully collected human and animal wastes and, like a priceless brew, carefully applied them to their private gardens. Because of the use of so dangerously infected a fertilizer, there was much typhoid. But starvation was rare.

[10]J. C. Wylie, *The Wastes of Civilization* (London, 1959), p. 124.

[11]Jacques M. May and Hoyt Lemmons, "The Ecology of Malnutrition," *Journal of the American Medical Association,* Vol. 207, No. 13 (March 31, 1969), p. 2403.

[12]Quoted in Nelson Manfred Blake, *Water for the Cities* (Syracuse, N.Y., 1956), p. 4.

from the dead carcasses of animals, from stagnant waters, and from every species of filth that can be collected from the city, thrown in heaps as if . . . to promote the purposes of death."[13]

The decade following 1790 saw repeated yellow fever epidemics sweeping through North American cities. In 1793, more than ten percent of the population of Philadelphia perished. A few years later New York was similarly afflicted. A few correctly guessed a relationship between the "clouds of musketoes" and the disease. Sheer fear stimulated the survivors to improve water supply and sewage disposal facilities. Large storm drainage systems had already been built. But these conduits had not been used for the disposal of human feces and urine. It was not until the nineteenth century that the idea of a water-carriage system of human excreta was accepted. This was "the major sanitary advance over the centuries."[14] By this means mankind could be separated from his disease-carrying waste.[15]

How did early educators view the increasing pollutions of their New World? Like the uneducated, they were annoyed. But did early college professors take a lead in the study of their major ecological problems? If the environment of the Colonial (and later) college campuses is an example, the good old days were not all that good. Much is made of the educational environment of the past. Sometimes deservedly. But how many historians remember that after a century of existence the Harvard library had yet to add the works of the dead Dryden, Johnson, Pope, and Swift?

Sometimes, food for the belly was as scarce as that for the brain. Nor was the former handled with much care. In the early nineteenth century it was common for underfed undergraduates at Harvard and Princeton to use a fork for more than eating. With it they would pin on the under surface of the dining table a few scraps of today's meat for tomorrow's dinner. Such property rights were rigidly respected by all but stray dogs. College cows often ate better than college men. They were pastured on most campuses, and at Harvard pigs were an animal garbage disposal system for commons. If college students turned up their noses in those days, there was, at least, good reason. Refuse was generally thrown out dormitory windows. The lower floors stank and, it is presumed, were reserved for freshmen and other wanderers.[16]

On the Spartan nature of early campus life

[13] *Ibid.*, p. 8.

[14] Abel Wolman, "Disposal of Man's Wastes," in William L. Thomas, Jr., ed., *Man's Role in Changing the Face of the Earth*, p. 808.

[15] Yet, at the same time as man learned to be rid of one waste, he created still another. On August 4, 1727, a German reporter in Paris wrote an article for his countrymen about "A certain mathematicus . . . [who] has invented a carriage for four persons, with which he will drive without horses through its own internal motion fourteen French miles in two hours." (Hermann Schreiber, *The History of Roads*, tr. by Stewart Thomson [London, 1961], p. 213.)
The Los Angeles-type smog was born.

[16] Christian Gauss, "How Good Were the Good Old Days?" in A. C. Spectorsky, ed., *The College Years* (New York, 1958), pp. 81–88.

The effluence of affluence

Now, almost two centuries later, the problems have changed but man's relationship to his environment has not improved; rather, it has deteriorated in proportion to the increase of his numbers and needs. For each pollution problem that was solved, another crucial one was created. More than a half century ago a distinguished university lecturer eloquently expressed a prophetic paradox. Mankind, he pointed out, had survived every disaster. He had endured devastating epidemics, wars, famine. Could he survive success? What experience lent him strength to endure progress?

"I do suspect," he told his class, "that many of you young gentlemen may live to see a time for which neither by tradition nor experience are we particularly well prepared, because the struggle of the future is going to be who will survive prosperity, not adversity. We have had a long racial experience on surviving adversity, but what do we know about surviving prosperity?"[17]

Radiation. Accidents. Noise. Pesticides. Water pollution. Air pollution. An increasing list of major environmental hazards besets man. For a long time his clutter and waste have been gathering. Can he live in harmony while his excess pollution remains uncontrolled? No. Mankind must be in balance with all else in his ecosystem. Only at his peril does man violate its fragile web. And the time for his reconsideration is dangerously short. It is here pertinent to call to mind a portion of an inscription long ago placed on the road to Vesuvius, some three miles from Naples. It is dated 1631, a year in which still another eruption killed four thousand people.

> *Posterity, posterity, this is your concern,*
> *one day enlightens the next, the next*
> *improves the third.*
> *Be attentive.*[18]

Water

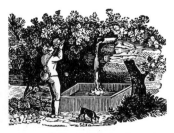

3-1 A fresh draught.

> *I am the Poem of Earth, said the voice of the rain,*
> *Eternal I rise impalpable out of the land and the bottomless sea,*
> *Upward to heaven, whence, vaguely form'd, altogether changed, and*
> *   yet the same,*
> *I descend to lave the drouths, atomies, dust-layers of the globe,*
> *And all that in them without me were seeds only, latent, unborn;*
> *And forever, by day and night, I give back life to my own origin,*
> *   and make pure and beautify it.*[19]

[17] Dr. Alan Gregg speaking of a lecture by Thomas Nixon Carver, quoted in William L. Thomas, Jr., ed., *Man's Role in Changing the Face of the Earth*, pp. 956–57.

[18] John Boyle, Earl of Orrery, *The Letters of Pliny the Younger with Observations on Each Letter*, 2nd ed., Vol. II, p. 59.

[19] Walt Whitman, "The Voice of the Rain," as quoted in *Scientist and Citizen*, Vol. 7, No. 2 (December 1964), p. 1.

The poet Walt Whitman thus described the eternal water cycle. The rainfall moistening the earth is gathered up as vapor by the sun's warmth. Air cools. Vapors condense. Clouds form. Then the rain falls again. During its life-giving stay on earth, some rainfall seeps into the ground. In sinking, it is slowly filtered through sand and cleansed. The American Indian understood this purifying action of filtration. He did not drink from a polluted stream. Instead he scooped a hole near its bank and drank the water that filtered into it.

Water purification

Water that does not seep underground flows from the mountains into rivulets and rivers, seeking—and eventually finding—the sea. In its course man draws from it. But first it must be made safe. In a water-treatment plant, this may be accomplished primarily by filtration and chlorination. Safe drinking water is one of the triumphs of modern public health. Even before chlorine was introduced into the United States as a water disinfectant (in 1908), filtration alone could provide considerable, though hardly enough, protection against water-borne disease. Among the most common of such diseases was typhoid fever. This infection is caused by a microbe that may be transmitted by human feces and urine. Pollution of drinking water or food by these human discharges resulted in frequent typhoid fever epidemics. At the turn of this century, the annual national typhoid fever death rate was about 35 per 100,000. Pittsburgh and Cincinnati still used unfiltered water. Their typhoid fever death rates were three times the national average. Chlorination brought bacteriological safety to a degree previously unknown. It does not cost much more to purify highly polluted water than relatively safe water.

Today, some two-thirds of the population of this country is served by a completely safe public water supply. For countless other millions of the world's city dwellers, however, safe water is a dream, water-borne disease the bitter reality. For example, nearly seven million people are packed into four hundred square miles of Calcutta.[20] Millions of Calcutta residents use unfiltered hydrant water for cleaning and drinking. As in Western countries two centuries ago, open sewers run through some streets. Cholera is common.

The uses of water

The Ancient Roman water supply, carried by a system of aqueducts more than 250 miles long, was the envy of the world. Sextus Julius Frontinus, the Roman water engineer, was well aware that a safe water supply made civilization possible: "With such an array of indispensable structures carrying so many waters," he boasted of the aqueducts, "compare, if you will, the idle Pyramids or the useless, though famous, works of the Greeks!"[21]

[20] By contrast, few of the two and a half million residents of Los Angeles' four hundred square miles think they have room to spare.
[21] Quoted in E. M. Winslow, *A Libation to the Gods* (London, 1963), p. 17.

The people of the United States use water lavishly. Swimming pools and lawn sprinklers help make Beverly Hills residents this nation's greatest per capita water consumers. But the average citizen is hardly parsimonious with it. He will use no less than five gallons a day to shave, wash, and brush his teeth. Flushing the toilet once requires five to seven gallons. A minute under a running shower spends five gallons. Almost thirty gallons are used in a home load of laundry.

Agriculture is a huge water consumer. To grow one pound of flour requires 375 gallons of water. It takes about 5,000 gallons to can 100 cases of peas or corn. A one-acre orange grove requires 800,000 gallons of water. But the thirstiest of all is industry, and it often demands water of high purity. The paper for the Sunday newspaper consumes 150 gallons. Brewing one barrel of beer uses 1,000 gallons of water. For the aluminum in a bomber, 29 million gallons are needed. Water does not only sustain life; it is also needed to maintain a way of life.

Waste reveals the era (and some tales of a tub)

Once used, urban water is a waste carrier. The character of that waste reflects the times. What can waste tell about the past? Are people of this civilization cleaner than their predecessors? Their remnant plumbing helps to tell. "There were more than one thousand baths in ancient Rome and that is more than were in London at the beginning of the last century."[22] Early urbanites of this nation found the opportunities for "all over" bathing extremely limited. The sixth president of the United States was no exception. In order to get a decent bath John Quincy Adams had to sneak away from the White House before dawn and use the Potomac River. In his later years, Benjamin Franklin had lived more luxuriously. His tub was shaped like a lady's slipper (see Figure 3-2). Under the heel was a place for a charcoal heater and on the instep the great Colonial philosopher could prop a book.

Perhaps the most sumptuous bath of all was described by Lord Bacon. In 1638, he prescribed a twenty-seven-hour bath. Among his suggestions were: "Oyle, and Salves . . . sit 2 hours in the Bath . . . wrap the Body in a seare-cloth made of Masticke, Myrrh, Pomander and Saffron . . . 24 houres . . . lastly . . . with an oyntment of Oyle, Salt and Saffron . . . anoint the Body."[23] Not even once was soap mentioned by his Lordship. Clearly the waste of his recommended bath would differ from the bath-waste of Benjamin Franklin or the modern bather. And detergents long ago replaced the strong lye soaps of another generation, as tissues have almost wholly replaced handkerchiefs. Leftovers from dinner, carefully preserved by the thrifty housewife of yesteryear, are now fed to the "electric pig." All this, and more,[24] finds its way into sewage pipes. All reveal a changing era. All bring new problems to waste disposal engineers.

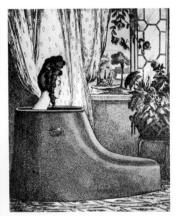

3-2 An early 19th-century English bathtub.

[22] J. C. Wylie, *The Wastes of Civilization*, p. 11.
[23] Quoted in Lawrence Wright, *Clean and Decent* (London, 1960), p. 75.
[24] An occasional crocodile ends up in a sewage system. Bought when small as pets, the crocodiles are flushed down the toilet when their owners tire of them. The crocodiles thrive on sewage and may grow to several feet in length.

In some areas waste is just collected by sewer pipes that lead it unpurified to the nearest river. At least this removes the problem from immediate sight. A better answer is the modern sewage treatment plant. From toilet bowl, laundromat, bathtub, shower, and sink, waste leaves the home by pipes leading to main sewer lines. By these routes it reaches sewage treatment plants. Here, body waste and other pollutions are removed. How? In the plant, sewage is first passed through a screen. Large objects, such as sticks and rags, are caught. Then the sewage may be passed through a tank. Within the tank, solids settle, and in the absence of oxygen, organic solids are broken down. The sewage may then be filtered. Then, by means of oxidation, sewage is further broken down to even simpler constituents. Finally, a disinfectant such as chlorine is added. Using these methods, only reasonably safe sewage need be discharged into a natural waterway. But even modern cities are frequently not advantaged by the best methods, or their methods are incomplete. At times, the demands of modern wastes are unmet. A major modern problem has developed—the vast and dangerous pollution of rivers, lakes, and streams.

What happens to urban waste?

But human wastes are not the only problem. In former times, animals providing man's food were widely distributed. When their waste was used for fertilizer it, too, was spread over a large area. Today hog and poultry production are concentrated, factory-like operations. Often cows are close to cities. "A cow generates as much manure as 16 human beings; one hog produces nearly as much waste as two human beings; seven chickens create as much of a disposal problem as one person does. In total, farm animals produce ten times as much organic waste as the human population"[25] Disposal of animal waste has become a problem not often handled satisfactorily. It is a topic of much federal Public Health Service concern.

Nonhuman waste pollution

To all these pollutions one must add over 500,000 different chemicals that find their way into U.S. streams. The dimensions of this nation's water pollution are indeed enormous. And the threat to water life is more than biological and chemical. Modern industry is now creating a dangerous physical change in aquatic ecosystems.

Rivers, streams, lakes, and other waters are now being used in certain cooling and condensing procedures in such industrial activities as the generation of electrical power. In these processes water temperature is raised, and in this way everything alive in the water is imperiled. Nuclear power plants require up to forty percent more cooling water than traditional power plants. Today the operational capacity of nuclear power plants is growing. By the turn of this century, the Atomic Energy Commission estimates that this operational capacity will have increased two-hundred-and-fifty fold. The threat to water life is apparent. In 1968, a

Thermal pollution

[25]"Restoring the Quality of Our Environment," report of the Environmental Pollution Panel, quoted in Philip H. Abelson, "Man-Made Environmental Hazards: How Man Shapes His Environment," *American Journal of Public Health*, Vol. 58, No. 11 (November 1968), p. 2046.

Senate subcommittee on air and water pollution opened hearings on the problem. They hope to prevent excessive thermal pollution "as well as to seek economically feasible solutions to the problem today emanating from the more traditional plants, fueled by coal, gas and oil."[26]

Of dirty waters   In the summer of 1842, the author of *The Scarlet Letter,* Nathaniel Hawthorne, visited a friend who was living by a quiet lake near Concord, Massachusetts. He was weary. The wooded stillness was good to him. Moreover, he enjoyed good company—some close friends. Among them was Ralph Waldo Emerson. In those days the lake was not yet famous. It was a small waterway called Walden Pond. Near its bank lived Hawthorne's friend, Henry David Thoreau.

"Walden Pond . . . is not very extensive," Hawthorne later wrote in his notebook, "but large enough for waves to dance upon its surface, and to look like a piece of blue firmament, earth-encircled." Hawthorne bathed in the pond. "A good deal of mud and river-slime had accumulated on my soul; but these bright waters washed it all away."[27]

Many such waters of this land have lost their brightness. They are filled with sewage. How does this dolorous condition of nature affect the condition of man?

The United States and Canada share a mutual blessing, the largest fresh-water reservoir on earth—the Great Lakes. In its basin live some fourteen percent of this country's population and almost a third of Canada's. Its vast waterway extends for two thousand miles, from the St. Lawrence River to Duluth. It provides transportation, hydroelectric power, and food. It is an unparalleled water playground. Its worst enemy is its greatest beneficiary—man.

City and industrial wastes have turned vast areas of the Great Lakes into a murky sewage pit. The dirtiest is the once sparkling Lake Erie. Geologically a young lake, it is, according to some experts, dying long before its time. Others already describe the lake as "a putrid corpse." Still others dispute that the pollution of Lake Erie is beyond remedy. However, nobody questions that it is seriously polluted. Since it is an average of 58 feet deep (compared to the 487 feet of Lake Superior), it is too shallow to dilute its pollutions. Huge industrial complexes and cities befoul it. The Detroit River, an enormous cesspool containing a variety of pollutants ranging from fecal bacteria to phenols and ammonia, spills filth into it. Lake Erie is an enormous receptacle for the garbage of industrial progress. Phenols and ammonia kill the fish. Waste decomposition diminishes the water's oxygen. Oxygen is further depleted by an overgrowth of countless algae. Algae are a group of plants, such as seaweed, widely distributed in both fresh and salt water. They thrive on the nitrogen and phosphorus

[26] Edmund S. Muskie, "Guest Editorial—Thermal Pollution," *New England Journal of Medicine,* Vol. 278, No. 12 (March 21, 1968), pp. 677–78.
[27] Nathaniel Hawthorne, 15 August 1842: *Note-Books* (1869), quoted in Holbrook Jackson, *Bookman's Pleasure* (New York, 1947), p. 130.

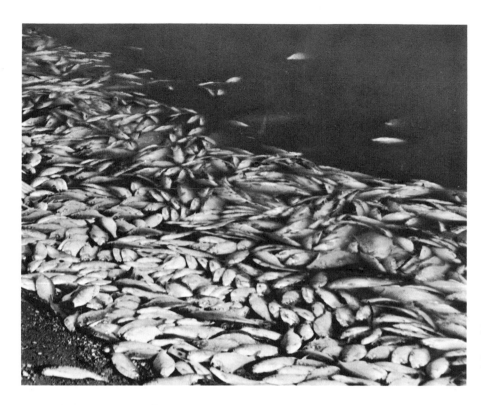

3-3 Water pollution. Sugar beet wastes dumped into this Ohio stream killed the fish.

provided them by pollution. And if these evils do algae some good, the algae do no good. As photosynthesis takes place within their cells, the algae create an excessively high oxygen level in the water during the day. During the night, oxygen levels fall markedly. Both conditions may kill many fish. When masses of the algae die and begin to decompose, the lake is further depleted of oxygen. This impedes the efforts of water-purification plants. To the nauseating stench of dead algae is added that of smothered fish. In 1936, Lake Erie yielded twenty million pounds of blue pike. Less than a generation later, the catch was under a thousand pounds. (Some observers feel that over-fishing has contributed to the biological imbalance in the lake.) It is as if a part of the Biblical prophecy of ancient Egypt's doom had today come true in these waters: "The fishers also shall mourn, and all they that cast angle into the brooks shall lament, and they that spread nets upon the waters shall languish" (Isaiah 19:8).

Man cannot change the exquisite balance of water ecology without risking the life within it. And if life within water is changed, so is bird life in the air and man's life on the ground.

More than a generation has elapsed since the late humorist Robert Benchley attended Harvard. One day, during an examination on American diplomatic history, he was asked a question on the rights to the New-foundland fisheries. Benchley worked around his ignorance this way: "This question has long been discussed from the American and British points of view, but has anyone ever considered the viewpoint of the fish?"[28] He gave that viewpoint and passed his exam.

Pollution of the waterways should be considered from the viewpoint of the fish. It is perhaps mankind's safest point of view, for the danger to fish is also one measure of man's danger.

Lake Erie is not the only spoiled waterway. The once beautiful Hudson River is an open sewer. In 1965, New York experienced a gross water shortage. As waiters doled out precious glasses of water, 30,000 gallons of the Hudson flowed by the city every second. To the New Yorker, Coleridge's lines had been realized: "Water, water, every where, / Nor any drop to drink." Why could the Hudson water not be used? Eight children had provided a pitiful answer. They ate a watermelon they found floating in the river. Within a short time, they had typhoid fever. Into the river from which that watermelon came, daily flow the feces and urine of over ten million people.

Oregon's Willamette River, too, is a "giant septic tank," according to the Public Health Service. A vast toilet, it is flushed by water released from federal dams. For half a century and more the Connecticut and Merrimac Rivers have not been safe for swimming. By the time the great Mississippi reaches its delta, it has been despoiled by the sewage of twenty million people. In 1969, the oily pollutions of the filth-ridden Cuyahoga River, near Cleveland, actually caught fire, damaging two bridges. To prod industrial research and investment in water purification equipment, the 1965 Water Quality Act was passed. A beginning was made, but only a beginning.

Detergents During the early sixties, the Indians south of Albuquerque had to find a new time to irrigate their fields. Wednesday was no longer suitable. On that day irrigation brought a flood of suds to their ditches. From the Monday wash of Albuquerque housewives, the suds came via the Rio Grande. These were not ordinary suds. They resulted when detergents reacted with the bacteria polluting the water. Ordinarily, soap and lye are broken down into simpler compounds by bacteria. Not so with the detergents then in use. Frothy yet somehow cheerless spreads of suds could be seen foaming on rivers. They showed up in sewage treatment plants. Sometimes a small amount of detergent, passing through a sewage system and a water treatment plant, brought a beerlike head of foam from a kitchen faucet. Too dilute to be harmful, the detergent did not even alter the taste of the water. It did, however, clearly demonstrate the imperfection of even the best water treatment plants. Finding a detergent that produced less stubborn bubbles required ten years and cost the soap industry 100 million dollars. The discovery did not come a moment too soon. By that time Wisconsin and Dade County, Florida, had passed antidetergent laws. But is the detergent pollution problem solved?

[28] Richard M. Dorson, "Campus Folklore," in A. C. Spectorsky, ed., *The College Years*, p. 281.

Not even a temporary solution is available to the thirty-four percent of U.S. homeowners using other than sewer-pipe systems. The new detergents do not readily break down in septic tanks.[29] Again, scientific discovery, in providing a seemingly immediate solution, has set only a long-term ecological trap. The detergents that had caused all the trouble are called "hard." They could not be broken down (biodegraded) by the bacteria of polluted water. The new, chemically "soft" detergents can be biodegraded. This "very biodegradability, however, makes it food for bacteria, and leads to characteristic organic pollution symptoms: high bacterial populations and subsequent higher levels of invertebrates with resulting low levels of dissolved oxygen."[30] So, soft detergents do not produce foam on rivers, but they may pollute them even more than the hard.

Detergent pollution continues to be a subject of wide and constant research efforts. Neither the soap industry nor government is unaware of the stakes. Together they are working hard to find a way of providing the U.S. housewife with both an effective laundry detergent and a more stable ecosystem.

What is being done to save water resources?

The total amount of the earth's water is not diminished by man's use of it. Nature's water cycle provides a constant supply. But water is unevenly distributed. In one part of the world, the people suffer drought. In another they fight flood. The western part of the United States is drier than the eastern. Los Angeles pipes water to its homes from hundreds of miles away. To obtain the water that daily drips from a leaky faucet in this country, a parched Asian, African, or Indian may need to walk a dozen miles. By keeping water pollution to a minimum and by reusing purified water, man can protect himself against the whims of nature.

The Ohio River Water Sanitation Pact (ORSANCO) is an example of a massive antipollution effort. Eight states have agreed to provide adequate sewage treatment facilities for almost all of the watershed population. Industry, too, is restudying its waste disposal processes. And it is making money doing it. Formerly dumped into the river, animal and fish-packing wastes are now used in pet-food preparations. Other industries use purified city sewage water. For almost thirty years the Bethlehem Steel Company plant at Sparrows Point, Maryland, near Baltimore, has used the processed and treated effluents of the sewage of almost a million people.[31] It is a magnificent example of waste water recycling that is beneficial to all—citizens and industry alike.

One of the most promising examples of water reuse, however, is provided by a small California community. Just thirteen thousand people live

[29] Barry Commoner, *Science and Survival* (New York, 1963), p. 22. A septic tank is one in which sewage is allowed to remain until purified by the action of certain bacteria flourishing in the absence of free oxygen. Such tanks must be periodically cleaned.

[30] Joe A. Edmisten, "Hard and Soft Detergents," *Scientist and Citizen*, Vol. 8, No. 10 (October 1966), p. 10.

[31] Abel Wolman, "Disposal of Man's Wastes," in William L. Thomas, Jr., ed., *Man's Role in Changing the Face of the Earth*, p. 814.

in Santee, California, and an annual average of only ten inches of rain falls upon them. A few short years ago Santee was known (if at all) as a small town thirty miles from the big city—San Diego. Today, it is studied and praised by water experts across the nation.

Water for Santee comes three hundred miles from the Colorado River. The distance of the source makes the water increasingly expensive. For years, like the residents of most other communities, Santee people bought, used, and then wasted water. In 1961, they decided to stop throwing their water money away. First, they carefully treated their sewage in a modern sewage treatment plant. Then they filtered the effluent through a deep stratum of natural sand. A lake was formed. Extensive laboratory tests proved the water safe. They stocked it with trout, bluegill, and bass. In this arid area, fathers took their children fishing. And the fish could safely be eaten. A huge swimming pool filled with reclaimed sewage water is today in use. With a federal loan, a new Santee waterworks is being constructed. Through a separate system, reclaimed sewage water will be used to irrigate urban and agricultural areas, to water a golf course, and to provide more lake water for boating, fishing and swimming.

The people of Santee are living the lines of Longfellow's *Evangeline:*

> *its waters, returning*
> *Back to the springs, like the rain, shall fill them full of refreshment;*
> *That which the fountain sends forth returns again to the fountain.*

Others are profiting by scientific reuse of water. Also in California, the Whittier Narrows water reclamation project is proving a safe source of water. After passing through a modern sewage treatment plant, used sewage water is lead to "spreading grounds." There, the used water is further purified as it percolates through soil, rock, and gravel to reach the underground water table. It is then pumped up again for use. In this way sewage water is transformed into safe drinking water.

Solid-waste disposal

The story is told of the indifferent housekeeper who, when asked what she did with her garbage, replied, "Oh, I just kick it around till it gets lost." Every year in the United States, 48 billion cans and 26 billion bottles are made; 86 billion pounds of paper products reach the market; 8 billion pounds of new plastics are produced; 6 million cars are scrapped and join the 25 to 40 million already stored in dumps.[32] Too often, much of this refuse just gets kicked around. The trouble is, it will not get lost. Getting rid of solid waste, moreover, is expensive. "It costs more to dispose of the *New York Sunday Times* than it does a subscriber to buy it."[33]

[32]Melvin W. First, "Urban Solid-Waste Management," *New England Journal of Medicine,* Vol. 275, No. 26 (December 29, 1966), pp. 1480–84.
[33]*Ibid.,* p. 1484.

Most solid waste consists of food wastes (garbage) and rubbish from households, institutions, and commercial establishments. Abandoned automobiles, dead cats, garden sweepings, radioactive materials, pus-laden hospital bandages, and refrigerators—all these and more, clog the ecosystem. In this country solid wastes do not usually transmit disease. True, their improper disposal breeds rats and insects and vermin associated with illnesses such as plague and gastrointestinal infections. But today's danger of inadequate solid-waste disposal lies in its pollution possibilities.

Open-dump burning of garbage promotes aerial garbage. To dump it into water merely aggravates an already serious mess. It has been used to fill land. Garbage fill has already transformed some steep hills and canyons of Los Angeles County into golf courses. The only hill in Evanston, Illinois, is a heap of garbage covered with layers of clay, dirt, and sod. In the winter it has provided some fine toboggan runs. But land to fill is limited and distant.[34] The farther it is, the greater are transportation costs. And an expanding population produces expanding garbage. What can be done?

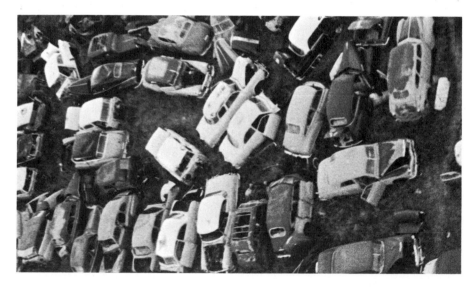

3-4 Solid wastes: an auto graveyard.

Solid waste may be controlled at the source or recycled. Both methods require a new look at the economic system. Reuse of the 26 billion bottles produced last year, for example, would help control this waste at its source. Automobiles may be recycled by being scrapped and then incorporated into steel production. An interesting idea is the "Cars for Peace"

[34] Nor is waste disposal into deep wells without danger. Many experts believe that "disposal of waste fluids by injection into a deep well has triggered earthquakes near Denver, Colorado." (J. H. Healy, W. W. Rubey, D. T. Griggs, and C. B. Raleigh, "The Denver Earthquakes," *Science*, Vol. 161, No. 3848 [September 27, 1968], pp. 1301–10.)

program. Old but serviceable cars, it is suggested, should be given to developing countries.[35] Surely some of the 25,000 automobiles yearly abandoned on New York City streets could be made to run again. In 1966 Congress passed the Solid Waste Disposal Act. It initiates research in solid-waste disposal and holds promise as an educational tool for local government officials.

The dirty, dangerous skies

O dark, dark, dark, amid the blaze of noon,
Irrecoverably dark, total Eclipse
Without all hope of day![36]

Two to four hundred centuries ago, some Paleolithic people decorated their cave walls with paintings of what they saw. In 1940, four French boys looking for a dog accidentally discovered their remarkable art. Thousands of tourists flocked to the cave at Lascaux in the French Perigord region. In less than twenty years, the cave paintings, previously inviolate for at least twenty thousand years, began to deteriorate. An ugly green fungus desecrated them. The damp air and the moisture from the visitors' breaths were blamed. These are natural pollutions. Air conditioning did not help. Neither did heavy bronze doors. The caves were closed to the public.[37]

"Cleopatra's Needle" refers to one of two Egyptian obelisks. Neither stone monument is in Egypt any more. One rests on the Thames embankment in London. The other, in New York's Central Park, is of present interest. Made in 1460 B.C., it was given to the city in 1881 by Ismail Pasha, the former khedive of Egypt. In less than a century, New York smog did what thirty-three centuries of Egyptian climate did not do—obscure the hieroglyphics on the obelisk.

Cleopatra's Needle is not the nation's only obelisk to be marred by polluted air. The discolored Washington Monument is dulled testimony to the aerial garbage that comes from the smoking District of Columbia garbage dump. There are other smog sources. There always are, whether the damage is to the Acropolis of Greece or to the Hilton of New York.

Some time ago a nagging question arose. If air pollution eats away stone, how does the seven to ten thousand quarts of polluted air each person inhales daily affect soft, friable lung tissue? In seeking an answer to this question, first consider the source and nature of this aerial rubbish.

It has been seen that living creatures are not the only creators of air pollution. Whether by a whipping sand storm or the gentle haze over

[35] Sheldon A. Mix, "Solid Wastes: Every Day Another 800 Million Pounds," *Today's Health*, Vol. 44, No. 3 (March 1966), p. 48.
[36] John Milton, *Samson Agonistes*, lines 80–82.
[37] Lucy Kavaler, *Mushrooms, Molds, and Miracles* (New York, 1965), p. 237.

blue-ridged mountains, nature pollutes. As both Pliny the Elder and the Younger (and others) learned at Pompeii, the ecological results of natural pollution may spell calamity. But the environmental imbalance from such pollution does not equal the peril that man has created for himself. Wrongly, he thought the air to be a limitless reservoir. Now his dirtying sky may yet become a tightening noose round his windpipe.

"A great city is a great desert," wrote the ancient Roman philosopher Seneca. He referred to urban man's loneliness. However, the Scottish essayist Thomas Carlyle made a less sensitive comment on city deficiencies when, in 1821, he wrote to his brother John, describing Edinburgh as "this accursed, stinking, reeky mass of stones and lime and dung." The nineteenth-century English poet Percy Bysshe Shelley loved London even less. He suffered from a pulmonary ailment; perhaps his affliction caused him to write that "Hell is a city much like London—a populous and smoky city."

What so troubled the ailing Shelley, and countless Londoners before and after him, is called *London-type smog*. The word "smog" probably originated from a 1901 scientific report attributing some 1,063 deaths in Glasgow and Edinburgh to "Smoke and Fog." London-type smog is not limited to the British Isles. It dims such industrialized communities as New York, Philadelphia, and Chicago. It is, as will be seen, quite different from Los Angeles-type smog, to be described below. However, it shares a basic feature with Los Angeles-type smog. **London-type smog**

In both types of air pollution normal cleansing of air is prevented by a phenomenon called *temperature inversion*. Ordinarily, temperature decreases with altitude. For each thousand-foot rise in elevation, the air temperature drops about five degrees Fahrenheit. So, under usual conditions, the air at ground level is warmer than the air above. It is this very difference in temperature that helps make possible the vertical air motion so necessary for cleansing man's ground-level air. But temperature inversion reverses (inverts) this ground-air cleansing situation. For a variety of meteorological reasons, a layer of warm air above traps a layer of cold air below. Over the affected area there is a blanket of warm air. In London-type smog this inversion layer of warmer air usually occurs at about three hundred or four hundred feet. In Los Angeles-type smog the warm-air blanket is higher—usually at a thousand feet and even more. The lower the inversion layer, the more severe the smog. Not until the cold layer of ground air is warmed enough by the sun to break the inversion, can the ground air escape and, with it, its accumulated pollutants. Thus it is temperature inversion that impedes normal dispersion of air pollutants. Temperature inversion phenomena cannot be controlled. Air pollution must be.

London-type smog came with coal. Smoking stacks meant employment. But coal burning released a product of its incomplete combustion, sulfur dioxide (SO_2) gas. Sunlight oxidized the SO_2 to sulfur trioxide (SO_3).

When the sulfur trioxide combined with air moisture (or fog), corrosive sulfuric acid (H_2SO_4) was formed. ($H_2O + SO_3 \rightarrow H_2SO_4$). There is an old laboratory ditty that has taken on a new relevance:

> *We often think of Willie.*
> *Alas he is no more.*
> *For what he thought was H_2O*
> *Was H_2SO_4.*

The recipe for London-type smog includes other poisonous gases such as benzopyrene and irritating particles of soot.

Los Angeles-type smog

Los Angeles-type smog ("oxidizing" or "photochemical" smog), unlike the London type, is a warm-weather irritant rarely associated with fog. It occurs in various regions of this country, as does the London type. Weather conditions and pollution (automobile and industrial) combine to produce it. Particularly during warm months, warm air enters the atmosphere at high levels. Caught beneath this warm blanket of air (the inversion layer) is the colder ground air. Every day four million cars in Los Angeles County consume eight million gallons of gasoline. And a car does not have to be running to emit smog-contributing chemicals. Fuel tank and carburetor evaporations add to the smog misery. Morning traffic begins. Into the trapped, cold ground air each car belches or evaporates its pollutants. The pollutants cannot penetrate beyond the thermal inversion. They are trapped beneath the warm air inversion blanket. The sun rises. It is indispensable for the smog that is brewing. Its ultraviolet light reacts with the pollutant pall.

Many chemicals comprise this pollution. In the formation of photochemical smog the two most important chemical groups necessary are the *hydrocarbons* and the *oxides of nitrogen*. In sunlight, nitrogen dioxide (NO_2) is dissociated into a simpler compound, nitric oxide, and oxygen. This oxygen readily combines with hydrocarbons to produce a series of reactions that in turn lead to the production of compounds of which poisonous *ozone* is one. Ozone is one of the four Los Angeles air contaminants that can cause a smog alert.[38] The other three are nitrogen oxides, sulphur oxides, and carbon monoxides. Sulphur oxides are primary to London-type smog. *Carbon monoxide,* although not related to the formation of photochemical smog, is nevertheless an important part of Los Angeles' air pollution. It is also largely a product of the gasoline-burning automobile. Every gallon of gasoline consumed results in three pounds of this deadly gas. It causes harm by inactivating the blood's hemoglobin—the oxygen-transporting pigment of the red blood cells.

---

[38] There are several stages to a Los Angeles smog alert, ranked according to danger. In 1955, Los Angeles County experienced fifteen first-stage smog alerts. Today, these are about one-third as frequent. Ozone is the only chemical compound in the Los Angeles atmosphere to have caused a first-stage smog alert level. At this level, the concentration of ozone is safe, but corrective action may be indicated.

Exposure to high levels of carbon monoxide can result in death. Depending on the length of time of exposure, a little more than one-tenth the lethal amount of carbon monoxide can risk the health of sensitive people. The headache, dizziness, and extreme fatigue noticed by traffic policemen in congested areas is not limited to them. Moreover, carbon monoxide is an added threat to both the cigarette-smoking driver and those about him. Cigarette smoke contains carbon monoxide. Heavy smoking and polluted air can combine to inactivate so much blood hemoglobin that driving functions are impaired. Still other chemicals are part of the Los Angeles-type smog. Some of these injure vegetation. (Los Angeles-type smog is causing an estimated $500 million damage to agriculture conducted near U.S. cities.) Other smog chemicals disintegrate rubber and women's nylon stockings. Still others occur in such low concentrations that they defy identification.

Charles Dickens opened his novel *Bleak House* (1852–53) with this description of nineteenth-century London: "Smoke lowering down from chimney-pots, making a soft black drizzle, with flakes of soot in it as big as full-grown snow flakes—gone into mourning . . . for the sun . . . Fog everywhere . . . Fog in the eyes and throats of ancient Greenwich pensioners wheezing by the firesides." There had always been a lot of fussing about "the black skullcap" that covers London. An occasional committee coughed through an occasional meeting. Nobody did much.

Some air pollution disasters

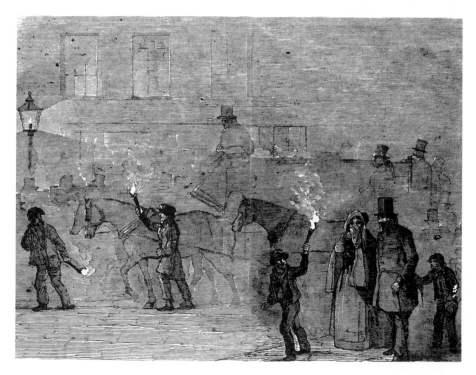

3-5 Dickens' London: smoke and fog (smog), 1847.

Then came December 5, 1952. On that day a strangling black fog lay on London. People fought to breathe. In less than a day many were dead. On December 9, the last day of the chill killer-fog, the London *Times* published a warm-hearted article about "the fogs of ancient Britons." It was a cheery piece: "The countryside dissolves under the spell into a parody of fairyland . . . The farmer hears news of the great city with a comradely smile. The fog has not forgotten to pay him a visit."[39] In his dying thoughts, many a city Englishman might have included a vain hope that the fog had been less attentive. Four thousand people perished in that fog. Most were sufferers from chronic respiratory disease who were over forty-five years old. In those several days, more Londoners died from the smog than from the nineteenth-century cholera epidemic.

There had been similar disasters. In December 1930, the Belgians of the Meuse River Valley endured a similar choker. They coughed and gasped. Thousands were seized by a constricting chest pain. Sixty Belgians, mostly the aged and the chronically sick, died. The substances thickening the gray fog were oxides of sulfur.

Evilly, fog had been curling, lurking about Donora's dank streets for some days, a pale yellow poison, before it snuffed out the life of its first victim. It was during October 1948. One-third of this Pennsylvania coal town's 13,839 population became ill. Seventeen died. Close by, the people of Pittsburgh looked on, horrified, apprehensive. A couple of years later (in 1950) a similar disaster visited the little Mexican oil-refining town of Poza Rica (population 22,000). Accidentally, some hydrogen sulfide gas was spilled. Within twenty-five minutes after the gas reached the people, its source was cut off. Nevertheless, three hundred and twenty people became ill. Twenty-two died.

What chemicals in the smog caused the London and Donora disasters? The findings give reason for somber concern. Dubos has noted that "no single smog component was present in unusually high concentrations."[40] He wonders if it could be that the smog, ordinarily breathed by everyone a day or two at a time without being harmful, could become injurious, even lethal, to many people when inhaled for a few days longer. Since these events took place, more disquieting data have been gathered. For those in Donora affected by the 1948 smog attack, illness and death rates are higher than would otherwise have been expected.

The breath of death   Since they were disasters, the tragedies in London, the Meuse River Valley, Donora, and Poza Rica are widely known. The average person is not so aware that there are other evidences of smog's lethal possibilities. In November 1953, an air pollution blanketed New York City. Not until nine years later did a review of vital statistics reveal a startling fact. During that 1953 episode two hundred more New Yorkers died than would

[39] Arie J. Haagen-Smit, "Atmospheric Ecology," *Archives of Environmental Health*, Vol. 11, No. 1 (July 1965), p. 87.
[40] René Dubos, *Man Adapting* (New Haven, Conn., 1965), p. 218.

have been expected to die in that period.[41] And during an episode beginning on January 29 and lasting through February 12, 1963, between two hundred and four hundred such "excess" deaths, presumably related to atmospheric sewage, occurred in New York City.[42] Other ominous data are being accumulated and analyzed. During and immediately following a 1966 Thanksgiving weekend attack of air pollution, there were 168 excess deaths in New York City.[43] Still another study points out that: "Examination of total deaths in New York City by day of occurrence shows periodic peaks in mortality which are associated with periods of high air pollution . . . fog is not a necessary part of this picture, and therefore the presence of these episodes is often not apparent at the time to most inhabitants."[44]

Confirmatory evidence that the Los Angeles-type smog is directly responsible for an increase in mortality is lacking. But there is much cause for concern. Emphysema (pages 427–28) is an example. Recent years have seen a marked increase in the deaths, both in California and elsewhere in the nation, from this crippling lung disease. Some of this increase is doubtlessly due to improved diagnosis, but certainly not all. Is better medical care allowing those suffering with emphysema to live to a somewhat older age, only to become victims of smog? Physicians recall that those who died in Donora in 1948, and in London in 1952, were older people suffering from chronic ailments of the bronchi and lungs. These were startling episodes. Is prolonged exposure to lower levels of smog producing less dramatic but no less damaging results? In the past twenty years, U.S. death rates from bronchitis and asthma have also risen sharply. The specific relationship between these rises and smog is unknown. But one fact is known: smog can kill.

Smog is not simply an irritating eyesore or a potential killer. It is an insidious presence, aggravating the illness of countless people who are already chronically ill. And to those not already so disadvantaged, smog may silently bring the beginnings of a serious sickness. Many people, particularly those with chronic respiratory diseases such as asthma, suffer painfully during a smog attack. Repeated epidemics of asthma in New Orleans between 1953 and 1960 were finally believed to be due to pollution from a garbage dump. In one week of an October episode, more than three hundred wheezing, gasping persons flocked to New Orleans' famed Charity Hospital emergency clinic. Nine died.[45] The night-cough, wheezing, and

Smog and sickness

[41]L. Greenburg, M. B. Jacobs, B. M. Drolette, F. Field, and M. M. Braverman, "Report of an Air Pollution Incident in New York City, November, 1953," *Public Health Reports*, Vol. 77, No. 1 (January 1962), pp. 7–16.

[42]L. Greenburg, F. Field, C. O. Erhardt, M. Glasser, and J. I. Reed, "Air Pollution, Influenza and Mortality in New York City, January–February 1963," *Archives of Environmental Health*, Vol. 15, No. 4 (October 1967), pp. 437–38.

[43]M. Glasser, L. Greenburg, and F. Field, "Mortality and Morbidity During a Period of High Levels of Air Pollution, New York, Nov. 23 to 25, 1966," *Archives of Environmental Health*, Vol. 15, No. 6 (December 1967), p. 694.

[44]James McCarroll and William Bradley, "Excess Mortality as an Indicator of Health Effects of Air Pollution," *American Journal of Public Health*, Vol. 56, No. 11, (November 1966), p. 1942.

[45]Robert Lewis, Murray M. Gilkeson, and Roy O. McCaldin, "Air Pollution and New Orleans Asthma, *Public Health Reports*, Vol. 77, No. 11 (November 1962), pp. 953–54.

shortness of breath of U.S. personnel assigned to the Tokyo-Yokohama industrial area ("Yokohama asthma") is probably an aggravation of previous infection and asthma.[46] In this country, one study emphasizes that "there can be no doubt that a considerable effect is exerted by pollutions on hospital admissions for certain disease groupings."[47] Another study suggests "that susceptibility to, or duration of, common viral respiratory infections is increased . . . by exposure to . . . air pollutants."[48] Yet another researcher writes that "a review of factors relating atmospheric pollution to lung cancer warrants its incrimination as one of the dominant agents . . . associated with the disease."[49] Various investigations point to an "association between urban residence and lung cancer" and implicate "the atmosphere as one dominant factor in . . . lung cancer."[50]

British research is no more encouraging. In one study of 3,866 children "upper respiratory tract infections were not related to the amount of air pollution, but lower respiratory infections were so related. The frequency and severity of lower respiratory infections increased with the amount of air pollution."[51] Other British research, and studies in Japan,[52] point to "a possible influence on respiratory disease of children."[53] Nor should it be thought that air pollution merely worsens the already sick. There is "clear evidence that oxidant air pollution has an adverse effect on athletic performance in healthy adolescent males."[54]

These are grim reports. However, another factor must again be emphasized. Time. Citizens complain about immediate discomforts. A burning sensation of the eyes, a night of coughing—these will prompt an angry letter to an editor or mayor. But what of prolonged, subtle exposure to low levels of pollution? Perhaps this is the far deadlier enemy: "the most important among the . . . deleterious effects of air pollution are slow in developing . . . continued exposure to low levels of toxic agents will eventually result in . . . misery . . . increasing the medical load."[55]

There remains yet another long-term effect to consider. Burning coal over the centuries and in such huge amounts concerns many ecologists.

[46]Rexford G. Haycroft, "Tokyo-Yokohama Asthma," *California Medicine,* Vol. 105, No. 2 (August 1966), pp. 89–92.

[47]T. D. Sterling, J. J. Phair, S. V. Pollack, D. A. Schumsky, and I. De Grott, "Urban Morbidity and Air Pollution," *Archives of Environmental Health,* Vol. 13, No. 1 (August 1966), p. 169.

[48]F. Curtis Dohan, "Air Pollutants and Incidence of Respiratory Disease," *Archives of Environmental Health,* Vol. 3, No. 4 (October 1961), p. 394.

[49]Paul Kotin, "The Role of Atmospheric Pollution in the Pathogenesis of Pulmonary Cancer: A Review," *Cancer Research,* Vol. 16, No. 5 (June 1956), pp. 375–93.

[50]Paul Kotin and Hans L. Falk, "Polluted Urban Air and Related Environmental Factors in the Pathogenesis of Pulmonary Cancer," *Diseases of the Chest,* Vol. 45, No. 3 (March 1964), p. 244.

[51]J. W. B. Douglas and R. E. Waller, "Air Pollution and Respiratory Infection in Children," *British Journal of Preventive Social Medicine,* Vol. 20, No. 1 (January 1966), p. 6.

[52]T. Toyama, "Air Pollution and Health Effects in Japan," a paper read before the Sixth Air Pollution Medical Research Conference, California State Department of Public Health, January 28–29, 1963.

[53]"Air Pollution and Respiratory Infection in Children," an editorial in *The Lancet,* No. 7452 (June 25, 1966), p. 1409.

[54]W. S. Wayne, P. F. Wehrle, and R. E. Carroll, "Oxidant Air Pollution and Athletic Performance," *Journal of the American Medical Association,* Vol. 199, No. 12 (March 20, 1967), pp. 901–04.

[55]René Dubos, "Adapting to Pollution," *Scientist and Citizen,* Vol. 10, No. 1 (January–February 1968), pp. 2–3.

It has been accompanied by a marked rise in atmospheric carbon dioxide (CO_2). Carbon dioxide absorbs the sun's infrared radiation. Then it radiates it back into the lower atmosphere. "As a result of such increases in atmospheric CO_2, the Antarctic icecap . . . could melt (from carbon dioxide warming) in four hundred to four thousand years . . . If 1,000 years were required to melt the icecap, the sea level would rise about 4 feet every 10 years, 40 feet per century."[56]

To some ecologists, therefore, vast flood disasters are within the realm of future possibilities.

What can be done?

To improve air, one must first find out what is polluting it. In areas troubled by the London-type smog, for example, the oxides of sulfur can be partly controlled with the cooperation of industry. Improvements in factory construction enable industrialists to dispose of sulfur pollutions without danger to surrounding populations. Moreover, various chemical processes may not only relieve the pollution problem but also benefit industry. From sulfur oxide gases, sulfuric acid and sulfur may be obtained and sold to a ready market.[57] Another possible solution would involve the development of power sources that would produce no harmful byproducts. As a smogless source of power, the nuclear power plant has no peer. Although much remains to be done to make these plants totally safe, they hold out a promise for a cleaner environment.

At the tip of Los Angeles County is San Pedro Bay. Local historians tell a rueful story about its discovery. Upon first observing it from aboard ship in October 1542, the Portuguese explorer Juan Rodriguez Cabrillo could only see the mountain peaks. The rest of the mountains were obscured by haze, perhaps by the smoke from Indian fires. "La Bahia de los Fumos"—The Bay of Smokes—he named the place, and sailed away convinced nobody could live there. More than four centuries later there are those who consider that he made a wise decision. But most of the residents of Los Angeles are trying to prove him wrong.

From its industries, varying from petroleum refineries to fish canneries, Los Angeles County has obtained a high level of cooperation. Every day, five thousand tons of more than fifty contaminants are kept out of the air.[58] It is now years, moreover, since the people of this sunny county burned trash or leaves. Not only the eyes but also the pride of Los Angeles residents has been stung by smog. More than twenty years ago, the state adopted a statute authorizing county air-pollution control districts. Intensive work with cooperating industries has helped; this work is being studied for application to other areas. Nevertheless, during the sixties Los

---

[56] Barry Commoner, "A Landmark in National Concern," *Restoring the Quality of Our Environment*, Report of the Environmental Pollution Panel, President's Science Advisory Committee, John W. Tukey, Chairman, The White House, November 1965, in *Scientist and Citizen*, Vol. 9, No. 1 (January 1967), p. 7.

[57] "Diminishing the Role of Sulfur Oxides in Air Pollution," an editorial in *Science*, Vol. 157, No. 3794 (September 15, 1967), p. 1265.

[58] S. Smith Griswold, "Community Control of Air Pollution," *Archives of Environmental Health*, Vol. 13, No. 2 (August 1966), p. 606.

Angeles air quality failed to improve. It was merely kept from worsening. The reasons are the usual ones—more population, cars, and industries.

In August 1968, sixty faculty members of the University of California Medical School at Los Angeles recommended, for those who had no compelling reason to remain, migration from "smoggy portions of Los Angeles, San Bernadino, and Riverside Counties to avoid chronic respiratory diseases like bronchitis and emphysema."

In June 1968, the governing council of the Los Angeles County Medical Association set forth the following protective measures that might be taken during severe smog conditions:

a. *Remain indoors whenever possible, especially from midmorning to midafternoon when the smog is usually the worst. Keep the doors and windows closed. Avoid dusts, smokes, fumes, sprays or other aerosols and particulates.*

b. *Use an air conditioner if possible, and recirculate the air inside only. Do not draw outside air in during the day. The best units combine an absolute filter with the activated carbon unit and the air conditioner. Electrostatic units do not remove chemical smoke and are inferior to the activated carbon units.*

c. *Obtain extra rest and sleep and avoid stimulating foods, drinks and medicines that increase metabolism. Avoid strenuous physical activity. Reduce to a minimum major cooking, cleaning and shopping activities.*

d. *Cigarette smoking should be stopped completely, or at least be drastically reduced, as this further aggravates the respiratory problem. It would be best to stop all forms of smoking.*

e. *Avoid driving the automobile if taking a depressant, tranquilizer or sedative drug. Avoid the freeways and sigalert conditions. [Sigalerts refer to congested or dangerous freeway traffic.]*

f. *Severe respiratory cripples living in smoggy areas should have facilities available for more intensive treatment. They should receive previous intensive treatment. They should receive previous instruction in the use of oxygen, bronchodilator drugs and respiratory assistance with intermittent positive pressure breathing devices.*

g. *If the individual becomes distressed or dyspneic [from the Greek dyspnoia, difficulty in breathing] the personal physician should be called.*

h. *Most of the radio and television stations carry the Air Pollution Control District smog forecasts. Keep informed on the daily air pollution conditions.*[59]

[59] "R for Heavy Smog Attacks," *Bulletin,* Los Angeles County Medical Association (October 3, 1968), p. 11.

The Federal Government has also become concerned with smog. The 1963 Clean Air Act provided funds to set up local programs as well as to control interstate air pollution. Amended in 1965, the Act now requires all new cars, beginning with 1968 models, to meet federal standards of exhaust control. Often, such federal regulations are inapplicable to local problems. Whether the Act's amendment will solve the Los Angeles smog problem, for example, remains to be seen.

Eighty percent of Los Angeles smog comes from motor vehicles. Four million autos crowd its streets. Every year that number increases by some ten percent. There is expert opinion that the federal standards for hydrocarbon and carbon monoxide emissions "will be inadequate ever to alleviate the problem of photochemical smog in Los Angeles County."[60] Other U.S. cities may also be in for serious trouble—Chicago (which has more automobiles per square mile than Los Angeles), New York, Philadelphia, and Detroit, for instance. Crankcase emissions are nearly controlled. There remain the problems of exhaust emissions and evaporative losses from the gas tank and carburetor. If these pollutants cannot be controlled, electric automobiles and mass transit systems may solve the problem by eliminating it.

Today, over 50 percent of this nation's 205 million people live in about one-tenth of its land area. By 1975, 75 percent of an estimated 235 million people will occupy the same space. By the turn of the century, 80 to 90 percent of the nation's 285 million people will be city dwellers. Air pollution most endangers its greatest producers—those living in concentrated areas.

If the present rate of fouling the air continues, by the turn of the century pure air could well require a greater public and private annual outlay than any other single resource category. It could become the "scarcest" natural resource in the sense of experiencing the most sharply increasing costs. Because of this, we will have to change our current conception of air as a "free good." It has been suggested that air will have to be regarded as a common domain to be managed under public tenure as the Bureau of Land Management administers many grazing lands in the West. Invasion of the domain by pollutors may then be regarded as trespass, and the cost of control assigned to the pollutors in a way that will motivate them to reduce noxious emissions.[61]

In 1969, President Nixon established a cabinet-ranked agency to study the environment. Among its major tasks: to find the answer to air pollution.

It must come soon, while there is still time and fresh air.

[60] "Inadequate Automobile Control But More Horsepower, More Chrome, and More Red Herring," an editorial in *Archives of Environmental Health*, Vol. 13, No. 2 (August 1966), p. 234.
[61] Harvey S. Perloff, "Modernizing Urban Development," *Daedalus* (Summer 1967), p. 792.

4

Man versus man: pesticides, radiation, noise, and accidents

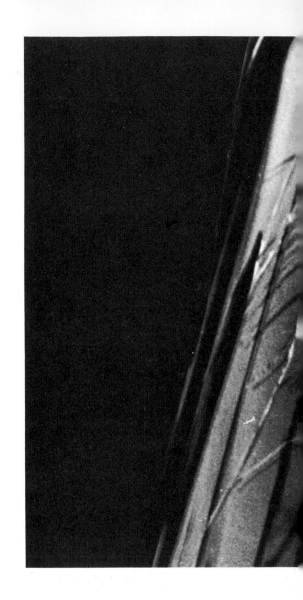

Pesticides

Suddenly the Maharaja Palden Thondup Namgyal sat up. He leaned forward in his camp chair beside the roaring Teetsa River. His eyes lit up with pleasure. He pointed to an orange and silver butterfly, a dazzling ephemera, lightly hovering above a delicately scented clematis blossom. "Maybe they are coming back to Sikkim," he murmured hopefully. "That's the fifth butterfly I've seen in an hour's time."

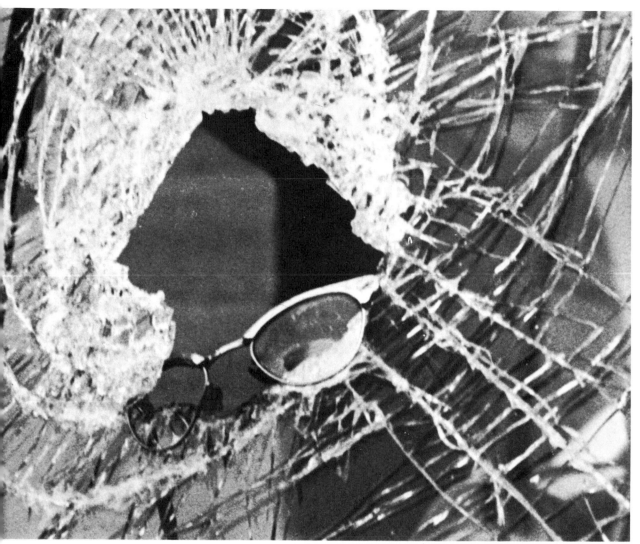

After the crash. The eyeglasses of an Indianapolis woman dangle from the smashed windshield. Damage to her head was severe. Upon arrival at the hospital, she was in fair condition.

Once Sikkim was a butterfly's paradise. Some native butterflies had a wing span of eight or nine inches. Now they are all gone. The Sikkim ecosystem had also included the malaria mosquito. DDT rid the tiny Indian protectorate of malaria, but the pesticide was unselective. The butterfly perished too.[1]

A few months before, in distant Cincinnati, Ohio, a great red cloud darkened the sky. The date was January 24, 1965. It was noon. In less than

[1]*The New York Times*, July 10, 1966, Sect. L., p. 15.

an hour the city lay in a shroud of red dust. Yet, nobody seemed to be harmed. Analysis proved the dust to be loaded with pesticides and other agricultural chemicals. Days, months, perhaps years before, they had been laid down on farms in Texas and Oklahoma. An unusual windstorm had lifted them high into the atmosphere and had carried them more than a thousand miles to be dumped on Cincinnati.[2]

In recent years the people of this nation have been involved in many an irksome "learning situation" regarding the effects of pesticides. There was, for instance, the Great Cranberry Crisis of 1959. The place of some national holidays, like the Fourth of July, is in the hearts of the people. With Thanksgiving, interest tends to shift to the stomach. Certainly thanks for the past and hope for the future are prayerfully expressed. But (quite properly) the symbol of the holiday is a table laden with stuffed turkey and all the etceteras. Indispensable to the feast is a rather acid fruit, the scarlet cranberry. Around Thanksgiving time it is big business. When, therefore, a few days before Thanksgiving, 1959, a high federal official announced that Thanksgiving cranberries might well be poisoned with cancer-causing chemical, the shock could be felt across the country. "What berries," people anxiously asked, "are involved?" How could the housewife tell whether the cranberries she purchased were safe? The official's answer: she couldn't.

The chemical was aminotriazole (ATZ). Improperly, it had been used as a weed-killer. Toxicity studies showed that rats that were fed tiny doses of ATZ developed tumors of the thyroid gland in about a year.

Quickly cranberries were stricken from menus and banished from grocery shelves. Sales collapsed. The Secretary of Agriculture went on television to do dignified battle with the Secretary of Health, Education, and Welfare, the official who had made the announcement. Cranberries, said he sturdily, would be on his Thanksgiving table. The confusion worsened. The cranberry growers opened a Washington office. Senators from cranberry-growing areas loaned them emergency staff. As the day of the feast approached, politicians from potato-growing states were doubly thankful.

The cranberry growers fought back. Uproar was added to confusion. At last, in the nick of time for Thanksgiving Day, a labeling program was developed. Cranberry lots were to be sampled by the Food and Drug Administration of the federal government. If free of the drug, they would be so labeled. Untested cranberries could appear in stores without the label. By observing the label, however, the purchaser could distinguish between tested and untested lots. For the growers, the cranberry season was a financial disaster. As compensation for their losses, they received about $10 million from the federal government.[3]

Was the poisoned cranberry experience unusual? Yes, but it was a warning. And such warnings keep the production, processing, and preser-

[2]Gladwin Hill, The New York Times, February 25, 1965, p. 68.
[3]Eugene Feingold, "The Great Cranberry Crisis," abr. by Sybil L. Stokes, in Robert M. Brown, ed., Project Director, The Dynamic Spectrum: Man, Health and Environment, National Sanitation Foundation Research Project on Fundamentals of Environmental Health, Monograph No. 5 (October 1966).

vation of foods safe. Whenever chemicals are used in any stage of food processing there is some risk. But in the case of food additives "the benefits greatly outweigh any hazard detected by present methods of toxicology and safety evaluation."[4] For agricultural chemicals, allowable limits, below which no human harm occurs, have been set. Rarely indeed are they exceeded. In 1964, the federal Food and Drug Administration analyzed 32,000 samples of raw agricultural products. Only 34 represented serious enough violations to merit legal action. When contamination does occur, both food industry officials and federal inspectors cooperate to keep the food off the market. How successful has this federal program of public protection been? "There has been no significant number of cases of poisoning resulting from contamination of food with agricultural chemicals in recent times.[5]

The cranberry crisis was rooted in a deeper crisis. It was one result of the inexorable war between man and those plants and animals that threaten his food supply. The wistful Maharaja of Sikkim, the dusty citizens of Cincinnati, and the bewildered U.S. housewives all reflect the increasing chemicalization of the world's ecosystems. Why has this occurred? Why does man use pesticides?

> **The competing insect: harbinger of hunger, bearer of disease**

Issa (1762–1826), perhaps the most beloved of all Japanese poets, wrote:

> Oh, don't mistreat
> the fly! He wrings his hands!
> He wrings his feet![6]

The kindly Issa notwithstanding, men everywhere seek to destroy insects. Implacably competitive, insects bring two calamities to man: starvation and sickness.

In *The Good Earth*, Pearl Buck tells about the first of these calamities:

> Then the sky grew black and the air was filled with the deep still roar of many wings beating against each other, and upon the land the locusts fell, flying over this field and leaving it whole, and falling upon that field, and eating it as bare as winter. And men sighed and said "So Heaven wills," but Wang Lung was furious and he beat the locusts and trampled on them.

Experienced with hunger, Wang Lung feared it.

From the nutritional standpoint alone, it would be idle to deny the benefits of pesticides. To the people of the United States, they have made possible a diet envied almost everywhere. Vitamin deficiency diseases (see Chapter 9) are not nearly as common as they were a generation ago. And

[4]Donald M. Mounce, "Standards of Safety for Foods in Relation to Public Health," *American Journal of Public Health*, Vol. 56, No. 6 (June 1966), p. 951.
[5]Bernard L. Oser, "How Safe Are the Chemicals in Our Food?" *Today's Health*, Vol. 44, No. 3 (March 1966), p. 62.
[6]Quoted in Harold G. Henderson, *An Introduction to Haiku* (Garden City, N.Y., 1958), p. 126.

4-1 A Moroccan farmer fights the eternal battle between man and insect. A swarm of locusts are denuding his land.

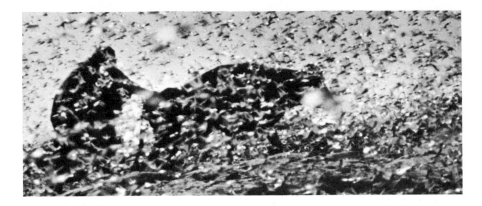

other diseases indicating poor nutrition are disappearing. Partly because of iodized salt, but also because of adequate food iodine, goiter (a thyroid gland disease) is no longer common in this country. In other parts of the world goiter is so common that the dolls are made with swollen necks. People there think the enlarged neck normal.

But pesticides have done more than help provide an abundance of better foods. Countless lives have been saved by them. Typhus fever may be either rat-flea-borne or rat-louse-borne. Following the First World War, more than two million Europeans died of the disease. As the Second World War wore on, typhus fever appeared in Naples. By dispensing louse-killing DDT at dusting stations, occupying U.S. military authorities aborted an epidemic of typhus. In many areas, the mosquito carrying the yellow fever virus has been virtually eliminated. In some countries of South America, for example, yellow fever has almost disappeared. And the nearby United States is safer as a result. A tiny threadworm threatens the sight of more than twenty million people of Africa and central South America. That threadworm is transmitted by a small black fly breeding in flowing water. DDT can kill the fly and thus eliminate river blindness from these areas.

Few diseases have so drained the strength and dwindled the numbers of man as malaria: "it has been accused of responsibility, directly or indirectly, for over one-half the world's mortality."[7] Since 1962, use of DDT has been intensified on a world-wide basis. In many previously malarial areas the consequent changes in the ecosystem have made the survival of the malarial mosquito impossible. The result: unparalleled prevention of sickness and great saving of life. Because of DDT, more than a billion people now live in malaria-free areas. Every year three million lives are spared. At last, entire countries have successfully brought malaria under control. Now they can hope for a better economy. Once it had been rightly said, "Whom malaria does not kill, it enslaves."[8] One official

[7]Louis L. Williams, "Pesticides: A Contribution to Public Health," in *Man—His Environment and Health,* a supplement to *American Journal of Public Health,* Vol. 54, No. 1 (January 1964), p. 34.
[8]Lewis Hackett, quoted in Louis L. Williams, "Pesticides: A Contribution to Public Health," p. 34.

mourned, "My people cannot work. They are either coming down with malaria or they have it or they are getting over it. They are too sick. They are dying." DDT changed all that. Malaria, typhus fever, river blindness, starvation, and malnutrition—these are but some of the blights of human-kind curtailed by pesticides. There are other benefits. In the more affluent industrial nations, such as the United States, pesticides have made possible a better quality of food for less cost. But what of the threat to the environment? Has mankind traded eventual catastrophe for temporary advantage?

More than 56,000 trade name pesticides are marketed today. Designed to kill insects, rodents, fungi, and weeds, they also find their way into people. How? By inhalation of contaminated air, by absorption through the skin, and by oral ingestion. The people in the greatest danger are those whose occupations involve the use of these chemicals, such as workers in pest control operations in agriculture and in malarial areas. In California, from 1954 to 1963, more than eight thousand cases of occupational disease were reported as due to pesticides.[9] But one need not work with pesticides to be exposed to them. They are now part of man's diet; well over three-fourths of his intake is ingested with his food. The air he breathes and the water he drinks also provide him with added measure-able doses. Because of the natural fats and oils in cosmetics, pesticides are a common, but generally harmless, contaminant of eye-shadows, lip-sticks, hair sprays, and hair dressings as well as creams and lotions. The possible accidental ingestion of some pesticides is not reduced by their sharing identical trade names with a mouthwash and a headache remedy. Asians (the people of India, for example) have much higher pesticide concentrations in their bodies than do Europeans (such as the English). This is because of the greater pesticide spraying programs in the developing countries.

Once absorbed, or during absorption, the pesticide may be broken down into simpler substances (which may then be rendered nontoxic by the liver), stored in various body tissues, or excreted in urine or bile. Fatty tissue is the major reservoir of pesticides. It has been found in such fat-containing tissues as the liver, brain, kidney, and gonads. People with severe kidney or liver diseases might be harmed by pesticide doses that are harmless to normal people. Thus, a man who works as a sprayer of one of these chemicals might become ill because his excretory processes are inefficient and the pesticide or its products are allowed to pile up in his body.

Some pesticides are more persistent than others in that they are more resistant to being broken down by the air, light, and water of the environment. Those who favor the use of the more persistent pesticides point

Pesticide problems

to the reduced cost of their application. Since only one or two applications a season of a persistent pesticide are necessary, labor costs are kept at a minimum. Complete abandonment of persistent pesticides in this country would promptly result in a marked increase in food bills.

DDT

Of all pesticides, DDT has been the most assiduously studied. It should be. Since its discovery, less than a generation ago, DDT has permeated living tissue everywhere. Its relatively low toxicity to mammals and intense toxicity to insects, combined with its small cost and availability as a dust, make it the most liberally used of all insecticides. All over the world is it found in the fatty tissues of man. It pollutes the strutting penguin of the Antarctic and the pheasant of California. Collecting in the North American earthworm, it kills robins. And there are high levels of DDT in the eggs and yolk sac of lake trout in New York State. Here, then, is one of its prime features. By wind and water, it *spreads* over the whole earth. No body, no thing escapes. (There is still another way that DDT gets around. Migrating birds and fish carry it thousands of miles.)

Where sprayed, DDT *accumulates*. It takes years for DDT to break down into its simpler constituents. Repeated sprayings, therefore, mean increasing residues. It is thus one of the more persistent pesticides. Recently, one group of investigators[10] sampled a marsh along Long Island's south shore. For twenty years, DDT had controlled mosquitoes in that area. The study revealed as much as thirty-two pounds of DDT per acre. True, that land was no longer fit for mosquitoes. But it was no longer fit for birds or man, either. Nor is repeated spraying necessary to threaten animal life. A single application of DDT in a forest will continue to be picked up by small mammals for nearly ten years.

DDT also *concentrates* in living tissue. That is why the robins die. The chemical accumulates astronomically in the earthworm—enough to destroy the birds of spring. How does DDT accumulate? To kill insects, DDT, or its related chemicals, may be sprayed over water. Or it may wash off adjacent plants. The amount in the water may be infinitesimal—perhaps a hundred parts per million. But the small aquatic mud animals helplessly collect it. They will contain thirty times as much as was in the water. The fish have ten times more than the small aquatic mud animals. And herring gulls will have almost thirty times as much as the fish. Oysters may store seventy thousand times the tenth-part-per-billion concentration in the surrounding water.[11] The oyster larva does not share the adult's ability to live with DDT. Only 0.05 parts DDT per million parts of water will kill ninety percent of oyster larvae.[12]

[10] George M. Woodwell, "Toxic Substances and Ecological Cycles," *Scientific American*, Vol. 216, No. 3 (March 1967), p. 31.
[11] *M.D., Medical Newsmagazine*, Vol. 9, No. 12 (December 1965), p. 115.
[12] Robert M. Paul, "Pesticides in the Wildlife Environment," *American Journal of Public Health*, Vol. 55, No. 7 (July 1965), p. 18.

Interference with reproduction is a fourth effect of DDT in the case of some animal life. The egg failures of one species of a DDT-polluted American hawk has almost eliminated this bird from the northeastern United States. DDT apparently interferes with their ability to handle calcium. As a result they lay eggs that are too thin-shelled. In the Midwest, the eagle has suffered the same way (Figure 4-2). But perhaps the most sinister of all the characteristics of DDT and its related chemicals is the development, by numerous insects, of a *resistance* to it. By mid-1968, insecticide resistance had developed in over two hundred insects, about half of which were known to attack man and animals. "The result is an escalating chemical warfare that is self-defeating."[13]

Are pesticides harmful to humans? Unusually high doses assuredly are. Twenty-five percent of the fatal poisonings of California children are due to careless storing of pesticides. Such data combined with the thousands of occupational poisonings due to mishandling are harsh testimony to the dangers inherent in these chemicals. But these instances are fortunately unusual. Is there too much pesticide in the average human ecosystem? Does the boy who eats too many apples in one day also eat too much pesticide? Does the woman applying lipstick also absorb and ingest a dangerous dose of an unwanted chemical? Certainly not according to any presently available evidence. DDT is one of the most persistent pesticides. Yet in the thirty years it has been used, there has never been a proved instance of death having resulted from its proper use. Moreover, even persistent pesticides are destroyed in the soil, albeit slowly. They are also normally broken down in the body and excreted. They do not pile up indefinitely. Nevertheless, at present concentrations in the United States, does prolonged exposure to pesticides make people sick?

In hasty alarm, some observers have pointed to the effect of DDT on the ability of the hawk to successfully reproduce its kind. But is the observation of the hawk egg applicable to the human embryo? Hardly. The bird embryo has no afterbirth. In this sense it is isolated from the mother. Human maternal defense mechanisms that absorb, detoxify, and excrete pesticides are unavailable to the bird embryo. To produce adverse effects in the embryos of experimental mammals, very large doses, compared to human exposure levels, are necessary. In discussing the value of animal studies as determinants of the safety of pesticide levels for human beings, two experts write: "How reliable is extrapolation of animal data to man? The honest answer to this question is that we do not know."[14] A species that in every respect handles pesticides like man does not exist. However, various species do exist that provide pieces of information that can be extrapolated to man with some confidence. These applications are of a highly technical nature. So because pesticides affect the hawk in one way and a small mammal like the chipmunk in another, it does not neces-

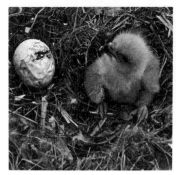

4-2 An eaglet and a damaged egg in a nest in Michigan.

[13] George M. Woodwell, "Toxic Substances and Ecological Cycles," p. 31.
[14] K. S. Khera and D. J. Clegg, "Perinatal Toxicity of Pesticides," *Canadian Medical Association Journal*, Vol. 100, No. 4 (January 25, 1969), p. 171.

sarily follow that a human being would be affected in the same way. Without dismissing the potential danger of pesticides, the informed individual will nevertheless do well to understand the limitation of much of the available data and to question the "scare" statements that are often based upon them.

At present levels of pesticide pollution in this country, there are no available data to indicate a harmful effect to the general population. But what about the chronic effects of continued, and possibly increasing doses over a long period of time? Little is known. This is the basic challenge of the pesticide problem. In 1963, to meet it, the federal Public Health Service began a full-scale study to learn about any cause and effect relationship between pesticide exposure and human disease. Until the results of this study become available, programs to prevent excessive pollutions are indicated. In the United States during the 1967 crop season, only half as much DDT was applied as in the peak year of 1959. And in November 1969 the Nixon administration announced that it would ban the use of DDT in this country except for essential purposes, such as the control of disease of epidemic proportions or of a major infestation of crop pests. The scientific community comprehends the problem of pesticides. What is it doing about it?

Nonchemical pest controls   Considerable research is being conducted to find ways of controlling pests without the use of chemical pesticides. More than half the pesticides used in this country are directed against unwelcome insect visitors who come to stay. *Ship fumigation* and *restriction of incoming agricultural products* have reduced the number of these insect immigrants. And *controlled intentional introduction of foreign pests* provides natural enemies to those already present. Over 150 such predators have been imported for domestic insect control.

Crop controls provide still other ways of combating insects. The development of insect-resistant crops is a significant result of prolonged cooperative studies between entomologists (Greek *entomo,* insects + *ology*) and plant breeders. Crops that are virtually immune to the ravages of such insects as the corn earthworm are now commonplace.

Simple *plowing* and *tilling* of soil control insects. Some insects cannot develop unless they are underground. Other insects, when exposed, fall victim to predators such as birds. *Avoidance of single crop planting* is another method of pest control. To suit his needs, man clears the land, thus destroying the ecological balance. Then he plants but a single crop. Only a species of insect suited to such a change survives. With competing predators gone, that species multiplies enormously; it overwhelms the ecosystem. If only cotton is planted, for example, the boll weevil loses all its natural predatory checks. It overruns the crop. (Deep in the cotton-growing South—in Coffee County, Alabama—a monument was raised in 1919 "in profound appreciation of the boll weevil." For the repeated destruction of their cotton crops, the citizens are grateful to the pest. It forced them into diversification and prosperity.)[15] The boll weevil still remains the most formidable competitor of the cotton grower. Thirty percent of all insecticides used in this country are directed against this insect.

Many insects, susceptible to *physical attractants* such as light and sound, may be lured to certain death by poisons. *Chemical attractants,* however, offer more promise. The Mediterranean fruit fly, for example, finds it hard to resist proteins from ripening fruit. Even more irresistible to male insects are the *sex attractants*. Virgin insect females possess but a tiny amount of these chemical substances. But a little of this goes a long way in the insect world. Some insect sex attractants are now synthetically produced in the laboratory. Used as a lure, they entice the male to annihilation.

Insect birth control is not without promise. First, the insects are sterilized by radiation. Their release into a sexually vigorous insect population results in many fruitless matings. A dramatic drop in insect birth occurs. Other sophisticated *genetic manipulations* enable scientists to breed sterile male insects. When they mate with normal females, nothing comes of the union. Enough competitive sterile males are released to outnumber the normal insects and crowd them out of the mating game. So the sterile insects do most of the mating but none of the reproducing. Repeated releases into normal insect populations of great numbers of sterile males may lead to complete elimination of a species. This insect birth control, a biological rather than a chemical insecticide, recently enabled the little Burmese town of Okpo to rid itself of the mosquito-borne deadly filariasis.[16] More programs of this sort are in the offing.

The insect's own *hormones* have also been turned against it. The development of most insects from larva to pupa is controlled by hormones. These must be secreted in exact amounts and at the proper time. If too much of a hormone is secreted or a hormone is secreted at the wrong time, the insect will not develop properly. Compounds that mimic the insect's own hormones can be turned into effective agents to disrupt insect life. Insects are also proving susceptible to various organisms not expected to be hazardous to other life. Insect *viruses* seem particularly promising, but much research needs to be done.

Radiation: the modern Janus

Janus, in Roman mythology, is the two-faced god. Radiation has become the Janus of modern times. One of its faces views a limitless beginning for mankind. Is the other face turned to the end of man? What is radiation? What are the origins of so encompassing a power?

[15]Adolph I. Cohen, Justin Frost, and Malcolm L. Peterson, "Pesticides, Series #1, Problems and Possibilities," *Scientist and Citizen,* Vol. 7, No. 5 (April 1965), p. 8.
[16]"New Genetic Technique Turns Insects Against Themselves," *Newsletter,* a news release from the Public Information Office, Pan American Sanitary Bureau, Regional Office of the World Health Organization (Washington, D. C., August 1967).

Atoms and their behavior

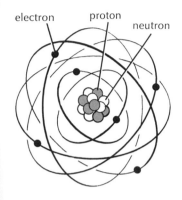

electron   proton   neutron

nucleus

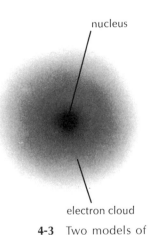

electron cloud

4-3 Two models of an atom: an atom of carbon 12, which has six electrons, six protons, and six neutrons (*top*) and a generalized model schematizing an electron cloud (*bottom*). The top diagram is highly simplified in that all the orbitals shown there are elliptical; actually, orbital shapes vary.

Everything in nature is made up of elements, and elements are made up of atoms.[17] The core of each atom is its *nucleus*. Within it are positively charged particles called *protons* and particles that have no charge, *neutrons*.[18] Surrounding the nucleus and dwarfing it like a star in space is a swirling cloud of negatively charged particles, *electrons*. Depending on where the electrons are whirling in their spacious orbitals, this cloud is more or less ball-shaped. Since the weight of this cloud of electrons is negligible, it is in the heavy nucleus that the protons and neutrons combine to give the atom almost all of its weight. For its size the atomic nucleus is the heaviest bit of matter on earth. In the cloud of each atom the number of negatively charged electrons cancels out or balances the electrical charge of an equal number of positively charged protons. Since the neutrons have no electrical charge, the electrically balanced atom is neutral. It has no charge.

The electrons whirling in the vast minispace of their thin orbital cloud determine the chemical behavior of an element. Food energy depends on these electrons, and so does the energy of fuel. But within the nucleus—the tiny, heavy nucleus—is leashed a source of energy unlike anything electrons provide. Although atoms of the same element have an equal number of protons and electrons, they can have an unequal number of neutrons. And because electrons determine chemical behavior and neutrons have weight (or mass), extra neutrons within an atom's nucleus will increase its weight but will not change its chemical properties. Atoms having the same number of electrons and protons (and thus the same chemical properties) but a different number of neutrons (and therefore different weights) are called *isotopes*. Almost all elements have more than one isotope.

Some isotopes are unstable. Their nuclei spontaneously disintegrate. Energy in the form of waves and particles is emitted from these unstable nuclei. This energy is called *ionizing radiation*, and the decaying isotope is a *radioactive isotope*.

One of the three major types of ionizing radiation that the nucleus of an unstable radioactive isotope may give off is the *alpha ray*. The individual particles of these rays are the *alpha particles*. An alpha particle is really the positively charged nucleus of a helium atom without its electron cloud. Surrounded by its orbiting electrons, the helium nucleus (and thus the helium atom of which it is a part) is a small and stable bit of matter. But when alpha particles stream as rays from decaying nuclei of larger atoms, those atoms are radioactive. Alpha particles can issue as rays from many large radioactive elements such as radium, uran-

[17]The following calculations have been made: if you are a person weighing 150 pounds, you are made up of some 6,700,000,000,000,000,000,000,000,000 atoms; and every time you lose or gain a pound you lose or gain this number divided by 150, or about 45,000,000,000,000,000,000,000,000 atoms. If you gain a pound in a month, you have gained at an average rate of approximately 17,000,000,000,000,000,000 (17 quintillion) atoms per second. (George E. Davis, *Radiation and Life* [Ames, Iowa, 1967], p. 4.)
[18]The hydrogen atom is an exception in that most hydrogen atoms have no neutrons in the nucleus. It should also be noted that there are numerous additional transitory subatomic particles in the nucleus; however, they are not appropriate to this discussion.

ium, and plutonium. And since these rays of particles are made up of charged atomic nuclei, loose to go into space (perhaps to collide with the electrons of another atom or enter and make the nucleus of another atom unstable), they are called *ions* (Greek *ion,* going). If the particles collide with electrons of other atoms and knock one or more of the electrons away, they make ions of these atoms, too. *Any* radiation that can do this is ionizing radiation. (If an atom *gains* extra electrons, it becomes charged, too, and is an ion.)

In addition to alpha radiation, two other forms of ionizing radiation are *beta rays* (or the *beta particles* of which they are composed) and *gamma rays.* Beta particles may be either positively or negatively charged. Negative beta particles are like high speed electrons. Surprisingly they come from disintegrating nuclei. Since electrons have been described to be the cloud surrounding a nucleus, how can this be so? Because neutrons in the disintegrating nucleus of a radioactive isotope decay into positively charged particles and negatively charged electrons of beta radiations.

The third form of ionizing radiation to come from the decaying nuclei of radioactive isotopes is a kind of ray that is not composed of particles, but of waves.[19] These are *gamma rays.* A different but similar kind of ray originates from electron disturbance in the orbitals—X-rays. So gamma rays are born in the nucleus of an atom and X-rays are born in the electron orbitals. These forms of wavelike radiation energy are called *electromagnetic radiation.* Other electromagnetic-wave radiations are radio waves, ultraviolet light waves, and ordinary light waves.

Sources of ionizing radiation

Ionizing radiation is a part of man's natural ecosystem. Radioactive materials in soil, rocks, air, food, and water, as well as in body and building materials, account for some fifty-eight percent of the radiation to which man is exposed. From outer space comes cosmic radiation to bombard everything on earth. Most cosmic radiation is blocked from reaching earth by the atmosphere, else man would perish. Man is constantly riddled by natural ionizing radiation but he has nevertheless flourished to make and use (as well as misuse) his own radiation. Man-made sources of ionizing radiation include X-rays, certain medical examinations, and industrial uses. These account for forty-one percent of man's ionizing radiation exposure. Fallout from nuclear weapons accounts for most of the remaining one percent.

The little burn of Becquerel: radiation damage

At the turn of the century, the famous physicist Henri Becquerel carried around in his vest pocket a tube of the intriguing new element radium, in a compound of radium salts. Before long he noticed a burn on his belly.

---

[19]Note, then, that some types of rays (alpha and beta rays) are composed of particles and others are not. Those rays not composed of particles are *waves.* A particle has weight or mass, and so, therefore, do the rays that are composed of particles. A wave without particles has no mass. Both forms of radiation can be measured by their effect on matter. For example, ultraviolet rays produce sunburn. Beta particles can also cause skin burn. But these forms of radiation energy are different.

To check Becquerel's observation, Pierre Curie (who, with his wife Marie, discovered radium) deliberately applied radium to his arm. Again a burn developed. The little burn of Becquerel has left its mark on mankind. Suspicion of damaging effects of radiation dates from such observations.

Like all other matter, human tissue is made up of atoms. Their nuclei are also surrounded by clouds of negatively charged electrons. How can ionizing radiations damage human tissue atoms? Consider these examples. A positively charged particle from a disintegrating atomic nucleus (alpha particles, positrons, protons) approaches the negatively charged electron cloud of a tissue atom. It is attracted (unlike charges attract). The damage then depends on its collision with the electrons of the cloud, affecting the chemistry of the atom (usually by removing an electron—ionizing the atom). When a negatively charged particle of a beta ray approaches a tissue atom, it will likely be repelled (like charges repel). But if the speed of the electron is great enough, it may overcome the repellent force and also collide with an electron in the atom's cloud. Because of the collision, the struck electron takes on increased energy and it speeds off to ricochet among the tissue atoms, ionizing some of them, too. What, then, occurs when an alpha particle or a high speed electron—or even a gamma ray— approaches a tissue atom? It can strike an electron in a cloud and, by increasing that electron's energy, send it off as an emissary to ionize nearby tissue atoms. Or the displaced electron can streak into a strange nucleus and affect it. Multiply this damage many times and there is body damage. If it is atoms in DNA molecules that have been assaulted, the DNA can no longer direct life's processes. Some of its own parts become ionized. The DNA is fragmented (see Figure 16-14).

In sum, then, when ionizing radiation collides with the various particles of tissue atoms or molecules, those tissue atoms or molecules are in turn ionized. Extensive damage can result. The radiation, causing the molecular disintegration of a cell's chemicals, interrupts cell function. Furthermore, the products of cellular destruction are believed to poison the cell. The general (somatic) body tissue cells and/or the specialized (gonadal) reproductive cells may be affected. Somatic cells may be grossly harmed or even killed by radiation. Damage to them may affect the lifetime of the individual exposed to the radiation, but damage to reproductive cells affects generations yet unborn—a cruel legacy for posterity. Radiation may change DNA structure directly or it may cause breaks in chromosomal structure that heal improperly. Here, too, toxic substances may be produced to poison the cell. Perhaps both chromosomal breaks and toxicity combine to violate the integrity of the DNA code and disrupt the cell. In a mutilated cell, ionized DNA sends improper messages. Abnormality is inevitable.

How much damage will radiation cause? This varies according to individual susceptibility, cell susceptibility, the kind of ionizing radiation, the radiation dose, and the length of time of exposure. Just as people vary in their sensitivity to pollen or smog, so they differ in their sensitivity

TABLE 4-1 _Radioisotopes of Major Biological Importance Occurring in Fallout_

ISOTOPE	HALF LIFE*	PATHS OF ENTRY	PART OF BODY AFFECTED
Iodine 131	8 days	Passed to man in dairy products (through surface contamination of plants cows eat.) Also inhaled by man.	Thyroid.
Barium 140	12.8 days	Passed to man in dairy products (through surface contamination of plants animals eat) or in grains and leafy vegetables man eats (through surface contamination of these plants).	Bone and bone marrow.
Strontium 89	53 days	Passed to man in dairy products (through surface and soil contamination of plants cows eat) or in grains and leafy vegetables man eats (which are also contaminated on the surface and through the soil).	Bone and bone marrow.
Strontium 90	28 years	Same as for strontium 89.	Bone and bone marrow.
Cesium 137	30 years	Passed to man in meat and in dairy products (through surface contamination of plants animals eat) or in grains and leafy vegetables man eats (through surface contamination of these plants).	Soft tissues, particularly muscles, also reproductive cells.
Carbon 14	5,600 years	Passed to man by ingestion (through food), by inhalation (through air), and by absorption.	Whole body, including reproductive cells.

*The time it takes the radioactivity originally associated with an isotope to lessen by half because of radioactive decay.

Sources: Dan I. Bolef, "Bomb Tests," _Scientist and Citizen_, Vol. 6, Nos. 9–10 (September–October 1964), p. 8; J. R. Arnold and E. A. Martell, "The Circulation of Isotopes," _Scientific American_, Vol. 201, No. 3 (September 1959), p. 90.

to equal doses of ionizing radiation. Also, tissue cells differ in their sensitivity and according to the type of ionizing radiation. Some ionizing radiation is more penetrating than others. Still other ionizing radiation has an affinity for specific structures because of its similarity to certain cellular constituents. Thus, strontium 89 and 90, closely resembling (bone) calcium, concentrate in bone and its marrow (see Table 4-1). The most sensitive cells to radiation are those of the stomach and intestines, bone marrow and lymph nodes (lymphocyte manufacturers), spleen, and reproductive organs. Large doses of all types of radiation will kill cells. But they must be delivered over a short period of time. Spread over many years, a person's exposure to radiation may amount to a considerable total. He will show few if any noticeable effects. Concentrated into a brief time (a split second, for example), the same ordinary total lifetime dosage may be fatal. Why? Given time, the body repairs or replaces many cells. It was the overwhelming dose delivered over a short time that resulted in the terrible events at Hiroshima and Nagasaki.

Ionizing radiation as man's benefactor

By means of nuclear reactors nuclear power can be converted to peaceful use on a world-wide scale.

Man-made radioisotopes may eventually replace natural fuels. The problems of the radiation hazards are being studied so that nuclear reactors will be safely controlled and shielded, and so that radioactive wastes can be disposed of without threatening future generations. Hopefully, in a world at peace, the problem of massive radiation will be confined to such projects as seeking new sources of energy for building dams, powering industry, lighting homes, and carrying technology forward. As will be seen below, agreement as to the best methods of accomplishing these benefits is not universal.

Perhaps more significant than the industrial potential of radiation are its medical uses. Radiation has provided new X-ray techniques for early diagnosis of cancer, and radiation has been used to treat cancers.

For example, radiation has provided new X-ray techniques for early diagnosis of breast cancer. To women with this illness as well as to thousands afflicted with cancer of the uterine cervix, radiation has brought years of life. X-ray methods also provide ways of viewing the heart and blood vessels (see Figure 4-4).

In an auto accident a man's kidney is badly damaged. It would best be removed. Can the remaining kidney carry the load of two? There is no time for prolonged laboratory tests. Into the patient's vein is injected a compound containing certain radioactive atoms of iodine. Over the kidney area of the patient's back a radiation counter is placed. This measures the radioactivity of the hopefully normal kidney. By the way the kidney handles the radioactive material, the physician can, in minutes determine whether the kidney is reliable. Injected, the radioactive iodine material revealed its position. It could thus be traced and measured. Such radioisotopes are called *tracers*.

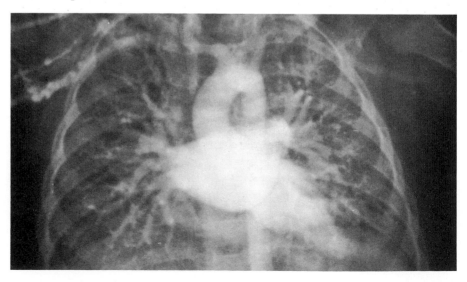

4-4 An X-ray photograph of a normal heart. The large looped vessel coming from the heart is the aorta, the largest of all arteries.

Another example: an anemic patient bleeds into the gut. His doctor wants to know how serious this bleeding is. He injects the radioisotope iron 59 into a vein. It is incorporated into the hemoglobin, the pigment of the red blood cell. If the patient is losing blood hemoglobin into the gut, his total radioactivity will be lost more rapidly than normal. Another patient has a brain tumor. In order to remove it, one must know exactly where in the brain the tumor lies. Inject the proper isotope. Multiplying tumor cells will take it up more readily than normal surrounding tissue. Radioactive scanning techniques locate the tumor.

Just as there is a biological risk to human life from natural radiation, there is the same risk in man's use of radiation. In terms of human life and in no other terms, it has been seen that the benefits of radiation can far outweigh the costs. Under proper conditions, diagnostic and treatment radiations are proper risks. Nevertheless, problems such as personnel shortages hamper inspection of X-rays used in both medicine and industry. By mid-1967, less than half of this nation's medical X-ray installations had met current state regulations or recommendations.[20] This is a dangerous loophole. For a considerable part of the population, X-rays and nuclear medicine have increased the average exposure to radiation as much as one hundred percent above the former rate.

The other face of Janus: radiation dangers

The dangers related to nuclear power plants[21] are similarly of growing concern. For example, their construction along some earthquake-prone California areas is being actively questioned by people who feel that an earthquake might so damage a nuclear power plant that excessive amounts of radioactive material would be let loose. One responsible scientist has urged that nuclear power plants be placed underground.[22] Research must lead "to complete development of defect-free processing and disposal methods before the public can be assured that the benefits of nuclear energy may not generate unacceptable risk."[23]

Two more recent man-made radiation sources need constant surveillance. Microwaves, used in a variety of ways ranging from military communications to food ovens, emit radiations that may be potentially harmful, especially to the eye. The same is true of laser-maser concentrated light-energy systems, which are finding use in industry and the military. So intense is the light energy of a laser that it can drill a hole through a diamond in moments—a process that, before lasers, took two days.

[20]L. H. Fess and L. Seabron, "Preliminary Results of 5,263 X-ray Protection Surveys of Facilities with Medical X-ray Equipment (1962–1967)," cited in James T. Terrill, "Microwaves, Lasers, and X-rays," *Archives of Environmental Health,* Vol. 19, No. 2 (August 1969), p. 269.

[21]To describe the nuclear-powered industrial complex of the future a new term—"nuplex"—is being used.

[22]"In principle, nuclear reactors are dangerous," Edward Teller, the "father of the H-bomb," said in 1965. "By being careful, and also by good luck, we have so far avoided all serious nuclear accidents . . . In my mind, nuclear reactors do not belong on the surface of the earth. Nuclear reactors belong underground." (Edward Teller, "Energy from Oil and from the Nucleus," cited in Sheldon Novick, *The Careless Atom* [Boston, 1969], p. 38.)

[23]Joel A. Snow, "Radioactive Waste from Reactors," *Scientist and Citizen,* Vol. 9, No. 5 (May 1967), p. 95.

Atomic accidents happen

In March 1954, unexpected winds picked up radioactive products of a nuclear test explosion on the island of Bikini and showered them on twenty-three unlucky Japanese fishermen on their boat, *The Lucky Dragon,* as well as on various Pacific islanders. It was not until ten years later that some of the children on the Rongelap Atoll developed thyroid nodules,[24] abnormal thyroid function, and signs of growth retardation. Thus the absence of early organ changes after exposure does not necessarily mean that the exposed person has escaped serious harm. Accidents involving atomic materials still occur too frequently. Nobody was hurt as a result of the nuclear plant accident at Windscale, England, some years ago. Nevertheless, an undue amount of radioactive iodine was released into this sparsely settled area. After the accident "authorities had to seize all milk and crops within 400 square miles of the plant."[25] By mid-1967 ten nuclear power plant accidents had occurred without known harm to anyone. Nor was anyone known to be hurt as a result of the seventeenth accident involving aircraft carrying nuclear weapons, in 1966. Nevertheless, the hazard exists and must be reduced to an absolute minimum.

A recent investigation into the worst fire in Atomic Energy Commission history at the Rocky Flats plutonium plant near Denver, Colorado, on May 11, 1969, does not help instill public confidence. Numerous smaller fires had preceded the May 11 holocaust at the Rocky Flats plant. Furthermore, over the years a considerable number of employees of this plant have been overexposed to radiation. The plant is operated for the processing of plutonium, a key ingredient in most atom bombs. Its employees are also involved in replacing defective bomb and warhead components. In this country today there are fifteen atomic power plants in operation and thirty-one are being built. Over forty more are being planned.[26]

The bomb

> I beheld the earth, and, lo, it was without form, and void; and the heavens, and they had no light.
> I beheld the mountains, and, lo, they trembled, and all the hills moved lightly.
> I beheld, and, lo, there was no man, and all the birds of the heavens were fled.
> I beheld, and, lo, the fruitful place was a wilderness, and all the cities thereof were broken down.

Thus does the prophecy of Jeremiah (4:23–26) tell of a destructive energy that suggests this most terrible of all inventions. Pressing the button of destruction at Alamogordo on the chill morning of July 16, 1945, men knew

[24]George M. Woodwell, "Toxic Substances and Ecological Cycles," p. 29.
[25]Roger Rapoport, "Secrecy and Safety at Rocky Flats," *Los Angeles Times,* September 7, 1969, p. 18.
[26]*Ibid.,* p. 12.

they had wrought the threat of their time. Almost twenty years later, J. Robert Oppenheimer, the director of the project that had developed the atom bomb, repeated the haunting appraisal of a scared security guard. "The long-hairs have let it get away from them."[27] For thousands of people, the threefold body assault by the bomb—burn, blast, and radiation—became agonizing reality. Until men live at peace, control of thermonuclear weapons will remain a consuming problem. The nuclear test ban is a step in the right direction. Not all nations have agreed to it.

Radioactive fallout

When a nuclear bomb explodes, radioactive material is let loose into the atmosphere. This material, falling to earth by gravity, is "fallout." Within a few hours, some of the particles settle to the ground. Within several months more descend. The lightest particles rise into the stratosphere and circulate around the world. Unless borne downward by rain or snow, they may not return to earth for months or years. Most fallout concentrates in the earth's Temperate Zone. In it lie the great cities of the world—London, Tokyo, New York, Moscow, Peking. And in this zone lives some eighty percent of the world's population.

"So well known has the BTS become that letters from children, addressed simply 'Tooth Fairy, St. Louis,' reach their destination at the CNI Office.[28] BTS means Baby Tooth Survey. CNI refers to the Greater St. Louis Citizens' Committee for Nuclear Information. The survey, started in 1958, is a splendid community-wide effort for measuring strontium 90 in baby teeth. It is just before and after birth that most strontium 90 is absorbed in the teeth of babies. So, baby teeth examined for strontium 90 reflect a situation seven to ten years old. The nuclear test ban occurred in 1963. By 1973, baby teeth should once more approach the nonradioactive state that existed before testing began. Someday, it may be hoped, there will be no need to do anything with such teeth except tuck them under pillows.

Epilogue: the St. Louis Baby Tooth Survey

The modern earache

"Noise," wrote the nineteenth-century German philosopher Schopenhauer not without his usual acrimony, "is the most impertinent of all interruptions."[29] Bitterly he railed against the "wanton, cursed, brain-paralyzing whine of the coachman's whip." Were he alive today, he might well remember the coachman's whip with nostalgia. Over ninety million

[27]Told by J. Robert Oppenheimer in the 1962 Whidden Lectures, at McMaster University, and cited in Henry E. Duckworth, *Little Men in the Unseen World* (New York, 1963), p. 110.
[28]Yvonne Logan, "The Story of the Baby Tooth Survey," *Scientist and Citizen,* Vol. 6, Nos. 9–10 (September–October 1964), p. 39.
[29]Arthur Schopenhauer, "On Noise," *The Pessimist's Handbook, A Collection of Popular Essays,* tr. by T. Bailey Saunders (Lincoln, Neb., 1964), p. 217.

automobiles, sixteen million trucks, and two-and-a-half million motor-cycles roar through the streets of this nation. Inside the home, such appliances as dishwashers, garbage disposals, and food blenders raise enough racket to threaten human hearing. Above, the skies shake from over twelve hundred jet aircraft.

While most people are disturbed by noise not of their own making, noise affects different people variously. The thrumming voice of a cello relaxes one person and distracts another. An epileptic seizure was the response of one sensitive Wisconsin housewife to the voices of three different radio announcers. (The successful treatment was the repetitious playing of tapes of the announcers' voices until they no longer affected her.)[30] Noise is unwanted sound. But what is sound?

Sound In a gust of wind, a heavy door swings. Its energy is expended in moving and in pushing air out of the way. The door slams shut. No longer can the moving door's energy be used in motion and pushing air. It is expended on the door frame and the walls. Immediately adjacent to the walls the air particles begin to vibrate. These, in turn, pass on their vibrations to the air particles next to them. This second group of particles cause a third group next to them to vibrate. So, starting from the vibrating air particles next to the shaking walls, vibrations are passed on from one group of particles to the next until the ear is reached. It is not the air particles that have moved from the wall to the ear. The air particles merely moved up and down, passing their vibrations along to their neighboring particles. It is the vibrations that have moved from the wall to the ear. The vibrations pass along in waves. Compare this phenomenon to a stone dropped in water. Ripples or waves spread out from the place where the stone fell. But the water itself merely moves up and down. A leaf in the water will move up and down with the disturbed water. It too will be disturbed but not moved along with the ripples or waves. In a like way, a slamming door will push air out of its way to make ripples or waves. These, combined with the air's vibrating particles, are the transmitted sound waves instigated by the energy of the slamming door. Over three hundred years ago, Galileo summed this up in his *Dialogues*: "Waves are produced by the vibrations of a sonorous body, which spread through the air, bringing to the tympanum[31] of the ear a stimulus which the mind interprets as sound." Since sound depends on air particles to travel, there is no sound in a vacuum or on the moon.

The ear For a sound to reach the brain for interpretation, each of the three main parts of the ear—*outer, middle,* and *inner*—must fulfill its purpose (see Figure 4-5).

The *outer ear* consists of the fleshy *external ear* (or *auricle*), which collects sound waves and directs them into the inch-long, funnel-shaped

---

[30]*Science News*, Vol. 93, No. 23 (June 8, 1968), p. 549.
[31]The *tympanum* is the cavity of the middle ear.

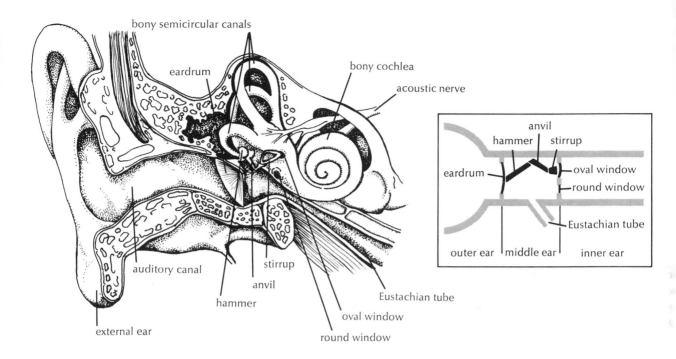

4-5 The ear: detailed and schematic views. Not visible in the illustration at the left is the membranous cochlear duct, which is housed in the bony cochlea. It is the cochlear duct that, in turn, contains the organ of hearing—the spiral organ of Corti. And it is the organ of Corti whose stimulated hair cells will induce the impulses on the surrounding acoustic nerve fibers. These impulses will reach the brain as sound.

auditory canal. This canal ends blindly. It is closed off by the outer wall of the middle ear, the *eardrum* (or *tympanic membrane*).

Except for the membranous eardrum, the walls of the middle ear chamber are bone. And it contains a connected chain of the three smallest bones in the body, named for their shape. The first is the *hammer* (or *malleus*). The handle of the hammer is attached to the inside of the eardrum. The second middle ear bone of the chain is the *anvil* (or *incus*), and the third is the *stirrup* (or *stapes*). Connecting the middle ear to the back of the nose is the *Eustachian tube,* named after a sixteenth-century anatomist, Eustacio. Ordinarily this tube is closed. With swallowing, however, it opens. Were it not for this tube, an increase in pressure in the auditory canal would force the eardrum into the middle ear; a decrease in pressure would draw it out. Air pressure changes within the auditory canal are small. To respond to such small changes, the average pressure on both sides of the eardrum must be kept the same. A loud noise, such as a cannon, can cause enough pressure within the auditory canal to rupture the eardrum. By keeping the mouth open, the pressure against the eardrum comes from both sides (auditory canal and Eustachian tube). This prevents this kind of damage. Those who fire cannon also often wear earplugs.

The inner wall of the middle ear is the outer wall of the inner ear. In this wall are two small openings—the *oval window* above and the *round window* below. The foot plate of the stirrup touches the thin membrane covering the oval window. As will be seen, the function of the tiny middle ear bones is to transmit the motion of the eardrum to the membrane of the oval window.

The *inner ear* is encased in bone. It consists of a series of minute and intricately tunneled bony canals, which contain membranous canals. Strands of connective tissue attach the membranous canals to their bony container. Within both the bony and membranous canals is a thin, limpid fluid. So the membranous canals are surrounded by this fluid and also contain it.

One part of the bony canals is molded into a pea-sized spiral passage making $2\frac{3}{4}$ turns; it is the *cochlea*. Its name is derived from the Latin word for "snail shell," which describes its shape. A second part of the bony canals are the *semicircular canals*. Within these bony semicircular canals fit the membranous *semicircular ducts*. The semicircular canals and their contained membranous ducts are concerned with balance. They have nothing to do with hearing.[32] It is the bony cochlea that is of present concern, for it houses the membranous *cochlear duct*. Within this duct, and attached to its floor, is a structure called the *spiral organ of Corti*. The organ of Corti contains sensory hair cells about which branch delicate fibers of the cranial nerve of hearing (the *acoustic nerve*). It is thus the organ of Corti that receives the stimuli of sound for transmission to the brain.

How hearing happens
Sound waves reaching the ear travel at about 1,100 feet a second. Compared to light waves they are very slow. That is why the puff of smoke of a distant train's steam whistle is visible long before the whistle is heard. Sound waves are caught by the external ear and are directed into the auditory canal. The waves strike the eardrum and set it to vibrating in time with the sound waves. The vibrations of the eardrum are conveyed by the bones of the middle ear to the oval window. The thin membrane of the oval window then vibrates. There the vibrations are converted into pressure waves in the fluid within the bony cochlea. These waves cause the membranous roof of the cochlear duct to vibrate. Waves are thereby set off in the fluid within the cochlear duct and these, in turn, set the membranous floor of the cochlear duct to vibrating. These vibrations stimulate the hair cells of the spiral organ of Corti attached to the floor

[32] The membranous and fluid-filled organs of equilibratory sense are the semicircular ducts and the *utricle*, both of which are inside the semicircular canals. Reflexes, initiated by stimulated nerves of the semicircular ducts, cause appropriate body movements to maintain equilibrium. Disease (such as infection) of these ducts soon produces dizziness. However, it is the nerve receptors of the utricle that are responsible in sea, car, and other motion sickness. The utricle is also involved with gravity. The marvelous ability of a falling cat to land on its feet is due to the function of its utricle.

of the cochlear duct. Finally, the stimulated hair cells of the organ of Corti induce impulses that are received by the surrounding fibers of the acoustic nerve and are carried to the brain for interpretation as sound. Thus is sound energy transmitted through air, bone, and fluid and converted, in the inner ear, into electrical nervous energy to be sent to the brain.

The round window is not directly involved in the transmission of sound energy. Located below the oval window, it is a membrane-covered window of adjustment. As the bones of the middle ear are stimulated by sound waves, the vibrating foot plate of the stirrup pushes the membrane of the oval window slightly inward. As was described above, this disturbs and displaces a small volume of the fluid within the bony cochlea. But fluid cannot be compressed. The displaced cochlear fluid must go somewhere. It is accommodated by the membrane of the round window. This membrane allows the fluid to push outward. When the foot plate moves outward, the fluid can move inward. So, the tiny membrane of the round window, by permitting the stirrup to move, permits hearing.

How sensitive is the hearing apparatus? The weakest sound that can be heard by the human ear causes its oval window to move no more than three-hundred-thousandths of a millionth of an inch. Comparing this amount of motion to the length of the ear canal is equivalent to comparing a thin sheet of paper to the distance between London and New York. No less remarkable is the range of pressures to which the ear is sensitive. The eardrum can withstand, without damage, the pressure of a loud noise that is fourteen million times greater than the pressure of the softest sound the ear can normally hear.[33]

Sound measured as a physical force

Sound waves traveling through the atmosphere cause changes of pressure within it. The smallest disturbance in air pressure that can be heard, under ideal conditions, by a young person is known as the *threshold of hearing*. It is from this threshold that sound levels in *decibels* are measured. What are decibels? They are the units of sound measurement—units of loudness. The "bel" in the word is named for the inventor of the telephone, Alexander Graham Bell. "Deci" is derived from the Latin *decem,* meaning "ten." Two sounds differ by one bel if their intensities are in the ratio 10:1. A decibel is thus one-tenth of a bel. As the number of decibels goes up from the threshold of hearing, the loudness increases as an exponent. One decibel is about the softest sound the human ear can usually hear. Ten decibels of sound is, thus, ten times louder, and a twenty-decibel sound is ten times louder than a ten-decibel sound. A thirty-decibel sound (a whisper) is ten times louder than a twenty-decibel sound. At one hundred feet a jet plane taking off is ten times louder than a pneumatic riveter, and it will hurt (see Figure 4-6). As decibels increase, sound energy multiplies in fantastic proportion. The greater this energy, the more the discomfort.

[33]Colin A. Ronan, The *Meaning of Sound* (New York, 1967), pp. 69, 71.

Unwanted sound: noise as an air pollutant

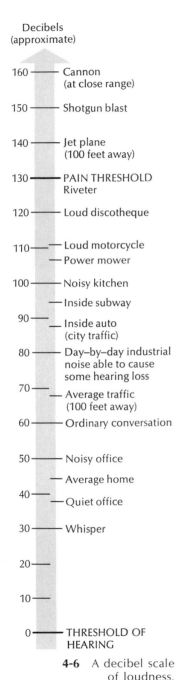

Decibels (approximate)

160 — Cannon (at close range)

150 — Shotgun blast

140 — Jet plane (100 feet away)

130 — PAIN THRESHOLD / Riveter

120 — Loud discotheque

110 — Loud motorcycle / Power mower

100 — Noisy kitchen / Inside subway

90 — Inside auto (city traffic)

80 — Day–by–day industrial noise able to cause some hearing loss

70 — Average traffic (100 feet away)

60 — Ordinary conversation

50 — Noisy office / Average home

40 — Quiet office

30 — Whisper

20 —

10 —

0 — THRESHOLD OF HEARING

4-6 A decibel scale of loudness.

That noise, like all other sound, is a physical force has long been appreciated. The Bible says that the people led by Joshua at Jericho "shouted with a great shout, that the wall fell down flat . . . and they took the city" (Joshua 6:20). The heat released by the energy of focused sound vibrations at an intensity of 170 decibels can kill a small animal or start a fire. Relatively short exposure to noise in excess of 130 decibels may do permanent damage to the ears of normal persons. Long exposure to a noise level of 100 decibels may permanently harm hearing.

In this culture, noise assaults the ear early in life, and escape is not always easy. Even the baby compartments of hospital incubators may be polluted by noise. One recent Chicago study found that "under the plastic hood of the incubators the noise spectrum fell well above the recommended acceptance level and, due to the prolonged exposure time, very close to the danger area."[34] And the incubator is not the only preserve of the child that is invaded by noise. In a downtown Boston school playground, a noise level of 78 decibels was recently recorded. In the Boston suburb of Wellesley, the noise level of a school playground was only 58 decibels. So the Boston city school children were exposed to noise a hundred times greater than the suburban children.

As people grow, their exposure to noise often increases. In one study, five members of a musical combo were studied before, during, and after a two-and-one-half-hour rehearsal session. Three of the group were nineteen years old; two were twenty. After the rehearsal all five musicians reported "ringing" or a sensation of "fullness" in the ears. All demonstrated some reduced hearing ability, presumably temporary. During the loudest period of the rehearsal session, sound intensity levels ranged from 120 to 130 decibels.[35] At the press site of a departing Saturn moon rocket, the decibel noise level rises to 120 decibels. Noise levels at two San Francisco discotheques peaked at 120 decibels.

Investigators recently surveyed hearing ability of three thousand Knoxville, Tennessee, school-age children. Only 3.8 percent of the sixth-graders had some impaired hearing. Among ninth-graders the percentage rose to 11. Twelfth-graders showed a prevalence of 10.6 percent.

The same investigators sought to discover whether rock 'n' roll music caused permanent damage to the ear (see Figure 4-8). A guinea pig was subjected to rock 'n' roll music adjusted to sound levels approximating those found in dance halls (about a peak of 122 decibels). Only the right ear of the guinea pig was exposed. The left ear was protected by a plug. Stimulation periods were varied according to observed exposure by teenagers to rock 'n' roll. Widespread irreversible damage to the hair cells in the cochlea of the exposed ear was noted.[36] Similar noise damage has

[34] Frank L. Seleney and Michael Streczyn, "Noise Characteristics in the Baby Compartment of Incubators," *American Journal of Diseases of Children*, Vol. 117, No. 4 (April 1969), p. 450.

[35] Ralph R. Rupp and Larry J. Koch, "Effects of Too-Loud Music on Human Ears. But, Mother, Rock 'n' Roll HAS to Be Loud!" *Clinical Pediatrics*, Vol. 8, No. 2 (February 1969), pp. 60–62.

[36] David M. Lipscomb, "High Intensity Sounds in the Recreational Environment: Hazard to Young Ears," *Clinical Pediatrics*, Vol. 8, No. 2 (February 1969), pp. 63–68.

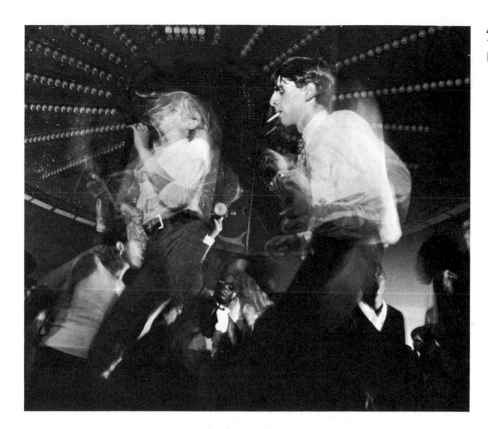

4-7 A discotheque. The decibel level here is about 120.

been observed in experiments with other laboratory animals as well. Although care must be exercised in applying results of animal experiments to humans, it is apparent that such damage may be occurring among young persons similarly exposed.

There is yet an added danger. During ordinary conversation at 60 decibels, only the lower hearing acuity levels are required. But the constant pressure of excessively loud sounds may first wear out the small beginning area of the delicate hair cells. That is why the early stages of deafness so often go unnoticed. A person who, according to an audiometer test, has a hearing impairment in both ears of forty percent may not even have noticed his deafness. Why? Because he can adequately hear speech. By the time a person is aware of his hearing problem—before he has trouble understanding speech—his hearing loss may already be considerable and permanent. He does not avoid damage to his hearing until much damage is done. So, insofar as hearing acuity is concerned, mere speech comprehension may be a cruelly deceptive measure.

One concerned medical specialist puts it this way: "The teen-agers' ability to 'turn us off' may change to a situation where they can no longer 'turn us on' again."[37]

[37]Alan R. Freedman, "Rock 'n' Roll Music: Harmful?" *Pediatrics*, Vol. 8, No. 2 (February 1969), p. 58.

a. Normal-appearing tissues in the organ of Corti of the protected ear (× approx. 850), showing supporting cells (SC), inner sensory hair cells (IHC), pillars of Corti (PC), and outer sensory hair cells (OHC).

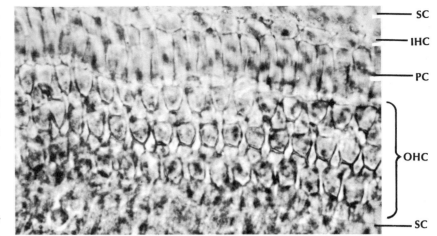

SC
IHC
PC
OHC
SC

4-8 Ear damage to a guinea pig from exposure to rock 'n' roll music. The animal's right ear was exposed; its left ear was protected by a plug.

b. Damaged inner sensory hair cells (top arrows) and missing or collapsed outer sensory hair cells (bottom arrows) in the unprotected organ of Corti (× approx. 935). Other damaged cells can be noted in the second and third rows of outer sensory hair cells.

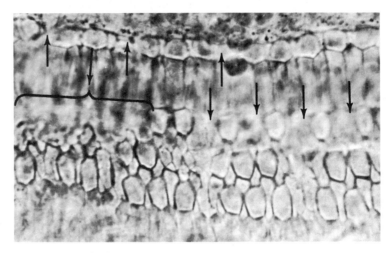

c. Torn segment of cochlear tissues from the unprotected ear. In this region of tissue, there was destruction across the entire breadth (arrow) of the organ of Corti (× approx. 935).

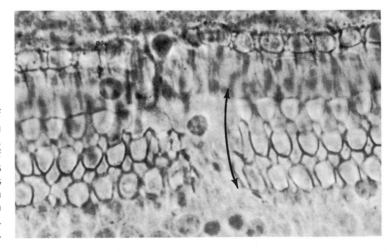

"Aged ears play truant at his tales," wrote Shakespeare in *Love's Labor's Lost* (II.i.74). Indeed, deafness has long been considered an inevitable disability of old age. To some extent, it may be. But among the Mabaan tribe in the African Sudan, for example, the aged hear about as well as the young. And old Mabaans hear better than old people in this country. Why? The environment of the gentle Mabaans is quiet—the sound level averages about 40 decibels. The Mabaans even sing softly. Their hearing mechanism is undamaged by noise.

To the city dweller in the Western world, noise may well be a cumulative hazard. Though on a day-to-day basis it may seem to be only an annoying byproduct of city life, like any other air pollutant it may become a health hazard to people who suffer prolonged exposure. The cost of noise is widespread deafness among older people. But that is not all. Studies conducted among the Mabaans verified earlier German research. With the Mabaans, blood "pressures remain essentially the same throughout life . . . whereas in our culture the blood pressure rises in the aging in apparently healthy individuals."[38] Loud noise may cause constriction of small blood vessels and a reduced output of blood from the heart. Some researchers believe that, because of this diminished output, less nourishing blood reaches the hearing nerves and that this deprivation promotes nerve cell abnormality and deafness. The possibility of continuous noise causing high blood pressure (even peptic ulcer) cannot be dismissed. However, a direct cause and effect relationship has not been proved.

Aged ears

> *An old lady who lived by the shore*
> *At length got so used to the roar*
> *That she never could sleep*
> *Unless someone would keep*
> *A-pounding away at the door.*

Weary ears

The exhausted city dweller may learn to sleep through noise, but does he rest? The most essential stage of sleep, the dream stage, may be ruptured by noise. Recent studies, moreover, suggest that excessive noise severely disturbs even a sound sleeper. Examinations of brain waves show that they may be grossly changed by noise.

Millions of people no longer expect rest, much less sleep, in their apartment homes. So noisy are many high-rise apartment houses that owners are as short of prospective tenants as their tenants are of sleep. Some tenants finally forsake their apartment houses for a hotel room and a good night of rest. No longer do desk clerks wonder why a room near an elevator is angrily rejected. Before renting an apartment, many weary prospective tenants bring their own testing equipment—a transistor radio. By playing the radio at various levels in an adjoining apartment, they can get a good indication of possible noise levels in the apartment they are

---

[38] Samuel Rosen et al., "Presbycusis Study of a Relatively Noise-Free Population in the Sudan, " *Annals of Otology, Rhinology and Laryngology*, Vol. 71, No. 3 (September 1962), p. 742.

considering. Recently, one Los Angeles house-hunter was shown a fine, but hard-to-sell home directly under the path of incoming airplanes. The roar was deafening. He could not hear the sales pitch.

"I can't hear you!" he shouted.

"What?" yelled the salesman.

The house-hunter waited. For a moment it was quieter.

"These airplanes . . ." he began.

"Oh, the airplanes!" the salesman cried ecstatically. "Where else could you buy a house just four hours from New York?"

One need not be directly under the flight path of a large jet to suffer noise distress. "When a 707-320 B jet is four miles from the point of brake release at the end of the runway, it has attained an altitude of 800 feet and the noise level on the ground one-half mile on either side of the flight path is approximately 85 decibels."[39]

Antinoise activity   Noise costs money. In lost production and accidents due to noise, the yearly cost to industry is estimated at four billion dollars. Annual compensation claims from deafness thought to be due to job noise amount to about two million dollars. Merely by changing an assembly-line operation from an area next to a boiler room to a quiet section of the shop, one factory manager markedly reduced costly errors. Another large company found office soundproofing a sound investment. Typing errors dropped 29 percent, machine operator errors 52 percent, absenteeism and employee turnover 37 and 47 percent respectively.[40] The management of one large New York bank tried to solve their noise problem in a roundabout way. Plagued by high employee turnover due to the insufferable noise, they finally resorted to hiring deaf people.[41]

In noise control, the Old World may yet show the New World the way. In France, transistor radios are forbidden in public places. Plastic or rubber lids cover the garbage pails of Paris. TV or radio noise outside a West German home may prompt a summons. Construction noise (a massive problem in this country) is limited by law in West Germany. Britain is developing similar antinoise legislation. Muscovites may not indiscriminately blow auto horns. Antinoise building codes limit racket in the new apartments of Britain, Germany, Russia, and the Low Countries.

In this country it is hard to control construction noise through legal codes. Such codes are local matters, and the thousands of cities and towns in the United States are fiercely protective of their own prerogatives. Nor does all legislation adequately control the problem. A 1967 California law permits a 50-horsepower motorcycle to make as much noise as four 300-horsepower Cadillacs. Ways are being studied in which noise-controlled construction would be required for structures built under FHA mortgages.

[39]Donald F. Anthrop, "Environmental Noise Pollution: A New Threat to Sanity," *Bulletin of the Atomic Scientists*, Vol. 25, No. 5 (May 1969), p. 13.

[40]*M.D., Medical Newsmagazine*, Vol. 10, No. 6 (June 1966), p. 122.

[41]"New York Employs Deaf," *Hearing and Speech News* (January 1967), p. 7, quoted in Robert Alex Baron, "Noise and Urban Man," *American Journal of Public Health*, Vol. 58, No. 11 (November 1968), p. 2061.

Many city administrators are considering the establishment of adequate antinoise codes. Such action is long overdue.

Some private dwellings are noise traps. Modern couples seeking a home often want transparency and continuity. These require an open floor plan and much glass. Acoustical nightmares may result. As with large buildings, home noise control depends on the construction plan and method. (It is, incidentally, quite possible to build a structure that is too quiet. The silence is intense. Even a slight noise—such as someone tapping a pencil—is then disturbing. An "acoustical perfume" or "white noise," such as soft music, may be installed to mask the intruding sound and to soothe the inhabitants.)

Many people endure deep disquiet from an explosive sonic boom. To them, fear of air accidents, compounded with a startling and foreboding bang from an unseen source above, is particularly unsettling. An airplane traveling faster than sound, tearing through the atmosphere, produces shock waves in its wake. These may be compared to water-wake waves produced by a speeding boat tearing through water. The shock waves caused by a supersonic airplane result in an air pressure wave that is the sonic boom. Dragging on the ground as a cone-shaped shock wave of sound, it causes a series of abrupt atmospheric pressure changes. First, there is a sudden rise. Then, just as suddenly, the atmospheric pressure drops. Finally, it shoots back to normal. The result: a double, closely-spaced, brain-quaking, earth-shaking thunderclap—the sonic boom.

In 1964, the people of Oklahoma City underwent an experiment. For more than six months military planes roared through their skies. In a sense, the experiment lacked complete objectivity. About one-third of the city's residents depend upon the aviation industry for a living. Nevertheless, 1,253 booms brought 12,588 complaints. Many people claimed damage to walls and windows. Babies wakened and wept, frightened. Dogs forgot their training. Careful investigation, however, revealed that the property damage was more imagined than real. By increasing the height at which planes are allowed to reach supersonic speed and by improving aircraft design, it is hoped that such noise will be diminished. Many airplane manufacturers have attached silencing devices to the exhaust ports of turbojet engines. Buffer zones separating airports from homes may prove useful.

In the summer of 1968, President Johnson signed a measure requiring the Federal Aviation Administration to control and abate aircraft noise. This agency has its work cut out for it.

The mobile epidemic

It doubtless never crossed his mind that his name would be inscribed in the record books. Yet, on September 13, 1895, when Mr. A. W. Bliss stepped off a New York trolley and was hit by a horseless carriage, he became the world's first auto fatality.[42] Since then, in this country alone, more than 1,600,000 people have died in car accidents. This is more than the total number of people that have died in all the wars of this nation's history.

The mathematics of death

According to the National Safety Council, 115,000 people in this country died because of accidents in 1968. Almost half of them—55,200—died in auto accidents.[43] In other words, on an average day, about 150 people died in motor-vehicle accidents. Auto accidents also account for about 2,000,000 disabling injuries a year.

Such large numbers often seem meaningless unless they are related to a personal experience. In Los Angeles, a twenty-six-year-old mother goes for a Sunday afternoon drive in the country with her husband and their two small daughters, aged three and five. There are two more children on the way, for next month this mother is due to deliver twins. Throughout his wife's pregnancy her physician husband has been amused at the idea of twins. The couple has bantered a lot and has had fun shopping for baby clothes. Now the mother is tired and a trifle impatient. "I can't be comfortable with these seat belts anymore," she tells her husband good-naturedly, and lets them fall unfastened. Then, as if reminded, she turns to be certain of the children's seat belts.

Soon they are in the country. It is a fine day. Suddenly somebody is coming over the hill on the wrong side of the road. They are hit head-on. In the hospital, the husband is repaired: seven stitches are needed for the scalp, five for his right cheek; some broken ribs are taped. Then he is told. The children are badly shaken up. That is all. But the wife has a crushing head injury. There is extensive brain damage. The twins are born and dead. That night the wife dies. She is, then, one of the 55,200 who died that year in an auto accident. So was the other driver. He was dead on admission to the hospital. The husband is counted along with the 2,000,000 disabled. That is part of the meaning of the numbers. Not the least interesting thing about them is how uninteresting they are to so many people.

How did it happen that this young woman was killed? One answer to this question is simply mathematical. There were two crashes, not one. Her husband was traveling 55 miles an hour. The first crash brought his car to a sudden halt. But for a fraction of a second the wife, unrestrained by a seat belt, continued traveling. She then became a projectile heading for a second crash. Her knees crumpled against the heater. Her chest hit

---

[42] *Guinness Book of Superlatives*, cited in G. Anthony Ryan, "Injuries in Traffic Accidents," *New England Journal of Medicine*, Vol. 276, No. 19 (May 11, 1967), p. 1066.

[43] National Safety Council, *Accident Facts: 1969 Edition.* Accidents in the home ranked second, with 28,500 fatalities. There were 20,500 accidental deaths in public (excluding motor-vehicle and work accidents in public places), and 14,300 Americans died of accidents that took place at work. These figures add up to more than the 115,000 total because of some overlapping: 3,200 work deaths involved motor vehicles and are in both the work and motor-vehicle categories; 300 motor-vehicle deaths occurred on home premises and are in both the home and motor-vehicle categories.

the dashboard. Her head struck the windshield, causing it to yield two inches. Her head collapsed two inches. Thus her head traveled four inches, or one-third of a foot, after hitting the windshield. What was the force of the impact? For this there is an equation:[44]

$$G = \frac{\text{miles per hour}^2}{30 \times \text{stopping distance in feet}} \text{ or } \frac{(55)^2}{30 \times \frac{1}{3}} = \frac{3,025}{10} = 302.5$$

The weight of that part of her upper body directly involved in the windshield blow is estimated at 20 percent of the weight of herself and her unborn babies (130 pounds) or 26 pounds. Multiplying 26 pounds by 302.5 G's equals 7,865 pounds—almost four tons. This was the average force with which her head impacted against the windshield.[45]

In this particular accident there was a lone driver in the opposite car. That he had been a heavy drinker for two years is the basic reason for the disaster. "It is known that well over half of all fatally injured drivers had been drinking; among drivers found to be responsible for the fatal crash, two-thirds had been drinking, and in the one-car fatal crashes, seven out of ten had been drinking."[46] A thirty-eight-month Michigan study of 96 fatal automobile accidents and a like number of controls revealed that the number of chronic alcoholic drivers in the fatal accidents outnumbered that in the controls by twelve to one (36 versus 3).[47]

The emotionally distressed driver

Further investigation of the accident involving the young mother revealed more about the lone drinking driver who was responsible for her death. Long subject to fits of depression, he had been referred by his family doctor to a psychiatrist some months before. (He had not kept his referral appointment.) As a teen-ager he had been somewhat impulsive but oddly conservative about driving. "He liked to go on these long rides," his father later grieved quietly. "Alone. All by himself. He'd say it relaxed him. Then he took to drinking. Then he wasn't good for driving or anything else."

This history is not unusual. The "graduation of the inexperienced, impulsive, but cautious beginner to a self-confident, financially independent, heavier drinking, and more dangerous young adult"[48] is an event that contributes to many an accident. In 1966, only 20 percent of the registered drivers in this country were under twenty-five. Yet, they were involved

[44] "Fighting Death on Wheels," *Roche Medical Image*, Vol. 8, No. 6 (June 1966), p. 8. G is the force developed in slowing an object, measured in terms of the force of gravity. In the formula, 30 represents a constant developed from the acceleration due to gravity (32.2 feet per second per second) and the measurement units used (in this case, miles per hour and feet).

[45] In Sweden, many car occupants now wear helmets. There is nothing in this equation that would make this practice anything but eminently sensible.

[46] H. Emerson Campbell, "Traffic Deaths Go up Again," *Journal of the American Medical Association*, Vol. 201, No. 11 (September 11, 1967), p. 861.

[47] Melvin L. Selzer, "Alcoholism, Mental Illness, and Stress in 96 Drivers Causing Fatal Accidents," *Behavioral Science*, Vol. 14, No. 1 (January 1969), pp. 1–10.

[48] Stanley H. Schuman *et al.*, "Young Male Drivers: Impulse Expression, Accidents, and Violations," *Journal of the American Medical Association*, Vol. 200, No. 12 (June 19, 1967), p. 102.

in one-third of the fatal accidents. Violent accidental death strikes young drivers harder than any other age group. In 1968, well over half the motor-vehicle fatalities (30,200 of the 55,200 total) were between the ages of fifteen and forty-four.

The close relationship between emotional illness and fatal accidents has long intrigued investigators. In one study, depressions, suicidal tendencies, and delusions of persecution were all found to be much more common among drivers responsible for fatal accidents than in a control group.[49] "It is clear," stated one health spokesman, "that an individual whose mind is filled with rage over a personal problem is not, at the moment, the best choice to drive a car."[50]

The emotionally sick, broken salesman in Arthur Miller's *Death of a Salesman*, speaks illuminatingly:

WILLY (with wonder). *I was driving along, you understand? And I was fine. I was even observing the scenery. You can imagine, me looking at the scenery, on the road every week of my life. But it's so beautiful up there, Linda, the trees are so thick, and the sun is warm. I opened the windshield and just let the warm air bathe over me. And then all of a sudden I'm goin' off the road! I'm tellin' ya, I absolutely forgot I was driving. If I'd've gone the other way over the white line I might've killed somebody. So I went on again—and five minutes later I'm dreamin' again, and I nearly—* (He presses two fingers against his eyes.) *I have such thoughts, I have such strange thoughts.*[51]

In studying two thousand safe drivers, the National Safety Council related careful driving habits to social adequacy.[52] All had splendid driving records in a variety of situations. On the average, what sort of people were they? They were 59 years old and married (few were divorced). They had one or two children. They had worked for the same company for some thirty-two years. Their major characteristics: stability and conformity. They did not seem to need anonymous expression, via their driving behavior, of hostility, discourtesy, or emotional conflict.

The increasing awareness of the relationship between accidents and emotional instability has led to much conjecture about the so-called accident prone individual. There is not enough scientific data to support this general term.[53] An individual may be likely to have an accident in one circumstance but not in another. People and circumstances vary too much to allow for this sweeping characterization.

[49] Melvin L. Selzer, Joseph E. Rogers, and Sue Kern, "Fatal Accidents: The Role of Psychopathology, Social Stress, and Acute Disturbance," *American Journal of Psychiatry*, Vol. 124, No. 8 (January 1968), p. 53.
[50] George James, former Commissioner of Health of New York City, quoted in "Chronic Disease, a Major Cause of Accidents," *Geriatric Focus*, Vol. 4, No. 4 (March 15, 1965), p. 1.
[51] Arthur Miller, *Death of a Salesman* (New York, 1949), Act I.
[52] M.D., *Medical Newsmagazine*, Vol. 12, No. 3 (March 1968), p. 188.
[53] "Accident Proneness," an editorial in *Canadian Medical Association Journal*, Vol. 90, No. 10 (March 7, 1964), pp. 646–47.

CAUSE OF FATALITY	SEAT BELT	SEAT BELT WITH SHOULDER BELT	SEAT BELT WITH DOUBLE SHOULDER BELT	COULD NOT BE SAVED	UNKNOWN	TOTAL
Ejection	25	1		1	1	28
Front door	2		2*	12	1	17
Steering assembly	4	8	2	14†		28
Instrument panel	2	3	2‡	2		9
Roof	2			6		8
Header (front part of roof over the windshield)	1	2				3
A-pillar (supporting pillar alongside the windshield)	4		1			5
Other	1	1		1		3
Totals	41	15	7	36	2	101

TABLE 4-2 *How Seat Belts Might Have Saved Drivers' Lives*

*In both cases, the right door collapsed but did not compromise the safety of the driver's compartment.
†In 11 of the 14 steering-assembly deaths, there was front-end collapse of the driver's compartment.
‡In one case, there was a collapse of the cabin area.

Source: Adapted from Donald F. Huelke and Paul W. Gikas, "Causes of Deaths in Automobile Accidents," *Journal of the American Medical Association*, Vol. 203, No. 13 (March 25, 1968), p. 1106.

Automobile accidents, like all other epidemics, must be considered in three interrelated aspects. The *host* or driver has already been discussed. Consider now the *agent* or automobile and the *environment* or roads. Some experts feel that the prevention of accidents should, insofar as possible, be taken out of the hands of the potential victim. Human frailty precludes the constant use of seat belts. Consequently, there is a newer emphasis on safer vehicles and roads. Yet, seat belts are lifesavers, and some facts about their value should be known.

Prevention of accidents: cars and roads

Seat belts

The experiments of Colonel Stapp in the New Mexico desert have demonstrated that an adequately restrained person is able to survive a 50-mile-per-hour head-on crash into a stone wall without injury.[54]

[54]Ross A. McFarland, "Injury—A Major Environmental Problem," *Archives of Environmental Health*, Vol. 19, No. 2 (August 1969), p. 253.

Like all accidents, the accident that killed the young mother and the drinking driver can teach. It is understandable that the young woman failed to fasten her seat belt. Yet, had she used seat belts she might have been one of the estimated 2,500 to 3,000 people in this country whose lives are annually saved by their use. (It is further estimated that a total of 8,000 to 10,000 lives would be saved each year if all passenger car occupants used seat belts at all times.) Lap and sash seat belts are more effective than lap belts alone.

A recent study of 139 fatal automobile accidents, in which 177 people were killed, shows how the use of seat belts might have saved the lives of 63 of the 101 drivers who were killed (see Table 4-2). Of the 28 drivers whose death resulted from ejection, 26 would probably have been saved by the use of the belts. Many facial injuries resulting from impact with the front door, steering assembly, and other parts of the car could also have been avoided. Nor, of course, were drivers the only victims who would have survived if they had used belts.

Tires

In this country nineteen manufacturers make some twenty dozen brands of tires in such a variety of fabrics, plies, and treads as to confuse any average buyer. Tires should be bought not according to price but according to intended use. A cross-country salesman will need a different set of tires than a truck driver, and the suburban shopper's needs are different yet.

Fabrics are built into the tire in plies (layers of fabric cords). It is not the number but rather the thickness of the plies or layers that determines fabric strength. And some kinds of fabric are safer than others. Rayon, an excellent cord material, is cheaper but not as strong as nylon. Polyester is almost as strong as nylon and, when combined with the fiberglass belt, is considered a superior safety tire. Also important for safety is the tire tread, the outer grooved surface of the tire. On wet roads effective tread patterns may be invaluable. Modern patterns wipe dry that wet portion of the road upon which the tire rests at any moment, thus reducing the chances of skidding.

For a car restricted to suburban errands, an 80-level[55] rayon or nylon tire is adequate. Freeway and family vacation travel requires at least a 100-level rayon or polyester tire. Fast drivers or those traveling long distances with heavy loads will do well to invest in nylon, fiberglass belt, or radial tires. High-speed tires have special nylon cord, thin-tread construction. They should not be confused with the extremely durable, 200-level, thick-tread tire, which is usually the best tire a company makes. Because these retain heat, they are unsuitable for high speeds. Among the safest of all tires is the "tire within a tire." Mandatory on a racetrack,

[55]Tires are still spoken of as quality level. A 100-level tire is one of a quality regarded as adequately safe for average driving.

it enables the driver with a puncture to get to a service station without further tire damage.

Correct air pressure is essential to tire care and safety. For the average car, 28–30 pounds are considered best. Lower pressures give softer but not safer rides. A slightly overloaded, underinflated tire traveling at 75 miles per hour will heat to 300 degrees! At 325 degrees rubber is a semi-liquid. Overinflation in a tire will carry one just as close to disaster. The blow of a road object cannot be properly absorbed. As a result the fabric tears and the tire may blow out immediately, or, if the damage is slight, fail days later. Wheel alignment checks prevent tire wear and provide greater safety, as do tire rotations. When is a tire beyond repair? Moulded into the patterns of most recently manufactured tires are tread-wear indicators. These are solid cross-bars between the grooves. If these show, the tire should no longer be in use. For tires without built-in indicators, a penny helps serve as an indicator. When the penny is inserted into the center groove, the date should not be visible.[56]

Other car safety factors

Growing public clamor is stimulating automobile safety design. "People don't really care about safe cars," some auto salesmen say. "That's a fact of life." But what people now know about the facts of death is prompting them to demand safer cars. Nothing does more to persuade a businessman than the opinion of the consumer. The recontoured and padded instrument panel, collapsible steering column, energy-absorbent materials in roof areas, securely fastened seats, rear windshield wipers and defrosters, improved seat locks, door locks with recessed handles, a stronger wall between the trunk area and the rear seat, removal of bumper projections, dual braking systems—these are some of the improvements being considered in reformed auto design (see Figure 4-9). Of considerable help in decreasing facial cuts is a new windshield (Figure 4-10). It has a plastic interlayer between the two panes of glass. Upon being struck, "the outer pane breaks first, reducing the immediate resistance to head impact forces. The . . . inner pane continues to flex, absorbing head impact energy before it [will] break into thousands of small, non-lacerating granules. The plastic interlayer is then free to 'balloon,' cushioning the head forces of the passenger."[57] After an accident, the granules of glass from the inner pane are found in a small pile on the instrument panel.

Roads

Safer automobiles must be matched by better road engineering. Seemingly insignificant matters have assumed new importance. Of twelve thousand motorists questioned on returning from a long trip, "one in three

[56]This section is based on an article by Don Macdonald, "All About Tires," *Westways*, Vol. 61, No. 3 (March 1969), pp. 28, 31, 47.
[57]A press release from the Corning Glass Works Public Relations Department, November 26, 1968.

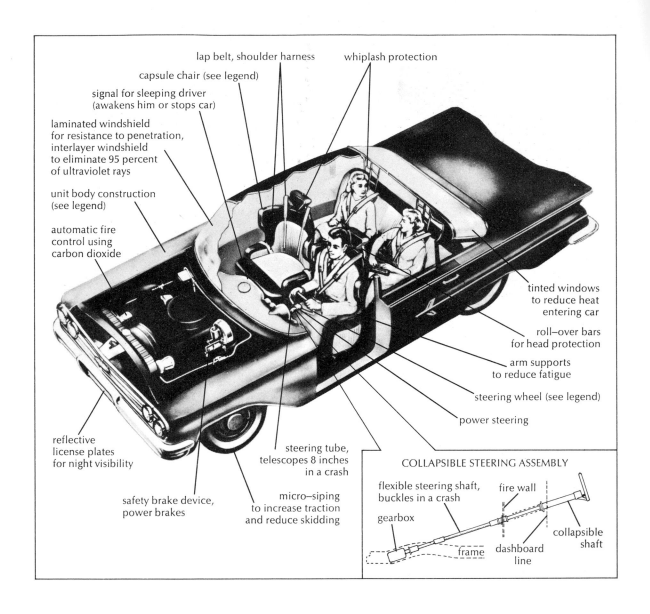

lap belt, shoulder harness

whiplash protection

capsule chair (see legend)

signal for sleeping driver
(awakens him or stops car)

laminated windshield
for resistance to penetration,
interlayer windshield
to eliminate 95 percent
of ultraviolet rays

unit body construction
(see legend)

automatic fire
control using
carbon dioxide

tinted windows
to reduce heat
entering car

roll−over bars
for head protection

arm supports
to reduce fatigue

steering wheel (see legend)

power steering

reflective
license plates
for night visibility

safety brake device,
power brakes

micro−siping
to increase traction
and reduce skidding

steering tube,
telescopes 8 inches
in a crash

COLLAPSIBLE STEERING ASSEMBLY

flexible steering shaft,
buckles in a crash

fire wall

gearbox

frame

dashboard
line

collapsible
shaft

4-9 Designed for safety. Many features of this car, which resulted from research by Liberty Mutual Insurance Company, are now standard in automobiles. The *capsule chair* restrains driver and passengers in a 30-mile-per-hour collision against a 5,000-pound blow and a deceleration force of 30 G's. The *unit body construction* has a high energy absorption factor. It will collapse and ruin the car at the moment of a severe impact but will protect passengers from injury. The *steering wheel* is constructed for improved maneuverability, turning ability, and drive stability. Its rectangular shape prevents breaking or bruising of knee-caps, and its reduced diameter increases driver visibility. Features not shown here include side reflection mirrors for greater driver visibility and a smooth hood over the engine to reduce injury to pedestrians who are hit.

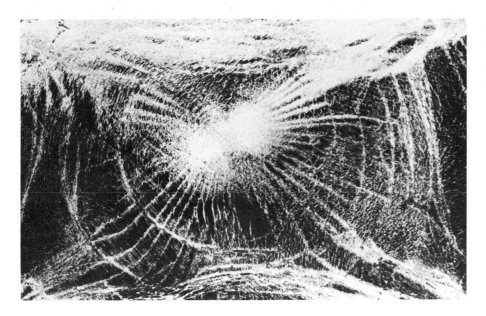

4-10 A safety windshield, which breaks into blunt-edged, nonlacerating granules.

felt he was on the wrong road at least once during the trip and one in every six *had* been.''[58] An uneasy feeling of being lost will hardly add to the sense of security so essential for safe driving.

Small highway improvements are often investments producing big dividends. By a program of such ''spot improvements,'' the County of Los Angeles has made driving safer for its millions of drivers. For example, in wet weather a section of the Hollywood Freeway was noted to be a skidding area. To combat this the pavement was regrooved. The result was almost a 90 percent reduction in accidents. A program in which locations of consistent accidents are studied and improved has spread throughout the state. Redesigned and relocated signs and land markings, adequate roadway widening, the construction of channeling islands— these are but a few of the spot improvements that in ''before and after studies'' have been shown to reduce accident fatalities by 53 percent and injuries by almost 25 percent. In 1969, almost one-fifth of the total California state highway construction budget was designated for such spot improvements.

Ninety-five million automobiles swarm over the highways of this country. Every year that number increases by nine million. One hundred and thirty-five million people are licensed to drive them. There is no dearth of advice on how to increase safety on the roads. One expert states that the fast driving of some women may be attributed to their high heels. ''They increase the leverage on the accelerator,'' he claims, ''when they 'sit up' very close to the wheel in order to avoid scuffing the backs of

Who should not drive?

[58]Slade F. Hulbert and Albert Burg, quoted in "Fighting Death on Wheels," p. 10.

their high heeled shoes."[59] Regardless of specific causes, it is undeniably true that the driving of some people is an accident on its way to happening. They should not drive.

"In Pennsylvania, a motorist was killed when he crashed into a tree. He was totally blind. An eight-year-old boy directed his driving."[60] This is an extreme. But it is also extreme to renew licenses by mail, as do thirty states. Some states require an eye examination only with the first issuance of the driver's license, not for license renewal. Surely this practice reflects an unwarranted optimism in the efficiency of aging vision.

What about drivers who are ill? "Half of the drivers who have heart attacks behind the wheel are unaware of their heart disease until the accident occurs."[61] A group of serious accident risks can and should be medically identified, if only to protect them against themselves. As for alcoholic drivers, a strictly punitive approach has been tried and has failed. What is needed is early identification of such drivers, who should then be given therapy and be denied driving privileges until they are cured.

Help for the wounded

Once an accident has occurred, how quickly does help come? The accident in which the young mother and her twins were killed happened in the open country, seventeen miles from a hospital. Emergency care was not quickly available. Rural areas are poor in emergency services. In an investigation of eight hundred California accidents, it was found that 90 percent of the fatally injured in rural areas died at the crash scene within an hour of the accident.[62] Only 37 percent of those fatally injured in urban areas were dead before they were moved by ambulance. Since rural accident victims often have to be transported twice as far as people injured in cities, more time elapses before they reach the hospital and receive treatment. And the length of time between injury and treatment may be a crucial factor in deciding the victim's fate.

During the First World War, the time lapse between injury and definitive surgical care was twelve to eighteen hours. During the Second World War, it was six to twelve hours. In Korea, only two to four hours elapsed before surgery. In Vietnam, the time has been reduced to one and one-half to two hours. During the Second World War, mortality of the wounded was 4.7 percent; in Korea, 2 percent; in Vietnam the estimate is 1 percent.[63] So, as the time lapse between injury and care is shortened, survival rates increase.

Pity the poor pedestrian

About twenty percent of traffic fatalities are pedestrians. Most are "relatively impaired for the task of walking in the presence of traffic. The

[59]*The New York Times*, March 14, 1965, Sect. L, p. 85.
[60]Joseph Kelner, "Highway Murder," *The New Republic*, Vol. 157 (September 2, 1967), p. 13.
[61]Julian Waller, "High 'Accident' Risk Among Middle-Aged Drivers and Pedestrians," *Geriatrics*, Vol. 21, No. 12 (December 1966), p. 134.
[62]John H. Rosenow and Robert W. Watkins, "What the Doctor Can Do to Cut the Traffic Toll," *Modern Medicine*, Vol. 35, No. 12 (June 5, 1967), p. 50.
[63]Ben Eisman, quoted in John H. Rosenow and Robert W. Watkins, "How Many Traffic Deaths Are Caused by Mistreatment and Mis-design?" *Modern Medicine*, Vol. 35, No. 10 (May 8, 1967), pp. 34–35.

very young and the very old have impairment of judgment and mobility associated with their age."[64] Decreased vision and intoxication also contribute to pedestrian deaths. In a pedestrian-auto collision, the pedestrian is not usually "run over."[65] He is lifted up by the car. It runs under him. His head hits the hood, or, while sprawled on the hood, he travels briefly along with the fast-moving vehicle, striking his head on the windshield and car roof. Cars without sloping hoods inflict more severe head injuries to a pedestrian than those with longer hoods. Similarly, cars with "gingerbread" projections are more injurious. The benefits of better safety design of automobiles are apparent, not only for the driver, but also for the pedestrian.

"Let go thy hold," wisely counsels the Fool in *King Lear,* "when a great wheel runs down a hill, lest it break thy neck with following it," (II.iv.72–74). Good advice, but not for modern motorcyclists. Too often they have no chance to let go. They are jarred loose and thrown.

Motorcycle hazards

There are almost three times as many motorcycle deaths and injuries today as there were in 1960. Experience is of critical importance for safe motorcycle driving. In a British study, Ryan found that drivers with less than six months' experience had a considerably higher accident rate than those with more experience.[66] Training in motorcycle operation is essential. Still another recent study revealed that auto-motorcycle accidents usually occurred when the car turned in front of the motorcycle.[67] (Ryan reports that bicycle-car accidents, on the other hand, seem to occur most often when a cyclist turns in front of a car.) More than half of the motorcycle accident victims sustain head injuries. Not all helmets are adequate. Ryan recommends "that the minimal standards for motorcyclist helmets should be British Standard . . . This provides for an all-enveloping shell, completely lined with energy absorbing material." Protective clothing on the legs and compulsory installation of crash (roll) bars on motorcycles have also been urged.[68]

"Be it ever so humble . . ."

"A child playing on the floor suddenly cries out in pain and immediately jumps to a standing position. Either the child or a nearby adult inspects the painful area and discovers a sewing needle partially penetrating . . .

[64]Julian Waller, "High 'Accident' Risk Among Middle-Aged Drivers and Pedestrians," p. 131.

[65]A tragic exception is the small child run over by a car backing out of a driveway. Every year three hundred children in this country are killed in this way. (National Safety Council, "Children in the Driveway: Family Safety," cited in Harvey Kravitz and Alvin Korach, "Deaths in Suburbia," *Clinical Pediatrics,* Vol. 5, No. 5 [May 1966], p. 266.)

[66]G. Anthony Ryan, "Injuries in Traffic Accidents," pp. 1069–72.

[67]"Motorcycle Accident Deaths Rising Rapidly," *Statistical Bulletin* of the Metropolitan Life Insurance Company, Vol. 48 (April 1967), p. 4.

[68]"Helmets Can Cut the Death Rate in Half," an editorial in *California's Health,* Vol. 25, No. 1 (July 1967), p. 6.

the knee."[69] This is a rare household mishap. But the fact that these writers carefully collected twenty-one cases of needle-in-the-knee does reflect the growing interest by medical people in household accidents.

Of the 28,500 people killed in the home in this country during 1968, just over half were very young (under five) or old (seventy-five or over). Falls account for fully 40 percent of deaths from household accidents, fires and burns for 20 percent.

Falls   The astronaut John Glenn managed to travel out of this world and back again without getting so much as a scratch. It was his crash landing on a bathroom floor that gave him dizzy spells for months. That year, he was one of the 4,300,000 citizens of this nation who were involved in accidents in the home.

In no age group are fatal falls more common than among the elderly. Arthritis, dizziness induced by poor blood supply to the brain, vision impairment—all commonly precipitate falls. Emotional stress or depression may be just as conductive to falling as a misplaced rug or a slippery floor. An elderly retiree may rise in the morning, out of sorts, still vaguely fatigued. He can think of no place to go. Not bothering to tie his shoelaces is but another sign of his discouragement. But if he stumbles down the stairs, he may lose his life. Railings, elastic shoelaces, night lights, luminous paint around light switches—these are among the devices wisely suggested to prevent falls by the elderly.[70]

Toddlers are a special problem. Only slowly do they learn to practice safety. While they are growing up, they must be protected—not frightened—from their normal curiosity. "About 15 children die daily as a result of needless accidents: this is more than die as a result of the five leading diseases combined (cancer, congenital malformations, pneumonia, gastroenteritis, and heart disease)."[71] Between 3 P.M. and 6 P.M. the preschooler is most tired and hungry and is most likely to have an accident. It is also the time when his mother is likely to feel that she is losing the footrace with her runabout child. The use of a babysitter for an hour or two—especially during the extra-busy early after-school hours—is often a surprisingly good investment.

Fire   When Longfellow wrote about a "martyrdom of fire," he was being painfully autobiographical. Years before, his wife had been preparing to seal some locks of their children's hair with wax when her flimsy dress had caught fire. She died. The poet had tried to save her; his face was badly burned in the process. It was probably to hide the scars that he grew his famed full beard.[72] The tragedy that befell him is still common.

[69]Robert H. Ramsey and Floyd G. Goodman, "The Sewing Needle and the Knee," *Journal of the American Medical Association*, Vol. 199, No. 1 (January 2, 1967), p. 23.
[70]Dorothy M. Sharp, "Safety in the Home," *Canadian Journal of Public Health*, Vol. 58, No. 1 (January 1967), p. 23.
[71]"Pediatric Briefs," *Clinical Pediatrics*, Vol. 5, No. 12 (December 1966), p. 12A.
[72]*M.D., Medical Newsmagazine*, Vol. 1, No. 4 (April 1957), pp. 42–43.

In Great Britain, a 1964 law requires all nightdresses for girls under fifteen to be made of flame-retardant materials. Few fire-resistant fabrics are presently used for clothing manufacture in the United States. Every year no fewer than 150,000 people in this country suffer burns because of clothing that catches fire. Thousands more are injured or killed by blazes in bedding or other household furnishings. Most of these terrifying experiences are preventable.

Wool is the most naturally fire-resistant of all fabrics. Cotton, viscose, and rayon burn quickly, but unless they are very sheer they can be made fire-resistant by the addition of chemicals without adverse changes in their texture. The Gemini space astronauts wore space-suits made of high-temperature–resistant nylon, as did all but one of the drivers in the 1966 Indianapolis "500" automobile race.[73] Glass textiles are permanently flame-retardant. Polyester can be made flame-retardant. Fiberglass Beta yarns are sheer and softly fine. They are now used in bedding, draperies, and home furnishings and soon will be added to some clothing. Saran is flame-retardant. Acrylic (which is better known by the trade names Orlon, Acrilan, Creslan, and Zafron) is very flammable. It can be combined with Modacrylic, a flame-retardant fiber. Mixed fibers may be dangerous. Clothing of a combination cotton and synthetic material can be most hazardous. Cotton and rayon support combustion. Some synthetic fibers, when afire, melt into sticky substances which cause grievous burns. Those who purchase play clothes for children should remember that denim burns slowly. Paper garments are best avoided.

Little girls are particularly susceptible to clothing fires because most girls are attracted to such hazards as ruffles, flounces, and bell-type sleeves. Women preferring these styles must exercise special care. Indeed, women's clothing, in standing further out from the body than men's, is more susceptible to catching fire.[74]

In the home, suffocations and poisonings of children occur with tragic frequency. Some children suffocate from regurgitation of food; consequently propping up the baby's bottle and leaving him to eat alone can be dangerous. Plastic bags and small metal objects constitute a distinct hazard. They fit nicely into a toddler's eager mouth and may clog his windpipe.

Suffocations and poisonings

The dimming vision of the elderly is responsible for many medication accidents. Clear labeling of bottles, adequate lighting in the bathroom, and corrected vision can combine to prevent many painful mistakes. But most accidental poisonings happen to children. Every year, in this country, about three hundred youngsters under the age of five die from ingested poisons. More poisonings occur between the ages of eighteen and twenty-four months than during any other six-month age-span. The most commonly ingested chemicals are aspirin, cleaning and polishing agents, and

[73]"Fabrics and Accidental Burns," an editorial in *Clinical Pediatrics,* Vol. 6, No. 8 (August 1967), p. 455.
[74]Manuel Castro, "Torch of Tragedy," *Michigan's Health,* Vol. 55, No. 3 (May–June 1967), pp. 6–9.

pesticides.[75] When rushing a possibly poisoned child to a physician for help, it is important to remember to bring along the poison container. A physician can telephone the nearest poison control center and be provided with immediate information about the poison and its antidote. Such centers exist in all major cities.

Dangerous fun and games

Some sportsmen get their pleasure from daring death. In this country, some thirty thousand people taunt it by racing automobiles. During three years (1964–66), more than a hundred racing drivers were accidentally killed.[76] Skydiving is another daredevil sport that is gaining popularity.

Perhaps a million people skin dive and scuba dive. Those with a history of illness, particularly if it is related to the heart and the lungs, should do neither. The experience of some physicians has led them to also apply this restriction to those with minor colds and moderately high blood pressure. As basic as medical fitness is training; few well-trained divers are ever endangered. The minimum beginning age sould be about seventeen. No diver should ever engage alone in the sport. A "buddy" should always accompany him. An important aspect of skin and scuba diving, rarely considered by amateur divers, is the quality of air. A few fly-by-night operators selling contaminated air can do much harm. The environmental health bureau of the local health department is the best source of advice about air.

In 1968, 7,400 people drowned in this country. Males drown six times as often as females. Moreover many more males than females drown as a result of water transportation accidents. Many studies attest to the estimate that fully "half the people in the United States do not swim well enough to cope with emergencies in water."[77] Nor are near-drowning victims immediately out of danger merely because they return to consciousness. Death from oxygen-shortage may still occur. All near-drowning victims should promptly be hospitalized for further care. Adequate water safety programs are long overdue. Most drownings, however, occur in water not specifically set aside for recreation. The old swimming hole is not as safe as a public beach.

Experienced skiers among this nation's two million skiers know the importance of adequate ski equipment, physical conditioning, and training. Particularly important is the proper adjustment of the boot's release-bindings so that when undue stress occurs the boot will easily release from the ski. Muscles both steer and brake the skier. Their condition is critically important. Preseason exercise programs are valuable, as are

[75] Henry L. Verhulst and John J. Crotty, "Childhood Poisoning Accidents," *Journal of the American Medical Association,* Vol. 203, No. 12 (March 18, 1968), pp. 1049–50.

[76] "Fatalities in Hazardous Sports," *Statistical Bulletin* of the Metropolitan Life Insurance Company, Vol. 48 (May 1967), p. 7.

[77] *Statistical Bulletin* of the Metropolitan Life Insurance Company, Vol. 49 (March 1968), p. 5.

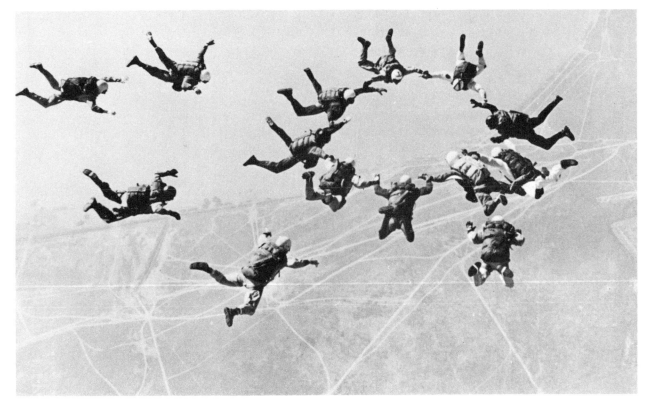

4-11 Skydiving. The goal is to get as many of the skydivers as possible into the circle or "star," and the five skydivers now outside the star are trying to get into it before they are so near the ground that they must pull their ripcords. As of September 1969, the record star consisted of sixteen skydivers.

warm-up periods before starting down a hill. Excessive fatigue should be avoided. Training in equipment use and skiing technique is essential, but such training does not supplant the wisdom of knowing one's limits on the slopes. The ski patrol, a splendid organization of experienced skiers devoted to first aid, should be supported by everyone interested in skiing, the most rapidly growing winter sport.

5

Disease and destiny

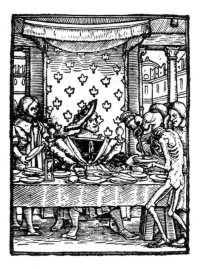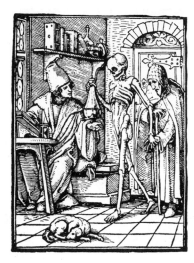

Prologue

ALCIBIADES.   *What is thy name? Is man so hateful to thee,*
That art thyself a man?[1]

Thirteen centuries ago (in 664) the Irish kings of Ulster and Munster called a meeting at Temora. Attending the council were the select lay and clerical leaders of their kingdoms. The problem besetting them was famine. The poor earth could not supply their growing populations. The starving people were unable to work and growing restive. What could be done?

The two kings agreed on a plan of action. Through devout prayer and a fast, a direct appeal was to be made to God. All would participate in these approaches to the Lord. In His infinite mercy, He would surely hear and help them.

Up to this point, there was harmony at the meeting. It was about the content of the prayer to the Lord that disagreement and debate arose. What the kings proposed to ask God for was a pestilence to kill the excess population, composed of "inferior" people. There would then be enough

[1] William Shakespeare, *Timon of Athens*, IV.iii.51–52.

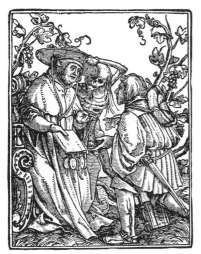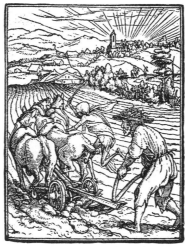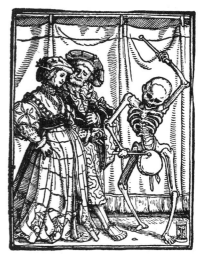

"The Dance of Death" (1538) by Hans Holbein the Younger (1497–1543). The dance of death was a major artistic theme, originating during the plagues and wars of the Middle Ages. Five of Holbein's forty-one woodcuts are reproduced here: "The King," "The Doctor," "The Cardinal," "The Husbandman," and "The Noblewoman."

food for the "superior" and "worthier" survivors. As to who would be included among the survivors, there seemed to be no doubt.

One man dissented. A few others joined him. Would it not be more in keeping with God's way, St. Gerald suggested, to pray, not for pestilence, but for more food? Certainly, it was just as easy. And the chances of being heard by a compassionate God would surely be greater. St. Gerald and his supporters moved to "supplicate the Almighty not to reduce the number of men till it answered the quantity of corn usually produced, but to increase the produce of the land, so that it might satisfy the wants of the people."[2]

But this motion failed to carry. In opposing it, St. Fechin gained favor with the lords and most of the clergy. The motion he supported carried. God was to be implored for a plague to rid the kingdoms of the lesser people.

According to the records of the Church at Mayo, however, God punished this wickedness. A pestilence did indeed visit Ulster and Munster. But it was not so discriminating as some had hoped. The kings and at least one-third of the nobles who had beseeched the Lord for the visitation were carried off by it.

[2] Edward Bascome, *A History of Epidemic Pestilences* (London, 1851), p. 28.

This immorality tale illustrates the grotesque vanity and indifference of those who enslave others. To the Irish tyrants, sickness and death were the expected due of their serfs. Sick societies are never free. Disease makes men susceptible to enslavement. Parents who see their babies die of hunger, who must prostitute their starving daughters for the family bread, who taste the dust of the land, will accept any promise, any hope. Men need to live with purpose and need to die for a purpose. Dead men, the ancient Chinese said, have indeed died in vain if live men refuse to look at them. If men die needlessly of disease, what does it mean to other men? "Am I my brother's keeper?" is an ancient question. In his seventeenth-century *Devotions* (XVII), John Donne replied in this way:

> *No man is an Iland, intire of itselfe; every man is a peece of the Continent, a part of the maine; if a Clod bee washed away by the Sea, Europe is the lesse, as well as if a Mannor of thy friends or of thine owne were; any man's death diminishes me, because I am involved in Mankinde; And therefore never send to know for whom the bell tolls; it tolls for thee.*

Modern leaders do not pray for the sickness and death of their people. A nation's vitality can only come from its people. In this age a nation prostrate with sickness can barely survive. Today, the world is small. The social convulsions of one nation are felt far beyond its borders. Whether in Biafra or Brazil, a sick man is the business of every man everywhere.

The philosopher George Santayana said, "Those who cannot remember the past are condemned to repeat it." That is why this chapter will explore the effect of disease on past events. For the sake of continuity, one major disease has been chosen: plague. Many others could be used as examples—typhus, malaria, smallpox, leprosy, syphilis, cholera. In addition, the effect of individual illness on the course of history will be discussed, with Napoleon serving as the major subject. "God was bored with him," wrote Victor Hugo. But if any one man can be said to have brought agony to his age, it is surely he.

Plague: what is it?

Throughout history, plague has killed an estimated 150 million people. It is primarily an affliction of rats and other rodents such as the squirrel and the chipmunk. In 1894 two men working separately, Shibasaburo Kitasato (a pupil of Koch) and Alexandre Yersin (a student of Pasteur), discovered its causative bacillus. This bacillus causes the several types of plague, of which the two most common are the *bubonic* and *pneumonic*.

Fleas transmit the bacillus of plague, *Pasteurella pestis*, from rat to rat and from rat to man. However, the bacillus may, under certain conditions, be transmitted directly from the respiratory tract of one person to that of another person by airborne droplets. Epidemics of plague pneumonia (pneumonic plague) can thus occur.

A flea takes a blood meal from an infected rodent. Plague bacilli get into its alimentary tract. There they multiply. In feeding on another rat or a human, the infected flea vomits the bacteria into the bite, thus transmitting the disease.

Usually several days after being bitten by an infected flea, the infected person becomes desperately ill. He develops a raging fever. His blood pressure falls. His pulse becomes rapid and irregular. Within hours, the patient is prostrate and incoherent. The pain in his neck, groin, or armpit (or in all three) is excruciating. In any or all of these areas swellings rapidly develop. Soon these swellings, called buboes (bubonic plague), abscess. Upon rupturing they discharge great quantities of pus. Extensive hemorrhages under the skin are common. The skin may become blackish-purple. It is this dread characteristic that gave rise to the medieval designation the "Black Death."

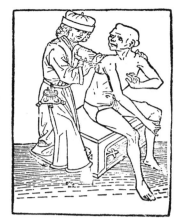

5-1 Lancing a bubo.

Plague and the Middle Ages

Historians disagree about when to date the beginning of the medieval era. Some have set it as early as 200 (the death of Galen). Others choose 800, the year in which Charlemagne was crowned Roman Emperor. But no matter which time is preferred, the whole period was marked by human migration and conflict. And always accompanying these two was epidemic disease.

As early as the fourth century, the migration of the barbarian Teutonic nations precipitated epochal European changes. Traveling westward and south across the line of the Danube and Rhine rivers, the fierce Germanic hordes of the north and far east, held at bay for two centuries, at last successfully poured through the Alpine passes. Storming past the Roman frontiers, they engaged and defeated the degenerate Romulus Augustulus and, in 477, established the first barbarian kingdom (Herulian) of Rome. Although this spelled the end of the Western Empire of Rome, the barbarians wisely preserved much of Roman culture. Indeed, Theodoric the Great, a king of the Goths (who in 494 had established the Ostrogoth Kingdom in Italy), maintained a government fundamentally Roman in character.

In the meantime, the Eastern Roman or Byzantine Empire remained undisturbed. By 527, Justinian had ascended the throne of the Byzantine Empire. It was during his reign that the plague came to Constantinople (now Istanbul). To some health historians this marks the beginning of the medieval period. And, the Middle Ages begin and end with the plague.

The plague of Justinian

The plague of Justinian was bubonic plague. Coming from the hinterlands of southwest Asia, it arrived in Constantinople, the capital of the Byzantine Empire, in about A.D. 532. Spreading west, it soon assaulted all Europe. A remarkable account of the epidemic at Constantinople is left by Procopius of Caesara. Plainly, he saw disease threatening civilization. "During these times," he wrote with horror, "there was a pestilence by which the whole human race came near to being annihilated."[3]

So accurately did Procopius describe the symptoms of plague that there is little doubt as to the disease. Within a few days—at the most five—of the onset of sickness, death occurred. Soon the burial places were exhausted. The dead littered the streets. Instead of being buried, many bodies were collected and piled one on top of the other in unoccupied buildings. The rats infesting these buildings became infected. They carried their infection to the people. In this way the contagion spread. "As a result of this," continued Procopius, "an evil stench pervaded the city and distressed the inhabitants still more and especially whenever the wind blew fresh from the quarters."[4]

The peoples of the greatest city of the Eastern Roman Empire were paralyzed. "The work of every description ceases . . . all the trades were abandoned by the artisans, and all other work as well."[5] How similar this comment is to the report of the modern Peace Corps worker: "They cannot work. They cannot learn. They can't do anything but be sick and die."

In explaining a cause for the calamity, Procopius forsook classical reasoning in favor of the religious fatalism so characteristic of the Dark Ages: "For this calamity is quite impossible either to express in words or to conceive in thought any explanation except indeed to refer it to God."[6]

With these words the intellectual night of the Dark Ages fell upon mankind.

Not until the end of the sixth century did the pandemic (world-wide epidemic) of bubonic plague come to an end.[7] Its effect was immeasurable. Italy was never the same. Roman civil administration ended. The Lombards replaced Roman law and administration with Germanic ideals. With the ascension of Gregory the Great to the papal throne (in 590), the Pontifical State became more powerful. In 565, Justinian died. He was the last and surely the greatest link between the East and the Roman Empire. The Eastern Roman Empire collapsed. Native Byzantines, not Romans, succeeded to power. Greek replaced Latin as the tongue of their rulers. Soon a new faith would find countless followers.

Further east, in Mecca, in 571, Mohammed was born.

The seventh century ushered in a new era. The plague was not the only cause of the death of the old era, but its effect on administrations, plots and plans, campaigns and counter-campaigns, cannot be denied. *Pasteurella pestis* had twisted the course of history.

[3]Procopius of Caesara, *History of the Wars*, Book II, The Persian War, Vols. XXIV and XXIII, tr. by H. E. Dewing (New York, 1914), p. 451.
[4]*Ibid.*, p. 469.
[5]*Ibid.*, p. 471.
[6]*Ibid.*, p. 453.
[7]During this period, even a sneeze was thought to herald certain death from plague. To mark this, there originated in sixth-century Italy the expression "God bless you." (Raymond Crawfurd, *Plague and Pestilence in Literature and Art* [Oxford, Eng., 1914], pp. 93–94.)

The Black Death

In 1333, a drought devastated China. Famine followed, then flood. In Kingsai, at that time the capital of China, some 400,000 people drowned. Deluge, locusts, earthquakes, famine—all followed one upon the other and spread across vast areas of the tormented land. Added to these sufferings was still another affliction—plague.[8] Starting somewhere in Central Asia, the scourge had spread rapidly to China and India. Finally the pestilence came to Europe. This is how.

In 1347, some Genoese merchants were making their way from China back to Europe. It had been a relatively safe seven-thousand-mile business trip. The violent attacks on Europe by Genghis Khan and Batu Khan had ceased the century before. Nevertheless, the merchants, returning with luxury items such as furs and silks, met their ancient enemy—the Tartars. Driven from the town of Tana on the River Don, they barricaded themselves in Caffa, a small fort on the Crimean Straits. There they stayed to resist the Tartar seige. Weeks passed.

One summer day, the Tartars suddenly hurled new weapons of destruction over the city walls. These weapons were the dead bodies of their own men who had died of the plague. This early attempt at bacteriological warfare was successful. The Genoese merchants were terrified. Many fell sick and died. The survivors expected momentary capture. But the besieging Tartars did not attack. They panicked. Hundreds of their men were being killed by the plague. Tartar bodies lay rotting in the sun. The Tartars fled, leaving the small fortress to its misery.

Those Genoese still alive boarded four small ships and set sail for Constantinople—that great meeting place of Asia, Europe, and Africa. Along the route, they saw great ships drifting aimlessly; all on board were dead of plague. In Constantinople the Genoese seeded the plague. The disease raced through Italy and then the rest of Europe.

In the constant competition between men and his parasites, it is the plague bacillus that has come closest to wiping out the human race. Like a wind of death, the disease bereaved the world.

Pope Clement VI (who kept the contagion from him by surrounding himself with two great fires) estimated the world loss of human life during this fourteenth-century pandemic at 43 million. The papal physicians considered the mortality in Europe to be between two-thirds and three-fourths of the population. Men thought the end of the world was at hand. Friar John Clyn, an Irish Franciscan, expecting death, left behind him this touching note (1349):

> So have I reduced these things to writing; and lest the writing
> should perish with the writer, and the work fail together with the
> workman, I leave parchment for continuing the work, if haply any

---

[8]The modern Chinese have repeatedly claimed that United States military planes drop fleas infected with plague bacilli into their country!

*man survive, and any of the race of Adam escape this pestilence
and continue the work which I have commenced.*

Here the sentence trails off. The writer lived to add but two more words:
"magna karistia"—great dearth. Another hand then briefly noted "here it
seems that the author died."[9]

SOCIETAL CHANGES   And so medieval Europe, terrorized by sickness, huddled under the repeated blows of the plague. As in the time of
Justinian, the societal changes were incalculable. To the modern student,
who sees whole populations in developing countries enslaved by disease,
an understanding of these changes is essential.

First, *moral standards* were lowered. The plague had killed many policemen and judges. The courts were always closed. The process of law
was stopped. Amorality became the rule. "Live today, tomorrow, death,"
was a way of existence. Debauchery and drunkeness were everywhere.
Thievery was rampant. For a short time, stolen goods could be obtained
at ridiculously low prices. Luxury items, such as jewelry and furs, were
bought in great quantities by those who had known nothing but grinding
poverty. The mortality resulted in a flooding of the market with a variety
of commodities. The dead left much property. Heirs awoke to find themselves suddenly wealthy. Much of the property was without owners. But
the time of low prices was short-lived. Disastrous *economic changes* followed. The surplus, accumulated as a result of plague deaths, was soon
gone. The death of large numbers of men from the disease reduced the
number of competent hands to do the work. This shortage of labor resulted
in higher prices. The twin economic spectres of diminished production
and soaring prices pushed Europe to the brink of ruin.

The *societal character* of medieval life also changed. The *nouveaux
riches* who were created by the plague did not result only from inheritance
and thievery. New opportunities became legally available and were
eagerly seized. Aristocratic holders of titles had died of the plague, many
of them leaving no heirs. Their lands and titles were dispensed by the
kings to newer favorites. But these new nobles were without tradition.
"The decay in manners in the last half of the fourteenth century is an
astonishing fact. The old fashioned gentility was gone; manners were
uncouth, rude, brutal."[10]

In addition, there were *changes in government and the Church*. Both
were to the detriment of the people. Again, excess death was the cause.
It had taken centuries to develop a competent governing corps with a
tradition of efficiency and service. In a short time, without warning, it
was gone. Positions formerly held by able men were now filled by incom-

[9]Friar John Clyn of the Convent of Friars Minor at Kilkenny, and Thady Dowling, Chancellor of Leighlin,
edited from the manuscripts by R. Butler (Dublin: Irish Archaeological Society, 1849), quoted in Charles
Creighton, *A History of Epidemics in Britain*, 2nd ed., Vol. I (New York, 1965), p. 115.
[10]James Westfall Thompson, "The Aftermath of the Black Death and the Aftermath of the Great War,"
American Journal of Sociology, Vol. 26, No. 7 (January 1921), p. 569.

petents and opportunists. From every quarter rose cries for reform. The Church suffered even more severely than did the government, for the people had already begun to doubt. Had not prayer failed to stop the dying? There are those who hold the view that the Black Death led to such questioning of the authority of the Church that it helped bring on the Reformation and, indeed, the Renaissance.

Remarkable as the effects of the Black Death were upon the economic, social, governmental, and religious structures, the effect on morals was even more astonishing. Insanity swept through Europe.

FLAGELLATION   Whipping, as a religious activity, had been vigorously practiced by the ancient Egyptians, Romans, and Greeks. Every February 15, at the fertility festivals, the ancient Romans flogged their women. Ostensibly, this was to guard them against sterility. In the eleventh century, the Church recognized flogging as a form of penance. During the Black Death of the fourteenth century, it developed into mass mania.

Woe filled Europe. Everywhere were death and suffering. To punish man for his sins God had sent the plague. Man's only salvation lay in doing penance.

In Hungary first, then in Germany, arose the Brotherhood of the Flagellants. In long lines they wove through the cities of Europe. They were robed as if in mourning. Red crosses marked their breasts, backs, and caps. In their hands they clutched triple whips, tied in three or four knots. In each knot were fixed points of iron.

On arriving at a chosen place of penance, the flagellants stripped off all their clothes except for a linen dress that extended from the waist to the ankles. They then lay down in a circle. The position assumed varied according to the sin. The adulterer kept his face to the ground. The murderer lay on his back. The perjurer lay on one side holding up three fingers. They were then castigated by the master. After they had lain on the ground long enough to say five paternosters, they rose and were whipped. All the while they sang psalms and prayed loudly for deliverance from the plague.

So powerful did the Brotherhood of the Flagellants become that they threatened the Church. However, the core of the movement had never been savory. Soon, crime and degeneracy crept in. Strict action by Pope Clement and the Holy Roman Emperor, Charles IV, heavily curtailed this gloomy sect. Not only had they helped spread the plague, they also played a part in spreading throughout Europe its vicious partners—suspicion and hatred.[11]

THE DANCING MANIA   Dancing and death have long been closely related. In primitive societies dances are held to celebrate the death of a tribal member. Dancing was part of the ancient Roman and Greek funeral. In his *Aeneid* Vergil depicted the joy of the dance in the land of the dead. The dance of death was a favorite subject of the medieval artist.

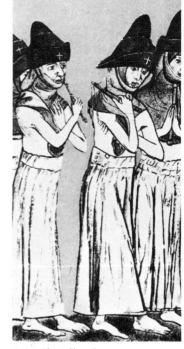

5-2 Flagellants in 1349. The cross on their hats earned these men and their fellow penitents the name Brothers of the Cross.

[11]To this day, there is, among the Indians of New Mexico, a group of flagellants called the Penitentes.

During the height of the Black Death, a dancing mania seized parts of Europe. Particularly in Germany, and to the northwest, strange assemblages of people behaved as if possessed. Holding hands at first, they formed circles. Then they would begin to dance. They danced with wild abandon, deliriously. Finally, exhausted, they collapsed. They lay and groaned as if in agony. This was a signal for swathing them in tight cloths, particularly around their waists. Apparently this relieved them. It is thought that their discomfort was due to the abdominal distension resulting from their exertions.

Sometimes the dancing mania (called the Dance of St. John or St. Vitus) began with a convulsion—with the afflicted falling to the ground and foaming at the mouth. Suddenly springing up, they would then begin to contort wildly.

THE PERSECUTION OF THE JEWS   Among the most grievous consequences of the Black Death was the pitiless persecution of the Jews. Since the Jews of the fourteenth and fifteenth centuries contributed many physicians to southern Europe, the maddened public suspected them of bringing about the plague. Jews were "put to the question." Upon denying that they were poisoning the population, they were put to the rack. Long and detailed confessions were thus obtained. The tortured admitted, finally, that poisons from spiders and owls, some of which were colored red and black, had been provided by rabbis for the express purpose of poisoning the wells. Other poison was smeared on the walls of buildings. Jews were accused of poisoning the very air. Hideous massacres took place. In Basle, Switzerland, all the Jews were enclosed in a wooden building, specially built for that purpose, and burned alive. Elsewhere, the Jews were handed over to the infuriated populace. So it was throughout Europe except in England, where most of the Jews had already been banished from the country. To those few remaining, there was little hostility.

ALAS, ALAS FOR HAMELIN!   The sad legend of the Pied Piper of Hamelin was again brought to life at the time of the Black Death.[12] The incident of the Pied Piper is thought to have occurred in 1284, a year after a violent plague epidemic. But now, over sixty years later, the story was retold again and again. Rats were associated with plague. Some droll piper may, indeed, have appeared at Hamelin so long ago and offered to charm the rats away with his music. He would come again, it was now whispered. And, in those times of lunacy, there is no reason to consider that his offer would have been rejected. Was it not possible that the children would be swept away on the crest of mass hysteria, even as children had joined a Children's Crusade in 1237, and had been lured away by a piper in 1284?

It was a time of mass madness, public whippings, wild dancing. It was a period of debauchery, decay, deprivation, and death. Robert Browning's wistful lines fit too innocently into those terrible times:

[12] James Westfall Thompson, "The Aftermath of the Black Death and the Aftermath of the Great War," p. 571.

All the little boys and girls,
With rosy cheeks and flaxen curls,
And sparkling eyes and teeth like pearls,
Tripping and skipping, ran merrily after
The wonderful music with shouting and laughter.

And now leave the Middle Ages. Enter into the early modern era. For the plague did just this. Like all communicable disease, it knew boundaries of neither nations nor time.

Plague in the early modern era

Plague and the bard of Avon

O, when mine eyes did see Olivia first,
Methought she purged the air of pestilence![13]

"Blessed be God; we live in fear, but we know not whether to flee, for to be better than we be here."[14] With these words ends one of a famous series of letters written in the fifteenth century by members of an English family, the Pastons. The letters describe the constant worry of the people of those times, for plague repeatedly afflicted not only London but the whole of Europe. In the three centuries between the Black Death of the fourteenth century and the Great Plague of London of the seventeenth century, hardly a year went by without the winnowing of the population of some European area by the illness.

As time went on, concepts of sanitation were developed and enforced. Of particular interest was a fine paid, in April 1552, by three good but careless citizens of Stratford-on-Avon. Adrian Quiney, Humfrey Reynolds, and John Shakespeare were fined for creating a new and unauthorized heap of garbage in Henley Street. John Shakespeare, the poet's father, was later to become mayor of the town.[15]

In 1592, strict measures were taken to prevent the spread of plague in London. Upon such regulations William Shakespeare plotted some of *Romeo and Juliet.* The law read, in part: "That in every howse infected, the Master, Mistris, governour, and the whole famulie and residentes therin at the time of such infeccon, shall remayne continuallie without departinge out of the same, and with the doores and windowes . . . shutt."[16]

Such an ordinance was used by the bard to set the tragedy of *Romeo and Juliet.* Friar Laurence tells Juliet (IV.i.93–94):

Take thou this vial, being then in bed,
And this distilled liquor drink thou off.

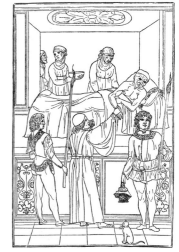

5-3 A 15th-century doctor smelling a pomander (a bag of aromatic substances thought to ward off infection), while examining a dying plague patient.

[13]William Shakespeare, *Twelfth Night,* I.i.19–20.
[14]Quoted in Charles F. Mullett, *The Bubonic Plague and England* (Lexington, Ky., 1956), p. 40.
[15]Charles Creighton, *A History of Epidemics in Britain,* 2nd ed., Vol. I, p. 327.
[16]R. R. Simpson, *Shakespeare and Medicine,* (Baltimore, 1959), p. 208.

The draught is to render her seemingly lifeless. Later she is to waken (IV.i.113–17):

> *In the meantime, against thou shalt awake,*
> *Shall Romeo by my letters know our drift,*
> *And hither shall he come, and he and I*
> *Will watch thy waking, and that very night*
> *Shall Romeo bear thee hence to Mantua.*

But the plot goes wrong. Juliet swallows the draught, and the good Friar Laurence gives a letter to Friar John that is to be delivered to Romeo. But the letter never reaches him because of the plague regulation. The tragedy continues (V.ii.2–16):

> FRIAR LAURENCE. *This same should be the voice of Friar John.*
> *Welcome from Mantua. What says Romeo?*
> *Or if his mind be writ, give me his letter.*
> FRIAR JOHN. *Going to find a barefoot brother out,*
> *One of our order, to associate me*
> *Here in this city visiting the sick,*
> *And finding him, the searchers of the town,*
> *Suspecting that we both were in a house*
> *Where the infectious pestilence did reign,*
> *Sealed up the doors and would not let us forth,*
> *So that my speed to Mantua there was stayed.*
> FRIAR LAURENCE. *Who bare my letter, then, to Romeo?*
> FRIAR JOHN. *I could not send it—here it is again—*
> *Nor get a messenger to bring it thee,*
> *So fearful were they of infection.*

Thus did a plague regulation prevent Romeo from knowing that the unconscious Juliet was really still alive. Thinking she was dead, he killed himself.

Eyam

The year 1664 had been good to the people of the ancient English village of Eyam. The passing of summer had been celebrated by the annual feast on St. Helen's Day. That August Sunday was to be the last happy holiday the villagers were to know for a long time. On that day scores of visitors had been added to the usual population of approximately three hundred. There had been dancing in the alehouses. The men had toasted one another. If anyone knew of the plague raging in London, a hundred and fifty miles away (which was unlikely in so remote a village), it did not dampen the enthusiasm of the celebration. Sheltered in the hollows of the Derbyshire hills, the rural winds of Eyam brought no thought of disease.

After the feast day, village life again became routine. It revolved around the church. The Reverend William Mompesson had recently come there, bringing his twenty-eight-year-old wife and their two children. The villagers respected him and liked his family.

Early in September a box of clothes arrived in Eyam from a London tailor. It was received by a village trader, Edward Cooper. George Vicars, a servant, opened the box. Remarking on the dampness of the tailor's samples, he hung them to the fire to dry.

This happened on the third of September. Three days later Vicars died in a delirium and with plague buboes swelling in his neck and groin. On September 22, Cooper's son was buried. The following day saw the funerals of Mary Thorpe and Sarah Lydall. Then two others died.

October began with two more funerals. That month twenty-two more villagers died. Like a slow stain, first apprehension, then terror spread in the village. "Pest families" were avoided on the street. The plague simmered. In November, only seven died of it. In December, nine. In January 1665, just four died. That month the villagers began to hope. Their hope was short lived. In February, eight died; in March, six. In April, there were nine.

In May, only three died. It was the best month in a long time and the villagers were desperate for some respite. Again there was hope, barely spoken.

But, by the beginning of June, seventy-four of the three hundred and fifty villagers of Eyam had died of the plague. Mrs. Mompesson implored her husband to send their children to Yorkshire. Reluctantly, he agreed. But he would not leave his people and she stayed with him.

It was in June that all the villagers began to think of flight. Some of the wealthiest had already left for other villages or the city. A few others had fled to the neighboring hills. Now the entire population wanted to run away.

At this point, the Reverend Mompesson spoke to his dwindling, stricken flock.

He told them this: In their hands lay the safety of the surrounding villages. Now they surely carried the disease. Spare the others, he implored them. He promised to seek help, to remain with them.

The villagers decided to stay.

An off-limits boundary, marked by stones and hills, was drawn, encircling all the land within half a mile of the village. Beyond this, nobody from Eyam would venture. North of Eyam was a rivulet. Today it is known as "Mompesson's Well" or "Mompesson's Brook." It was one of several places where articles were deposited for the villagers. From nearby villages people delivered provisions and placed them beside the brook and fled. Money for payment was left in the water in the hope of purifying it. On Mompesson's request the Earl of Devonshire also sent provisions.

Towards the end of June, the plague grew worse. Nineteen perished. Yet the living stayed.

July was a month of indescribable suffering. Each family began to bury its own dead or to hire Marshall Howe, who had apparently recovered from the disease and now seemed immune. His pay consisted of the possessions of the deceased. For many years after the plague, parents of Eyam stilled unruly children by threatening to send for Marshall Howe.

In July, fifty-seven were lost. Yet the ordeal was not over. August was an utter desolation. Every thought was of death. Seventy-eight perished. One woman dug graves for her husband and six children. On the twenty-second, Catherine Mompesson, the reverend's wife, died. Towards the end of that harrowing summer month, eighty percent of the village had been killed by the plague. And still they stayed.

At last, by September, the plague began to abate. Only twenty-four perished that month. With the death of fifteen more in October, the plague was finished with Eyam.

Thirty-three of the original three hundred villagers of Eyam were left. (Mompesson did not die. Because he had walked among so much death, he lived to be ostracized by another village.)

What did the people of Eyam accomplish? Two things. First, they demonstrated rare fortitude. Second, they demonstrated the terrible price of medical ignorance.

By isolating themselves with their rats and fleas and bacilli, they condemned themselves. Had they all left Eyam soon after the appearance of the plague, leaving their possessions behind and submitting to isolation until dissemination of the illness was no longer possible, deaths would have been cut by ninety percent.[17] The error was as ancient as the ignorance. When, during the plague of Justinian, more than a thousand years before, the panic-stricken citizens of Constantinople piled their dead into buildings and locked the doors and windows, they guaranteed the spread of the disease.

Even as the villagers of Eyam doomed themselves, so was London, at the same time, shutting up infected people in their houses, thereby spreading the plague.

The Great Plague of London, 1665

> O let it be enough what Thou has done,
> When spotted death ran arm'd through every street.[18]

Of the numerous descriptions of the 1665 Great Plague of London, none are so celebrated as Daniel Defoe's *Journal of the Plague Year* (1722) and the *Diary and Correspondence* of Samuel Pepys.

Defoe, author of *The Surprising Adventures of Robinson Crusoe*, considered his *Journal* sheer history. So masterfully is it written that generations of readers have believed him an eyewitness. He was not, nor is

[17] W. G. Bell, *The Great Plague in London in 1665* (London, 1924), p. 297.
[18] John Dryden, *Annus Mirabilis*, verse 267, line 1065.

his *Journal* a historical document. At the time of the epidemic, Defoe was six years old. His observations were influenced by the Plague of Marseilles (in 1720). He used only one major source for the *Journal:* "Orders Conceived and Published by the Lord Mayor and Alderman of the City of London concerning the Infection of the Plague, 1665." In his reliance on this single source, he erred twice. He assumed that the orders were carried out, and he believed that the orders gave an accurate picture of London activity during the plague year.

A more realistic account of the London plague is provided by the robust English diarist Samuel Pepys. He sallied forth into the midst of the Great Plague of 1665, noting everything, truly touched by nothing. As his fellow Londoners suffered and perished, he worried about his wig. On September 3, 1665, he notes: "And it is a wonder what will be the fashion after the plague is done, as to periwigs, for nobody will dare buy any hair for fear of infection, that it had been cut off the heads of people dead of the plague."

When Pepys first saw two or three plague houses in Drury Lane "marked with a red cross upon the doors" and a notice, "Lord have mercy upon us," he was so distressed he "was forced to buy some roll-tobacco to smell and to chaw, which took away the apprehension."

On September 30, he notes in his diary: "But Lord! What a sad time it is to see no boats upon the river; and grass grows all up and down White Hall Court, and nobody but poor wretches in the streets!"

But in his diary on September 30, 1665, he is in a better frame of mind:

I do end this month with the greatest content, and may say that these last three months, for joy, health, and profit, have been much of the greatest that ever I received all my life in any twelve months, having nothing upon me but the sickliness of the season to mortify me.

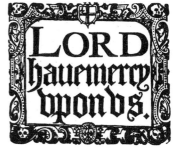

5-4 Heading from a 1636 Death Bill, a list of plague victims and health measures.

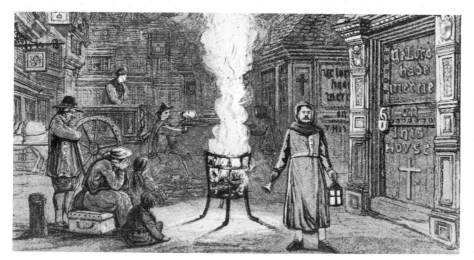

5-5 London during the Great Plague, 1665. Fires were built in the streets; it was thought that the smoke might drive away the plague. Over a century later, such fires were built in the cities of the New World to drive off epidemics.

Pepys ends his review of the tragic desolation of the plague year in his diary cheerfully:

> *Thus ends this year, to my great joy in this manner. I have raised my estate . . . Pray God continue the plague's decrease! For that keeps the court away from the place of business, and so all goes to rack as to public matters, they at a distance not thinking of it.*

How can one account for such destructive epidemics of plague during this time? Poor sanitation and poor personal hygiene combined with overcrowding always promote community infection. Rats seek garbage. The filth of both people and rats provided a fertile soil for pestilence. Both man and animal were the abode of vermin. They, and their surroundings, were unspeakably dirty. People bathed infrequently, if at all. The little available water was needed for drinking and cooking. Among the well-to-do, perfumes were used to mask body odors. Soap was a rare commodity. Seventeenth-century English judges wore wigs to cover their heads, shaved (as with the ancient Greeks) "as far as the louse." Throughout the centuries vermin and rats had continued to multiply appallingly. In 1170 monks recovered the body of the murdered Thomas à Becket to reverently prepare it for burial. As the fathers undressed the body this is what they saw:

> *The dead Archbishop was clothed in an extraordinary accumulation of garments. Outermost there was a large brown mantle; next, a white surplice; underneath this, a fur coat of lambs' wool; then a woolen pelisse; then another woolen pelisse; below this the black cowled robe of the Benedictine order; then a shirt; and finally, next to the body, a tight-fitting suit of coarse hair-cloth covered on the outside with linen, the first of its kind seen in England. The innumerable vermin which had infested the dead prelate were stimulated to such activity by the cold that his hair-cloth, in the words of the chronicler, "boiled over with them like water in a simmering cauldron."*[19]

Rats, it is known, will desert a sinking ship and vermin a cold dead body. This maxim explains, in one sense, how they spread disease.

The surroundings of the early modern era were no cleaner than their inhabitants. Erasmus (1466–1536), the celebrated Dutch scholar, wrote of the medieval English hovel in this way: "The floors are commonly of clay, strewn with rushes, which were occasionally removed, but underneath lies unmolested, an ancient collection of beer, grease, fragments of fish, spittle, the excrement of dogs, cats and everything that was nasty."[20] One can only imagine the filth that accumulated when plague patients were, according to the practice of the times, locked up in their houses.

[19] Sir William MacArthur, quoted in Arthur Swinson, *The History of Public Health* (Exeter, Eng., 1965), p. 19. During the medieval years of the Black Death, human cleanliness was not fostered. In some quarters it was a mortal sin to view one's own body. It became easier to whip it than to wash it.
[20] Quoted in Edward Bascome, *A History of Epidemic Pestilences*, p. 206.

Even the floor of the presence-chamber of Queen Elizabeth was covered with hay. (The Queen, incidentally, in 1564 had a gallows erected in the marketplace of Windsor to hang anyone who came there from plague-ridden London. On pain of hanging, nobody could even bring wares from London.)

Samuel Pepys may have had a good year in 1665, but few other Englishmen could say the same. In this, "the poor man's plague," over a hundred thousand Londoners lost their lives. Nor was the English countryside spared. Entire towns were depopulated or deserted. When plague came to a town, those who could afford it left first. This departure of the rich impoverished the poor even more. The rich had provided jobs. With their absence unemployment spread.

The constant presence of death, always somehow unexpected because it was so quick, sapped the moral strength of the Englishman and drained his vitality. Trade, industry, and agriculture suffered. With the decrease in productive enterprise (which might have bolstered a flagging economy), expenditures on welfare and relief increased. Prices rose. Stores, offices, warehouses, ships—all were without workers. Because those with money feared to risk it, investment was at a low ebb. Although, as Pepys amply shows, English life continued, government administrative routines were either halted or greatly slowed. In times of war, societies plan for better times, meanwhile carrying on societal functions. But during the 1665 London plague, the machinery of society worked erratically. True, the social disorganizations in the wake of the fourteenth-century plague did not now recur. The moral, political, economic, and religious convulsions of the earlier period were not characteristic of Pepys's time. Yet it is apparent that widespread sickness helped change the age and thus the course of human history.

Nonetheless, the plague was an ill wind that blew some good. From the enormous disorder came a degree of order. Dire need caused attention to improving sanitation. Hospitals were constructed. Straw for bedding and floors (in which vermin could breed) fell into disuse. Brick replaced rotting wood for buildings. Because planners could start anew, the Great Fire of London made possible a better organized city. Crowding was diminished. As the eighteenth century approached, England took a long, deep breath of air. *Pasteurella pestis* was gone. But a new plague, air pollution, had replaced the old (Chapter 3).

The tiniest enemies of Napoleon

"What a nuisance an unemployed conqueror can be," complained Thibaudeau, the nineteenth-century French politician. He referred to the restless Bonaparte, the conqueror of Italy. So France decided to send her famous general against England. A direct attack, Napoleon argued, was out of the question. He would attack England through Egypt. By ruining English trade with the Orient, Napoleon would, in due time, make England ripe for his picking.

In less than a month he captured Egypt. Meanwhile, however, Nelson craftily destroyed the French fleet. Napoleon could then neither expect reinforcements from his homeland nor return to it. He decided, therefore, to take Syria, then Constantinople, overthrowing the Turkish Empire. Then he would establish his own kingdom and get home via Austria, subduing it on the way. It was a typically brilliant plan, full of bravado, turning problems into successes, hardly considering the possibility of defeat. It had one flaw. Napoleon was a poor sanitarian. He thought his only enemies were men.

He beseiged the Turks at St. John of Acre, an ancient city near Jerusalem. Opposing him was Phillipeaux, his old schoolmate. The Turks resisted bravely. They were helped by Admiral Sir Sidney Smith who continually supplied them with food. Then Napoleon's rear was lashed by an unexpected enemy—*Pasteurella pestis*. His men fell ill with plague. The resistance of the Turks and the help of Admiral Smith, combined with the ravages of plague, forced Napoleon to abandon the seige of St. John of Acre. It was his first major setback. Years later, he recalled this experience. "A grain of sand stopped me," he mused.

In haste, Napoleon retreated to Joppa (now Jaffa). The sick and dying were everywhere. French soldiers were demoralized. The general saw his dreams shattered by an invisible enemy. He went to the hospitals, walking among the sick, touching the festering buboes, saying quietly, "You see, it is nothing." Apprehensive doctors warned him, worrying lest he too would be infected. "It is my duty," he replied. "I am the general in chief."

5-6 Detail from "Napoleon at the Pest House at Jaffa" (1804) by Antoine Jean Gros (1771–1835).

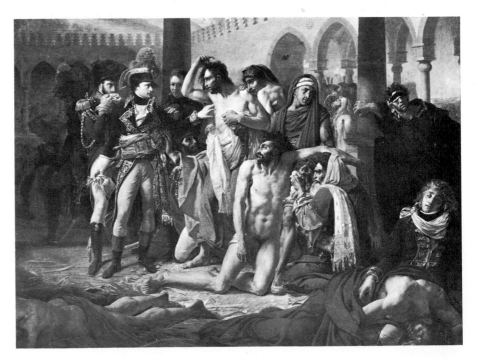

A letter by Comte d'Aure related that Napoleon even helped carry one French soldier, covered with foam and pus, from a doorway to his bed. Napoleon's secretary, Bourrienne, however, denies that Napoleon touched the infected. Indeed, Bourrienne relates a rather different incident. Fearful that plague-infected soldiers would infect the rest, Napoleon, after discussion with his staff, decided to poison the sickest. Considerable research has been done on this story. Apparently, Napoleon did suggest that seven or eight men should be put out of their misery. Napoleon, at St. Helena, defended this on the ground of humanity, but denied wholesale poisoning of soldiers.[21] For the massacre of three thousand Turkish prisoners who were taken at Joppa and who were killed because there was not enough food for them,[22] Napoleon never felt any need to explain.

Up to this point, the effect of plague on the course of history has been considered in relation to the distant past.

Plague in more recent times

In this century, however, one finds that the plague bacillus still abounds in India, Africa, and even in South America. And it still menaces this country. In the United States, as late as 1924, the threat became reality. That year, the same plague bacillus, the same flea, the same rat that combined to produce the epidemics that slew the innocents of Justinian's time, demoralized Europe in the fourteenth and again in the sixteenth century, depopulated little Eyam, and helped stop Napoleon at St. John of Acre, were working together to kill people in Los Angeles, just as they had, around 1900, already killed in Oakland and San Francisco.

The plague infects Los Angeles

As certain diseases—smallpox, poliomyelitis, typhoid fever, diphtheria, and yellow fever, for example—disappear in developed countries such as the United States, increasing numbers of young physicians have only a textbook acquaintance with them. This situation is of some concern to health officers. For, despite every precaution, disease can be imported into this country. Every epidemic starts with a first case infecting an inadequately vaccinated person. That is why only one case of smallpox in this country would make national headlines.

In view of this limiting factor in medical education, one can hardly be critical of the physician who telephoned the communicable disease section of the County of Los Angeles General Hospital on an October day in 1924. He was puzzled and was glad to share his problem with the resident expert in communicable diseases.

On Clara Street, in the Belvedere district of Los Angeles County, he had just examined an extremely sick elderly Mexican-American woman. The patient had a high fever and a severe pain in the back and chest. A young man in the house, as well as other neighborhood people, had

[21]Raymond Crawfurd, *Plague and Pestilence in Literature and Art*, pp. 210–11.
[22]Ralph H. Major, *Fatal Partners, War and Disease* (New York, 1941), p. 112.

similar symptoms. The illness could easily be contagious. Would it not be best to hospitalize the patients and then seek a definite diagnosis? The resident agreed. Ordering an ambulance, he went along to Clara Street to help.

Arriving at the address, the resident found the patient to be feverish. She was coughing and crying. Lying on a couch along the wall was a young man, perhaps thirty, who also seemed to be very sick. Neither patient spoke English. A neighbor offered to act as interpreter.

The young man had been sick all day. First he had had a pain in his chest. Within a few hours he had a backache and a fever. Now there were red spots on his chest.

The old woman had been stricken a few days before the man and in about the same manner. For two days she had been coughing. Now she was breathing heavily and coughing up large amounts of bloody sputum.

As the two patients were being placed into the ambulance, the interpreter asked the hospital resident if he would be willing to look at some other people in the neighborhood who were sick in the same way. In another house, the doctor found a man in bed. He had a high fever and complained of a terrible pain in the back and chest. His young wife, in an adjoining bedroom, had similar symptoms. On a settee in the front room, sat a young girl. She was holding her head in her hands. Her face was flushed, but she insisted that she was not sick. "I'm just tired," she said. "Awfully tired."

Three days later the man was dead and his young wife was dying. The young girl also lay dying in the hospital.

At this time, however, the resident made plans for their immediate hospitalization. Another ambulance would soon come, he told them. He turned to leave. Again the interpreter approached him. He thought the doctor should know that not more than two weeks before the mother and father of the young man who was being taken in the ambulance had died in the hospital. They had been sick the same way as their son now was. Someone had said they had died of pneumonia. Furthermore, the interpreter continued, there were four boys in the neighborhood—relatives of these sick people—who also had this sickness. The doctor went to see the boys and that night they were brought to the hospital. On the following day six more patients were admitted. Each of the six had severe pneumonia. They spat blood. Their skins turned blue. During the first day of hospitalization three died.

An autopsy of one of the patients who had so died was performed. Lung smears showed the presence of the plague bacillus. It was October 31.

On that day a nurse was admitted to the hospital. She had cared for the first patient during his few remaining hours of life in the pneumonia ward. She had plague. The next to be admitted to the hospital was the forty-eight-year-old priest, who had administered the last rites to a boy ill with the plague. He was followed by one of the ambulance drivers. Of the three, only the nurse survived.

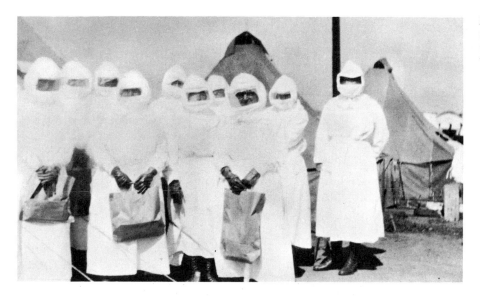

In rapid succession thirty-three people died of the plague. Of the thirty-one people who had pneumonic plague, twenty-nine died; of the six with bubonic plague, four died.

And so, most people who got the plague in Los Angeles that autumn died. It has been seen that plague can become widespread, affecting whole cities, like London, depopulating entire countries, like Italy, sweeping across continents, indeed over the world.

In India, twenty-five years previous to the Los Angeles epidemic, the English were loath at first to admit that plague had come to the country. Such an admission would have hurt the tourist trade. A few years later, San Francisco similarly permitted politics and greed to impede the efforts of health department plague fighters. Los Angeles profited from these costly mistakes.

How was the plague stopped in Los Angeles? Known cases were immediately isolated in the hospital. They were seen only by those who were taking care of them. Seven blocks surrounding the Clara Street address were promptly quarantined. The entire area was roped off. Seventy-five officers were assigned to patrol its boundaries. Until the situation was under control, none of the sixteen hundred persons inside were allowed to leave the area. At one point, some of those quarantined attempted to break through the barriers. Sawed-off shotguns were provided to some of the quarantine guards. The residents stayed. To prevent gatherings of people, the theatre and dance hall were closed. After special instructions, selected health department nurses and inspectors entered the area. Street clothes were not worn. "The nurse has to wear cap, mask, gloves, and gown," ordered the health officer. "Also each nurse will please wear trousers and puttees provided, and high shoes if possible." This last was to protect against contact with rats. Day after day the nurses visited homes

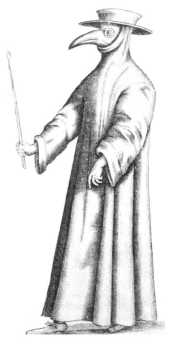

5-8 Physician as a plague fighter in Marseilles, 1720. The beak contained herbs thought to prevent infection.

PLAGUE: WHAT IS IT? **141**

where they knew people had been exposed to see if any of them were sick. Those who were ill were promptly hospitalized. For those who were not, other necessary help was brought. In those days there was no known cure for the plague. It was dangerous work. Still another precaution was instituted. All undertakers were instructed not to embalm the body of a person from the plague-stricken area who had died suddenly or of undetermined causes until the body was examined by a health department physician.

Meanwhile, inside the lines and in the neighboring areas, health department workers were trying to stop the plague from spreading. A house-to-house canvass was begun. All lumber had to be elevated eighteen inches above the ground. Garbage and rubbish were collected and burned. The whole area was subjected to a general cleanup. Rats were killed by the thousands. Many rats were found to be infested with the flea that carries the plague bacillus. A direct attack on the flea was mounted by the use of chemical sprays and lime. Squirrels also carry plague. Three men were constantly occupied in shooting squirrels found in the city limits.

Among most of the quarantined, there was general cooperation. Mr. E. J. Bumiller, a health department sanitarian, reported: "Many of the people complied, even before our men served notices upon them, for they apparently realized the necessity of thorough cooperation." Then the sanitarian added, "I have insisted that my inspectors sell public health and not rely on prosecutions."

What a contrast between Bumiller's approach and Queen Elizabeth's Windsor gallows! And how different from the piling up of the bodies in buildings in ancient times and the sealing of "plague houses" during the days of Skakespeare! The County of Los Angeles Health Department had also "sealed off" an infected area. But the people were not locked in with the infected human cases and other possible carriers of the plague, and a massive campaign to exterminate rodents and fleas was carried on.

To this day the County of Los Angeles Health Department maintains vector control specialists. It is their job to combat the rat. Vigilance buys freedom from plague—and from all communicable disease.

Some other pestilences

> *So, naturalists observe, a flea*
> *Hath smaller fleas that on him prey;*
> *And these have smaller still to bite 'em;*
> *And so proceed ad infinitum.*[23]

This narrative has shown that one disease, plague, played a major role in the drama of human history. Soon after 1665, the disease disappeared from London. During the eighteenth century, it left Europe. It then lashed

[23] Jonathan Swift, "On Poetry, A Rhapsody."

at this continent. Even today, it lurks in the wildlife of the West. In these pages, the broad review of its havoc has surely pointed to the international character of disease and its capacity to affect the course of human events. The rat that carries plague has found its way to every port. It has exerted as great an influence on history as any politician or general.

But plague is not the only pestilence that has affected man's destiny. Today, the defeat of epidemic disease holds great promise for the future of the world's developing nations. So it was with this country. For example, without conquering the mosquito that carried the *yellow fever* virus to man, the Panama Canal could never have been built. This country had been hit early by the disease. In 1793, Philadelphia, at that time the nation's capital, became literally a ghost town because of the illness. Poor advice on how to control epidemics persists and travels long distances. In 1665, during the Great Plague of London, the boys at Eton had been forced to smoke or be whipped. A hundred and twenty-eight years later, cigar smoking was thought by Philadelphians to prevent yellow fever.

In the nineteenth century, *cholera* decimated the armies of the Crimean War, the American Civil War, and the Austro-Prussian War. In his 1866 campaign, Bismarck lost more men from cholera than from war wounds. Recently, cholera attacked Asia and Africa. The masses of India still suffer from this disease, so completely preventable by adequate sanitation.

Many experts believe *typhus* to have been the disease that helped destroy the "glory that was Greece." With the Spartans laying siege to Athens, in 420 B.C., an epidemic attacked the Greeks, the impact of which is described by Thucydides:

> The crowding of the people out of the country into the city aggravated the misery . . . the dead lay as they had died, one upon another, while others hardly alive wallowed in the streets . . . the temples . . . were full of corpses . . . there were . . . forms of lawlessness . . . men who had hitherto concealed what they took pleasure in, now grew bolder . . . and they resolved to enjoy themselves while they could, and to think only of pleasure.

Because of the plague the Athenians could not resist. Nevertheless, the Spartans fled rather than be exposed to the diseased city. However, the Athenians never recovered to again become so elemental a force in world affairs.

So did the ancient Greeks, in those terrible days of the Peloponnesian War, have cause to recall a prophetic verse that had been current among them long before:

> A Dorian war will come and a plague with it.

Whether typhus was or was not the disease that caused the Athenian calamity is not a basic interest of this chapter. What *is* relevant is the effect of an overwhelming disease on the culture of the times. The scales of more than one war have been tipped by typhus—that disease of armies. Soldiers of the past were particularly prone to become victims of typhus. Sanitation was poor; personal hygiene, almost impossible. Crowding was inevitable. The microbe-carrying flea or louse could easily transmit the disease from rat to man. The early sixteenth century saw the beginnings of a long struggle between Francis I of France and Charles V of the Holy Roman Empire. It culminated in a seige by the French at Naples in the spring of 1528. Suddenly typhus broke out among the French troops. A mere handful lived to retreat. Francis and Charles then merely quarreled with one another until, in 1547, Francis died and with him, his ambition to conquer the Holy Roman Empire. Typhus also accompanied the soldiers into the notorious Thirty Years' War. Between 1618 and 1630, it decimated the troops in the area of operations. After 1630, the plague took over to beleaguer these same troops.

Coming and going, Napoleon's armies in Russia were tormented by typhus. During the 1845 potato famine in Ireland, it will be remembered, this disease added to the general misery. But perhaps the most devastating toll that typhus ever took of human life took place in Russia following the Revolution of 1917. Disease has always spread with great population movements. After the revolution, masses of Russians were on the move in search of food. Their sufferings were piteous. In some areas even cannibalism was practiced. From the starving cities streamed the Mechotniki or "sack carriers." They wandered from place to place hoping to find a crust of bread to put in their sacks. Instead they found typhus, and death. They also spread the disease. From 1917 through 1921, an estimated twenty-five million Russians developed typhus fever. Three million died.

In 1910, during a Mexican outbreak of typhus, two American doctors, Dr. Howard T. Ricketts and Dr. Russell Wilder, confirmed the transmission of the disease by the louse. They also described microscopic organisms, much smaller than ordinary bacteria, as a possible cause of the disease. During the outbreak Ricketts died. It remained for Von Prowazek, in Serbia, to identify the organisms as the cause of typhus. In 1915, Von Prowazek, too, died of the disease. The causative microorganism of typhus is named *Rickettsia prowazeki* in honor of these two investigators who died so far one from the other in distance, but not in purpose.

This chapter so far has been dealing with the historic consequences of epidemic diseases. Can individual health problems also affect the course of history?

Individual illness and history

The steward and loyal follower of Joan of Arc testified that Joan never menstruated. Was this indeed true? If so, what relation did this simple physiologic fact (a not infrequent problem in the gynecologist's office) have on her hearing voices to the effect that she was to remain a virgin? And does this help account for her chasing away the women who followed the men of her armies, smiting and actually killing one with her sword?[24] (Upon hearing of Joan's action King Charles is said to have asked, reasonably enough, "Would not a stick have done quite as well?") Did Henry VIII really have syphilis, and did he, indeed, transmit the disease to his various wives? If so, this could have been the reason that some of them were disposed to miscarry or to have stillborn babies. Frantically Henry searched for a wife who could provide him with an heir. When he suspected that a wife would fail him, he divorced or executed her and manipulated still another marriage. His desire to divorce his first wife, Catherine of Aragon, led to his quarrel with the Church and to the establishment of the Anglican faith. Had Peter the Great perished of smallpox, in 1685, would his ambitious sister, Sophia, successfully have taken control of Russia? What effect did the emotional disorder of George III, first noted early in 1765, have on the restrictive English policies towards his angered American colonies?[25] Had Marat's inflamed skin itched less, would he have been more tolerant, and would the cruelties of the French Revolution have been eased, and its bloody course changed? What effect did Robert E. Lee's diarrhea, disabling him for two critical weeks, have on the Civil War? What would have happened to the national economy if the news had leaked out of Grover Cleveland's two highly secret operations for mouth cancer? Had Woodrow Wilson not been crippled during his last presidential years, what would the era following the First World War have been like? It has been written that his stroke was followed by episodes of paranoia.[26] After also suffering terribly from delusions of persecution, the first U.S. Secretary of Defense, James Forrestal, committed suicide in 1949. This may have affected history.

But of all the aches and pains of the powerful, those of Napoleon Bonaparte most intrigue footnote historians. History is a culmination of events; it has many aspects of varying consequence. And the sickly Napoleon Bonaparte lends credence to this concept. Consider the effects of his illnesses on his Russian campaign.

The Battle of Borodino was Napoleon's great opportunity to finally conquer Russia. Not only had a French Grande Armée been collected for the purpose, but also in the Corsican's ranks were unwilling Germans, Italians, Poles, Austrians, Swiss, and Hollanders. They wheeled through Prussia and Poland, a vast conglomeration of men and arms. Pillaging their way past Kovno, Vilna, Vitepsk, Smolensk, and Viasma, they were, within three months, at Borodino, fifty miles from Moscow. Napoleon could taste victory. In all of Europe nobody had a more rapacious appetite for it.

Napoleon at Borodino

[24] It was customary for droves of women to accompany the armies. During the seige of Troy, they were present in great numbers. The armies of Alexander tolerated a considerable female following, as did the Crusaders. These prostitutes frequently numbered into the thousands.

[25] His particular symptoms are today thought to have been associated with a hereditary disease of body chemistry.

[26] Robert E. Kantor and William G. Herron, "Paranoia and High Office," *Mental Hygiene,* Vol. 52, No. 4 (October 1968), pp. 507–11.

At Borodino, on September 5, 1812, the Russian general, Kutusoff, turned to face Bonaparte. Here he would fight it out. He waited for the onslaught. But for two days Napoleon did nothing. Why?

It has been said that Napoleon did not attack either on the fifth or sixth of September because he had a cold. The truth is, he had more than a cold. He suffered from an old ailment, dysuria; he could not pass his urine without great pain. (Some cynics claim that Napoleon's grim expression, as he rode his white steed in Russia, may well have been caused by this factor rather than true concern for his troops.) By the time Napoleon's bladder eased, he had developed a sore throat and was so hoarse that he could not dictate his orders. His hand shook as he was forced to write them.

At Borodino Napoleon failed to destroy the Russian army. Later that army returned to hound him. Some historians lay this failure to his limited ability to make decisions at Borodino. The Russian army escaped to the East. In escaping, it battered the French army with its parting shots and retreated to return at a more opportune time. Always before, Napoleon had based his success on quickly conquering a country and then living off its wealth. Had he not successfully done this in his earlier Italian, German and Austrian invasions? Had he not taken a ragged French army and, by quick victories, rewarded them with the wealth and women of the conquered?

The Russians provided neither him nor his army with these comforts. When the French Emperor and his army entered Moscow, they found a bleak, bitter, and burning capital. Was the course of history changed because Napoleon could not pass his urine? Or because he had a cold?

In his novel *War and Peace*, Tolstoy rejects the notion that Napoleon's illness affected the outcome at Borodino:

If it depended on Napoleon's will . . . to make this or that arrangement, then it is evident that a cold, which had an influence on the manifestations of his will, could have been the cause of Russia's salvation, and that, therefore, the valet who on the 24th forgot to hand Napoleon a pair of water-tight boots was the savior of Russia.

Tolstoy goes on to wisely emphasize the psychological state of the Napoleonic army at Borodino. The "Borodino slaughter of eighty thousand men did not take place by will of Napoleon"—Napoleon only thought this was so. True, Napoleon made the major decisions in choosing to assail rather than to dislodge the Russian army. However, once that decision was made, the mood of his army was such that he could not have rescinded it under any circumstances. Men who must endure a leader's decisions may not long suffer his indecisions. Even if it were true that the discomfort or sickness partly molded his decisions, sickness hardly explains the vast, cataclysmic events that brought the sensitive urinary bladder of the French dictator to the chilled winds of Borodino.

From the Tsar, dislodged to the East, came no word of surrender. In Moscow, Napoleon awaited evidence of peace overtures. None came. He offered an armistice. It was treated with cold contempt. Moscow was a black ruin. Morale was low, and so were supplies. In the streets, the men bickered among themselves or stood silently, longing for home. A Russian winter was coming. On the way to Moscow, typhus had plagued Napoleon's soldiers. Now it broke out with increasing severity. An apocalyptic air hung over them all. There was nothing to do but get out.

On October 19, Napoleon ordered his men to leave Moscow for home. In the long, sad annals of human conflict, there is no more ghastly story than that grim retreat. Men starved and froze. Napoleon's military genius never did encompass a medical corps. He failed to understand the importance of sanitation for an army. Repeatedly his men paid for this. Even the experience at St. John of Acre had taught him little. Now typhus broke out anew. The loss of life was appalling. And, meanwhile, in a sort of hit and run operation, the intact armies of Tsar Alexander kept hitting him, harassing him. With Napoleon trapped in the cold vastness of Russia, time and space became the enemies of the invaders, the allies of the Russians. Disease, hunger, and cold scourged the remnants of the Napoleonic army. The living robbed the dying. There were endless desertions. Men wandered aimlessly about the countryside. Starving, they gnawed on the bones of horses and the frozen roots of plants.

Some ended up in Polish Vilna. Conditions there were unspeakable. The living stumbled over the dead and dying, feebly beseeching help. Gangrene was prevalent. Typhus, and now an epidemic of typhoid, were killing Russian victors and French prisoners alike.

The Tsar came to Vilna. To those men of Russian Poland who had sided with the invaders, he granted an amnesty. Every effort was made to relieve the agony. Hospitals were established. The remnant Napoleonic forces were well treated. It will be remembered that men of several countries served under Napoleon in Russia. The rulers of these countries sent money to help relieve the suffering. Only one man sent nothing—Napoleon.[27]

Napoleon at autopsy

"Look, Doctor," said Napoleon to his physician as he came naked out of his room after an alcohol rub. "Look what lovely arms! What smooth white skin, without a single hair! What rounded breasts! Any beauty would be proud of a bosom like mine."[28]

Joan of Arc had heard voices inspiring her. Her notion was that a virgin would save France. Napoleon needed no visions to inspire his belief in himself as the savior of Europe. Until he was forty, he had been remarkably successful. At that age, however, Napoleon underwent a remarkable physical change. When he should have been at his peak, he was a has-been.

[27] Hereford B. George, *Napoleon's Invasion of Russia* (London, 1899), p. 398.
[28] W. R. Bett, "An Hypothalmic Interpretation of History," *Bulletin of the History of Medicine,* Vol. 27, No. 2 (March–April 1953), pp. 128–32.

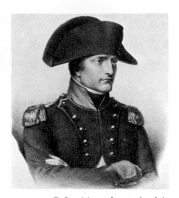

5-9 Napoleon in his early thirties, when he was First Consul of France.

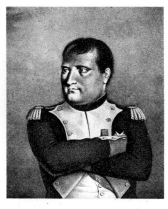

5-10 Napoleon as Emperor, between the ages of thirty-five and forty-five.

As a young man, Napoleon had been thin. His eyes were piercing. He had an eager look. His movements were quick, his manner imperious. Sleep was a waste of precious time.

At forty, he was fat and slow. His eyes were dull, his expression placid. His hair, previously thick, became thin. It was curiously silken. He waddled a trifle. His body developed feminine tendencies. "He has a roundness of figure not of our sex," Count Las Cases once remarked, perhaps nervously. Napoleon began to suffer from an overwhelming need for sleep. The story is told that, at the battle of Leipzig, French soldiers retreating over a bridge, were killed when, through an error, the bridge was blown up too early. Napoleon, it seems, was awakened by the explosion.

On Saturday, May 5, 1821, Napoleon died. On the following afternoon, at 2 P.M., seventeen people, English and French, assembled on St. Helena for the autopsy. The dissection was performed by Dr. Antommarchi, Napoleon's personal physician. Upon removal of the heart and stomach, a wave of sentiment welled up in both General Count Bertrand and General Montholon. They had been part of the Emperor's staff at St. Helena. Now they begged for the heart. The English were not so sentimental. The heart was placed in a silver vessel. As a preservative, some spirits of wine were added. Antommarchi, who had contributed little to Napoleon's health in life, requested the cancerous stomach. In this way he could prove that nobody could have successfully treated the Emperor. The stomach, however, was deposited in another vessel. Both vessels were left in the sealed coffin. In later years, there was to be some disagreement between Dr. Antommarchi and an English doctor, Rutledge, as to who sealed the vessels and, indeed, how. Rutledge claimed to have sealed the vessel containing the heart with a silver shilling bearing the head of George III. Antommarchi heatedly denied this final victory over Napoleon. It might be interesting to have a look.

Scientific shenanigans aside, three separate autopsy reports were made. Part of one, written by the English observer Dr. Henry is singularly revealing:

> *The whole surface of the body was deeply covered with fat . . . the skin was . . . particularly white and delicate as were the hands and arms. Indeed the whole body was slender and effeminate. There was scarcely any hair on the body and that of the head was thin, fine and silky. The pubis much resembled the Mons Veneris in women . . . the shoulders were narrow, the hips wide . . . the penis and testicles were very small, and the whole genital system seemed to exhibit a physical cause for the absence of sexual desire and the chastity which had been stated to have characterized the Deceased.*[29]

So did the colossal Corsican conqueror appear in death.

[29] James Kemble, *Napoleon Immortal: The Medical History and Private Life of Napoleon Bonaparte* (London, 1959), p. 282.

Some think that Napoleon, at about forty, had developed Fröhlich's syndrome or adiposogenital dystrophy. This is a disease of the hypothalamus, a small area at the base of the brain near the origin of the pituitary. Among its many functions is the regulation of the activity of the pituitary gland. It is, thus, intimately involved in growth and reproduction. If Napoleon did indeed have this rather rare disease, it would surely be fair to wonder about its effect on world history. It is, however, important to indulge in such speculations only within their proper perspective.

The great medical historian Sigerist has written:

Concluding thoughts

> History is made by individual human beings, to be sure, and whether they are healthy or sick, sane or insane, makes a difference. Yet the place an individual holds, the power with which he is invested, and the use he is permitted to make of his power are determined by a great variety of factors, by social and economic conditions first of all, but also by hopes and fears, ambitions and frustrations and other psychological factors . . . disease of an individual and even a deadly disease does not alter the course of history. A cause may collapse when the leader dies but not because of his collapse. It collapses only when the forces that carried the leader have lost their momentum. Otherwise, his death may activate the cause, as history has demonstrated more than once.[30]

Tolstoy and Sigerist agree on the relatively limited effect on history of individual sickness. Concerning past events this is indisputable. But it need not apply to the future. Nor did either Tolstoy or Sigerist refer to tomorrow's risks. What can the illness of past leaders teach those who plan for the future?

Leadership is an exhausting ordeal. A Washington correspondent aptly wrote:

> It would be hard to overestimate the physical and nervous tension on the men at the top of this government.
> They are on the go 18 hours a day, and in the President's case, often longer: endless conferences, constant testimony on Capitol Hill, a succession of tedious ceremonial dinners, pressure for more bombing, pressure for less bombing—all this, and a constant drumfire of criticism at home and abroad. The Johnson system here is based on the assumption that men can do whatever they have to do . . . It is a dubious assumption.[31]

Leaders need help and health. It is not only their responsibility but also the obligation of those they lead, to make certain that they have both.

[30] Henry E. Sigerist, *Civilization and Disease* (New York, 1944), pp. 127–28.
[31] James Reston, "A Tired, Tense Administration," quoted in Robert E. Kantor and William G. Herron, "Paranoia and High Office," pp. 507–11.

Epilogue

There is no national science, just as there is no national multiplication table; what is national is no longer science.[32]

Malaria, smallpox, influenza, typhoid fever—these and other enemies of man have killed him and taught him. But have they taught him enough?

The surest safeguard against the spread of communicable disease, whether it be smallpox or Asian influenza, is control of the disease in the country of origin. In the absence of such internal control, a next safeguard is a worldwide communicable disease intelligence program geared to early detection of epidemics—and the attendant possibility of international transmissibility.[33]

This basic statement calls for a degree of international maturity more often seen in health than in other aspects of world politics. It is doubtful that man, by his own efforts, will ever completely eliminate communicable diseases. However, he is slowly conquering and controlling them. Constant vigilance is essential. Nonetheless, one cannot gainsay the virtual disappearance of malaria, smallpox, plague, yellow fever, cholera, and typhus from vast, formerly devastated areas. And the picture will improve. In many areas of the Western world, measles and poliomyelitis are also disappearing diseases. The realization by developing societies that sickness grievously impedes their development—the sure knowledge that a community, riddled by malaria, for example, cannot take its place in the modern world—is a local stimulus for improvement. To those whose societies already benefit from disease control, helping to create such a stimulus in other countries is an opportunity. Those who seek a better world, who seek bridges, not walls, between nations, must understand the paramount necessity of controlling disease. This is the fundamental proposition of this chapter—a proposition whose meaning has been made abundantly clear by history.

The United States, through its Agency for International Development, the Peace Corps, the International Health Division of the Public Health Service, the World Health Organization, and its armed services, is combining with a massive effort by such voluntary agencies as the Ford and Rockefeller Foundations, in making an enormous health contribution to the world's developing areas. Whether it be through a technical health expert in Sierra Leone, or a medic in Vietnam, or a child health project of the Ford Foundation, or a Peace Corps worker in northern Brazil, the contribution is palpable and important. Moreover, the World Health Organization is promoting medical research on an international level.

[32]From *The Personal Papers of Anton Chekhov.*
[33]Lenor S. Goerke, "Preface: Graduate Training for Responsibilities in International Health," in Lenor S. Goerke, ed., *Proceedings of the Los Angeles World Health Conference* (Los Angeles, 1962), pp. 2–3.

Such an effort promises even more than new knowledge about such health enigmas as cancer. From such international undertakings there develops a dialogue between nations that surely promotes understanding and peace between war-weary peoples. Is it too much to hope that the health worker will yet show the way to the greatest health of all—peace?

Disease knows no boundaries. This is a harsh historic experience. Even in wartime, countries have cooperated in health matters. In 1800, France and England were at war. At that time, Jenner's vaccination against small-pox was being tested in England. French doctors wanted to learn about it. Special arrangements were made by the French Foreign Minister, Talleyrand. An English physician came to France, was treated with great regard, and vaccinated French children with English vaccine. Is there better proof of hope for mankind?

Only a short time ago, a group of sixty eastern U.S. college students were asked to list the six largest (in population) cities of America. Only five included Mexico City. It is a long road from such parochialism to a sympathetic knowledge of the customs of other societies, but this kind of knowledge is being acquired. The good international health worker no longer tries to impose his culture on others. He understands that other cultures have developed other ways to handle problems than those to which he is accustomed. Among the Majingaye Saras of the Chad Republic, a boy who behaves badly during his initiation ceremonies to manhood is destroyed: "If he panics and wants to go home to his mother, the others drive a stick into his head."[34] Cruel? To the Westerner, yes. But the entire social structure of the Saras tribe depends on the paternal principle. This is how these particular primitives maintain their social edifice.

To assist those of a more primitive world, to improve their condition, one must first learn to appreciate their social edifice. This is one of the wise principles on which the Peace Corps is based. But there is a paradox in this. One may rightly ask: is my world truly better? Is it really preferable to theirs? Do we not lose by needless heart attacks what we save by penicillin? Whose disease, whose destiny is better? Is it not best to leave them alone?

But no longer can anyone depend on being left alone. One can but work so that each culture will gain, and not suffer, from the others. For although the scientist can distinguish innumerable ecosystems, the world is one all-inclusive ecosystem that is shared by every man.

Failing to learn this, men have failed to learn anything.

[34] Tanneguy de Quénetain in an interview with Robert Jaulin, "What I Learned from My Tribal Initiation in Africa," *Realities,* No. 199 (June 1967), p. 75.

6

Man's smallest enemies: the agents of communicable sickness

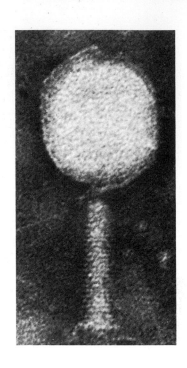

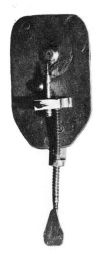

6-1 A three-inch-long Leeuwenhoek microscope (back view). The lens is in the small hole in the circular bulge.

The "little animalcules" of van Leeuwenhoek

"Dear God," wrote Anton van Leeuwenhoek, "what marvels there are in so small a creature!" It was autumn of 1693. The Dutch cloth merchant and microscope maker had achieved a magnification of 270. With growing excitement, he explored a "wee" world, a new ecosystem. Under his lenses he placed his own blood, the saliva of friends, a cow's urine. In his own excrement he found "animalcules a-moving very prettily." Describing his own semen, he cautioned, "What I investigate is only what . . . remains as a residue after conjugal coitus." The first to completely describe red blood cells, to see protozoa and bacteria, the mild Dutchman made a path on which no proper signpost would be placed for another two hundred years. For not until 1870 did Robert Koch prove that bacteria could cause disease. Then, Koch, joined by a host of other investigators (including his unfriendly rival Louis Pasteur), began a great search to find man's tiniest adversaries—disease-causing organisms. Only by identifying the enemy could one destroy it.

A microorganism is a minute, usually microscopic, living organism. When such an organism invades the body, lives off it like a parasite, and

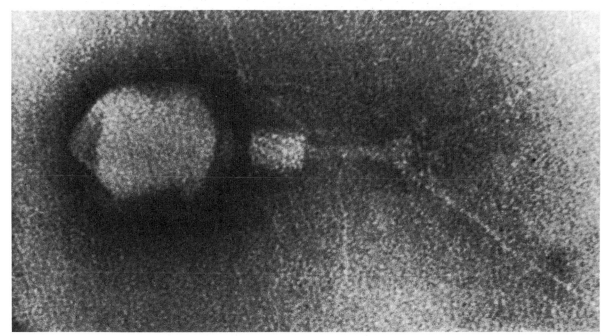

A biotic drama. Left: An "untriggered" T2 virus (×324,000). Within its six-sided head lie coiled its genes—its infective DNA (not shown). The virus' tail is surrounded by a screw-shaped sheath. *Right:* The virus has met with a bacterium (not shown). A bacterial substance caused the sheath to contract, releasing its tail fibers. The "triggered" virus (×340,000) has injected its DNA into the bacterium. (See also Figure 1-3, on page 15, and page 185.)

causes disease, *infection* results. For infection to occur, then, there must be a causative organism (the *parasite*) invading a receptive individual (the *host*) in an ecosystem, or *environment,* in which all interact. Some organisms are more likely to cause disease than others (*virulence*). Some individuals are better able to ward them off (*resistance*). With infection there is active combat between the invading parasite and the host.

When the infection can be transferred from one person to another, it is *communicable.* Some infectious diseases are more communicable than others. For example, regular measles, which is spread via droplets in the air, is much more communicable than a form of leprosy that is usually spread by skin contact. With time, an infectious disease may even lose its ability to be communicable. Untreated, syphilitic infection may persist in the body for years, even a lifetime, silently attacking circulatory and nervous systems. But after the first two years of the initial infection, the period of active communicability is usually over. The microorganism causing the disease does not surface to the skin to be transferred. It remains deep in the body. There is no danger to anyone else.

Not all organisms causing infection are too small to be seen by the naked eye. Some *helminths* (parasitic worms) such as the tapeworm can be seen without a microscope (their eggs, however, are microscopic). The helminths are the largest of the organisms that may enter the body and cause infection. Other organisms, the *ectoparasites,* such as fleas, lice, and mites, may also be easily observed without aids. Smaller than these, and in the order of their decreasing size, are *fungi, protozoa, bacteria, rickettsia,* and *viruses.* These are the *etiological agents* (Greek *aitia,* cause + *ology*); these are the organisms that cause infectious disease.

The variety of etiological agents

Helminths, the parasitic worms, are responsible for a wide variety of world-wide infections, including tapeworm, hookworm, and pinworm.

The mite causing *scabies* (the "itch"), an example of an *ectoparasite,* invades only the outer skin. The male of the species causing this illness is hard to see, but the female is twice as large as the male and she can be seen. The female burrows into the superficial skin to deposit her eggs.

Fungi are plants. They include the *molds* and the *yeasts.* Many of them cause disease. Molds, for example, cause ringworm and athlete's foot. One category of mold, *Penicillium,* produces penicillin. (Another mold, appropriately named *Penicillium roqueforti,* is responsible for Roquefort cheese.) Maladies caused by yeastlike fungi include a lung infection called *valley fever,* and *thrush,* a disease (usually of children) characterized by whitish spots in the mouth. Among the illnesses caused by one-celled *protozoa* are malaria and amebic dysentery.

Bacteria that are rod-shaped are called *bacilli.* Spherical bacteria are *cocci,* and those that are spirals are the *spirilla.* Bacilli cause such illnesses as tuberculosis and diphtheria. The meningococcus and gonococcus, causing meningitis and gonorrhea, respectively, are perhaps the best-known spherical bacteria. The *Spirochaeta pallidum* (*Treponema pallidum*), the bacterium that causes syphilis, is an example of a spirillum. Some bacteria (tetanus bacilli, for example) have the capacity to form spores—protective shells that shield them, for years if necessary, against a hostile environment such as soil. When these bacteria come in contact with a more agreeable ecosystem, such as human tissue, they revert to their active, disease-causing state.

Rickettsia, classified between viruses and bacteria, have characteristics of each. Like viruses, they are found within cells. Unlike viruses, but like bacteria, they are visible under an ordinary microscope. Their discoverer, Howard T. Ricketts (1871–1910), died of typhus fever, a rickettsial disease.

There are some two hundred *viruses* of importance to man. These smallest of all infectious agents cannot multiply outside a cell. They are responsible for a host of man's ailments ranging from the "cold sore" to poliomyelitis.

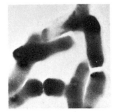

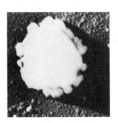

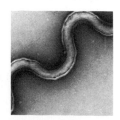

6-2 Bacteria: *Corynebacterium diphtheriae,* a bacillus (*top*); *Neisseria gonorrhoeae,* a coccus (*center*); *Treponema pallidum,* a spirillum (*bottom*).

Because they are the most common causes of communicable disease in this country, the bacterial and viral disease agents will be the major concern of this chapter.

How microbes leave one home and find another

Contagion has this illness widely spread;
And, I feel sure, will further spread it yet. [1]

Microbes have a number of ways of moving from one host to another. The material from an open lesion (perhaps the sore of syphilis or an open staphylococcic skin sore) may be directly transmitted from one person to another. In the nineteenth-century hospital of the Hungarian physician Ignaz Semmelweis, direct contact between the pus-stained hands of doctors (who had just left the autopsy rooms) and mothers laboring in childbirth meant infectious death to many a trusting woman. (Semmelweis' proof that the fatal fevers of these mothers was caused in this manner made him a pioneer in the safer care of mothers.)

Transmission of infection may be indirect. A child with measles coughs. Within the droplets, forcibly expelled from the respiratory tract, swarms the measles virus. The infected droplets hover suspended in the air, wafted about by its currents. Numerous susceptible persons may inhale them. Or, instead of air, some inanimate object may act as the transmitting agent. Examples are a handkerchief (contaminated, perhaps, with the hardy bacillus of tuberculosis) and food (such as milk, in which the typhoid bacillus thrives so well).

The indirect routes of spread may be still more circuitous. A person who has recovered from typhoid fever may continue to harbor its bacillus for a long time. He is, therefore, a "carrier" (see page 181). Occasionally, he excretes the typhoid bacillus in his stool. If he fails to wash his contaminated hands he may contaminate someone else's food. Scores of typhoid fever outbreaks have occurred in this way.

Insects and other animals may carry disease. A person shaking with malaria may infect stray female mosquitoes feeding on his blood. After an interval, the mosquitoes inoculate other people. A rabid animal may inoculate another animal or person by biting him.

The routes by which infection enters and leaves the body and the ways of its transmission are thus numerous and often devious. An outbreak of communicable diseases often has all the elements of a mystery. The public health detective must know that gonorrhea is directly spread through sexual intercourse or that an outbreak of typhoid fever may have

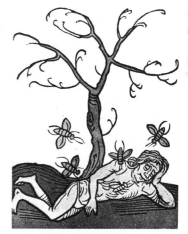

6-3 Mosquitoes and man, from a 15th-century book on natural history.

[1] Juvenal, *Second Satire*, quoted in Heinrich Oppenheimer, *Medical and Allied Topics in Latin Poetry* (London, 1928), p. 78.

been caused by water or food contaminated by human feces; these are critical bits of information that give him his leads to the source of the disease and to their control. By charting the routes of communicable disease a microbial culprit may be found, the linked chain of spread broken, and a new chain of prevention forged.

Body resistance to microbial invasion

Broken skin will admit microbes to start an infection. Intact, the skin is a natural fortress against countless organisms. Nevertheless, hookworm larvae and the spirochete of syphilis may penetrate even the unbroken skin. The intact mucous membrane also resists infection. Yet, the mucous membrane of the respiratory tract may fail to resist and be overcome by the diphtheria bacillus; in the same manner the gonococcus may infect the urogenital system. If the mucous membrane of the mouth, pharynx, stomach, and intestine is intact, the tetanus organism may be swallowed harmlessly. Indeed the human intestine is a common habitat of this organism. It is when the tetanus organism finds an abrasion on the skin or on the mucous membrane of an unimmunized person that this serious disease can occur. Within the intestine, the colon bacillus usually (but not always) lives in ecological balance with man. But should it escape through a ruptured appendix into the abdominal cavity, it would be cause for concern. Saliva has some bacteria-killing power, and stomach acid has even more. So, despite some vulnerability, the body does possess mechanical and other barriers to fight infection.

Should invading microbes penetrate these first lines of defense, the body rushes certain white cells to attack, engulf, and destroy the invader. This white-blood-cell resistance to infection is called *phagocytosis* (Greek *phagein*, to eat + *kytos*, hollow vessel). Malnutrition, fatigue, poor general health (including other infections), anemia—all these promote poor resistance. All favor infection. Even one's anatomy influences the struggle between invading microbe and body resistance. The short, straight Eustachian tube (see page 99) of the child provides an easier route for infection of the middle ear than does the curved and longer tube of the adult.

But these are *nonspecific* aspects of resistance. There is also *specific* resistance, a resistance resulting from the body's exact response to each separate specific invader. This is *immunity*.

Lady Montagu's harsh lesson about immunity in the community

Mary Pierrepont was only eight years old in 1697, but she was already so exquisite that the members of her father's literary club toasted her as the beauty of the year. Forming gracefully into womanhood, she did not disappoint them. A fine fair complexion and great eyes made her a striking English beauty. At twenty she married well, if impulsively, and settled down, as Lady Mary Wortley Montagu, to a life of taste and wit.

Then, at twenty-six, she contracted smallpox. Her long eyelashes were lost forever. Deep angry scars pitted her skin. In a poem, she mourned "my beauty is no more!" Unable to hide her visible wounds, she nevertheless bore her invisible hurt well. She accompanied her husband to his new post as ambassador extraordinary to the distant Turkish port of Constantinople. To a friend, she sent an excited letter. "I am going to tell you a thing that I am sure will make you wish your selfe here," she wrote. "The Small Pox, so fatal and so general amongst us, is here entirely harmless by the invention of ingrafting."[2]

What was "ingrafting"? From the pustular sores of a mild case of smallpox, old Turkish women would collect matter and place it in a walnut shell. They would then visit family parties, often held for smallpox ingrafting. For those seeking to avoid severe smallpox, the operation was simple. With a needle a vein was opened. A small amount of matter was then inserted into the vein. The wound was bound. The ingrafting was complete. In a week, the recipient was sick and feverish. At the inoculation site, running sores developed. On the face about twenty-five pustules appeared. But in about another week, there was complete recovery. There was no scarring. Best of all, resistance or *immunity* to the disease seemed complete.

How did the immunity come about?

Smallpox is caused by a virus (see pages 183–95). Like all microorganisms, the basic chemical substance of viruses is protein. But each specific virus has its own protein chemical structure, its unique arrangement and number of protein building blocks. The arrangement and number of proteins, the chemical genetic formula, of the smallpox virus is different from that of the chickenpox virus, which, in turn, is different from that of the measles virus, and so on. (The principle of genetic difference is true of all life forms.)

The old Turkish ingrafters had inoculated a small amount of smallpox virus protein into people susceptible to the disease. To the body cells of those recipients, that protein was an unacceptable foreigner, an invading stranger. Unchallenged, it would continue to multiply, consume, overwhelm, and finally destroy the host. How could overwhelming invasion by the foreign protein be resisted? By deliberately giving a susceptible individual a mild case of the disease. The Turkish ingrafters did not know why a mild case of smallpox apparently prevented later severe smallpox; all they knew was that it did. (They were not the first to discover the value of this procedure. Thousands of years before, the Chinese had used powdered smallpox scabs as snuff to prevent smallpox.) Those eighteenth-century Turks who were inoculated with the smallpox virus did not even become sick during a smallpox epidemic. Those not inoculated frequently

[2] Quoted in Hubert A. Lechevalier and Morris Solotorovsky, *Three Centuries of Microbiology* (New York, 1965), p. 9.

sickened and died. Why? For several reasons. The matter used by the ingrafters was taken from mild cases. Carried about in nutshells, some of the virus probably weakened in time and some died. So the inoculated dose was doubtless smaller and weaker than that inhaled. Also, local inoculation gave the body precious time to build resistance against the invaders.

But what is the mechanism of resistance? How does mild smallpox infection prevent later smallpox reinfection? There is some relatively recent, still incomplete, information.

Antibodies and their generators

Special body cells accept the challenge of invasion by any foreign protein microbe by producing a protein to neutralize it. This produced protein is called *antibody*. Any substance stimulating these special cells to produce antibody is an *antibody generator* or an *antigen*. In the body, microorganisms are antigens. When a microbial antigen enters the body, the far-flung production centers of the blood's white cells—spleen, bone marrow, lymph nodes—begin to produce specialized *plasma cells*. Stimulated by the uniquely specific antigen, the plasma cell's genetic mechanism instructs it to produce antibody appropriate to the invading antigen and to no other.

So exact in chemical structure are the stimulating antigen and the generated antibody, so specific is one to the other, that their protein building blocks are arranged to exactly fit into one another. They actually have combining sites. Specific antibody molecules "lock into" the very antigen molecules that generated them (and into no other). Plasma cells can produce any one of thousands of different antibodies, each one of which is specifically made to neutralize a specific invading antigen. By what mechanism had the Turkish ingrafters achieved resistance, or immunity, to smallpox? Antibodies that had been generated by the deliberately induced mild smallpox virus infection (the antigen) had "locked into," and thus neutralized smallpox virus antigen that was later inhaled.

But how is this accomplished? What happens when a person who has been previously exposed to antigen and who has already made antibodies to successfully attack it, is reexposed to the same antigen? The first exposure left the individual with immature or *precursor cells,* which, upon stimulation by the second invasion of the antigen, became mature plasma cells. And these, again instructed by their genes, in turn manufacture a second massive number of antibodies to meet the antigenic threat. The precursor cells are called "memory cells" and the entire process is called "immunological memory."

Thus, the early Chinese (and other ancients) had practiced a concept known to the eighteenth-century Turks but learned too late by the scarred Lady Montagu. Its principle: although resistance to smallpox might be gained by accidentally contracting a severe form of the disease, it could also be accomplished by deliberately contracting even a mild form of it. Lady Montagu vowed to import this knowledge to England. Before a group of famed London doctors (one of whom had failed to save her beauty), she had her three-year-old daughter inoculated. After further experimental inoculation of some Newgate prisoners and orphaned children, the royal children were protected. This set a fashion for vaccinating the high-born. Fashion, it turned out, was more helpful to the wealthy minority than to the average Englishman. It was 1721. An epidemic of smallpox raged in England.

A mercy expedition of antigens

Slowly smallpox inoculation grew in popularity. In 1803, Francisco Xavier de Balmis, physician to the Spanish court, set sail from his homeland on a "Vaccination Expedition" to the New World. His orders from the King were to vaccinate from "arm to arm to all that may come, furnishing it free to the poor." He realized that a live agent was necessary to transmit the disease. On board the ship there were doctors and nurses, twenty-two orphaned children, and some material containing dried but live smallpox virus. But who could tell how long the dried stuff would be useful? So every week two children were inoculated with matter taken from the arm sores of children who had been inoculated the previous week. Healthy children were thus used as a living chain to propagate the virus. In this way fresh live virus reached the New World and was used for vaccinations. On April 8, 1806, the provincial governor of Texas at Bexar (now San Antonio) received from de Balmis a "vial with the vaccine fluid and the paper full of scabs of smallpox which accompanied it." In this still lived enough virus to begin the first smallpox vaccination in Texas.[3] Not long afterwards, a Los Angeles physician substituted material taken from sailors instead of children. Much to his dismay, a number of his patients came down with syphilis.[4]

Jenner gives cowpox to prevent smallpox

But several years before the Vaccination Expedition set out on its merciful course, a better way to protect against smallpox had been found. As a teen-age surgeon's assistant, Edward Jenner had heard a milkmaid's memorable answer to the suggestion that she might be developing smallpox. "I cannot take that disease," she said, "for I have had the cowpox." Jenner never forgot that remark, and on May 14, 1796, he vaccinated a small boy, James Phipps, with material from a cowpox pustule taken from the wrist of Sarah Nelms, a milkmaid (see Figure 6-4). Six weeks later Jenner tested the ability of cowpox virus to prevent smallpox virus infection. He deliberately inoculated the boy with matter taken from a smallpox pustule on the body of a patient. The boy had no reaction; he was immune. In the years that followed, Jenner so tested "poor Phipps" (as

[3]The separated scabs of smallpox can remain infectious for years.
[4]Richard Dunlop, *Doctors of the American Frontier* (Garden City, N.Y., 1965), pp. 51, 56.

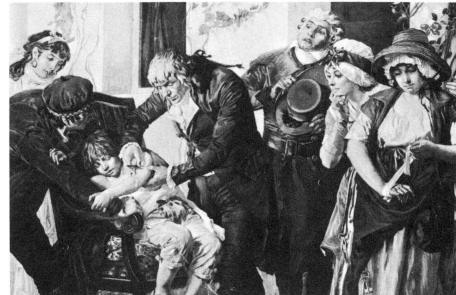

6-4 Jenner vaccinates "poor Phipps," while the milkmaid Sarah Nelms binds her cowpox sores.

6-5 Chambon, a Brooklyn physician, uses his ready source of cowpox virus, while the patients in his parlor wait to be vaccinated.

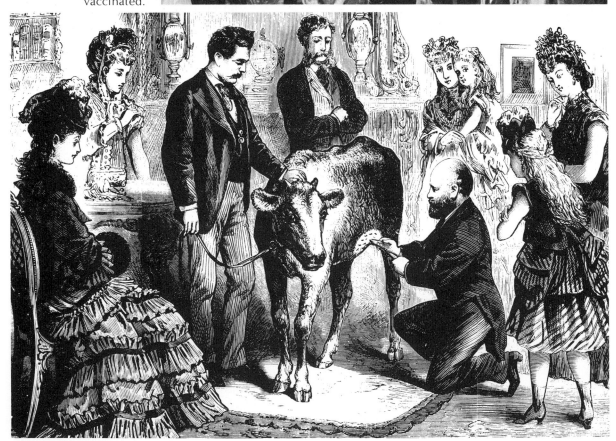

he called him) almost two dozen times. Nothing significant ever happened. The case was proved. Illness from cowpox resulted in prolonged immunity to smallpox. But how is this fact related to smallpox vaccination?

Cowpox is a viral disease of cattle. Smallpox is a viral disease of man. Cowpox virus and smallpox virus are genetic cousins and belong to the same family, the *poxvirus* group. To humanity's good fortune, Jenner found that cowpox could be transmitted to man as an extremely mild infection and that this cowpox infection in humans would prevent infection by the smallpox virus. In the years following Jenner's discovery, the arm-to-arm transmission of (probably weakened) smallpox virus (the method used by de Balmis) was replaced by arm-to-arm transmission of cowpox virus. As this was done, the cowpox virus doubtless became contaminated with smallpox and other viruses. Still it remained wonderfully useful. Today the material used for vaccination against smallpox is *vaccinia* virus (Latin *vacca,* cow), a laboratory-developed virus related to both the smallpox and cowpox viruses. Live vaccinia virus stimulates antibodies in humans that are effective against smallpox virus. Although prolonged, the immunity is not lifelong. The vaccination must be repeated (see Table 6-1).

To summarize: to be immune to smallpox virus antigen, one must have, circulating in the blood, enough antibodies specific to that particular antigen. These antibodies will "lock into" and thus neutralize the specific antigen. In the case of smallpox, a person's antibody production may be stimulated in two ways:

1. *By having the disease.* This may be deliberately accomplished by inoculation with a weakened smallpox virus, the method of the Turkish ingrafters, or it may be achieved by accidental inhalation or ingestion, as occurs in outbreaks of the disease.

2. *By being vaccinated.* The second way of stimulating smallpox antibody is surely the best—that is, by vaccination with the smallpox virus' laboratory-produced first cousin, vaccinia virus. A mild disease prevents a serious one. It is a good bargain. The vaccinia virus vaccine—now routinely used in industrial countries—needs to be still more widely used. Still commonly seen in twenty-seven countries of Africa, Asia, and South America, smallpox is frequently imported into other countries otherwise free of it. Eighty such introductions were reported in the years between 1946 and 1968. Great Britain alone has seen thirty-two of these. Not since 1950 has the United States reported a valid case, but travel poses a constant threat. The best protection is a high level of community immunity.

In 1885, Pasteur developed a rabies virus vaccine. Until the 1930's, the vaccinia and rabies vaccines were the only two virus vaccines in use. The first protective vaccines against smallpox and rabies had been produced without knowledge that a virus was the specific causative agent. Modern scientists are not so handicapped.

TABLE 6-1	Immunization Becomes More Acceptable . . .			
DISEASE	VACCINE TYPE	AGE AT WHICH IMMUNIZATION MAY BEGIN	NUMBER OF BASIC DOSES	BOOSTERS
Smallpox[a]	Viral (vaccinia virus) (infective)	1 year	1 vaccination	On entry into school; then every 10 years. Every 3 years for high-risk groups (nurses, doctors, travelers).
Regular measles (rubeola)	Viral (infective attenuated)	1 year	1 injection (sometimes accompanied by gamma globulin)	None.
German measles (rubella)	Viral (infective attenuated)	1 year	1 injection	Need for booster not established.
Poliomyelitis[a,b]	Viral (infective attenuated—Sabin vaccine)[c]	6 weeks for either	Under age 18: 2 oral doses 6–8 weeks apart; 3rd oral dose 8–12 months after 2nd	One oral dose on entry into school.
	Viral (noninfective, killed—Salk vaccine)		All ages: 3 injections 1 month apart; 4th in 6–12 months	Every 2 to 3 years, as recommended by physician.
Influenza[d]	Viral (noninfective, killed)	Considered at any age with certain chronic debilitating conditions	Adults: 2 doses 6–8 weeks apart Infants: as determined by physician	Yearly, in the fall. Must contain the current strain(s) of the virus.
Mumps	Viral (infective attenuated)	1 year	1 injection	Need for booster not established.
Diphtheria Tetanus Pertussis (whooping cough)	Toxoid Toxoid Bacterial (noninfective) } DTP	6–8 weeks	3 injections 1 month apart; 4th 1 year later	On entry into school. After age 6 booster every 10 years.[e]

[a] Smallpox vaccination and poliomyelitis live attenuated virus vaccine may be given together. All other infective (live) virus vaccines are now separated from one another by one month.

[b] Routine immunization for adults residing in the continental U.S. is usually unnecessary except in epidemic situations.

[c] Many physicians prefer to use the Sabin vaccine only, and at all ages.

[d] Influenza virus vaccine is not routinely given during childhood.

[e] Pertussis vaccine is not included in the booster given after age 6 because of undue reactions. The diphtheria fraction of the booster is, moreover, much lessened in amount.

Source: *Morbidity and Mortality Weekly Report,* Vol. 18, No. 43 (October 25, 1969), in the *Supplement: Collected Recommendations of the Public Health Service Advisory Committee on Immunization Practices.*

No matter how a virus (or any other infectious agent) enters the body, the plasma cells must themselves actively react to the intruder. They must produce their own protective antibody. The body actively produces its own immunity. This process of reacting to the invader is called *active immunity*. The plasma cells do not borrow. Stimulated by the foreign microbial antigen and according to their own genetic instruction, they actively work for and earn their immunity. And, like money that is earned and banked, active immunity lasts a long time.

A vaccine contains living or dead organisms, and it is these organisms that act as antigens to stimulate antibody formation. All vaccine antigens stimulate active immunity. Table 6-1 shows those immunizing agents most commonly used in the United States. With the exception of diphtheria, whooping cough, and tetanus, all the diseases they prevent are caused by viruses. Few benefits of science have so successfully prevented sickness and death as have vaccines. Table 6-2 shows, for selected years, the number of reported cases in the United States of certain previously common communicable illnesses. For all of them, effective vaccines are available. Much progress has been made. More work needs to be done.

Vaccination with live vaccinia virus to prevent smallpox has already been discussed. Now consider the remaining vaccines in common use.

The active immunity of individual effort

TABLE 6-2 . . . *and History Records the Changes*						
Reported cases in the United States of selected diseases preventable by immunization*						
YEAR	SMALLPOX	REGULAR MEASLES	POLIOMYELITIS (ACUTE)	DIPHTHERIA	WHOOPING COUGH (PERTUSSIS)	TETANUS
1945	346	146,013	13,624	18,675	133,792	Figures not available.
1950	39	319,214	33,300	5,796	120,718	486
1955	2†	555,156	28,985	1,984	62,786	462
1960	0	441,703	3,190	918	14,809	368
1965	0	261,904	61	164	6,799	300
1967	0	62,705	40	219	9,718	263
1968	0	22,527	57	186	Figures not available.	159

*Figures include Alaska from 1959, Hawaii from 1960.
†These cases do not fulfill the generally accepted criteria for diagnosis of smallpox.

Sources: For 1945 and 1950, *Weekly Morbidity Report,* Public Health Service, National Office of Vital Statistics, Vol. 2, No. 53 (February 17, 1953). For 1955 and 1960, *Morbidity and Mortality Weekly Report,* Public Health Service, U.S. Department of Health, Education, and Welfare, Vol. 9, No. 53 (October 30, 1961). For 1965 and 1967, *Morbidity and Mortality,* Annual Supplement, Summary, 1967, Vol. 16, No. 53 (November 1968). For 1968, unofficial, hand-tabulated data from *Morbidity and Mortality Weekly Reports.*

The viral vaccines

It has been seen that the injection of a virus, even weakened (attenuated), causes specific antibody production and, consequently, immunity. The injection of dead viruses has the same effect. A weakened virus vaccine causes a mild infection but no significant sickness. A vaccine in which the microbe is killed causes no infection.

TWO VACCINES TO PREVENT POLIOMYELITIS AND ONE AGAINST MUMPS Salk's *killed poliomyelitis virus vaccine* contains virus that, although killed by a chemical (formalin), retains the ability to generate antibodies. Sabin's *attenuated poliomyelitis virus vaccine* contains live poliovirus weakened in the laboratory.[5] So unaccompanied by paralysis or symptoms is the mild poliomyelitis infection it produces, that it is one of mankind's safest vaccines. Although serious permanent complications from mumps are uncommon, the illness does cause considerable discomfort and disability. A safe and effective *attenuated live mumps virus vaccine* is available. It may be administered after one year of age. Children approaching puberty, adolescents, and young adults (especially males) who have never had mumps are particularly benefited.

TWO VACCINES TO PREVENT TWO DIFFERENT KINDS OF MEASLES Two different kinds of measles, caused by distinctly different viruses, are regular measles (*rubeola*) and German measles (*rubella*). By entering the blood stream of a susceptible pregnant woman, the latter can harm the unborn child. The *live attenuated regular measles (rubeola) virus vaccine* is so weakened by laboratory procedures that it can no longer cause significant illness. It does however, cause a relatively minor infection followed by a durable immunity. Vaccination against regular measles has brought about a resistant population in which the virus is not able to survive (see Figure 6-7). Soon regular measles will be relatively rare. Before the vaccine was available, almost everybody had regular measles as a child.

But today a considerable number of pregnant women have not had German measles (rubella). Infection with German measles virus is a serious threat to unborn babies (see page 192). Since late 1969, a safe, effective, *attenuated live German measles virus vaccine* has been generally available. In this country it is not being given to pregnant women for fear that the live virus in the vaccine will harm the unborn child. Whether to give the vaccine to any presumably nonpregnant woman will be decided individually by the family doctor. There is some evidence that it is possible for a vaccinated girl to later be exposed to the virus and unknowingly carry it in her blood (subclinical infection). Only experience and careful evaluation of vaccinated girls will tell if the German measles vaccine will permanently prevent a vaccinated girl from someday giving birth to a child harmed as a result of a subclinical German measles infection. But

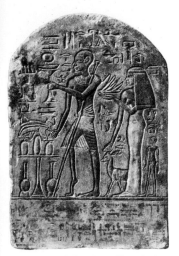

6-6 A polio victim in ancient Egypt.

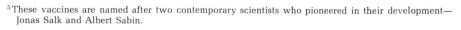

[5]These vaccines are named after two contemporary scientists who pioneered in their development—Jonas Salk and Albert Sabin.

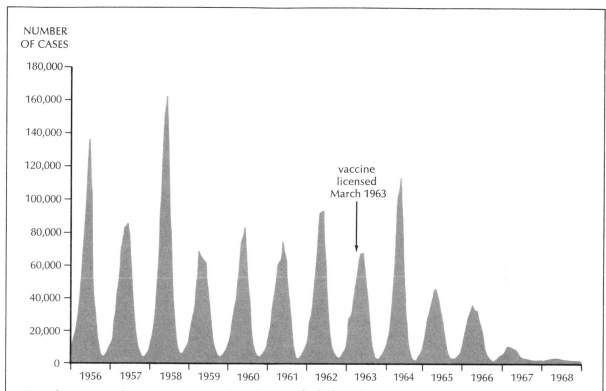

NUMBER OF CASES

Note the recurrent late winter-spring peak each year. The high peak in 1964, occurring after the introduction of the vaccine, reflects an unknown admixture of German measles, which was epidemic at that time.

Source: *Morbidity and Mortality Weekly Reports*, Public Health Service, U.S. Department of Health, Education, and Welfare.

6-7 Regular measles: reported cases in the United States, 1956–68.

it should be emphasized that all susceptible children should be vaccinated against German measles. Only in this way may the pool of virus in a community be diminished and the disease defeated.

THE INFLUENZA VIRUS VACCINE   In this vaccine, as in Salk's, the virus is killed and so cannot cause infection and disease. The killed virus nevertheless retains the ability to stimulate antibody production and, therefore, to produce a resistance. Occasionally people who have received the influenza vaccine injection complain of aftereffects—fever, backache, and sore arm. These mostly result from vaccine impurities not from the killed virus. Improved procedures have produced an influenza vaccine with many fewer side effects.

Influenza virus vaccine presents a special problem. Genetically speaking, the virus does not stand still. Influenza virus contains RNA.[6] From generation to generation, the RNA carries the genetic chemical structure. But,

[6]For a discussion of viral genetics, see pages 183–89.

too often, a mishap occurs. The chemical arrangement of influenzal RNA of a succeeding generation is then not the same as the RNA that preceded it. When this occurs, there is a new influenza virus. The virus antigen has shifted. This *antigenic shift* accounted for an influenza type A0 virus in 1933, an A1 subtype in 1947, and an A2 subtype in 1957. Furthermore, each of these broad groups contains numerous minor genetic changes or shifts. Influenza virus vaccine manufacturers are in a dilemma. An influenza virus vaccine (the antigen) that is effective for one season may change and thus be ineffective for the next.

In mid-July, 1968, an influenza A2 epidemic suddenly broke out in Hong Kong (see page 25). Implacably, the virus continued on to the Philippines. By the end of August, Taipei, Taiwan; Malaysia; and Singapore had been affected. In September came similar reports from Vietnam and Bombay. In that month, at Teheran, one-third of over a thousand delegates to the International Congress on Tropical Medicine and Malaria fell sick with influenza. They had come from all parts of the world to share their information about communicable diseases. In this country, there was growing concern. Why? A mutation had occurred. The antigenic components of the 1968 influenza virus were different from any previous influenza A2 virus (1957, 1961, or 1966). Previous vaccines, containing earlier strains of the influenza A2 virus, were relatively ineffective. A new vaccine was needed. But it takes time to manufacture a new vaccine that meets scrupulous scientific requirements. Feverishly, U.S. drug companies labored to produce enough vaccine. Meanwhile, by sea and air, travelers carried the virus to this country, seeding it in the population. Between the virus and man a race developed. Could sufficient vaccine be made in time to avert an epidemic?

Man lost.

Influenza virus type changes cannot always be incorporated into vaccines in time for an anticipated outbreak. However, medical personnel are kept advised about the effectiveness of vaccines so that they can respond to virus changes with maximum possible speed.

The scientific servants of mankind have good reasons to seek methods of making a better influenza vaccine. An estimated twenty million people throughout the world died of the disease and its complications during the 1918–20 epidemics. In the United States, the 1957 A2 influenza epidemic sent some twenty-two million people to bed. In the winter of 1963, an estimated fifty-seven thousand more deaths occurred in this country than would have been expected in the absence of an influenza epidemic. During a 1967–68 winter influenza epidemic in the United States, excess deaths were reported in all parts of the country except on the West Coast. During such epidemics, those who die are usually the elderly or chronically ill (especially people with heart disease, hypertension, diabetes, and tuberculosis).

TO SUMMARIZE   Viruses, as antigens generating specific antibodies, account for a variety of effective vaccines. Attenuated (weakened) living poliovirus vaccine (Sabin), as well as attenuated living regular measles, German measles, and mumps viruses vaccines, result in mild infection. Thereby, they actively stimulate effective antibody production (active immunity). Vaccinia virus vaccine causes a mild infection in human beings that prevents smallpox. Nonliving viral vaccines (Salk killed poliovirus vaccine and killed influenza virus vaccine) cause no infection, yet retain the ability to stimulate antibody production. Immunity from living viral vaccines is more prolonged than that from the nonliving.

But not all antigens are viral. There are *bacterial antigens,* which may be used to prepare *bacterial vaccines.* Like the viruses in viral vaccines, the bacteria in bacterial vaccines may be weakened or killed in the laboratory. In both cases the ability to stimulate antibodies is retained. There is still another special type of vaccine, which prevents diphtheria and tetanus. This type is made not from the bacterium itself but from the toxic products resulting from bacterial multiplication.

A vaccine of living attenuated bacteria

The BCG[7] vaccine is useful in preventing tuberculosis, but it has found less favor in this country than abroad. Why? Because it causes a positive skin text (*Mantoux test*) for tuberculosis. A positive Mantoux test may mean either active tuberculosis or a former tuberculosis that has healed. In either case, it is a signal that the person has been infected by someone else. The infectious source must be sought, found, and treated. The Mantoux test has great value in finding possible cases and screening suspected sources. But if everyone were given the BCG vaccine, almost everyone would have a positive Mantoux test, and the test would lose its detection value. Still another advantage of the Mantoux test that would be lost is that the test could no longer be used as an indicator for treatment of selected individuals who react positively to it. People without active tuberculosis who show a positive Mantoux test have a markedly greater chance of developing active disease. These risks are much reduced by preventive treatment. Without a way of separating those infected by ordinary routes and those infected by BCG vaccination, a large program of prophylactic therapy against tuberculosis would be impossible (see page 178). Tuberculosis specialists in this country have accomplished as much without widespread BCG vaccination as have specialists in other countries where such vaccination is routine practice. In this country, however, some physicians strongly recommend BCG vaccination, particularly for unduly exposed groups: doctors and nurses,[8] personnel serving in Vietnam and other tropical countries, slum residents, and people who live with a tuberculosis patient.[9]

[7] Bacille (bacillus) Calmette Guérin, named after the French scientists Albert Léon Charles Calmette (1863–1933) and Alphonse François Marie Guérin (1816–95).
[8] "BCG Vaccination," a letter to the editor drafted by W. H. Oatway, Jr., and cosigned by twenty other physicians, in *American Review of Respiratory Disease,* Vol. 96, No. 4 (October 1967), pp. 830–31.
[9] David T. Smith, "Diagnostic and Prognostic Significance of the Quantitative Tuberculin Tests," quoted in *Modern Medicine,* Vol. 36, No. 5 (February 26, 1968), p. 110.

Vaccines of nonliving bacteria

Another way of using bacteria as antigens is to kill them with heat or chemicals. Thus rendered noninfectious yet retaining their ability to stimulate antibodies, they are used as vaccines. The *whooping cough (pertussis)* and *typhoid fever vaccines* are prepared from dead bacterial cells that retain their power to generate antibodies.

On the uses of bacterial poisons

The principle that certain body cells produce a substance to combat poisons is hardly modern. Clearly the idea had occurred to the first-century Roman epic poet Lucan. In writing of the resistance of some Africans to snake poison he says:

> *Them not the serpent's tooth nor poison harms.*
> *Nor do they thus in arts alone excel,*
> *But nature too their blood has tempered well,*
> *And taught with vital force the venom to repel.*[10]

That the repeated injection of small doses of snake venom by bite or by needle into an individual (or an animal) produced immunity to the poison (or *toxin*) was known by Emil A. Von Behring (1854–1917). The venom, or toxin antigen, stimulated the body to produce protective antibody antitoxin. This knowledge helped the German Nobel Prize winner to develop concepts of diphtheria prevention and treatment that have saved generations of children.

As snakes produce poisons, so do some bacteria produce toxins as they multiply. As microbial agents stimulate the body to produce antibodies, so do toxins enter the body as foreign proteins to stimulate plasma cell production of antitoxins. When certain toxin-producing bacteria invade the body, it is not they per se, but rather their toxin liberated into the body tissues as they multiply that causes sickness. The diphtheria bacillus multiplies in the respiratory tract; the bacillus of tetanus in a wound. Locally, each produces a toxin. Carried by the blood, the toxin may affect distant organs. With tetanus the central nervous system is irritated. Fatal diphtheria often results from an affected heart. The toxin is the antibody generator, the antigen. How can it be used to prevent disease?

TOXOID: ACTIVE IMMUNITY FROM MODIFIED TOXIN ANTIGENS Grow the tetanus or diphtheria bacterium on a rich culture medium and it produces toxin. Filter the laboratory culture. The fluid portion passing through the filter contains the toxin. The toxin can do two things: cause sickness and produce antitoxin. How can one reduce the first and conserve the second? Add formalin, which is a 40 percent solution of gaseous formaldehyde. The toxin antigen is modified. Its toxic properties are de-

---

[10]Lucan, *Pharsalia*, quoted in Heinrich Oppenheimer, *Medical and Allied Topics in Latin Poetry*, pp. 285–86.

stroyed, but injected into the body, it can stimulate the production of antibody antitoxin. It is now called *toxoid*. Diphtheria toxoid and tetanus toxoid can be added to killed pertussis (whooping cough) bacterial cells. A triple antigen is produced—the *diphtheria, tetanus,* and *pertussis (DTP) vaccine* (Table 6-1). Injected, it stimulates active immunity against all three diseases.

ANTITOXIN   Inject a small measured amount of diphtheria or tetanus toxin antigen into a horse. Each day, for some days, slowly increase the injected dose of toxin antigen. The horse obligingly responds to the foreign protein toxin antigen by producing antibody antitoxin. The horse produces his own (active) immunity. Bleed the horse. In the laboratory, isolate the antibody antitoxin from the blood. The antibody antitoxin can be used to neutralize toxin antigen—to render it harmless. How?

Circulating in the blood of a child desperately sick with diphtheria or tetanus is the killing toxin antigen specific for the disease. The toxin stimulates the child's cells to produce antitoxin. But the process is too slow. An emergency exists. Antitoxin is needed immediately. Can borrowed horse antibody antitoxin be used to neutralize the toxin antigen? Yes. Injected into the child's vein, the horse antibody antitoxin neutralizes the child's circulating toxin antigen. Used in time, the injection will save the child's life. Horse tetanus antitoxin, once so useful, has been replaced by a human blood product—*tetanus immune globulin—TIG*. Since it is not so foreign, it causes few of the disagreeable and even serious side effects so common with the horse product. The immunity achieved by using another person's or animal's antibodies is called *passive immunity*. What does that term really mean?

Passive immunity is borrowed immunity. Through vaccination or disease, another creature (man or animal) must first earn active immunity—must first be stimulated actively to make his own antibodies. Then that creature is bled. From the blood the actual antibody is obtained. It has been seen that horse blood containing antibody antitoxin can be borrowed to treat diphtheria and tetanus. But sometimes human blood, containing antibodies, can similarly be borrowed. *Gamma globulin* is the part of the human blood that is the antibody.

Human gamma globulin may be used to prevent rubeola and infectious hepatitis. For example, an individual, susceptible to rubeola, is exposed to the disease. Used within six days of the exposure, the injection of enough gamma globulin (somebody else's earned antibodies) will prevent the disease. Another person is exposed to a case of infectious hepatitis. He has shared the same home, the same meals, and may have ingested the virus. An injection of gamma globulin within about a month of the time of exposure may prevent jaundice in the contact. Although the gamma globulin is merely borrowed antibody, it is enough to meet the circulating virus antigen, to "lock into" it, and to render it harmless before visible sickness can occur. Within about two to six weeks, the used bor-

Passive immunity: the temporary resistance provided by borrowed antibody

rowed antibodies are excreted. So borrowed immunity is like borrowed money. It lasts but a short time.

Passive immunity that passes through the placenta, from mother to baby, is also temporary. A newborn will lose his mother's polio antibodies in about six weeks. The mother's measles and mumps antibodies remain with the baby for only a year (or slightly less) after birth. The family physician does not vaccinate a child against polio until he is six weeks old. And he waits until the first year before vaccinating against measles and mumps. Otherwise the mother's antibodies in the child interfere with the injected antigen (vaccine).[11]

Bacterial competitors in the human ecosystem

The venereal diseases   *Historical notes*

"Because the daughters of Zion . . . walk with stretched forth necks and wanton eyes . . . the Lord will smite with a scab the crown of the head . . . and . . . will discover their secret parts," (Isaiah 3:16–17). Long ago, then, the ancient Hebrews considered venereal disease (probably syphilis) a divine punishment for sexual transgression. "Thy bones are hollow," wrote Shakespeare, somewhat piously, many centuries later, "impiety has made a feast of thee." [12] In the bard's bawdy day, the houses of prostitution were located in London's theatre district. Elizabethan plays made frequent mention of syphilis. The "French pox," it was often called. French writers preferred the word "venereal" (Latin *venereus*, pertaining to Venus, the goddess of love). But they were outnumbered. Outside of France, the "Gallic Disease" was perhaps the most common medical reference to the malady.

Syphilis gives still more evidence that microbes know no borders. Two years after Columbus discovered America, Charles VIII of France (1470–98), seeking a Byzantine Empire, invaded Italy and laid siege to Naples. At that time the port city was being defended by Spaniards. Like all armies of that era, the Spanish army was accompanied by a host of harlots. Many of these women, it was thought, had been infected by sailors formerly with Columbus. If the account of the sixteenth-century anatomist Fallopius is to be believed (and it is not by everyone), the Spanish deliberately sent their debauched women to meet the French army. This unmilitary maneuver succeeded. The soldiers of the French army lost no time in meeting the harlots. They caught syphilis.[13]

Too diseased to fight, the French army retreated. In dispersing, they spread their disease throughout Europe. The Italians and Spanish called

[11]Chickenpox and shingles are caused by exactly the same virus and, if given in time, a special gamma globulin (shingles antibodies) can prevent chickenpox in those exposed.
[12]*Measure for Measure*, I.ii.60–61.
[13]Gabriel Fallopius, *On Gallic Disease*, quoted in Herbert Silvette, *The Doctor on the Stage* (Knoxville, Tenn., 1967), p. 196.

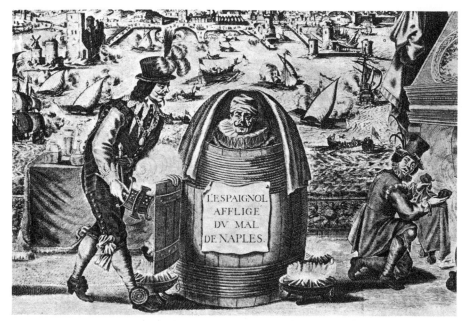

6-8 A Spaniard afflicted with Neapolitan disease: a French satire of 1647.

the affliction the "French disease." To the French, it was, at first, the "Neapolitan disease" (Figure 6-8) and then the "Spanish sickness." The Germans named the malady the "Polish pocks." The Poles retaliated with "German pox." Bitterly remembering the Crusades, the unforgiving Turks called it the "disease of the Christians." To others, it could only be the "Persian fire." Finally, in 1530, an Italian medical man and poet, Girolamo Fracastorius, wrote of a shepherd, Syphilus, who aroused the ire of the sun god by worshiping at an altar of his king. In jealous anger, the sun god sent a plague to earth. Syphilus was its first victim. The disease was thus named, if not claimed.

Often contracted together, syphilis and gonorrhea were, at first, incorrectly thought to be different manifestations of one disease. An eccentric eighteenth-century Scotch surgeon, John Hunter, did not help matters. Deliberately, he infected himself. "Two punctures were made on the penis with a lancet dipped in venereal matter from a gonorrhea."[14] Apparently he got more than he experimented for. Developing both gonorrhea and syphilis, he carefully and wrongly described them as one disease. Another—less heroic—Scotch physician, Benjamin Bell, inoculated his students and learned from them that the diseases were clinically different. In Dublin, William Wallace inoculated healthy patients to prove that the rash of syphilis was contagious.[15] Not until the gonococcus was identified (in 1879) and the *Treponema pallidum* discovered (in 1905) were gonorrhea and syphilis proved to be diseases caused by different microorganisms.

[14]Greer Williams, *Virus Hunters* (New York, 1959), p. 18.
[15]R. S. Morton, *Venereal Diseases* (Harmondsworth, Eng., 1966), p. 21.

TABLE 6-3 *Natural History of Acquired Syphilis*

DISEASE	RESERVOIR FOR AGENT	CAUSATIVE AGENT	INCUBATION PERIOD	MODE OF TRANSMISSION	IMMUNITY
Syphilis	Man	*Treponema pallidum* (a spirochete)	10–90 days, usually 21 days following exposure.	Direct physical contact, usually during sexual relations.	A vaccine to prevent syphilis recently proved successful in rabbits. Hopes are high that a successful vaccine to prevent human syphilis will soon be available.

THE DISEASE PROCESS

Syphilis The first sign of *primary syphilis* is a single, painless lesion or sore called a chancre. Most often it appears at the place where the germs enter the body—the genital area. Sometimes this chancre does not appear or is overlooked, especially in women. If it does appear, it disappears without treatment in about two weeks. In a short time, which may vary from a few weeks to six months, *secondary syphilis* signs appear. The disease is then no longer local. The entire body is infected. Although different people have different symptoms, the most common are lesions, which may be few or many, large or small, and which may appear on various body areas. There may be a widespread rash. This rash, and the chancre that preceded it, teems with spirochetes. Whitish patches in the mouth or throat, "moth eaten" or "patchy" falling hair, low fever, painless swelling of lymph glands, and pain in bones and joints may all be signs of secondary syphilis. While the *primary* and *secondary* manifestations persist, the disease is highly contagious. Lesions in moist body areas, such as the mouth, anus, or genitals are most contagious. Without treatment, the secondary symptoms disappear in less than a month.* The disease then enters a period of *early latency*. The degree of communicability associated with *early latent syphilis* is governed by the recurrence of secondary lesions. Because of such a possibility, the disease is considered communicable for approximately two years following initial infection. The final category, *noncommunicable late latent syphilis,* may eventually cause heart disease, insanity, paralysis, blindness, or death. These end results of untreated syphilis may not take place until ten to thirty years after the primary infection.

*The chancre of primary syphilis and the signs and symptoms of secondary syphilis disappear by themselves without treatment. This accounts for the "success" of the quack. His phony treatments "cure" these signs and symptoms. But the patient is left with the destructive living spirochetes in his body.

Source: Gerald A. Heidbreder, Health Officer, County of Los Angeles Health Department.

The two major venereal diseases

There are five different venereal diseases. In this country, the most important are syphilis and gonorrhea. They are described in Tables 6-3 and 6-4. The other three—chancroid, lymphogranuloma venereum, and granuloma inguinale—are infrequently seen in this country.

TABLE 6-4 *Natural History of Acquired Gonorrhea*

DISEASE	RESERVOIR FOR AGENT	CAUSATIVE AGENT	INCUBATION PERIOD	MODE OF TRANSMISSION	IMMUNITY
Gonorrhea	Man	*Neisseria gonorrheae,* the gonococcus (a bacterium)	Within 5 days (often less) following exposure for 85% of males; 2–8 days for females.	Usually sexual intercourse. Practically never from toilet seats, towels, or other objects.	There is no available immunizing agent (vaccine) against gonorrhea. An attack of the disease does not afford protection against reinfection.

THE DISEASE PROCESS

Gonorrhea is a local disease of the body parts affected. Unlike syphilis, it is usually not a body-wide or systemic disease. In the *male,* the disease manifests itself as a burning on urination and a discharge of pus. The disease is quite painful. Usually, discomfort forces the male patient to seek medical attention. Although not very common, *chronic* male gonorrhea may lead to involvement of other portions of the urinary or generative system and may, if not treated early, produce sterility. In the *female,* the early symptoms of gonorrhea are less pronounced. There may be slight discomfort associated with infrequent urinary symptoms. This rarely motivates the infected female to seek early treatment. Progression of the disease often leads to infection of the Fallopian tubes, ovaries, and lower abdomen. In this event, pain is severe. Due to scarring and closure of the tubes, or to emergency surgery, sterility often results. Rectal infection can occur in both sexes. It is seldom recognized because its symptoms consist only of a sensation of wetness or itching around the anus.

Source: Gerald A. Heidbreder, Health Officer, County of Los Angeles Health Department.

The extent of the V.D. problem today

In 1943, it was demonstrated that a single massive dose of penicillin cured most early syphilis as well as gonorrhea. This led to a de-emphasis of previously energetic venereal disease control programs. When an individual has a venereal disease, it is essential to seek the source of his infection as well as those he may have infected. Such contact tracing, the search for the source and spread of new infections, was no longer considered of paramount importance. Penicillin alone, it was thought, would eventually eliminate venereal disease. That turned out to be a grievous error. For some years there was a downward trend. But by 1959 the downward trend was reversing itself. With renewed effort it was, in the case of syphilis, maintained. However, gonorrhea has been increasing steadily (Table 6-5). Since 1957, in Los Angeles County, for example, the rate of gonorrhea has increased four-and-a-half times as much as the rate of population increase. In 1969, it outnumbered all other reportable diseases combined.

TABLE 6-5 *Syphilis and Gonorrhea*

Reported cases and rates in the United States*

| | SYPHILIS | | | | GONORRHEA | |
| | TOTAL SYPHILIS† | | PRIMARY AND SECONDARY SYPHILIS | | | |
YEAR	Number of cases	Rate (per 100,000 population)	Number of cases	Rate (per 100,000 population)	Number of cases	Rate (per 100,000 population)
1947	372,963	271.7	106,539	75.6	368,020	275.0
1950	229,723	154.2	32,148	21.6	303,992	204.0
1955	122,075	76.0	6,516	4.1	239,787	149.2
1960	120,249	68.0	12,471	7.1	246,697	139.6
1963	128,450	69.3	22,045	11.9	270,076	145.7
1964	118,247	62.9	22,733	12.1	290,603	154.5
1965	112,842	58.7	23,338	12.2	324,925	169.3
1966	105,159	54.5	21,414	11.1	351,738	181.5
1967	103,546	53.2	21,090	10.8	375,606	193.0
1968	98,195	49.9	20,182	10.3	431,380	219.2

*Fiscal year data are shown for all years except 1965 and 1966, which show calendar year data.
†Total syphilis refers to all reported stages of the disease, including late latent and congenital.

Sources: *V.D. Statistical Letter* and *V.D. Branch Annual Reports*, Public Health Service, U.S. Department of Health, Education, and Welfare.

What age group is at greatest risk?

In 1969, more than half the infected cases of venereal disease were reported in persons under twenty-five years of age. "The greatest increase of infections has occurred among boys and girls between 10 and 14 years of age and among teen-agers 15 to 19 years of age."[16] In this respect, Table 6-6 is revealing.

It is abundantly clear that gonorrhea is increasing among Los Angeles teen-agers at twice the rate of other age groups. That this is in part due to changing sexual attitudes of many teen-agers can hardly be questioned. Moreover, both the Los Angeles and San Francisco areas have experienced a migration of essentially transient teen-agers who are alienated from society. Among these young people gonorrhea is epidemic. The

[16] Walter H. Smartt, "Venereal Disease," in Lenor S. Goerke *et al.*, eds., *Mustard's Introduction to Public Health*, 5th ed. (New York, 1968), p. 282.

TABLE 6-6   *Gonorrhea*

Reported case rates for ages 15 to 19 and all other ages
per 100,000 population in Los Angeles County—1959–68

YEAR	15–19 YEARS	ALL OTHER AGES
1959	258.0	144.9
1960	287.0	155.3
1961	347.0	180.2
1962	407.0	196.0
1963	534.0	224.5
1964	523.0	232.1
1965	595.0	248.4
1966	643.0	253.5
1967	808.0	336.8
1968*	1,004.0*	448.5*

*The highest ever recorded in Los Angeles County. By December 1969, special efforts to combat gonorrhea had cut the rate of increase of the disease by almost two-thirds. However, the rate of primary and secondary syphilis had increased more than thirty-four percent compared to a like period in 1968.

Source: Records and Statistics Division, County of Los Angeles Health Department, May 1969.

health departments of both cities have established clinics to try to meet the most pressing problems of these young people, and since early 1969 it has been legal for a California physician to treat the venereal infection of any minor beginning at age twelve without parental consent. Another reason for the rise in reported gonorrhea is improved physician reporting of these infections to the health department. This is essential. The best hope of controlling the epidemic does not lie in merely treating the known case. The infected female reservoir, who usually has few or no symptoms early in the disease, must be found and treated. Otherwise the silent reservoir of infection can only grow. By no means should it be surmised that gonorrhea is increasing only among this teen-age group. Health workers from all the nation's large cities report a rapid rise in the incidence of gonorrhea among all age groups and in all segments of the population.

Syphilis and gonorrhea as a special risk to the female

Both syphilis and gonorrhea are more commonly reported in the male. Although the primary sore, or chancre, of syphilis does not hurt him, he can see it. He can usually see a gonorrheal discharge, and his pain on urination will help drive him to a physician.

The infected female is less fortunate. Unlike the male, she may easily miss a syphilitic infection. Many primary syphilitic chancres are located on the cervix. The cervix has no nerve supply. A painless lesion that is not visible to the patient gives no warning of its presence.

Gonorrheal infection gives the female even less warning than syphilis. Usually the female urinary system is not involved. Severe urinary symptoms, then, are not common. Her infection is most often within the opening of the womb, in the cervix. Without knowing it, she may remain a reservoir of infection for years. An inflammation of one or both Fallopian tubes often ensues. Without treatment sterility may result. Chronically inflamed Fallopian tubes and ovaries are a frequent complication of prolonged, untreated gonorrheal infection. For the exposed female, early examination and treatment are essential. The need for surgery to cure illness due to an old gonorrheal infection is still not uncommon.[17]

Venereal disease infection of children

A child born of a gonorrhea-infected mother, in passing through the cervix and vagina, may pick up the disease. His eyes may become infected. For this reason, forty-seven states make it mandatory to apply either a silver nitrate solution or penicillin ointment to a newborn infant's eyes. After the seventeenth week of pregnancy, a syphilitic mother can infect her unborn child. By that time, the mother's spirochetes can pass through the placenta. But even late in pregnancy, adequate treatment of a mother can prevent syphilitic infection of her unborn child. Several states still lack laws requiring premarital and prenatal blood tests for syphilis.

On helping to find those who need help

People who have a venereal disease almost always got it from someone. And frequently they give it to others. The sick must be immediately and adequately treated. In addition, public protection demands a thorough investigation of the source and spread of every new case. Without active contact tracing, the reservoir of the venereally infected in a community grows; and with it, a spreading sea of chronic sickness and despair. The venereally infected individual who refuses to name his contacts is not being chivalrous. He is refusing information (held, both by law and practice, in absolute confidence) that will spare others endless pain. "Fools alone their ulcered ills conceal," wrote Horace. This ancient thought of the Roman poet might well be applied to modern venereal disease control.

Undetected venereal disease can become epidemic. Both in 1968 and in 1969, to help combat an epidemic of gonorrhea, Los Angeles County government officials wisely allocated a large emergency fund. The reservoir of unfound cases of gonorrhea in the female population was estimated to be at least 35,000. One recent study investigated sixty-nine venereal

---

[17] By no means are all discharges from the penis or vagina gonorrheal. In many male discharges a microbe is not found (*nonspecific* urethritis, or inflammation of the urethra). *Vaginal thrush* is caused by a fungus. It causes a creamy white vaginal discharge and itching. Men with thrush may note irritation at the tip of the penis or under the foreskin. Both conditions may be transmitted sexually. Treatment of both partners is then necessary. There are various causes for sores about the genitalia and anus as well as discharges from these areas. They are not always venereal but should always be promptly investigated and treated.

disease outbreaks eventually involving almost 10,000 people in twenty-eight states. "One man infected with syphilis initiated the ultimate exposure of 274 other persons resulting in 42 additional cases of infectious syphilis within a relatively short period."[18]

It pays to investigate. And to cooperate.

Tuberculosis

"Mounting the stairs made her breathe very quick . . . she coughed troublesomely sometimes." Thus does Emily Brontë describe a character who is soon to die of tuberculosis. Emily's sister Charlotte also knew only too well what she described in *Jane Eyre* as "the sound of a hollow cough." Pitifully, all the Brontës knew tuberculosis intimately. Charlotte, Emily, Anne, Maria, Elizabeth, Bramwell—all six Brontë children died of the disease. Maria and Elizabeth did not even live to teen age.

Tuberculosis infection may involve almost any part of the body but it is far most common in the lung. When the bacillus causing tuberculosis first invades the lung, the inflammation that occurs in that organ is called a primary infection. Within about two to eight weeks from the time of infection, the person will show a positive reaction to the Mantoux (tuberculin) skin test for tuberculosis (see page 167). Many such primary cases of tuberculosis heal without treatment and may never again recur actively. Some, however, do recur. Such *reinfection* tuberculosis may occur under two circumstances. Because of a reduced resistance, an original lesion may break down and thus become activated or the person may be exposed to another dose of bacilli. Even such reinfections may heal without treatment. However, many progress until the lesion breaks into a bronchus (see page 424). It is then that the case of tuberculosis is "open." For with coughing or sneezing, indeed with a forced expulsion of air, myriads of the infecting bacilli escape into the air. The symptoms of early chronic tuberculosis may be so mild as to be hardly noticeable—perhaps no more severe than a cold. Among the more common symptoms are loss of weight, night-sweats, and chronic cough. It is the unknown case of tuberculosis that is the greatest danger both to the affected individual and to his community. Early modern drug treatment heals his tuberculosis lesion rapidly and decreases his cough and the number of bacilli in his sputum so quickly that he soon becomes noncommunicable.

Today, the Mantoux test is a routine part of medical examination of young children. The physician will first do this allergy test when the child is about six months of age. Infection with the bacillus of tuberculosis causes an individual to be allergic to its growth products, *tuberculin*. A positive tuberculin test means that infection has occurred, although the disease may be self-healed and thus not active. Should the child's Mantoux test be negative, it would be regularly repeated. A positive Mantoux test may indicate the need for treatment. For the individual, the

---

[18] The Association of State and Territorial Health Officers, the American Public Health Association, the American Venereal Disease Association, and the American Social Health Association: A Joint Statement, *Today's VD Control Problems*, cited in Walter H. Smartt, "Venereal Disease," p. 290.

TABLE 6-7	*Deaths Due to Tuberculosis in the United States*	
YEAR	DEATH RATE (per 100,000 population)	
1900	194.4	Sources: Adapted from *Historical Statistics of the United States, Colonial Times to 1967,* U.S. Bureau of the Census (1960). Also, *Statistical Abstract of the United States* (1965). Figure for 1967 is from *Morbidity and Mortality,* Annual Supplement, Summary, 1967, Public Health Service, U.S. Department of Health, Education, and Welfare, Vol. 16, No. 53 (November 1968).
1910	153.8	
1920	113.1	
1930	71.1	
1940	45.9	
1950	22.5	
1960	6.1	
1968	3.3	

Mantoux test is a diagnostic tool. For the community, it is a tool for surveillance. Why? If positive it raises a question that the physician and health department must seek to answer: where did the child get the infection? To find and treat the case, to find and treat the source, to seek out all possible close contacts, and thus prevent further spread—these are among the essential concepts of tuberculosis control (see BCG vaccine, page 167).

In the past few years the Mantoux test has taken on added importance. In this country, more than twenty-five million people are Mantoux positive. The vast majority of them do not have active tuberculosis. They have been infected and presumably have recovered from the disease. Nevertheless, recent studies prove that every positive reactor has a greatly increased risk of developing active tuberculosis. Ideally, everyone with a markedly positive Mantoux test should take the preventive drug isoniazid. The tablets would be taken daily for a year. People who take them must have regular check-ups to make certain that they do not react adversely to the drug, although such reactions are rare. To provide isoniazid tablets to all positive tuberculin reactors is beyond the resources of health departments. Therefore, priorities have been established. These are largely based on the relative risk of developing tuberculosis and infecting others. Both family physicians and local health officers closely cooperate in selecting priorities for preventive treatment. [19]

In these ways repetitions of the Brontë tragedy can be avoided. At the turn of this century the U.S. death rate from tuberculosis was 194.4 per 100,000 population. By 1968, it had decreased to 3.3 (see Table 6-7). Slowly, tuberculosis has diminished remarkably in this nation. Other countries

[19] Gordon M. Meade, "Chemoprophylaxis of Tuberculosis," *GP*, Vol. 38, No. 3 (September 1968), pp. 113–19.

are less fortunate. World-wide, it is estimated that more than one hundred million people harbor, and are spreading, virulent tuberculosis bacilli. Every year, between two and five million of the world's people die of the disease. "Tuberculosis is a disease of poverty," Robert Koch had said. The discoverer of the tuberculosis bacillus, he knew that wherever there was the stress of grinding poverty, of malnutrition, and of overcrowding, there people perished in great numbers from tuberculosis.

Antituberculosis tools are available—drugs, such as isoniazid and streptomycin, tuberculin tests, X-rays, BCG, programs of treatments, and prophylaxis, and methods of case finding. These, plus constant effort and, above all, a better standard of living, will someday bring mankind relative freedom from "the white plague."

A streptococcus attacks the U.S. Air Force Academy

Sickness from food contamination

Never before had physicians at the hospital clinic of the U.S. Air Force Academy seen anything like it. April 28, 1968, was a Sunday. On this one relatively free day cadets rarely came to the clinic complaining of illness. This Sunday over 600 cadets did just that. Their throats were sore. Their fevers were high. Many complained of severe dizziness and weakness. Most had a splitting headache. Later that evening 360 more cadets were treated in the dormitories. Within the next thirty-six hours, 76 required admission to the hospital. In the gymnasium an emergency hospital was soon set up for 28 others. During the epidemic, about 1,200 cadets became ill and 111 required hospitalization. The sick were treated with an antibiotic. Although over 2,000 cadets did not report sick, they were, nonetheless, given a preventive antibiotic. Within eighteen hours, preliminary tests from throat swabs showed the presence of virulent streptococci in more than half the tested cadets. On the following day came confirmatory laboratory results.

The explosive outbreak pointed to a single source—a noon meal consumed the previous Friday. Why was this meal suspected?

1. The time between the ingestion of the suspect noon meal (the exposure) and the onset of symptoms fitted the type of strep infection with which the cadets were afflicted.

2. Of twenty-eight visitors and Air Force personnel who shared only the moon meal with the cadets, nine became ill.

3. In a separate dining area, eight of twenty-three civilian employees ate the same meal as the cadets. All eight became ill.

4. A flight-training class of sixty-one cadets provided another piece of critical evidence. They had not partaken of the noon meal. Within the time period from exposure to illness of the others, not one of them became ill. Five of them did get sick but not until they had well passed the incubation period of the others. It was reasonable to assume that they had contracted their infection, not from the noon meal, but from fellow cadets. So the microbes had been spread in two ways—first by food, and then

TABLE 6-8	Two Ingredients of Illness: Staphylococcus and Salmonella				
TYPE OF ORGANISM INVOLVED	MODE OF ACTION	INCUBATION PERIOD	COMMON SYMPTOMS	COMMON FOOD SOURCES	FOOD-HANDLING CAUTIONS
Staphylococcus	Toxin	Under 6 hours (usually 2–4 hours)	Vomiting (in almost all cases) Cramps Diarrhea No fever (temperature may be below normal)	Pastries Custards Salads, salad dressings Sliced meats	Cook food thoroughly. Refrigerate food. (Staphylococci grow rapidly at room temperature, producing toxin. Salmonellae grow rapidly at temperatures between 60°F to 120°F.) Be scrupulous about personal hygiene (especially handwashing). Protect food from animal excreta.
Salmonella	Bacterial infection	6–48 hours (usually 12–24 hours)	Abdominal pain Diarrhea (in almost all cases) Vomiting Fever	Poultry Raw eggs Egg products Raw milk Meats, meat pies Fish Lightly cooked foods	

by the infected individuals. Further investigation indicated that boiled eggs, included in a tuna salad, were responsible. Throat cultures for bacteriological examination were taken from 229 food handlers employed in the mess hall. Of these, three yielded the type of streptococcus that had made the cadets ill. None of the three had been sick. Of those three, one man had directly assisted in the preparation of the ninety-six dozen boiled eggs used in the salad.[20]

Salmonella attacks a hospital

Many other microbes, using food as a convenient medium, can cause illness. Salmonellosis, caused by a group of microorganisms called *Salmonella,* can live and grow in the intestinal tract. A continuous infecting cycle is thus established. The organism may be spread from animal to man, man to man, and man to animal. There are more than twelve hundred species of the genus *Salmonella.* Many cause disease in man. (The *typhoid* bacillus is but one of the salmonellae.) Some years ago, fifty-three hospitals in thirteen states experienced a serious outbreak of salmonellosis of one species. In each hospital the causative salmonellae were isolated

[20]This account is drawn from Harry R. Hill, Robert A. Zimmerman, Gordon V. K. Reid, Elizabeth Wilson, and Major Roger M. Kilton, "Food-Borne Epidemic of Streptococcal Pharyngitis at the United States Air Force Academy," *New England Journal of Medicine,* Vol. 280, No. 17 (April 24, 1969), pp. 917–21.

in patients, staff employees, and contaminated raw and undercooked eggs. The outbreak ended when raw and undercooked eggs were no longer used in meal preparation. The infection was being transmitted both by the eggs and by hospital personnel handling the food and careless about personal hygiene. Since salmonellae in no way affect the taste, smell, or appearance of food, their presence was not betrayed until sick people got sicker.

Another important genus of microbes found in contaminated food is called *Shigella*. Now under study is a vaccine to prevent infection against one type of shigellosis.

Staphylococcal food poisoning is a true poisoning. Why? Because while growing in food, the staphylococcus produces a toxin. It is the toxin, not the staphylococcus that, upon ingestion, causes the illness. This is not the case with most bacterial illness associated with food. In the hospital-salmonella infections, it was the bacteria, not the toxin liberated in the food, that caused the symptoms. Table 6-8 presents some basic differences between staphylococcic *intoxication*[21] and salmonella *infection*. One can readily see how judicious interrogation about such points as what time the symptoms began and what foods the victim had eaten can lead an investigator to the cause of an outbreak of food poisoning.

One type of meningitis, its "carrier state," and the closing of schools

In the food-borne outbreak of streptococcic sore throat, discussed above, it was noted that three foodhandlers carried in their throats the microorganism that had caused all the sickness. But they were not ill. It is quite possible that the foodhandlers were *carriers*. A carrier, then, harbors the specific organisms of a disease without himself having the symptoms. Probably unaware of this, he innocently spreads his infection.

The carrier state of no disease is more misunderstood than that of *meningococcic meningitis* ("spinal meningitis"). A few years ago, a seventeen-year-old southern California high school senior was diagnosed as having the disease. Not twenty-four hours before, he had complained of only a headache and a mild cold. Now he lay desperately ill. Panic swept through the school. Almost everybody seemed to remember some "close contact" with him the day before. Frantic parents besieged private physicians and health department officials demanding "a shot of penicillin." A delegation of mothers excoriated school officials for not closing the schools. Then, suddenly, came a numbing blow. The young patient died. In front of the health department building the lines were three blocks long. One reporter seized a shoddy opportunity. "As many as five percent, and even more, of the people in this town can carry this killer bug," his newsy article proclaimed.

Together, medical men and school officials joined with the health department to bring the truth to the community. What are some of the facts?

---

[21] *Botulism* is also caused by a toxin which is produced by the growth of its microbe in improperly canned or preserved foods. Fortunately, it is rare. Its toxin, and that of tetanus, are perhaps the most poisonous known.

1. Outside of its host, man, the extremely fragile meningococcus dies speedily. Common germicides, cold, drying, sunlight—all rapidly kill it. Contracting the disease indirectly, as from an infected mattress, is hardly likely.

2. The microbe is transmitted from person to person by intimate contact. So close must this contact be that infected nose and throat secretions of one person must ordinarily reach, quite directly, the nose and throat of another individual. That is why outbreaks occur in crowded quarters, such as army barracks.

3. It is quite true that, at any time and even between epidemics, between five and twenty percent of the healthy persons in a given population might be harboring the organism in the nose and throat.[22] But that by no means suggests that all of these carriers will get the disease. In years of higher incidence of the disease, not one in ten thousand individuals, in that part of the general population carrying the microbe, will become ill. During years of ordinary incidence, the risk is often closer to one in twenty thousand, even less. Why do so many individuals harbor the microbe without developing the disease? Nobody knows for sure. Some people may harbor just a few of the microbes and so may be able to resist them. Other people may have slowly built up resistance as a result of having been exposed to the microbe in small numbers over a period of time. Los Angeles County health officials have noted a relationship between several influenza epidemics and a subsequent increase in reported cases of this type of meningitis. With some people it is possible that influenza diminishes resistance to the meningococcus. The ecological balance between the microbe and the host may be upset by the host's previous infection.

4. In view of the enormous number of normal carriers, it would be both foolish and dangerous to attempt to provide penicillin or sulfadiazine prophylaxis to the casual contacts of a case of meningococcic meningitis. The hazard from adverse reactions to either drug is, for the ordinary contact, doubtless greater than the danger of coming down with the disease. Preventive drugs should be considered for extraordinarily close contacts (such as barracks mates) of this type of meningitis victim.

5. Those who demand closing of schools should consider this: no urban epidemic (or outbreak) has ever been controlled in this manner. Worse, closed schools disperse students from the watchful eye of the school health workers (and these include teachers) to the unsupervised corner drug store and movie house. Consideration should be given to closing schools only when (a) there is an inadequate number of teachers, nurses, and physicians to observe the students and exclude the sick and (b) well students will strictly isolate themselves one from the other. These conditions are likely only in highly rural communities.

Tetanus   On a vacant lot in a suburban town two boys scuffle. One pokes at the other's arm with a stick. He succeeds in hitting him, causing a small,

---

[22] The carrier state is true of many host-microbe relationships.

penetrating wound. There is hardly any bleeding. In a day or two the wound is healed, forgotten. Yet, ten days later, the scratched boy lies critically sick. His back is arched. His hands are clenched. His face is fixed in a ghastly grin of agony. Utterly exhausted, he cannot rest. He cannot move normally. For every muscle contracting one way, another contracts in the opposite way. As one observer has remarked, "he is pitted against himself." Worried doctors work to relieve his contractions and racking pain. They know that his chances of survival are a tossup. The stick had been contaminated with soil containing the tetanus organism. Tetanus (lockjaw) is a completely preventable disease (see pages 168–69).

The symptoms of tetanus are caused not by the bacterium but by the deadly toxin liberated by it. Indeed, so unaffected is the original wound that it is often hard to find. In this country, tetanus still occurs with disturbing frequency (see Table 6-2). In the past dozen years, almost three-fourths of all tetanus in New York has occurred among heroin abusers, who doubtless inject themselves with the tetanus organism via dirty needles. In developing countries, where immunization levels are low and sanitation is poor, tetanus is common. Tetanus of the newborn is a frequent baby-killer in many of these countries. Immunization of the mother may prevent this tragedy.

Viral competitors in the human ecosystem

Most viruses (the smallest microbes) are visible only under the electron microscope.[23] The simplest viruses are chemically composed of a tightly packed central core of nucleic acids within a protein overcoat (see Figure 6-9). The central core of nucleic acids (the genes of the virus) is responsible for the infection. The protein overcoat determines the specificity of the virus as an antigen; its structure decides which specific antibody the virus will cause to be produced.

How may viruses be known?

The central core of viral genes is of two types: RNA (ribonucleic acid) or DNA (deoxyribonucleic acid). Viruses contain either RNA or DNA but never both. (Cells of higher organisms, whether bacteria or people, do contain both.) Viruses differ from one another in their *size*. The influenza virus, for example, is ten times bigger than poliovirus. Viruses also vary in *shape*. The "cold sore" (herpes simplex) virus is spherical. Other viruses are shaped like bricks, still others like threads.

In one major respect all viruses are identical. They cannot multiply outside a cell. As obligatory parasites, they may cause disease. But this feature also makes it possible, in the laboratory, to grow and study them in a culture of cells.

---

[23] To give an idea of their size, the virus of tobacco-mosaic diseases is "300 millimicrons long by 15 wide, or 60/5,000,000 of an inch by 3/5,000,000," according to Greer Williams, *Virus Hunters*, p. 104.

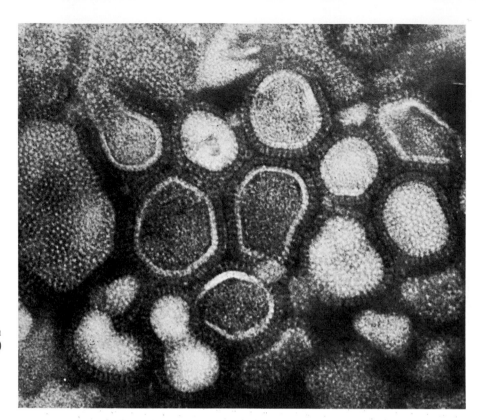

6-9 Asian influenza virus. ($\times$ 250,000)

Cell culturing

This process is a modern scientific achievement of paramount importance. Live cells are placed in a container of specially prepared "soup." There they are nourished and multiply. Waste collects. So some of the cellular growth is transferred to another container of fresh nourishment. These transferred cells multiply in turn. Another transfer in made and then still another. In this way chicken heart cells were kept functioning for thirty years. In all that time they lost neither vitality nor reproductive power. Some years ago, cancer cells from a patient's uterine cervix were obtained and, by transfer, repeatedly cultured. Tons of cells, originating from this one person's original cervical cancer cells, have been distributed to virus laboratories throughout the world. There are many other sources of cells in which to grow viruses. Among them are surgically excised human tissues, monkey and dog kidney tissue, and placental tissue. When viruses gain entrance into a cell, whether it be of a plant or laboratory animal or a human being, they may cause it to sicken (see Figure 6-10).[24] How? By interfering with the manner in which a normal cell uses nutrients to live.

[24]This is called the *cytopathogenic* effect (Greek *kyto*, hollow vessel (cell) + *pathos*, disease + *genesis*, production).

Normal cellular protein manufacture: a brief account

The manner in which a normal cell makes protein is described in Chapter 16, pages 528–32. The nuclear DNA bears the master plan of genetic characteristics for protein manufacture. But the DNA cannot leave the nucleus. So a molecule of messenger RNA, by apposing itself to the nuclear DNA, incorporates within itself the proper message for protein manufacture. It becomes a working copy. Then the messenger RNA leaves the nucleus and enters the surrounding territory, the cellular cytoplasm. Throughout this cytoplasm are located the ribosomes—the workbenches at which protein will be manufactured. Ribosomal structure also depends on the DNA. As a form of RNA, it had left the nucleus to be established in the cytoplasm. Messenger RNA, carrying from the nucleus the DNA instructions, attaches itself to a ribosome. At the ribosome the RNA instructions for making protein are then followed. How does protein building material get to the ribosome? A third RNA, transfer RNA, leaves the nucleus. Its job is to bring cytoplasmic amino-acid building blocks to the ribosome for protein construction. (Thus, several kinds of RNA originate from the DNA—ribosomal, messenger, and transfer.)

A virus invades a bacterial cell in one way, an animal cell in another. **Viral infection** When a virus invades a bacterium it first attaches itself to the bacterium and then erodes the covering cell membrane. Then, through a tiny hole in its tail, the virus ejects its nucleic acid core, or genes, into the bacterium. In this case, the protein overcoat, left outside the bacterial cell, is washed away. Viruses that infect bacteria and destroy them are called *bacteriophage* (bacteria + Greek *phagein*, to eat; see pages 152–53).

The complex animal cell reacts differently to viral infection than does the simple bacterium. But, like a bacterium, an animal cell infected with a virus is sick. In its sickness it can be affected in four ways and with four results:

1. The invading virus uses the animal cell to make more viruses. First, virus particles attach themselves to a cell, and then they penetrate it (see Figure 6-10). The virus enters the cell, protein overcoat and all. A cell with virus in it is infected. Once in the cell, the virus undergoes an "uncoating phenomenon"; that is, the protein coat opens, the virus disrobes (or is disrobed, it is not known which), and the nucleic acid molecules are released "naked" into the cell. When they are thus freed in the cell, the viral nucleic acids interrupt the cell's normal DNA mechanism. How the invading virus accomplishes this is not yet completely clear. However, what happens to the different kinds of infected cells depends on whether the invading virus contains DNA or RNA.

If, following the uncoating phenomenon, it is viral DNA that is released into the cell, it follows that the cell is burdened. Normally it is geared to contain only cellular DNA. Now it contains two kinds of DNA—cellular DNA, which is designed to make protein for more cells, and viral DNA,

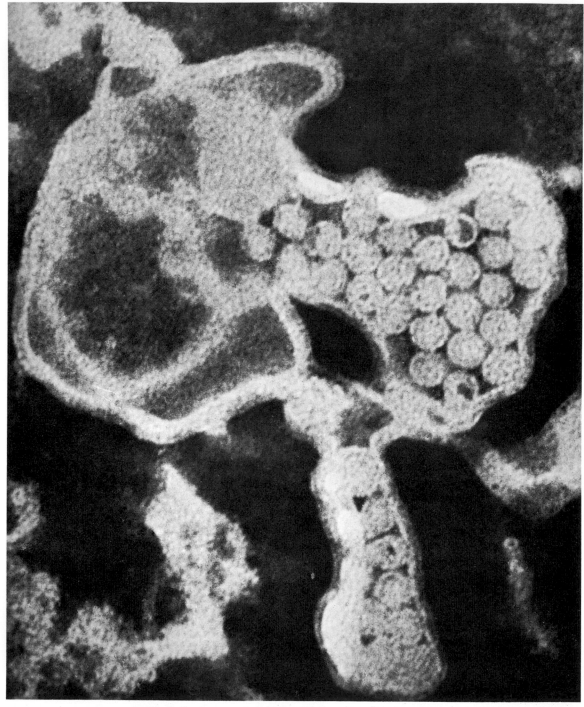

6-10 Poliovirus particles (the clustered round objects) inside a fragment of a cell. (×320,000)

which is designed to make more virus. For a while they may exist together without harm to the cell. Usually, they compete promptly. The viral DNA does not tell the cell's DNA what to do. Viral DNA merely uses the available servants and the housekeeping equipment normally used by the cell's DNA. For example: to operate normally for protein production, the cell's DNA must use ribosomes. Viral DNA also uses the ribosomes but to make more virus. To make protein, the cell's DNA must use cytoplasmic amino acids. Viral DNA also uses the cell's amino acids. In normal cell protein production, cellular DNA directs the synthesis of cellular enzymes and messenger RNA and both participate in the manufacture of cell proteins. In viral production, viral DNA directs the cell to synthesize enzymes and messenger RNA that will participate in the manufacture of viral proteins and more viral DNA. The intruding viral DNA "crowds" the cell's normal DNA. Within the cell there is a "chemical overpopulation." The usurped cell sickens and dies. But not before viral nucleic acids, exactly like those that were within the original invaders, have been assembled at its ribosomes and clothed in new overcoats. Dying, the cell ruptures and the new virus escapes to seek other cells.

What happens when the invading virus contains RNA instead of DNA molecules? The viral RNA can act as its own messenger. Carrying its own coded message to the ribosome, it seduces the cell into making enzymes that, in turn, favor the production of viral RNA and viral protein instead of cellular RNA and cellular protein. Where do the amino acids that are destined to become viral protein come from? They are picked out of the cytoplasmic pool. How do they reach the ribosome at which the viral RNA waits with its instructions? Whether a form of viral RNA is created to accomplish this or the regular cellular RNA works for the creation of virus protein is not known. But the viral RNA can itself act as a template and use the cell's servants and housekeeping equipment to make more RNA like itself. Some normal cellular RNA continues to be made. However, viral RNA soon overwhelms the cell. As in the case of DNA viral infection, the cell breaks open. The newly created virus is released. But the virus cannot tolerate freedom. Away from the cell its ecosystem is utterly inadequate. It must quickly find more cells in which to multiply and prosper. The irony is this: if the virus kills enough cells, the host dies. Then, the virus, trapped in a host of dead cells, must find a new host or also die.

2. A second consequence of viral infection is that the cell may be instructed to decrease its speed of multiplication and growth. This is the "reverse cancer effect." An unborn baby, up to three or four months after conception, can be secondarily infected by the mother's infection with the German measles (rubella) virus (see pages 164 and 192). The virus takes over the genetic mechanism directing the fetus' rapidly multiplying cells. The rate of cellular multiplication is slowed down. Fewer cells are formed. Twenty percent of such children are born with an inadequate number of cells; these children may be blind, deaf, or retarded, or they may have heart and other defects.

3. For many years after viral infection, even for a lifetime, the viral nucleic acid may remain in the cell and, in some unknown way, remain in balanced harmony with it. During this ecological balance, no apparent harm results. Often, however, stimulated by an added infection (another virus perhaps) or by some mechanical stimulation (such as sunburn or radiation or a chemical), the viral nucleic acids may be triggered and viral multiplication is initiated. Cells fall ill. They are inflamed. Some shrink and die. One example of this is the "cold sore" (herpes simplex). Many persons harbor the cold sore virus most of their lives. It is manifested only when irritated into multiplication. This "switching on" of a dormant virus may help explain how some cancers occur. It is possible, for example, that a virus in ecological balance with a bronchial cell may be "switched on" by a chemical in tobacco smoke.

4. The virus can cause animal cancer (see pages 202–04). The viral DNA or RNA captured in the cell may send messages of malignancy. There is a "cancer effect." The capacity for controlled growth (previously so inherently a part of normal DNA and RNA function) is lost. Tumor results (see page 199). It has been proved that viruses may cause animal cancers, but that they cause cancer in humans has not yet been proved.

Interferon

The time: 1960. The place: a capsule hurtling through space. It is all very dramatic. Four of Flash Gordon's members lie dead. Then another falls sick. He sinks into a coma. Then still another crew member succumbs. But then, in the nick of time, enter interferon!

It works. The rest of the crew is saved.

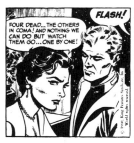
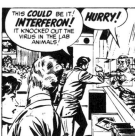
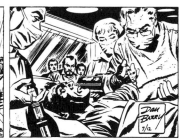
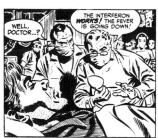
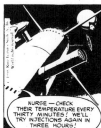
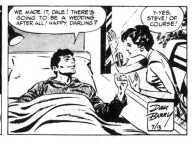

6-11 Enter interferon!

Interferon is not, however, the product of cartoonist Dan Barry's imagination. It is the product of British scientists Alick Issac and Jean Lindenmann's labor. What is interferon?

It is a protein. As was just noted, virus-infected cells may be instructed to produce more virus. In some way, as yet not clearly revealed, the viral nucleic acid is responsible for the production of interferon within infected cells. Interferon does not protect the cell that is already infected and that, indeed, is producing it. It is thought to prevent the infection of as yet uninvolved adjacent cells. Thus, strangely, the virus not only corrupts the cell into making more virus, but also provides a way, via interferon, of preventing exactly that from happening in adjacent cells. Interferon so produced may be capable of preventing infection by many other viruses attacking the host. Growth of microscopic agents other than viruses is also inhibited. Indeed, interferon has recently been shown to inhibit the growth of a malarial parasite of rats and the microbe of parrot fever (psittacosis), both of which grow only in the host's cells.

FOR HELEN   A cell may be stimulated to produce interferon by substances other than viruses. One interferon stimulator was found under unusual circumstances. In the summer of 1945 the Second World War slowly drew to its ominous close. All over the world, the dispersed forces waited to be sent home. Seated at a desk in his lonely quarters on Guam was Navy Commander Richard E. Shope. He was looking at a picture of his wife. On the picture's isinglass cover he noticed a speck of mold. Most men would have scraped it off and forgotten it. But Dr. Shope sent it to the laboratory. The report identified it as *Penicillium funiculosum*. On being discharged, Dr. Shope took the mold with him to his New York laboratory. He discovered that as it grew, it produced a liquid. And this liquid, he found, protected mice from encephalitis virus and pneumonia virus. He named the liquid *helenine,* "largely out of recognition of the good taste shown by the mold producing the substance in locating on the picture of my wife, Helen."[25]

Helenine induces cells to produce interferon. Thus, viruses are not essential for interferon production. Not only helenine but some bacteria stimulate interferon, as do some bacterial toxins, as well as RNA and DNA. Among the synthetic chemicals inducing interferon, one called poly I:C is of special interest because it is not so toxic. This drug has already stimulated interferon that cures rabbits of a fatal viral eye disease. Poly I:C may be tried on consenting terminal cancer patients at the hospital of the National Institutes of Health. If a way is found to produce interferon in large amounts and if interferon does indeed impede virus production, perhaps man will have a new way of preventing viral disease.

The search is on.

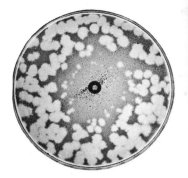

6-12 Virus-infected chick embryo cells in a Petri dish. Interferon applied in the center diffused outward. The clear area shows where infected cells were destroyed.

[25] Richard E. Shope, "Antiviral substance from penicillium funiculosum; effect upon infection in mice with swine influenza virus and columbia SK encephalomyelitis virus," quoted in *CA—A Cancer Journal for Clinicians*, Vol. 18, No. 1 (January–February 1968), pp. 40–41.

Drugs versus viruses

Because viruses multiply in cells, most known drugs are generally helpless against them. Most drugs that kill viruses kill cells too. The problem then is to kill the virus without harming the cell. Bacteria do not enter the animal cell. They attack it from the outside. That is why drugs that are able to differentiate between bacterial and animal cells are effective against bacterial diseases. By February 1970, only four drugs were known to be effective against human viral disease without serious harm to the human host: a compound called *IUdR* is effective against a viral infection of the cornea of the eye; Symmetrel (or amantadine) seems to prevent influenza A2 (British and Russian studies suggest it is effective against the Hong Kong strain too); rimantadine also apparently prevents (and perhaps treats) A2 influenza; and Marboran (methisazone) seems to prevent smallpox if taken during the incubation period of the disease. A new antibiotic, rifampicin, also appears to be effective (in the test tube) against several viral enemies of man. Most (not all) of these drugs enter the cell to interfere with viral multiplication. Amantadine prevents the influenza A2 virus from entering the cell. Mankind's future attack against the virus world will probably be by a combination of vaccines, interferon, and drugs.

The common cold: the vagrant viruses

A cold is not, in the traditional sense, a disease. It is a collection of signs and relatively mild symptoms. Sometimes these lead the way to more severe symptoms and serious disease. Symptoms of a cold may be caused by a wide variety of microorganisms ranging from viruses to fungi.

An example: an unvaccinated person who has never been infected with poliovirus is susceptible to it. Assume such an individual is invaded by the virus. If his resistance is adequate, he shows no symptoms. This is usual. With less resistance he will have cold symptoms. This is occasional. Rarely he will develop paralysis and even die. In such an instance, resistance was indeed poor. This is unusual. These stages are caused by the same poliovirus. At any stage the body resistance may overcome the poliovirus. The body is then immune to that specific virus. Later, another virus attacks. This time it may be a rubeola virus. Then a person with inadequate resistance and without previous vaccination may develop cold symptoms (respiratory symptoms always involve the lower as well as the upper respiratory tract), a velvety, itching rash, and, once in a thousand cases, serious brain inflammation (measles encephalitis). With infection, therefore, the forces of resistance are in combat with the forces of the infecting agent. The stage of disease called the cold may or may not occur, depending on the powers of the host's resistance.

With scores of other viral infections (perhaps a hundred or more) the same spectrum of stages occurs. Influenza virus may cause no symptoms, or cold symptoms, or pneumonia, or even death. But viruses are not alone in causing cold symptoms. A serious bacterial disease, such as tuberculosis, may also be heralded by mild symptoms of a cold. The same may be said for some fungus diseases such as "valley fever."

Crib death—the sudden and unexpected death of an infant left alone in a crib—is a particularly tragic circumstance that is worth noting here. The child, usually two to six months of age, is unaccountably found dead in his crib. Why? the agonized parents ask. The reason for these deaths is not known. Certainly there is no correlation whatsoever between crib deaths and the adequacy of parental care. "The most convincing hypothesis at this time would tend to suggest that the baby's first experience with respiratory viruses may be overwhelming and that a 'cold of the lungs' is sufficient to interfere with vital and essential ventilation, leading to sharply reduced supplies of oxygen and sudden unexpected death."[26] Other studies have emphasized the possibility of a slowly developing allergic reaction to milk.[27]

THE TREATMENT OF COLDS   A cold vaccine that would include all the microorganisms that can cause the signs and symptoms of a common cold may never be developed. Vaccines are, however, available for some illnesses for which a cold is introductory or in which it is a transient phase (see page 164). Vaccination against measles or mumps, for example, will protect not only against these diseases, but also against the colds that are an early stage of them. An *adenovirus*[28] *vaccine* (developed in 1958) now effectively prevents the colds that, between 1942 and 1945, sent many thousands of soldiers-in-training to the hospital.[29]

Colds are hard to prevent and they may be equally hard to get rid of. Present-day antibiotics, such as penicillin, are helpless against viruses. (They can often, however, destroy secondarily invading bacteria, such as staphylococci or pneumococci. This explains their occasional use in some severe respiratory infections.) In mice, interferon—the virus fighter naturally produced by cells—accumulates in greater amounts in the presence of fever. Perhaps this explains why fever is often associated with recovery. Fever-reducing aspirin (or its numerous associated compounds) should, therefore, be used only with the family doctor's advice. Research has shown that vitamin C, in the form of fruit juice, however pleasant, is useless in preventing or shortening colds. Alcohol, by causing nasal and pharyngeal congestion, may prolong and worsen a cold. To ease the symptoms and shorten the seige of an ordinary cold, one should drink enough fluids, eat what is desired, but moderately, and get extra rest. Some medical advice for the treatment of colds four centuries ago is still appropriate: "The beste and moste sure help in this case is not to meddle with anye kynde of medicines, but to let nature worke her operacio."[30]

[26]John M. Adams, *Viruses and Colds: The Modern Plague* (New York, 1967), pp. 103–04.
[27]Daniel Stowens, "Sudden Unexpected Death in Infancy," *Clinical Pediatrics*, Vol. 5, No. 4 (April 1966), pp. 243–54.
[28]A group of viruses found in adenoid tissue. Colds are but one of a variety of disease syndromes produced by adenoviruses.
[29]Greer Williams, *Virus Hunters*, p. 373.
[30]Thomas Phaire, *The Boke of Chyldren* (The Book of Children), quoted in John M. Adams, *Viruses and Colds: The Modern Plague*, p. 135.

German measles (rubella)

In most of the United States except the West, winter and spring of 1963–64 were marked by widespread rubella. The same seasons of the following year saw a similar epidemic in the Pacific States. As a result of these infections, many malformed babies were born.

About twenty percent of women of childbearing age have not had rubella. They are therefore susceptible to this highly infectious disease. Should a woman contract the disease just before or during the first twelve weeks of her pregnancy, the risk of bearing a malformed child is about twenty percent. Abnormality of the child has, however, been reported with maternal infection in the second three months of pregnancy.

A wide range of abnormalities has been described, including defects of hearing and vision, cardiac problems, and mental retardation. In addition, the affected child (as well as an apparently normal child exposed in the uterus) remains contagious for months after delivery. Such a child must be isolated, particularly from pregnant women and from susceptible babies.

Gamma globulin may curtail the mother's symptoms of the disease. Its effectiveness in preventing rubella infection, and resultant infant disability, is not proven. Many physicians feel that, if desired by the parents, abortion is indicated if maternal rubella has occurred in the first fourteen to sixteen weeks of pregnancy. Factors of consummate importance include religious belief, the age of the parents, and the number of children they already have.

An effective vaccine for rubella is available (see Table 6-1).

Other viruses affecting the unborn

Various other viral diseases occasionally threaten a pregnancy. In this country, smallpox is at present nonexistent. Some evidence indicates that vaccination of a pregnant woman against the disease may harm the child within her. Except under unusual circumstances, therefore, smallpox vaccination is best deferred until after delivery. Although maternal chickenpox may terminate a pregnancy, there is no evidence that its virus causes malformations. Children of mothers who develop chickenpox in the last week or two of pregnancy may be born with the disease or develop it soon after birth. This is rarely serious. For an adult, the "cold sore" virus produces a common and mild infection. Fortunately, it rarely infects the unborn child. When it does, it may end the pregnancy.

In this country, the menace of regular measles virus to children, born and unborn, should disappear in the wake of the effective vaccine. Before the vaccine was available, regular measles killed between four hundred and five hundred children every year. Every epidemic, moreover, left an army of the physically and mentally retarded. Some expert opinion suggests that it was also responsible for the intrauterine infection and malformation of some children.

CYTOMEGALIC INCLUSION DISEASE   The name of this disease is descriptive of some aspects of the illness. *Kyto* (Greek, a hollow vessel) denotes relationship with a cell. *Megalic* is derived from the Greek *megaleios* (meaning magnificent) and refers to the unique large cells associated with the disease. The word "inclusion" describes the unusual inclusion bodies found within those cells. This illness, usually noted in the first month of life, is due to cytomegalovirus infection. In the adult the disease is usually so mild that it is not detected. When transmitted from pregnant women to fetus, it often manifests itself by a wide variety of malformations in the newborn child. As with German measles, children with the disease may be contagious for months after delivery. They should be isolated, particularly from pregnant women.

A relationship beteen mumps and fetal disease has not been established. The possibility that infectious hepatitis has a deleterious effect on the unborn child has been suggested. A growing suspicion that many other viruses may affect the child within the uterus indicates the need for more research in this field.[31]

Mumps

Although, during mumps infection, virus is carried by the blood to all body tissues, several organs most frequently show manifestations. Commonly, but not always, the salivary glands swell. As a maximum, about twenty percent of all male mumps patients thirteen years of age or over develop swelling (as a result of inflammation) of the testicle (*orchitis*). Young soldiers are frequently attacked. During both world wars, mumps was a frequent cause of sickness.

The incidence of sterility from testicular swelling is in dispute. It most certainly is rare. Public apprehension on this account is understandable, but unjustified. The third most common mumps manifestation is inflammation of the brain and its linings. In between 30 and 50 percent of all cases of mumps, there is laboratory evidence of some central nervous system involvement. Ninety-nine percent of all such cases recover and ninety-five percent show no aftereffects. Mumps meningitis is perhaps the mildest of the meningitides. Despite these facts, many silly old wives' tales have been spun around the horrid effects of mumps on the testicle, ovary, and brain. The infection is not known to cause impotence, although a parent's distress with a young son's swollen testicle may leave the child with psychological problems. Although death from mumps is of the greatest rarity and serious complications are quite uncommon, the illness does cause considerable temporary discomfort and disability. The attenuated live mumps virus vaccine (see page 164) is effective and safe.

Viral hepatitis

There is some opinion that a single virus (called the *Australia antigen*) may be responsible for the two most common types of hepatitis (inflam-

---

[31] Janet B. Hardy, "Viruses and the Fetus," *Postgraduate Medicine*, Vol. 43, No. 1 (January 1968), pp. 156–65.

mation of the liver)—*infectious hepatitis* and *serum hepatitis*. The symptoms of these two distinct diseases may be indistinguishable. They include loss of appetite, a variable amount of fever, nausea, joint stiffness, and pain in the upper right abdomen. As either disease progresses, the urine becomes dark and the stool light. With the occurrence of jaundice, the affected individual may become depressed. The jaundice may persist for about six weeks. As long as three months may be required for recovery. Chronic liver problems sometimes result from hepatitis.

The virus of infectious hepatitis is usually incidental to overcrowding, inadequate sanitation, and poor hygiene. It is generally transmitted by hands contaminated with infected feces. An individual who is careless about hand-washing may, therefore, spread the infection. Neither pasteurization nor chlorination destroys the virus. Thus health departments have added infectious hepatitis to their list of water-borne diseases that merit careful attention.

The virus of serum hepatitis is usually transmitted by contaminated equipment used for injections or by similarly dangerous blood or blood products.

In the past several years a few areas in this country have experienced a striking increase in viral hepatitis—both infectious and serum. Since 1965, California, for example, has had a two-fold increase in infectious hepatitis and a six-fold increase in serum hepatitis. This epidemic is confined to the teen-age and young adult segment of the population. Widespread drug use combined with crowded and insanitary living conditions as well as poor personal hygiene are considered to be responsible.

Lacking a vaccine, the best tool for prevention of either type of hepatitis is cleanliness. This is not always easy. The infectious hepatitis fostered by the unavoidably difficult conditions of some army installations is an example of such a circumstance. Armies on the move often suffer epidemics of infectious hepatitis. Sterilization of needles, syringes, and other equipment used in blood or intravenous work is essential to the prevention of viral hepatitis of either type. Frequent victims of serum hepatitis are drug abusers and those exposed to contaminated tattoo needles.

Gamma globulin (which provides passive immunity) will effectively prevent exposed persons from developing jaundice. Vast amounts of this material are now being used for U.S. troops in Vietnam. For this purpose gamma globulin is only effective for two to six weeks.

Infectious mononucleosis

This is a viral disease manifested by fever, fatigue, swollen neck lymph nodes (lymph nodes throughout the body may be involved), and sore throat. There is a marked increase in the number of lymphocytes (a variety of white blood cell) in the blood. This cell is manufactured in lymph nodes. Enlargement of the spleen and liver is common. Very occasionally the sick person may have a rash or be jaundiced. Serious complications, such as brain and heart inflammation, are thankfully rare. Some recovered individuals may become easily fatigued for months. Recent work suggests a relationship between the virus causing infectious mononucleosis and other illnesses, but this is as yet unclear.

Unless abetted by direct and intimate contact, the disease is not readily transmitted. The illness is not uncommonly diagnosed in (but hardly limited to) college students. For this reason it has been variously called the "college" or "student's" or "kissing" disease.

Infectious mononucleosis lasts from one to three weeks. However, it can be prolonged for months. The incubation period is usually between one and two weeks, sometimes longer. It is probably communicable before symptoms begin. It may remain communicable until the fever and sore throat are gone. Recovery is the rule.

In industrial countries, progress against communicable diseases has removed ancient terrors. In developing nations, health workers still labor to provide their people with proven methods of prevention and cure. But no matter what the stage of success, the greatest enemy is laxity. A single case of plague in New Mexico, an outbreak of typhoid in New York, an epidemic of gonorrhea in Los Angeles—these warn against a false sense of security. Only constant vigilance buys freedom from the communicable diseases.

7

Of structure, function, and chronic impairments thereto: part I

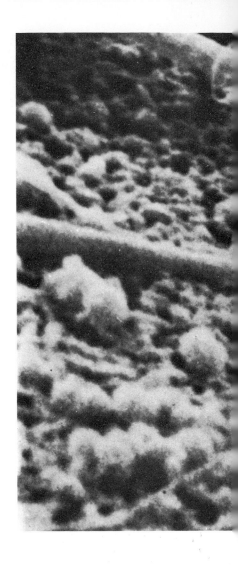

Beautiful is what can be seen, more beautiful what can be under-stood, by far the most beautiful is that which we don't know.[1]

Chronic disease: the price of success

At the turn of this century, infectious diseases were the primary health menace to this nation. Acute respiratory conditions such as pneumonia and influenza were the major killers. Tuberculosis, too, drained the nation's

[1] Neils Stensen (1638–86), quoted in Chandler McC. Brooks and Paul F. Cranefield, eds., *The Historical Development of Physiological Thought* (New York, 1959), p. 38.

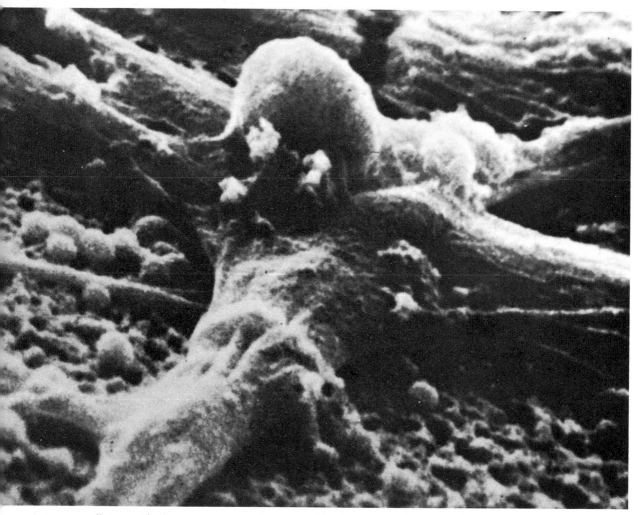

A cancer cell (magnified over 3,500 times) spreads like the roots of a tree and can invade normal tissue.

vitality. Gastrointestinal infections decimated the child population. A great era of environmental control helped change all this. Water and milk supplies were made safe. Engineers constructed systems to handle and treat perilous human wastes and to render them safe. Food sanitation and personal hygiene became a way of life. Continual labors of public health workers diminished death rates of mothers and their infants. Countless children were vaccinated. Tuberculosis was brought under control. True, new environmental hazards replaced the old (Chapters 3 and 4). But people survived to suffer them. In 1900, the average person in the United States barely eked out fifty years of life. Some twenty years have since been added to this life expectancy.

But each generation is saddled on the last. Yesterday's success often brings tomorrow's challenge. The longer life span—a mark of progress—intensified another group of health problems and made them predominant, the *chronic degenerative diseases:* "chronic," because they linger; "degenerative," because they may cause progressive deterioration of tissues. As a group they share certain characteristics: their causes are frequently unclear; often, they are a long time developing; the disability they bring may be relatively prolonged; usually they leave some residual impairment; and their treatments, because they are long-term, are costly.

That the chronic diseases have become the nation's major health problem is apparent from a few statistics: at the turn of this century, one in seven deaths was due to heart disease and stroke; today, that ratio is one in every two. Cancer has joined heart disease and stroke in a destructive assault on the middle and advanced years. But chronic illness is also a major concern of youth. For most chronic diseases, cure, as it is generally understood, remains unlikely. But suffering stimulates research, and the search into the unknown begets knowledge. In this there is hope, and this is the meaning of Stensen's statement that opened this discussion.

In this chapter, cancer, allergies, joint disorders, and the structure and disorders of the nervous system and the endocrine and exocrine glands will be discussed. The next chapter will deal with the structure and disorders of the circulatory system and the kidneys.

Cancer: the lawless cells

Anarchy, anarchy! Show me a greater evil!

So cries Creon, King of Thebes, in the great Sophoclean tragedy *Antigone*. Cancer is cellular anarchy. Its microscopic, greedy lawlessness, contemptuous of body government, "destroys man in a unique and appalling way, as flesh of his own flesh, which has somehow been rendered proliferative, rampant, predatory, and ungovernable."[2]

In Chapter 16, the momentous destiny of the fertilized egg—the zygote —is described. Under genetic direction, it divides. There are then two cells and these divide to produce four cells. Each of these divides, and so on. As cells grow in number, they migrate. Some divide here, others there. All the while their DNA is active. To obedient RNA molecules, DNA imparts codes to construct proteins. The proteins are destined to play their vital part in the structure of various tissue, whether brain or liver or skin or any other. So cells differentiate. Nourished in the womb's wall, the disciplined cluster of cells is alive. But how is it held together? Cells lay down nonliving substances between one another. They spare salts, for example, long ago borrowed from the seas, for bone construction. This cellular division, migration, and differentiation, this laying down of frame-

---

[2] Peyton Rous, "The Challenge to Man of Neoplastic Disease," Nobel Prize acceptance speech delivered in Stockholm, December 13, 1966.

work, is not haphazard. A rhythmic miracle, rivaling the movements of the celestial bodies, it is a directed plan for growth. This is body government. When this government is usurped, there is anarchy, chaos, cancer.

At birth all organs are differentiated. But growth continues, and so does cell division. With adolescence a special spurt of cell division occurs in the sexual organs. At twenty the average person is full-grown. Normally, he will be a harmonious ecosystem of cells, and each of his many trillions of cells will be an ecosystem too.

Some cells stop dividing, but not all. The neurons in the adult brain and spinal cord no longer divide, but the cells of their supporting tissue do. Some cells divide only when necessary. Liver, kidney, and endocrine gland cells divide to replace those killed by infection or other injury. (There are cells that do not divide but grow. In this way the woman's uterus and breasts respond to pregnancy.) Still other cells divide throughout life. Blood cells continually need to be replaced because they are buffeted about and destroyed during their extensive travels. So blood cell division continually goes on in bone marrow and lymph nodes. Surface skin cells and those of the linings of the respiratory, gastrointestinal, and urinary tracts also undergo harsh treatment. Hence, the destroyed cells are constantly replaced. It is estimated that the entire mucous lining of the gastrointestinal tract is replaced about twice a week.[3]

The basic difference between normal cells and tumor cells is that normal cells are controlled. Tumor cells have escaped normal body controls. They are instructed by the genetic material to divide. But, as will be seen, the management has been taken over. Tumor cells are in ecological imbalance with the body that feeds them. Thus, they are doomed, as, too often, is their host. How this occurs is described below.

Tumors, as indicated above, are masses of cells resulting from uncontrolled growth.[4] *Benign tumors* are not cancers. Of themselves, they do not kill. Only by incidentally interfering with function (for example, by obstructing the bowel) can they cause death. Such tumors are regularly defined and encapsulated. They are a localized cellular overgrowth. A surrounding capsule keeps them within bounds. As they grow, they do not penetrate tissues; they push them. Surgically, they can be shelled out of their capsule; cure results.

Malignant tumors are the cancers. By the very nature of their behavior, they can kill. Crab-shaped (Greek *karkinos,* crab), they behave like crabs. Not withheld by a capsule, they project into normal tissue, clawing their way, destroying whatever cells are in their path. Often they travel in other ways. They *metastasize.* Cancer cells may reach other organs, near or far, in three basic ways. (1) By penetrating the delicate lymph channel walls,

The benign tumors and the malignant cancers and how they spread

[3] As would be expected, adult cells that do not divide, such as the neurons of the spinal cord, do not become tumors. The supporting tissue cells of the adult central nervous system can become tumors. Most susceptible to becoming tumors are the cells that constantly divide. Cells dividing when needed for repair or for a new function also go out of control, but less frequently.
[4] The late distinguished U.S. physician James Ewing called tumors "an uncontrolled new growth of tissue."

they set up secondary cancer depots in nearby and distant lymph nodes (see page 255). (2) In addition, they may invade the veins, which are less resistant than the arteries. Following the circulatory routes, they then set up secondary tumors in remote places. That is why cigarette smoker's cancer is so often fatal. Deluded that his cough is a "cigarette cough," that the pain in his chest is temporary, the smoker may not see a physician until his lung cancer has been long dispersed to the body's vital centers.[5] (3) Cancer cells may break off from an original location and migrate to the fibrous sacs enclosing the intestines, the lungs, or the heart. Then, after penetrating the sac, they may float in its enclosed fluid, finally settling down on an organ. They may then start a secondary cancerous growth.

Not all metastases cause early death. The traveling cells of some tumors end in the lung, for example, and there they die. Others go to some distant bone (as do cells of some breast cancers). They may stay there without causing disease for many years. Nobody knows why.

The tissues from which malignant tumors (cancers) arise

One of the most widely accepted hypotheses in cancer research is that the initial event leading to malignancy is a change in a single cell. Following this, there may be a series of events within succeeding generations of cells, finally culminating in many malignant cells which may develop into a mass as a "solid" tumor or may be at once widespread throughout the body, such as occurs in the leukemias.

Carcinomas are the most common form of cancer. They arise from epithelial cells, important as a covering or lining tissue, which exists in numerous forms. Skin is composed of one kind of epithelium; when it becomes cancerous, it is designated as skin carcinoma. Other carcinomas arise from the glandular organs, such as breast, which are composed of different epithelial tissue, as are the smooth, shiny mucous membranes such as those that line the mouth, stomach, and lungs.

Sarcomas occur less frequently. They are a more heterogeneous group of cancers, arising from fibrous (connective) tissue and from muscle, bone, and cartilage. Together, the carcinomas and sarcomas have been classified as "solid" tumors.[6]

The causes of cancer

There are four basic groups of cancer causes: *physical, chemical, genetic,* and *viral.*

---

[5] It was recently estimated that of 61,000 people in the United States who contracted lung cancer in 1968, close to 75 percent would be dead within one year, 93 percent within five years. Of 100 lung cancer patients medically examined, 50 to 60 would be beyond chance for cure. Of the remaining 40 to 50, only half are operable. "Of the 20 to 25 with operable growths, only 5 to 8 live 5 years after surgery." Of these, almost one-fourth recur. (Bernard Roswit, cited in "Medical Science Notes," *Science News*, Vol. 94, No. 3 [August 1968], p. 112.) These figures are not included in cigarette advertising.

[6] *Progress Against Cancer 1969: A Report by the National Advisory Cancer Council,* National Cancer Institute, U.S. Department of Health, Education, and Welfare, pp. 52–53.

Physical causes

As was discussed in Chapter 4, some substances emit cancer-causing radiations as they degenerate. Examples of radiation-produced cancers are the lung cancer of Colorado uranium miners, the increased leukemia rates among Hiroshima and Nagasaki survivors (the leukemia incidence among them is five times that of the rest of the Japanese population[7]), the increased incidence of female breast cancer (two to four times) among these same survivors,[8] and the higher leukemia rates among X-ray workers. The sun's ultraviolet light radiation is responsible for most skin cancers[9] (see page 208).

Chemical causes

That chemicals can cause cancer was first noted in 1775 by an English surgeon, Percival Potts. He correctly attributed the frequent scrotal cancer of chimney sweepers to soot exposure. Many an orphaned six-year-old, recruited to work in the chimneys, also slept in them. Sometimes chemicals combine with other injuries, particularly burns, to cause cancer. Poor nineteenth-century natives of the Kangri area in India often developed skin cancer of the abdomen. They warmed themselves by keeping baskets of live coals in their clothes. Burns plus the chemical products of coal combustion diseased them. In Panama, washerwomen still smoke cigarettes with the lit end inside the mouth. Mouth cancers among them are frequent.

Today, potential chemical *carcinogens* (cancer-producing substances) surround man. Smog is an example. But despite considerable research "no final conclusion about the effect of atmospheric pollution is yet possible."[10] Some sprays and drugs may be cancer producers. Deaths from cancers of the mouth, pharynx, larynx, and esophagus are associated with heavy drinking.[11] Creosote, used to preserve garden fences, causes cancer in mice. Prolonged exposure to insecticides containing arsenic, to crude oils, and to chemicals used in the rubber and cable industry can result in human cancer. With their constant testing program, the Food and Drug Administration does extensive work in public protection. But the effect of atmospheric and food pollution requires more research. Not enough is known about the long-term effect of many of these pollutants.

Genetic causes

Heredity is of enormous importance in cancer of laboratory animals. Mice have been bred that invariably develop a particular cancer. Such genetically dependable pure strains, produced by brother-sister matings

---

[7] R. J. C. Harris, *Cancer* (Baltimore, 1962), p. 50.
[8] C. K. Wanebo et al., "Breast Cancer After Exposure to the Atomic Bombings of Hiroshima and Nagasaki," *New England Journal of Medicine*, Vol. 279, No. 13 (September 26, 1968), pp. 667–71.
[9] Robert G. Freeman and John M. Knox, "Skin Cancer and the Sun," *CA—A Cancer Journal for Clinicians*, Vol. 17, No. 5 (September–October 1967), p. 235.
[10] Richard Doll, *Prevention of Cancer: Pointers in Epidemiology* (London, 1967), p. 62.
[11] *Ibid.*, p. 81.

of twenty or more generations, have provided a laboratory creature that is indispensable to research. These mice help man, for heredity plays a role in human cancer. Exactly what that role is remains, as yet, unclear. Exceedingly few cancers are strictly genetic or hereditary. Among them are an uncommon tumor of the retina and another of the nervous system, each of which is determined by a specific gene. The familial aspects of female breast cancer are discussed later in this chapter (page 209).

Viral causes

In 1933, a young Iowa physician noted that wild rabbits near his home had skin warts. A farmer's son caught some of the rabbits for him. The physician, Richard E. Shope, subsequently became the first to prove that a virus could cause a solid tumor in a mammal.

Dr. Shope died of cancer on October 2, 1966. In a magnificent scientific paper, published in that year, he wrote of "the sly and indirect processes" of "some animal tumor viruses."[12] He emphasized, nevertheless, that "it is no longer realistic to contend that human cells are different from the cells of other species of animals in their capacity to react to cancer-causing viruses."[13]

Investigations such as Dr. Shope's, indicating a viral cause of tumors, were not new. Some twenty years earlier, in 1911, Peyton Rous had shown that chickens developed connective tissue tumors from viruses. But scant attention was paid to either Rous or Shope. Years later, a virus that was recovered from a mouse produced cancers in rats, guinea pigs, hamsters, and other species. A new research race was on. And perhaps to mark it, fifty-five years after his original work, Rous was awarded the Nobel prize. By the beginning of 1970, no human cancer had been proven to be caused by a virus.

HOW INFECTING VIRUSES CAUSE ANIMAL CANCERS   It is understandable that the solution to the cancer riddle is being sought in the laboratories of the virologists. It has been seen that cancer is a disease of the cell. And in Chapter 6 it was pointed out that viruses are obliged to multiply in living cells. The viruses that can cause animal cancers, like all viruses, consist of a protein overcoat and a core of nucleic acid. The protein overcoat is the part of the virus that gives it specificity as an antigen. It is the core, however, that causes cellular infection. That core of the virus is composed either of RNA or DNA, but never contains both types of nucleic acid. Within the nucleus of the animal cell there is also DNA, and it is DNA that directs the formation of RNA. So the core of the virus contains the same basic chemicals as the nuclear core of animal cells.

It will be recalled (Chapter 6) that a virus attaches itself to an animal cell, penetrates it, and undergoes uncoating to free its nucleic acid mole-

---

[12] Richard E. Shope, "Evolutionary Episodes in the Concept of Viral Oncogenesis," *Perspectives in Biology and Medicine*, Vol. 9, No. 3 (Winter 1966), p. 273.
[13] *Ibid.*, p. 270.

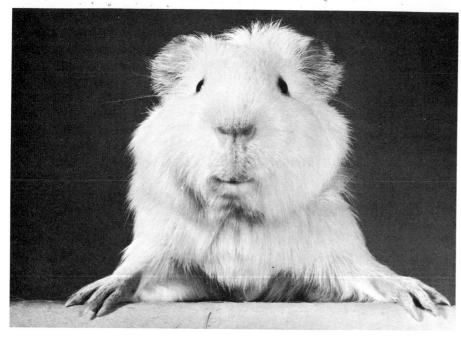

7-1 A hero of cancer research: the guinea pig.

cules. Four things may then happen to the animal cell: (1) The viral nucleic acid may subvert the cell into making more virus. (2) The speed of cellular multiplication may be retarded by the viral nucleic acids (a "reverse cancer effect"). (3) Nothing that is apparent may happen until the viral nucleic acids, lurking in the cell and biding their time, are stimulated into action, perhaps by an irritant such as radiation or a second virus. Or (4) (in the animal at least) the viral nucleic acid may induce a cancerous multiplication of cells (see pages 184–85). (Interestingly, viruses that can cause cancers in animals do not always do so. Often they merely infect the animal cell to cause the production of more virus.) What determines whether a virus will cause a cell to produce more virus or become a cancer? This is not known.

Animal studies have revealed much about the virus-cancer relationships. All is by no means known. But the process depends on which viral genetic structure, RNA or DNA, invades the cell. Consider these separately. *If the invading cancer-causing virus contains RNA,* the laboratory investigator can find the RNA in the cell. What is it doing there? It is thought that the viral RNA successfully competes with the work usually performed by the cell's messenger RNA. As a result, not as much normal messenger RNA is created within the cell. Subverting the cell's household equipment (such as its ribosomes) and its materials (such as the amino acids of the cytoplasmic proteins), the cancer-causing viral RNA causes the cell to lose the controls that maintain its normal relationships with other cells. *If, however, the cancer-causing virus contains DNA,* the virus invades the cell and, like all viruses, sheds its coat. But then the naked

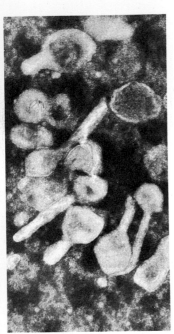

7-2 The virus causing mouse leukemia (×75,000).

viral DNA disappears. Unlike viral RNA, viral DNA cannot be found in the invaded cell by the laboratory worker. It "hides" by actually becoming incorporated into the cellular DNA. (That is why investigators fail to find a separate causal viral DNA for animal cancer.) How, then, does the virologist know the viral DNA is there? Because the viral DNA leaves chemical "footprints"[14] as evidence. By means of highly sophisticated laboratory techniques, the virologist can detect its presence. So not only does the cancer-causing virus containing DNA move into the animal cell, occupy it, plunder it, and direct it to disaster, it also becomes a part of it. It is the supreme imposition.

This usurpation of the prerogatives of the cell's DNA by viral DNA robs the cellular DNA of its normal ability to direct the making of cellular protein. Usurped, corrupt, the cellular DNA can now send only messages of malignancy. Malignant cells divide into daughter cells that carry the new and deadly instructions of their parent cells. Helplessly, they carry and transmit the capacity for uncontrolled growth. A cancer is born.

Does this mean that viruses causing animal cancers are contagious? Certainly, those viruses proven to induce cancer in animals are. But they apparently need something (what, is not entirely determined) "to turn them on," to activate them. Are human cancers contagious? It has not yet been proven that viruses cause human cancer. (Interestingly, some viruses infecting humans can cause animal cancers.) In some way viruses are involved in the process of some human cancer. Exactly what that involvement is in human beings remains unknown. Perhaps they too need to be potentiated by a cancer-producing substance, such as may be found in cigarette smoke. One human tumor is known to be caused by a virus. It is the common *wart.* Another human tumor, called *molluscum contagiosum,* is probably caused by a virus. (*Molluscum* is a Latin word meaning "soft," and the disease is manifested by soft, round skin tumors.) Both warts and molluscum contagiosum are contagious but neither is a cancer. They are benign tumors. There is nothing in the pattern of occurrence of human cancers to indicate that they are communicable, as that term is understood today.

Progress against leukemia

The search goes on slowly, as research must. As a cancer of the blood, leukemia has provided an excellent opportunity for study. When a cancer of the tissue that produces white blood cells occurs, an excess of those cells is found in the blood. This condition, called *leukemia,* is widely distributed, occurring in a great variety of animals, including the cat, dog, and cow. Milk from leukemic herds has yielded particles of virus. A vaccine, prepared with mouse leukemia viruses (see Figure 7-2), can now prevent leukemia in certain laboratory animals. Particles resembling mouse leukemia viruses (that they are viruses is hardly certain) have been found in children's blood. Too, these particles have been found in the pet

[14]Fred Rapp and Joseph L. Melnick, "The Footprints of Tumor Viruses," *Scientific American,* Vol. 214, No. 3 (March 1966), pp. 34–41.

dogs of leukemic patients. Of course, this may be coincidental. But how about human leukemia? Here again there has been progress. Although cures are still not possible, the use of drugs has led to increasing periods of remission (temporary disappearance of all or most signs and symptoms) in a significant number of children suffering from acute leukemia. As of 1970 many leukemia sufferers were surviving, on the average, more than twice as long as they did only a half-dozen years before.

In laboratories throughout the world scientists are solving the virus-cancer enigma. As Shope wrote in his last paper, there is no reason to believe that man is unique in this respect. If certain viruses can cause cancer in animals, in some way some viruses must cause it in man. Are other agents involved with them? If so, what are they? If viruses do indeed cause cancer in man, will it be found that there are many kinds, as is the case in animals? And if such viruses are unmasked, will it be shown that human cancer-causing viruses cause disease in such a way that an effective vaccine will be possible. Only the future will tell. But that future is no longer so distant.[15]

More hope

Today, cancers are treated by *surgical removal, radiation,* and *drugs.* The uses of radiation are limited because the amount needed to destroy all cancer cells also destroys normal tissue. Some drugs act specifically on some tissues. A variety of these have brought years to many leukemia sufferers. Results from a combination of two or more cancer treatments, such as radiation and surgery, are encouraging. New X-ray techniques provide a means of early diagnosis of breast tumors long before they can be felt. Moreover, new laboratory tests promise earlier detection of cancers than ever before. Recently, for example, some Canadian workers isolated a foreign substance—an antigen— from certain bowel tumors that do not appear in normal tissue. A test has been developed to detect as little as one billionth of a part of this antigen in the blood. This holds hope for a diagnostic test for bowel cancer. In addition, it has been found that nearly all animal tumors and some human tumors have antigens on their cell surfaces. These antigens are specific, that is, each tumor has its own set of antigens. It is such new information that offers hope, albeit reserved, for a vaccine for some cancers someday.[16]

For thirty years cancer has been the second leading cause of death in the United States. At present rates, more than fifty million people in this country, one in four, will get cancer. Figure 7-3 shows the cancer incidence by site and sex. In late 1969 the American Cancer Society made its

Extent of the cancer problem

[15] Indeed recent work suggests that an infectious agent called the C-type RNA virus is possibly the underlying cause of all cancers, whether spontaneous or induced by chemical or physical agents. This virus, it is postulated, may be transmitted from mother to child by ordinary genetic processes as if it were a gene (or oncogene, a cancer-causing gene). Such a dormant or covert or latent gene could be "switched on" or triggered, as it were, by some stimulus such as radiation, chemicals, or even another virus.

[16] Barbara J. Culliton, *Science News,* Vol. 95, No. 19 (May 10, 1969), pp. 457–59.

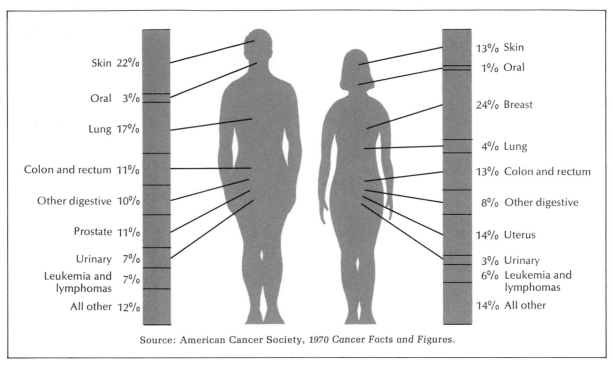

Skin 22% — 13% Skin
Oral 3% — 1% Oral
Lung 17% — 24% Breast
Colon and rectum 11% — 4% Lung
Other digestive 10% — 13% Colon and rectum
Prostate 11% — 8% Other digestive
Urinary 7% — 14% Uterus
Leukemia and lymphomas 7% — 3% Urinary
All other 12% — 6% Leukemia and lymphomas
— 14% All other

Source: American Cancer Society, *1970 Cancer Facts and Figures.*

7-3 Cancer: the incidence by site and sex.

annual—and usually devastatingly accurate—predictions of cancer deaths (Table 7-1).

Yet, as has been suggested above, all is not gloom. First, the figures may, in a sense, be viewed as a price of success. At the turn of the century millions died before they could develop cancer. And some 1,400,000 people of this nation have been cured of cancer. ("Cure," when one is speaking of cancer, means that the person shows no evidence of cancer five years after diagnosis and first treatment.) Thirty years ago 25 percent of cancer patients were cured. By 1960 the figure had crept to 33 percent. In mid-1969 it was 40 percent. That adds up to more than 53,000 saved lives yearly.

A program for cancer prevention
Using health education techniques as a common denominator, any disease prevention program is concerned with the prevention of its occurrence and, failing in this, prevention of its progression. Three basic ways are available to prevent the occurrence of cancer: (1) avoidance of those ecological factors associated with a high incidence of certain malignancies; (2) the removal of lesions that, although not yet malignant, may become cancers; (3) discouragement of marriages that might produce children with a high risk of developing cancers. As is emphasized below, such "hereditary" cancers are exceedingly rare.

TABLE 7-1 Cancer: The Casualty Figures, Warning Signals, and Safeguards

SITE	ESTIMATED NEW CASES 1970	ESTIMATED DEATHS 1970	WARNING SIGNAL (WHEN LASTING LONGER THAN TWO WEEKS SEE YOUR DOCTOR)	SAFEGUARDS	COMMENT
Breast	67,000	29,000	Lump or thickening in the breast.	Annual checkup; monthly breast self-examination.	The leading cause of cancer death in women.
Colon and rectum	73,000	46,000	Change in bowel habits; bleeding.	Annual checkup, including proctoscopy.	Considered a highly curable disease when found early during routine physical examinations.
Lung	68,000	62,000	Persistent cough, or lingering respiratory ailment.	Prevention: heed facts about smoking; annual checkup; chest X-ray.	The leading cause of cancer death among men, this form of cancer is largely preventable.
Oral (including pharynx)	14,000	7,000	Sore that does not heal; difficulty in swallowing.	Annual checkup.	Many more lives should be saved because the mouth is easily accessible to visual examination by physicians and dentists.
Skin	112,000	5,000	Sore that does not heal, or change in wart or mole.	Annual checkup; avoidance of over-exposure to sun.	Readily detected by observation, and diagnosed by simple biopsy.
Uterus	42,000	13,000	Unusual bleeding or discharge.	Annual checkup, including pelvic examination and Papanicolaou smear.	Mortality has declined 50% during the last 25 years. With wider application of the "Pap" smear, many thousands more lives can be saved.
Kidney and bladder	32,000	15,000	Urinary difficulty; bleeding, in which case consult your doctor at once.	Annual checkup with urinalysis.	Protective measures for workers in high-risk industries are helping to eliminate one of the important causes of these cancers.
Larynx	7,000	3,000	Hoarseness; difficulty in swallowing.	Annual checkup, including mirror laryngoscopy.	Readily curable if caught early.
Prostate	35,000	17,000	Urinary difficulty.	Annual checkup, including palpation.	Occurring mainly in men over 60, the disease can be detected by palpation and urinalysis at annual checkup.
Stomach	17,000	16,000	Indigestion.	Annual checkup.	A 40% decline in mortality in 20 years, for reasons yet unknown.
Leukemia	19,000	15,000	Leukemia is a cancer of blood-forming tissues and is characterized by the abnormal production of immature white blood cells. Acute leukemia strikes mainly children and is treated by drugs that have extended life from a few months to as much as three years. Chronic leukemia strikes usually after age 25 and progresses less rapidly.		
			Cancer experts believe that if drugs or vaccines are found that can cure or prevent any cancers they will be successful first for leukemia and the lymphomas.		
Lymphomas	23,000	18,000	These diseases arise in the lymph system and include Hodgkin's disease. Some patients with lymphatic cancers can lead normal lives for many years.		

Source: American Cancer Society, *1970 Cancer Facts and Figures.*

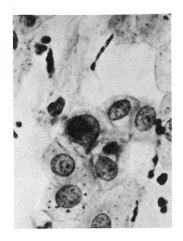

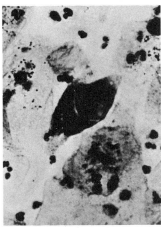

7-4 Slides of Pap smears for microscopic detection of cancer of the uterine cervix: normal cervical cells (*top*) and cervical cancer cells (*bottom*).

Consider the *ecological factors.* Excessive sunlight is a major cause of *skin cancer,* especially among fair people.[17] Although it is a highly curable cancer (with a 92 percent cure rate), it is the most common and still causes about five thousand deaths a year in this country. It usually occurs in people over fifty. However, one-third to one-half of the total lifetime exposure to the sun occurs in the first twenty years of life. The family physician can suggest the most effective sunscreen preparations. Two factors associated with an increased incidence of *cancer of the uterine cervix* (see Table 7-1) are continuing sexual activity at an early age and poor hygiene of the external genitalia.[18,19,20] Promiscuity and too-early marriage account for the first of these. Poor personal hygiene, particularly in the uncircumcised male, results in the collection under the covering penile skin fold (the prepuce) of a thick, creamy, ill-smelling secretion called smegma. With the female it may collect around the clitoris. Smegma has been shown to cause cancer in animals.[21] Some (but not all) cancer experts agree that women whose husbands are circumcised (and are, therefore, able to practice more thorough personal hygiene) have a much lower incidence of cervical cancer than women whose husbands are not circumcised. A simple, painless examination of vaginal fluid, the Papanicolaou test—named after its originator, Dr. George Papanicolaou—provides excellent diagnostic information about cervical cancer. The Pap test (its familiar name) has become a routine part of a physical examination (see Figure 7-4). Women can easily obtain their own cervical cells without going to a physician.[22] Though not as reliable as those obtained by the physician, these cells can be examined by laboratory specialists recommended by him and can be of great diagnostic value.

Cigarette smoking is a cause of *lung cancer.* It is, moreover, associated with an increased incidence of other malignancies, such as those of the mouth and urinary bladder. Cigarette smoking is killing people, and it should be condemned (Chapter 12). Much has been accomplished in *removing cancer-causing agents from the workers' environment.* Workers occupationally exposed to asbestos fibers and uranium miners exposed to ionizing radiation both have increased lung cancer rates. These are but examples of the added preventive work yet to be done.

Precancerous lesions always indicate an immediate, often lifesaving visit to the family physician. The warning signals listed in Table 7-1 may indicate not cancer, but a cellular change that may become malignant if neglected.

[17] Robert G. Freeman and John M. Knox, "Skin Cancer and the Sun," pp. 231–37.

[18] K. S. Moghissi and H. C. Mack, "Epidemiology of Cervical Cancer," *American Journal of Obstetrics and Gynecology,* Vol. 100, No. 5 (March 1, 1968), pp. 607–14.

[19] I. D. Rotkin, "Sexual Patterns and Cervical Cancer," *American Journal of Public Health,* Vol. 57, No. 5 (May 1967), p. 815.

[20] Clyde E. Martin, "Marital and Coital Factors in Cervical Cancer," *ibid.,* p. 803.

[21] William M. Christopherson, "Sex Activity and Cancer of the Cervix," *CA—A Cancer Journal for Clinicians,* Vol. 15, No. 6 (November–December 1965), pp. 278–82.

[22] W. A. D. Anderson and Samuel A. Gunn, "Cancer of the Cervix. Further Studies of Patient-Obtained Vaginal Irrigation Smear," *CA—A Cancer Journal for Clinicians,* Vol. 17, No. 3 (May–June 1967), p. 102.

The extremely rare precancerous and cancerous tumors that are caused by *gene abnormalities* have been mentioned on page 202. Is *cancer of the female breast* solely hereditary? No. It is true that a genetically determined predisposition to a particular cancer may occur in some families. But this genetic predisposition is complicated by many other factors. Studies of cancer incidence in identical twins (that is, with identical genetic constitutions) have shown that the same cancer rarely occurs in both members.[23] It is, however, true that there are a number of instances of breast cancer in identical twins. Moreover, there is evidence of an inherited susceptibility to breast cancer. Statistically, female relatives, particularly sisters, of breast cancer patients have two to three times the tendency to the disease. But the high-risk group also includes those who started menstruating early, have been menstruating for more than thirty years, have never been married, have done little or no breast feeding, have had few or no pregnancies, and have had some previous breast disease.[24] Thus, a host of variables are involved. One could hardly suggest that a woman to whom one or more of these variables applies will inevitably develop breast cancer. Like all other women, however, she should ever be on guard against this scourge. At the end of each menstrual period (but continuing after the menopause), self-examination of the breast is an essential part of every woman's health regimen. This is the procedure:

Step 1: Sit straight before a mirror, first with the arms relaxed at the sides and then raised high above the head. In each position, observe whether any change has occurred in the size or shape of the breasts, especially any abnormal puckering or dimpling of the skin.

Step 2: Lie down, place a folded towel under the left shoulder, raise the left arm and place the hand under the head. With the flat of the fingers of the right hand feel gently the inner half of the left breast, from nipple line to breast bone, and from top to bottom. Less than 20 percent of cancers occur here.

Step 3: Bring the arm down to the side and feel gently the outer half of the breast. Since this is the area of maximum danger, it should be examined with special care. Give particular attention to the upper outer section where most cancers of the breast occur—some 47 percent.

Follow steps 2 and 3 for the right breast.[25]

Any lump or thickening merits immediate consultation with the family physician. Early breast cancer is usually painless. These routine self-examinations supplement, but do not replace, the periodic physical examinations by the family physician. New X-ray techniques are available which can detect breast tumors that are not ordinarily palpable.

[23] P. C. Koller, "Chromosomes: The Genetic Component of the Tumor Cell," in E. J. Ambrose and F. J. C. Rose, eds., *The Biology of Cancer,* (London, 1966), p. 48.
[24] Catherine B. Hess, "Some Epidemiological Aspects of Breast Cancer in Need of Further Investigation," *CA—A Cancer Journal for Clinicians,* Vol. 18, No. 1 (January–February 1968), p. 28.
[25] These directions are provided by the National Cancer Institute, in *Breast Self-Examination,* Public Health Publication No. 48 (Washington, D.C.).

The major element preventing the progression of any cancer is early diagnosis. The most common internal cancers are those of the *rectum* and *colon*. Delay may mean death. Early diagnosis means cure. Using a recently improved appliance for visualizing the affected area with little or no discomfort to the patients, doctors can now diagnose almost three-fourths of these conditions early.

Early diagnosis is similarly crucial with *Hodgkin's disease*. The outlook used to be hopeless for people who had this tumor of the lymph nodes, spleen, and general lymphoid tissue. Today, early intensive treatment promises cure.

In the race for life, cancer always has a head start. It need not win. It is delay, often based on fear, that so often ends in despair. "Through early diagnosis and prompt treatment of cancer, the present survival ratio could be one in two."[26]

The danger signals are summarized in Table 7-1. They are worth repeating and expanding:

1. Any sore that increases in size or does not heal, particularly on the lips, tongue, ears, eyelids, or the genital organs.

2. Any lump or thickening that persists, especially in the breast, tongue, lips, neck, armpit, or groin.

3. Bleeding or abnormal discharge from any body opening, especially the mouth, rectum, vagina, or bladder.

4. A change in bowel habits, particularly after the age of forty, or difficulty in passing urine.

5. Persistent indigestion.

6. Persistent cough, hoarseness, sore throat, or difficulty in swallowing.

7. Unintended loss of weight, continued unexplained fever, or a feeling of weakness.

8. Progressive changes in the color or size of a wart, mole, or birthmark.

9. Persistent headache, or difficulty in seeing.

These signs and symptoms do not necessarily mean cancer. They do require an immediate visit to the family doctor. All physicians have endured the quiet pain that comes when making a cancer diagnosis too late to help. Every physician has a high index of suspicion. He often needs to embark on a time-consuming but always worthwhile investigation. If a cancer is localized, he can hold out hope. If it has escaped from its origin, if there is regional involvement, hope diminishes. In Figure 7-5, note, for example, that if cancer of the breast is localized, the five-year survival rate is 83 percent. Only 52 percent of the women with regional involvement are alive at the end of five years.

But should one unconcernedly await signs and symptoms? No. If cancer is found in symptomless individuals, the outlook is brightest. Every family doctor's office is a cancer detection center. His physical examinations save lives. Moreover, numerous communities sponsor cancer detection pro-

[26] *CA—A Cancer Journal for Clinicians*, Vol. 18, No. 1 (January–February 1968), p. 13.

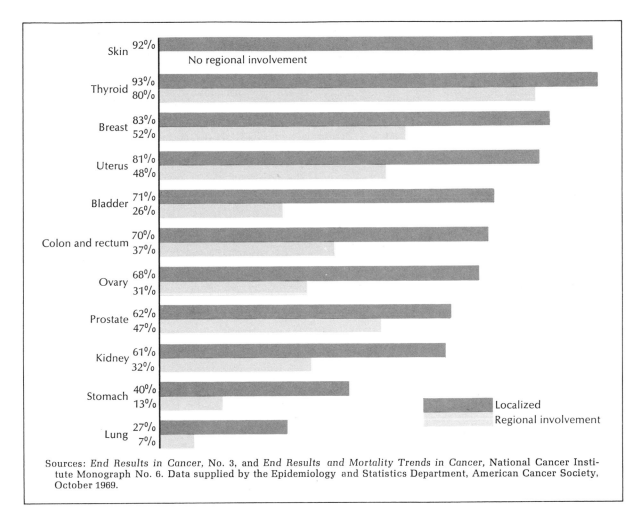

Skin	92%	No regional involvement
Thyroid	93%	
	80%	
Breast	83%	
	52%	
Uterus	81%	
	48%	
Bladder	71%	
	26%	
Colon and rectum	70%	
	37%	
Ovary	68%	
	31%	
Prostate	62%	
	47%	
Kidney	61%	
	32%	
Stomach	40%	
	13%	
Lung	27%	
	7%	

Localized
Regional involvement

Sources: *End Results in Cancer*, No. 3, and *End Results and Mortality Trends in Cancer*, National Cancer Institute Monograph No. 6. Data supplied by the Epidemiology and Statistics Department, American Cancer Society, October 1969.

7-5 Five-year cancer survival rates for selected sites (adjusted for normal life expectancy). Diagnosis before the cancer spreads is lifesaving.

grams. These provide routine cancer examinations for those without symptoms. When found, symptomless cancer patients have a better than average chance for a five-year cure. For example: in a cancer detection center, a woman without symptoms is discovered to have a breast cancer. Her chances of cure are increased as much as 34 percent. Another individual has an early, still symptomless cancer of the colon. His chances of cure are over 35 percent higher than they would be if he had been diagnosed late enough for symptoms to occur. A cancer detection program, provided for all, could save approximately 80,000 lives a year in this country.[27]

[27] Emerson Day, "Value of Regular Medical Examinations," in Ronald W. Raven and J. C. Roe, eds., *The Prevention of Cancer* (London, 1967), p. 367.

Allergy: a swelling

How allergy occurs

Whatever turns your skin to scum,
Or turns your blood to glue,
Why that's the what, the special what,
That you're allergic to.[28]

To be allergic to a causative substance, a susceptible individual must encounter it at least twice. The initial time he is sensitized to it. Later he reacts to it.

At the first encounter, the foreign substance—the antigen—stimulates the body cells to generate specific antibodies to it. The individual shows no symptoms. At the second encounter, the antigen reacts with the very antibodies it had previously caused to be formed. Thus has the reaction of an individual to a specific stimulus been altered. This altered reaction is allergy.

An antigen-antibody reaction on a cell injures the cell. This injury causes the release of histamine and histamine-like substances. When liberated, they cause the dilation of local capillaries and arterioles. More blood rushes to the scene. The injured cells are fed more oxygen, more nourishment, more of life's healing alchemy. With allergy there is an excess influence of histamine and an abnormal dilation of capillaries and arterioles. In overabundance, blood fluid leaks into the tissue spaces. There is swelling. This may occur in a small body organ, or the entire respiratory tree may be involved. In this latter instance, excessive swelling of the lining of the bronchioles (one of the smaller subdivisions of the branched bronchial tree) results in narrowed airways and difficult breathing. In the skin, it is swelling that produces hives. It is swelling that is responsible for all the manifestations of allergy.

"I have gout,[29] asthma, and seven other maladies," wrote Sydney Smith (1771–1845) lugubriously, "but am otherwise very well."[30] The two maladies he names are more than enough.

The kinds of allergic reactions

The various types of allergy are legion and are endured by legions of sufferers. There are the nasal allergies manifested by sneezing, runny stuffed nose, itching, tearing eyes, and dulled hearing, taste, and smell. The sneezing season varies in different areas. In some parts of the East, for example, the sources are trees in March, grasses in May, and weeds in August. Some people, often children, are troubled all year.[31] Commonly, secondary superimposed infections plague them. *Asthma* is an evil manifestation of bronchial allergy. In chronic cases, the constantly irri-

---

[28] Ogden Nash, "Allergy Met a Bear," in *I'm a Stranger Here Myself* (Boston, 1938), p. 125.
[29] See page 213.
[30] *A Memoir of the Reverend Sydney Smith, by His Daughter, Lady Holland, with a Selection of His Letters*, Mrs. Austin, ed., 2nd ed., Vol. I (London, 1885), p. 285.
[31] It is a grievous irony that ragweed, an herb tormenting innumerable asthmatics, is of the genus *Ambrosia*—a word that may also refer to a delicious, fragrant food or drink.

tated, thickened muscle fibers of the smaller breathing tubes go into constricting spasm. The channels of the breathing tubes, already decreased by swollen linings and plugged by thick secretions, are further narrowed. The sufferer coughs, wheezes, struggles for breath. Asthma can debilitate and it can kill. It may require constant medical attention.

The itching raised areas of *hives* may be a skin manifestation of food or drug allergy. *Eczema,* a chronic skin disease, is now considered an allergic illness. A common manifestation of skin allergy is termed *contact dermatitis.* The classic example is poison ivy. However, perfumes, hair bleaches, and similar products are frequent offenders. Some physicians consider the dreadful headache of *migraine* to be caused by an allergy to various foods or inhalants. There is frequently a strong emotional component to these episodes.

The treatments of allergy

The treatments of allergies depend largely on *avoidance of the cause* and, perhaps, *hyposensitization.* In this latter procedure, small, but increasing, doses of the offending agent (antigen) are injected into the susceptible individual. As a result, the patient slowly builds a tolerance to the antigen. Thus, he is able to endure higher doses of exposure before symptoms are precipitated. An example: an individual has symptoms from exposure to small amounts of grasses. By injection he receives small doses of the symptom-causing factors of those grasses. He develops a tolerance to them. Unless exposed to grasses in much larger amounts than ordinary, he then will not have symptoms. The patient is less sensitive. He is *hypo*sensitive.

Treatment with drugs, such as antihistamines, is effective with some patients. They do neutralize histamines and relieve symptoms. But they do not prevent cellular injury. Thus, although treatment of hay fever patients with antihistamines alone is temporarily effective, without added treatment it may be dangerous. Why? Such inadequately treated individuals may develop asthma or bronchitis. Individuals with hay fever should, therefore, seek total treatment from their physicians. Self-medication with over-the-counter antihistamines gives relief, but it is only transient.

Some chronic muscle and joint disorders

"And I have a rheum in mine eyes too, and such an ache in my bones that, unless a man were cursed, I cannot tell what to think on 't."[32]

Gout

When the greatest physician of the seventeenth century, Thomas Sydenham, described the treatment of gout, he did so ruefully. Having himself suffered this agonizing joint affliction for thirty years, he expected his recommended treatments to be greeted with reserve. Unfortunately, this was not the case. The poor advice of great men may live longer than

[32] William Shakespeare, *Troilus and Cressida,* V.iii.104–07.

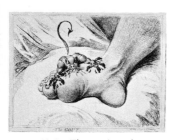

7-6 The pain of gout: a fanciful rendition.

their wisdoms. For two centuries, it was, in part, his opinion that banished the use of the drug colchicum in the treatment of gout. This left gout sufferers with little else but pain.

Sydenham's therapeutic error may even be considered a contributing cause of the American Revolution. More than once, William Pitt rose on his swollen foot in the House of Commons to defend the colonists. "The Americans," he declared, "are entitled to the common rights of representation and cannot be bound to pay taxes without their consent."[33] A particularly violent attack of gout, forcing the English statesman to be absent from the House, made it possible to pass a colonial duty on tea. The Boston Tea Party of 1773 resulted.

The painful, hot, swollen, blue-red joint of the gout sufferer has long and wrongly been attributed to overindulgence in food and drink. In the blood and other body fluids of gout victims there collects an excess of uric acid. This is deposited, as crystals, in the joints and other tissues. The disease runs in families, is rare in women, and is most common in people thirty years of age and older. In this country some 350,000 people are afflicted with it. Elevation of the extremity, rest, drugs, and diet are the best treatment. The diet is partly outlined in these lines:

> *At last the happy truth is out—*
> *Port wine is not the cause of gout;*
> *Far more responsible for pain*
> *Are kidneys, liver, sweetbread, brain—*
> *The Clubman should by any means*
> *Avoid anchovies and sardines.*[34]

Gout is but one of almost fifty *rheumatic diseases*. All have one common denominator: connective tissue is involved. This includes not only the delicate scaffolding between cells, but also the tendons and ligaments, cartilage and fat that provide, along with the bone, the support and shape for the body. In the rheumatic diseases it is usually the muscles and joints that are involved. *Arthritis* (Greek *arthron*, joint + *-itis*, a word ending denoting inflammation) is not a specific disease. It is a joint inflammation causing pain, swelling, and stiffness.

About three-fourths of people with rheumatism have one of two conditions: *rheumatoid arthritis* or *osteoarthritis*.

Rheumatoid arthritis

The use of the word "arthritis" should not mislead one into considering this illness a mere joint inflammation. The connective tissue throughout the whole body is involved. Nobody knows the cause. It is not an infection and is, of course, not communicable. A wide variety of circumstances seem to trigger the disease. These include exposure, surgery, infection,

---

[33] W. S. C. Copeman, *A Short History of the Gout and the Rheumatic Diseases* (Berkeley, 1964), p. 96.
[34] A poem by Sir Alan Herbert, quoted in W. S. C. Copeman, *Arthritis and Rheumatism* (London, 1967), p. 75.

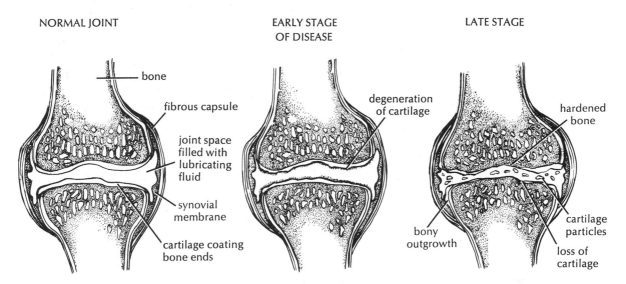

bone

fibrous capsule

joint space filled with lubricating fluid

synovial membrane

cartilage coating bone ends

degeneration of cartilage

hardened bone

bony outgrowth

cartilage particles

loss of cartilage

7-7 A normal joint and early and late stages of osteoarthritis.

cold, and emotional distress. It attacks women more often than men. No other chronic disease disables more people during the working years. Although even infants have the disease, about 80 percent of the cases occur between those vital years, twenty and fifty.

The joints hurt most, the smaller hand joints (particularly the knuckles) most often. If the joints of one hand are affected, the corresponding opposite joints are usually soon involved. In early stages, the individual may experience temporary periods of improvement. It is then that he is most susceptible to quackery.

The outlook is hopeful. The total crippling of another day is now rare. Rest is the most important aspect of treatment. Splints, proper exercise, and physical therapy help to prevent deformity. About one-fourth of the cases of rheumatoid arthritis seem to recover completely. Another half have considerable periods of freedom from the disease. But treatment must be continuously planned. And drugs are the least important aspect of that treatment.

Osteoarthritis is a degenerative joint disease, not an inflammation (see Figures 7-7 and 7-8). The *-itis* is thus unjustified. It is surely the most common of all joint ailments. After forty, almost everyone has it to some degree. Most people, diagnosing their own "arthritis," more likely have degenerative joint disease. Animals are also susceptible. Because of it, more than one racehorse has been put to pasture.

In this chronic condition, cartilage, a specialized fibrous connective tissue, gradually deteriorates. So does bone. This occurs because of the constantly repeated small injuries of weight-bearing. Chronic joint irrita-

Osteoarthritis

7-8 An X-ray of a hand diseased by osteoarthritis. The light areas on either side of the arrow represent increased bone formation, which is partly in response to loss of cartilage in the joint. This joint—the junction of the thumb and wrist—is the most common site of osteoarthritis in the hand.

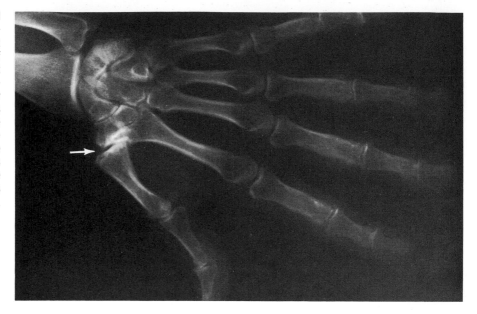

tion due to obesity, poor posture, old damage from infection, dislocation, or fracture—all these promote osteoarthritis. Healing is slow (cartilage is the slowest healing body tissue). Unlike rheumatoid arthritis, with osteoarthritis the damage is local.

There is no cure. However, progression can be arrested. Orthopedic appliances (when necessary), weight reduction, physical therapy, and mild drugs to mitigate discomfort all help.

Rheumatism not involving a joint

A wide variety of rheumatic disorders, involving various body parts other than joints, come under the heading *nonarticular* (Latin *articularis,* of a joint) *rheumatism.* One of these is *fibrositis,* an inflammation of the body's white fibrous tissue, particularly the tissue sheathing muscles. Muscle soreness and stiffness are major symptoms. However, neither joint swelling nor bone damage occurs. Fibrositis is often associated with emotional disorders. It can also be precipitated by strain, cold, and fatigue. *Lumbago* means back pain. It may be a local fibrositis or it may be due to the much more serious rupture of one of the discs between the bones of the spinal column. Each disc is made of *fibrocartilage* (a specialized connective tissue with a considerable groundwork of fibrous tissue). These *intervertebral discs* act as shock absorbers. When damage occurs to the ligaments holding them in place, they slip and bulge. This condition requires expert care. Surgery may be indicated. The pain of *sciatica,* extending along the large branching nerve to the leg, may be caused by a "slipped disc."

Aspirin, injections of anesthetics, heat, massage, light exercise, and hot baths are all useful in treating most of these conditions. If the patient cooperates, the outlook is excellent.

The nervous system: ease and disease

By means of his nervous system man perceives his ecosystems, relates to them, and communicates with other people within them. To deprive him experimentally of almost all environmental stimuli leads to hallucinations, space-time disorientations, even panic. It is perhaps not entirely coincidental that the brain's cerebral cells "are the most sensitive to arrest of circulation, beginning to die within five minutes. The whole brain may be considered dead in 15 minutes."[35] So, although the peripheral nerves live longer, the brain can no longer receive and perceive their messages. That is one reason why victims of threatened heart stoppage or near-drowning need extremely rapid emergency treatment.

The complexity of the nervous system

A mother leans to her baby. Lightly she strokes his cheek, tickling him. His pleasure is intense. Without such love, but no less gently, a stranger tickles the child. The reaction: fear. The tickler, then, must be a familiar person. To enjoy the caress, the infant must associate it with a giver of pleasure, must know that the tickler means no harm, must sense the difference between being tickled pink and tickled to death. So the tickle is more than a pressure stimulus to local skin nerves. Higher brain centers are involved.

Since tickling is but an itch that moves,[36] consider the itch. Only in its immediate relief is there pleasure. Yet first there is pain. A severe itch (as occurs with some skin disorders) insists on virtual violence. The scratch must be enough to tear off the whole upper layer of itching skin, including some of the network of tormenting nerves. So the itch, the itch that moves (the tickle), and skin pain are related. Indeed, all three are thought to be mediated by the same group of nerve cells. They are differentiated high in the brain. But the itch, the tickle, and the skin pain all originated peripherally, as variously intense skin pressures. How did the stimuli reach the brain? By means of the basic working unit of the nervous system, the *neuron*.

The neuron: basic unit of the nervous system

Over ten billion neurons coordinate man's body. Yet the structure of one is typical of them all. Figure 7-9 is a diagram of a neuron. Like other cells, its *cell body* contains a nucleus and other structures. Unlike other cells, its cellular material extends at each end into nerve *fibers* (see body chart 8 in the color section). It is these fine, threadlike extensions of the cell bodies that transmit information from one part of the nervous system to another. A bundle of thousands of nerve fibers constitutes a *nerve*. At one end of the cell body the nerve fiber extensions are the many-twigged *dendrites*. They pick up sensory impulses and transmit them *toward* the cell bodies. From the other pole of the cell body extends the

---

[35] "The Moment of Death," an editorial in *World Medical Journal*, Vol. 14, No. 5 (May 1967), p. 133.
[36] Thomas Mintz, "Tickle—The Itch That Moves," *Psychosomatic Medicine*, Vol. 29, No. 6 (November–December 1967), pp. 606–11.

7-9 A neuron.

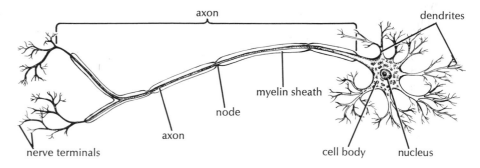

longer, single *axon*, which carries impulses *away* from the cell bodies. Most (but not all) axons are sheathed in a whitish substance called *myelin*, which probably acts as an insulator. The degeneration of this myelin sheath results in *multiple sclerosis* (page 229). *Nodes* are constrictions of the myelin sheath at regular intervals. They behave as relay stations to improve conduction of a nerve impulse. The axon terminates in many branching filaments or *nerve terminals*. However, the myelin sheath disappears just before these branches occur.

The transmission of a nerve impulse

What happens when a stimulus—such as a tickle, an itch, or a skin pain—is received by a sensory nerve terminal? At that point the energy of the stimulus is converted into an electrochemical process. The electrochemical change then progresses along the nerve fiber, causing a small, but measurable electric current—a *nerve impulse*. The impulse is usually transmitted in one direction—from the dendrites of one neuron, through its cell body, along the axon, to the dendrites or cell body of a second neuron or to a muscle or gland.

In considering the process of nerve impulse transmission several concepts should be kept in mind.

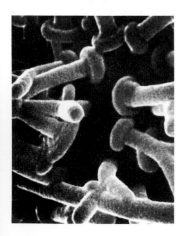

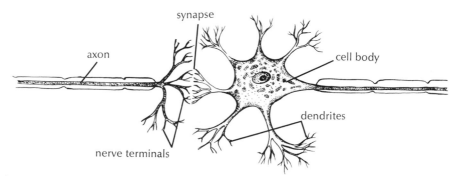

7-10 Two views of the synapse: a diagram (*above*) and one of the first photographs of nerve fibers and synaptic knobs (*left*). It is believed the knobs pass nerve impulses from one cell to another.

1. The place where the nerve terminals of an axon meet the dendrites or cell body of a second neuron is called a *synapse* (Figure 7-10). A synapse is a tiny space. When a nerve impulse reaches the end of an axon, a chemical is released into the synaptic space. This chemical acts as the intermediary between neurons, making possible the transmission of nerve impulses between them.

2. Neurons do not necessarily have a simple one-to-one relationship. The axons of hundreds of neurons can make synaptic junctions with the dendrites and cell body of a single neuron.

3. Neurons vary enormously in length. Remarkably, a single neuron may extend from the tip of the finger to the spinal cord. Or, in the brain, a single neuron may be but a microscopic fraction of an inch in length.

1. The *afferent* or *sensory neurons* (Latin *ad,* to or toward + *ferre,* to carry) conduct messages *toward* the brain and spinal cord from the sensory *receptor organs* of the body (see Figure 7-11). A sensory receptor organ is a sensory nerve ending that responds to stimuli of various kinds. The five senses, of course, are sight, hearing, taste, smell, and variations of touch. In the *skin* there are five general kinds of receptors: those sensitive to touch, pressure, pain, cold, and heat. When stimulated, these are activated to relay information to the spinal cord and brain. Various combinations of skin receptors combine to give more complex skin sensations such as burning or tickling. Receptors of messages that stimulate nerves are also found in the muscles, tendons, and joints. These are involved with the sense of body position and with muscle movements. Many sources may stimulate man at the same time. He must react with coordinated and integrated harmony. He touches a pot of percolating coffee. Not only are most of the receptors of the five primary skin senses stimulated, but those of hunger are stimulated as well.

2. *Efferent* or *motor neurons* (Latin *ex,* out + *ferre,* to carry) conduct impulses *from* the central nervous system to the muscles, glands, or blood vessels. Organs functioning as a result of such nerve impulses are called *effector organs.* They include the muscles and glands.

The three types of neurons

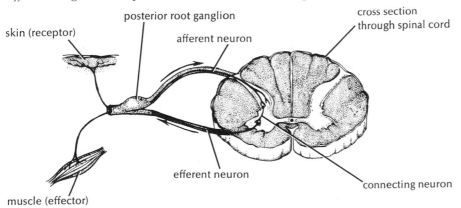

skin (receptor)

posterior root ganglion

afferent neuron

cross section through spinal cord

efferent neuron

connecting neuron

muscle (effector)

7-11 Transmission of a nerve impulse. Illustrated here is the path of a stimulus received by skin and carried to muscle.

THE NERVOUS SYSTEM: EASE AND DISEASE **219**

3. The *connecting neurons* are those between other neurons. Most of them are in the brain and spinal cord.

During evolution, as neurons increased in man's brain and their interconnections became more complex, man became less a creature of instinct and more a creature of reflection. He began to associate, to differentiate, to question his instincts. It is by using these neurons that he thinks to pick up a stone on the moon and to learn about it rather than to kick it out of the way. Rigidly inherited neuron patterns send birds on their migrations. But in man these have evolved into unique complex cerebral neurons used in thought. They compel him to think: "Here I will stay. This I will do. It is my duty." Even as a child, man had neurons associating, differentiating. For that is how the baby "decides" that the mother's caress is pleasurable and the stranger's tickle frightening.

New explorations of the brain

"Oh the brain, the brain! . . . oh the nerves, the nerves," wrote Charles Dickens, "the mysteries of this machine called man!"[37] Much of this machine remains a mystery. But not all.

Recently a Yale physiologist reported the case of an eleven-year-old boy institutionalized because of uncontrollable epilepsy and destructive behavior. Drugs were inadequate. To direct brain surgery that was being contemplated, electrodes were implanted in the boy's brain for several days. It was found that electrical stimulation of a certain brain convolution made the boy friendly and more communicative. In the past, the outlook for this young patient would have been dim. But today there is hope:

> In human beings, implanted electrodes are now used in major hospitals for the diagnosis and treatment of difficult cases of epilepsy, involuntary movements, organic pain, anxiety, and other illnesses. The presence of electrodes in the brain is not harmful or even uncomfortable, and patients lead normal lives in their own homes, going to work and returning to the hospital from time to time for ambulatory therapy.[38]

Such benefits for human beings have resulted from continuing animal experiments. Stimulation of specific brain centers by radio signals has brought about reactions ranging from halting a charging bull (see Figure 7-12) to inducing a mother monkey to ignore her infant. With electrical stimulation in one brain area a cat will purr happily at an approaching mouse. Stimulation in another area precipitates rage at a friend. So modern science is reaching into the complexities of the nervous system to help mankind. What is the gross structure of this system? What are some of its afflictions?

---

[37] Charles Dickens, *Christmas Books* (London, 1954), p. 129.
[38] José M. R. Delgado, "Radio-Controlled Behavior," *New York State Journal of Medicine*, Vol. 69, No. 3 (February 1, 1969), pp. 413–14.

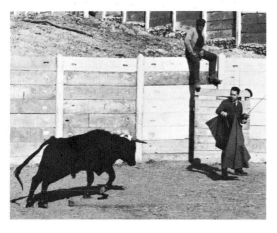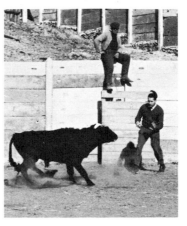

A radio-controlled "bull-fight." The charging bull (*left*) is stopped short (*right*) when the experimenter presses a button on the radio transmitter he is holding. The transmitter sends a mild current to electrodes that were planted into specific places in the bull's brain.

The entire nervous system has been seen to be a complex arrangement of neurons designed to bring about appropriate responses to internal and external environmental stimuli. The stimuli are picked up by body's far-flung sensory receptor organs. The impulses are then conducted, via sensory nerve pathways, to the brain and spinal cord, where they are sorted. They are then transmitted by efferent nerves to responding effector organs. The main divisions of the nervous system are the *central nervous system* and the *peripheral nervous system*. The central nervous system consists of the *brain* and *spinal cord*. The remainder of the nervous system is peripheral. It includes the *cranial* and *spinal nerves* as well as the *autonomic nervous system*. (See Figure 7-14 and body charts 7 and 8 in the color section.)

A general view of nervous system structure

The central nervous system

The brain and spinal cord act as a clearing house for receiving, classifying, and appraising information from the environment. Having done this, they instruct the more than six hundred muscles and the glands how to respond. Completely surrounded and bathed by a protective cushion of clear fluid, enveloped by three membranes (*meninges*) and encased in bone (the skull's *cranium* and the spine's *vertebral column*), the brain and spinal cord directly or indirectly affect every one of the trillions of body cells.

Not all stimuli reach the brain for decision. Some simple, local reflexes, such as the knee-jerk, are handled in the cord. But the brain is the body's ruling organ. At birth the human brain weighs about one pound, approximately one-seventh of the baby's total body weight. The average adult male brain, which weighs about three pounds, is some five and one-half ounces heavier than that of the female. Within the same species, there is no relation between brain weight and intelligence. The largest brain ever recorded belonged to an imbecile. There is, however, a relation between species and brain–body-weight ratios. The delightful dolphin (the large species) has a brain that weighs more (3.5 pounds) than man's,

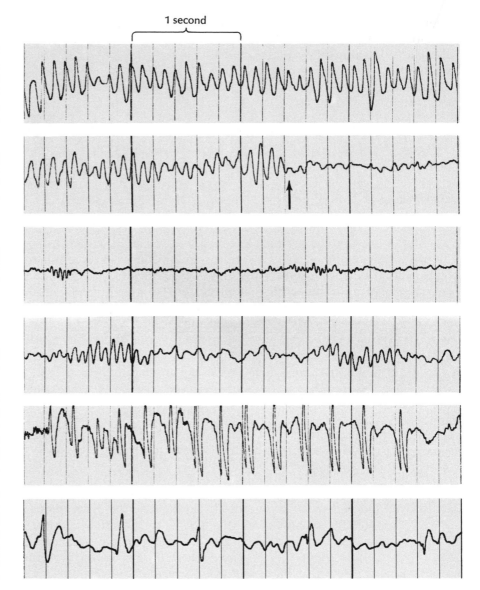

a. Normal rhythm (about 10 cycles per second). Such regular brain waves, characteristic of the relaxed state, are called alpha waves.

b. Alpha brain wave activity is here blocked when the subject opens his eyes (arrow).

c. Brain waves during rapid eye movement (REM) sleep.

d. Brain waves during moderately deep sleep.

e. Alternating spiked waves and slow waves characteristic of epilepsy, generally petit mal but also grand mal (page 228).

f. Spiked waves from one part of the brain, indicating epilepsy of local origin. When the discharges spread to both brain hemispheres, grand mal may occur.

1 second

7-13 Electroencephalograph recordings from the scalp.

but its body weight is twice as great as man's. Man has the highest brain-body-weight ratio of all creatures.

Body chart 7 in the color section shows a cross section of the human brain and a portion of the spinal cord. The brain consists of a *cerebrum*, *cerebellum*, and *brain stem*. The cerebrum is divided into left and right cerebral *hemispheres*. The wrinkled surface of these hemispheres is the *cerebral cortex*. In it are the complexities of humanness, for it is responsible for the distinction that is man. The *cerebellum* is a coordinator, being responsible for muscle tone, body balance, and the rhythms of body movements. The *brain stem* supports the cerebral hemispheres. It contains pathways to and from the cerebral cortex as well as nerve centers controlling a wide variety of body functions including the heartbeat, breathing, digestion, body temperature, and blood pressure.

Electrical energy is constantly produced in the normal brain. This electrical activity can be traced in definite patterns, or waves, on an *electroencephalogram* (EEG). When the brain has been excited, brain waves are rapid and of small amplitude. Brain waves show characteristic changes in various stages of sleep (see Figure 7-13, c and d). People with head injuries, tumors, infections, and hemorrhages may show electroencephalographic changes. Epileptics usually reveal abnormal electroencephalograms. The electroencephalogram is a valuable, painless diagnostic tool. However, emotional disorders are generally not detected by the EEG.

The spinal cord is continuous with the brain stem and is that part of the nervous system enclosed in the bony vertebral column. It is, however, much shorter than its bony protector and ends in a group of tail-like nerves that go to the organs within the pelvis and to the lower extremities.

The *cerebrospinal fluid* circulates not only around the outside surfaces of the brain and spinal cord but also around their internal surfaces. By inserting a needle through a space between two vertebral bodies of the vertebral column, a small amount of this cerebrospinal fluid may be withdrawn for examination (*spinal tap*). In this examination the needle does not touch spinal cord tissue. Spinal taps are important in the diagnosis of certain neurologic diseases. For spinal anesthesia, an anesthetic is introduced into the space filled with cerebrospinal fluid.

The peripheral nervous system

The *peripheral nervous system* is composed of all nervous structures not included in the brain and spinal cord. It brings environmental stimuli to the central nervous system and relays instructions from it to the body's effector organs.

Twelve pairs of peripheral nerves issue directly from the brain. They are called *cranial nerves* and chiefly supply the head and neck. However, one of the pairs of cranial nerves (the *vagus* nerve) extends to the heart, blood vessels, and other internal organs (see body chart 7 in the color section). Other cranial nerves include the *acoustic* (hearing), *optic* (seeing), and *olfactory* (smelling) nerves. There are cranial nerves controlling balance, eye motion, speech, taste, and other functions. The thirty-one pairs of *spinal nerves* carry impulses between the spinal cord and the skin and muscle below the brain level.

Part of the peripheral nervous system, the *autonomic* of "self-controlling" *nervous system,* has the specialized task of regulating body functions over which an individual has no control. Heart rate, circulation, part of the sexual function, digestion, respiration—all these self-regulatory body activities that are not governed by the will are controlled by the autonomic nervous system.

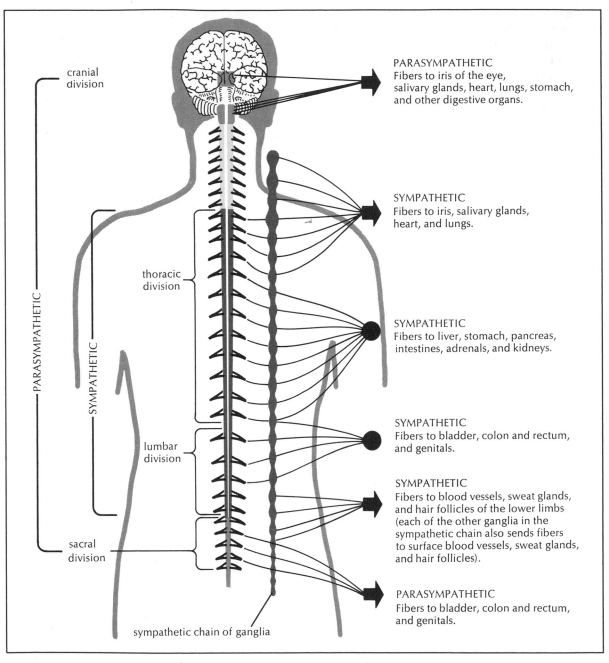

cranial division

PARASYMPATHETIC
Fibers to iris of the eye,
salivary glands, heart, lungs, stomach,
and other digestive organs.

SYMPATHETIC
Fibers to iris, salivary glands,
heart, and lungs.

thoracic division

SYMPATHETIC
Fibers to liver, stomach, pancreas,
intestines, adrenals, and kidneys.

PARASYMPATHETIC

SYMPATHETIC

lumbar division

SYMPATHETIC
Fibers to bladder, colon and rectum,
and genitals.

SYMPATHETIC
Fibers to blood vessels, sweat glands,
and hair follicles of the lower limbs
(each of the other ganglia in the
sympathetic chain also sends fibers
to surface blood vessels, sweat glands,
and hair follicles).

sacral division

PARASYMPATHETIC
Fibers to bladder, colon and rectum,
and genitals.

sympathetic chain of ganglia

7-14 The autonomic nervous system. The sympathetic system is characterized by chains of ganglia on either side of the spinal cord as well as by other large ganglia (represented here by large circles). The parasympathetic system has its ganglia (not shown) nearer the organs stimulated. Only half the autonomic nervous system is shown here; it is duplicated on the other side of the spinal cord.

The autonomic nervous system has two divisions, the *sympathetic* and *parasympathetic* (Figure 7-14). The sympathetic division is composed of nerve fibers and masses of cell bodies called *ganglia,* which are located on either side of the spinal column (see body chart 7 in the color section). Sympathetic nerves are concerned with emotions. When a person is under stress, the sympathetic division takes over from the parasympathetic division, which predominates when the person is relaxed.

A soldier is about to attack. Suddenly, he is overcome by anxiety. The sympathetic nerves have gone into action. His heart is "in his mouth." Why? Its rate has greatly increased. He feels weak and needs energy. To help, the liver releases sugar into his blood. The muscular contraction of his intestine decreases. By constricting the intestinal blood vessels, the sympathetic nerves diminish the intestine's blood supply. Sympathetic nerve action dilates the pupils of his eyes and causes his sweat of fear.

The attack is over. He has survived. Now he rests, even relaxes. The parasympathetic division of the autonomic nervous system has taken over. It constricts the pupils of his eyes, decreases his heart rate, permits the liver to again store sugar, dilates his blood vessels, and increases the involuntary movements of his intestine.

Sometimes the two autonomic divisions work together. In the male sexual act, erection is parasympathetic in origin; ejaculation, sympathetic.

The Boston arm

The electrochemical nature of nerve impulses has afforded help to the disabled. By 1961 the Russians were using electrical signals from muscles to operate an open-and-close artificial hand. In this country, using electrical signals stemming from muscle tension, a motor-driven elbow has been developed. From this has been invented the artificial "Boston arm" (Figure 7-15). An amputee who has lost an arm can, nonetheless, cerebrally will it into action. The ennervated stump muscle discharges the same signal as an arm would discharge. In the Boston arm, this electric signal is amplified. The amplified electric current controls a battery-powered electric motor in the arm. (The battery is worn in a belt around the waist.) The motor sends the arm into action. Ten pounds can be lifted with the Boston arm. Fifty pounds can be held back. And, to repeat, its control is willed by the user, through neurons high in the brain.[39]

Some disorders of the central nervous system

A basic fact about the central nervous system is that neurons in the adult central nervous system do not divide. That is why some spinal cord injuries are permanent. That is also why early treatment is so important in nervous system diseases. Early removal of a brain tumor, for example, can prevent widespread, hopeless dysfunction. Early treatment of syphilis infection precludes irreversible nervous (and other) damage. So it is with other assaults to the nervous system, such as those occurring from poisoning (alcoholism, for example) and malnourishment (beriberi, for example).

[39] *Hospital Tribune*, October 7, 1968, p. 8.

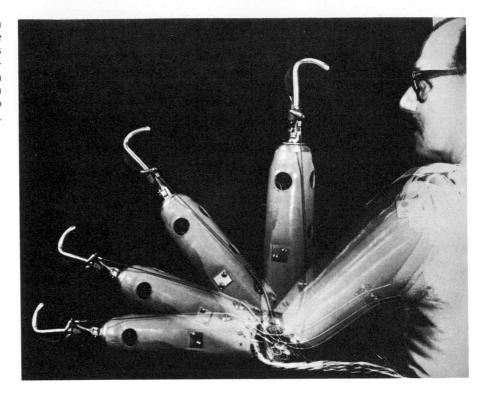

7-15 A stop-action photograph of the "Boston arm." This is the first above-the-elbow artificial arm that an amputee can literally will into action.

The loss of function from a nervous system disease—such as a tumor or infection—depends on where the lesion is and how severe it is. One brain tumor will produce only a pressure headache; another may advance to a withering affliction in which few functions are spared. A few of the more common nervous system diseases are briefly discussed here.

Encephalitis

Encephalitis (Greek *encephalos*, brain + *-itis*), or inflammation of the brain, may be caused by a direct infection (usually a virus) or by a complication of another infection. The encephalitis that may follow mumps rarely has serious consequences. That following regular measles (rubeola) may kill or result in permanent mental and physical retardation. Encephalitis is usually accompanied by a *meningitis,* or inflammation of the meninges, the membranes that envelop the brain and spinal cord.

Stroke

When the blood supply to the brain is impeded, the resultant lack of oxygen causes death of tissue. This *cerebrovascular disease* is called *stroke* (see pages 256 and 265). It may be precipitated either by the formation of a clot in a cerebral vessel or by the rupture of such a vessel that has been weakened by disease. Paralysis and anesthesia (loss of feeling) result. Since each cerebral hemisphere controls the opposite part of the body, right-sided paralysis indicates left cerebral involvement and vice versa. With most people the left side of the brain is the area controlling the learning of speech. Damage to that side may deprive a person of the ability to talk. If there has been bleeding, some of the clot may be absorbed. The pressure on the brain is then relieved, and there is some recovery. Unlike the nerve fibers of the peripheral nervous system, the fibers of the adult central nervous system do not repair, and some permanent damage is not uncommon.

Strokes may be considered from both preventive and rehabilitative aspects. About three-fourths of stroke patients have warning signs and symptoms. Weakness of one or more extremities, speech difficulties, dizziness—these may herald an impending stroke. They are "little strokes." By early treatment of little strokes, big strokes can often be prevented. The great majority of stroke sufferers survive their first major episode. The stroke victim can learn to use undamaged nerve pathways and to strengthen weak muscles. Early and intensive rehabilitative treatment can do much to return stroke victims to useful lives.

Spinal cord tumor

As has been seen, the spinal cord, snugly protected within the bony vertebral column, connects the brain with the spinal nerves. In addition to pain, a wide variety of symptoms may result from a spinal cord tumor because of sheer compression of the spinal cord against its bony container. None are easy to bear. Leg weakness, paralysis, spasticity, and disturbance of sensation may all occur. Such a spinal cord tumor is, if possible, surgically removed.

Epilepsy

The ancients considered those who suffered seizures (Greek *epilepsis*, seizure) divine. Hippocrates, however (late 5th century B.C.), rejected his contemporaries' concept that epilepsy was a *morbus sacer*—a holy disease. And the description of epilepsy by the Roman poet Lucretius (96?–55 B.C.) was hardly spiritual: "Ofttimes with vi'lent fits a patient falls, / As if with thunder struck; and foams and bawls."[40]

On various occasions Shakespeare, too, refers to the condition. In Othello (IV.i.51–52), Iago tells Cassio: "My lord is fall'n into an epilepsy / This is his second fit, he had one yesterday."

Today, between four and six of every one thousand people in this country have epilepsy. It is a mark neither of unusual intelligence nor of mental retardation. Nor is it a disease as such. It is but a sign of a disorder of brain electrical activity. Thus, it can often be diagnosed with

---

[40] From *On the Nature of Things,* quoted in Heinrich Oppenheimer, *Medical and Allied Topics in Latin Poetry* (London, 1928), p. 302.

the electroencephalogram (see page 222). Even between seizures many persons with epilepsy will show abnormal EEG patterns. The causes of the seizures (such as trauma or infection) are known in less than half the cases. Rarely, seizures are precipitated by flashing lights of a suitable frequency, such as those emanating from a flickering television picture.

The most common types of epilepsy are *petit mal* (French, "little illness"), *grand mal,* and *psychomotor. Petit mal* episodes are manifested by momentary blackouts of consciousness and muscular twitchings. They may occur dozens of times a day. *Grand mal* seizures are more severe. Usually the affected person falls and is unconscious for some time. He may froth at the mouth or bite his tongue or lose control of bowel and bladder. *Psychomotor epilepsy* is manifested by unusual behavior. The individual smacks his lips or picks at his clothes. Often, he is confused and restless. A nameless terror may accompany such a seizure. Following all this, there is no memory of the attack.

Many absurd superstitions still surround epilepsy. For the vast majority of epileptics, research has made possible normal life and employability. To more than fifty percent of all epileptics, various combinations of modern medications have brought literally complete convulsion control. Another thirty percent lead almost normal lives; their convulsions are relatively infrequent. There is a genetic predisposition to most forms of epilepsy. Those concerned about marrying a person with epilepsy will find genetic counseling helpful (see page 554). However, the great majority of epileptics are just as dependable parents as anyone else.

Cerebral palsy

Well over half a million people in this country have cerebral palsy. Every year, ten thousand more are born with the condition. The brain lesion causing cerebral palsy may occur before birth as a developmental failure. It may follow such infections as whooping cough and measles. It may be rooted in a blood incompatibility involving the Rh blood factor (see page 546). Head injury may be the cause. Thus, not all cerebral palsy results from birth injury. Moreover, brain damage can vary from mild involvement, with few, hardly discernible symptoms, to a widespread spastic paralysis (associated with severe tremor) and poor coordination.

Usually, there is more than one handicap. In half the cases speech defects occur. So do visual defects. About twenty-five percent have hearing problems. Another twenty-five percent have convulsions. About half of those with cerebral palsy are retarded.

It is a tragic truth that many thousands suffering cerebral palsy are unable to put to use the abilities they do have. Shortages of community facilities combine with indifference, even hostility, to deprive them of opportunity. Early diagnosis, combined with active treatment, rehabilitation, and education, can provide the willing community with many useful citizens.

Multiple sclerosis

In *multiple sclerosis* (Greek *skleros*, hard) hardening of nerve tissue is distributed throughout the brain or spinal cord or both. Neither the cause nor the cure of this disease is known. Nor is present treatment adequate. However, modern physical therapy and other rehabilitative efforts today hold out the promise of years of productive life to these patients.

In this country an estimated quarter-million people have this progressive disease. For reasons unknown, it occurs more often in cold climates than it does in warm climates. The rate and degree of progression vary with individuals. The onset age is during the prime years—twenty to forty. The basic lesion is a patchy loss of *myelin*, the fatty covering that protects and insulates the nerve fibers of the brain and spinal cord. The myelin is replaced by scar tissue. One area may lose its myelin, unaccountably seem to improve, and then degenerate further. (It is during such periods of remission that the patient, believing himself permanently improving, may become prey to a quack.) Eventually, widespread patchy degeneration results in a host of distressing symptoms such as weakness, numbness, double vision, tremor, and slurring of the speech. There may be loss of bowel and bladder control. Paralysis slowly develops. Occasionally the disease will progress rapidly.

Present arduous research offers hope for this difficult disease. It has been noted that human multiple sclerosis and scrapie (a nervous system disease of sheep caused by a virus) are similar. This does not mean that multiple sclerosis is viral or communicable. However, it is a clue worth pursuing.[41] Other sophisticated studies, aimed at a better understanding of the myelin mystery, have led to incidental information about other previously unknown factors of this nerve disease. Knowledge of the cause of the degenerative change may yet lead to its prevention and cure.

"The shaking palsy": Parkinson's syndrome

In 1915, the war-harrassed Romanians reported an alarming sleeping sickness epidemic. It was not until 1917 that a Viennese neurologist, Constantine von Economo, identified the causative illness. By 1918, the epidemic had left Europe reeling. (That unhappy continent was still suffering from the war and influenza.) It then reached American shores.

It is thought that this inflammation of the brain (believed to be viral) left many with the residual lesions of *Parkinson's syndrome*. Note the word "syndrome"—a complex of symptoms. Described a century and a half ago by a London doctor, James Parkinson, the disease is associated with the lack of a body chemical called dopamine. The lesion is deep in the brain. The limbs and trunk become rigid, the face masklike. The patient, usually elderly, may, to his embarrassment, drool. At rest, he has a four-to-six

---

[41] Robert W. Leader, "The Kinship of Animal and Human Disease," *Scientific American*, Vol. 216, No. 1 (January 1967), pp. 110–11.

per second shaking tremor of the hands. When he moves, the tremor improves. He may well be depressed. But his mental ability is unaffected.

A promising new drug, L-dopa, is under present investigation. This drug is changed by the brain cells to yield the lacking chemical, dopamine. In a recently reported trial with the drug at the Cornell University Medical College, two-thirds of patients with Parkinson's disease showed improvement rated either "good" or "excellent."[42] In selected cases, a unique surgery may relieve those whose tremor is worse on one side of the body. A lesion is purposely placed on the side of the brain supplying the more affected side. On the operating table, the patient may notice the dramatic diminution in tremor. Physical therapy also helps.

Sight:
a special sense—
order and disorder

"The light of the body is the eye" (Matthew 6:22).

The blind poet John Milton wrote these poignant lines:

> *Why was the sight*
> *To such a tender ball as th' eye confin'd?*
> *So obvious and so easy to be quench't,*
> *And not as feeling through all parts diffus'd,*
> *That she might look at will through every pore?*[43]

To substitute for the lost vision, the blind do indeed learn skillful use of other body parts. The dependence of actual seeing, however, on "such a tender ball" starkly emphasizes the constant need of preventive protection. The anatomic delicacy of the eye lends to its inordinate vulnerability. Like enemies of the night, some vision disorders develop stealthily, insidiously. Before one is aware enough to act, the damage is done and, often, permanent. Hence, the importance, at all ages, of routine, frequent eye examinations. With a five-year-old, for example, even mild nearsightedness (see Figure 7-19) is important. Like other eye conditions, this has a tendency to worsen with time. Early attention can prevent much vision loss.

Eye problems are rampant among school children. One survey[44] of some 200,000 Philadelphia school children from kindergarten through the twelfth grade revealed almost one in five with defective vision or eye strain. Older people suffer an even more appalling vision loss:

> *About 3.5 million people in the United States have some chronic*
> *or permanent visual impairment, in addition to those with refractive*
> *errors correctable to the extent that they have no trouble seeing.*

---

[42] "Parkinson Mobility, Gait Improved with L-Dopa," *Medical Tribune*, Vol. 10, No. 72 (September 8, 1969), pp. 1, 22.

[43] Quoted in Kester Svendsen, *Milton and Science* (Cambridge, Mass., 1956), p. 185.

[44] Walter H. Fink, "Ocular Defects in Preschool Children," *The Sight-saving Review*, Vol. 24, No. 4 (1954), pp. 196–200.

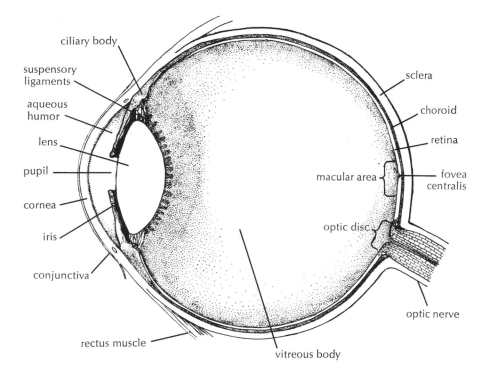

ciliary body
suspensory ligaments
aqueous humor
lens
pupil
cornea
iris
conjunctiva
rectus muscle
vitreous body
sclera
choroid
retina
macular area
fovea centralis
optic disc
optic nerve

Half of these are 65 or over, and 2 of 3 of those with severe visual impairment are in this age group.[45]

Eye structure and function

The fluid of the eyeball is contained by a three-layered wall. These three layers, or coats, are the *sclera, choroid,* and *retina.* The tough *sclera,* the outer layer, sheaths the whole eyeball except the *cornea.* The sclera helps maintain the shape of the eyeball. It is the white of the eye and it protects the eye's delicate inner structure.

It is this fluid under pressure, regulated by a tiny system of canals, that keeps the ball of the eye normally tensed. Behind the lens, the jellylike *vitreous body* (99 percent water) fills the rear of the eyeball (see Figure 7-16). The *aqueous fluid (aqueous humor),* smaller in amount, fills the space in front of the lens. The aqueous fluid is constantly provided by filtration from, and through, capillaries. Normally it is drained off into the blood through a canal around the cornea.

Only the front center of the eye, the transparent cornea, which is a continuation of the sclera, is the true "window of the eye." It is so clear that it seems to be without structure. Actually it is composed of at least five layers of flat cells. Each layer is cemented on the other, like sheets

---

[45] Harry J. Bakst, "Prevention in Geriatric Practice," in Duncan W. Clark and Brian MacMahon, eds., *Preventive Medicine* (Boston, 1967), p. 722.

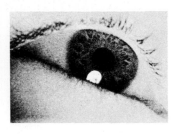

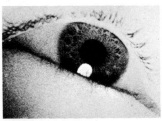

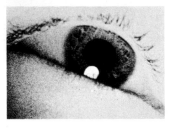

7-17 Pupil response of a man looking at a picture of a pretty woman. These three photographs show (from top to bottom) a 30 percent increase in pupil size over a period of 2½ seconds. Pupils dilate with other pleasant stimuli and constrict with unpleasant stimuli.

of plate glass. Damage to the cornea may scar it. A severe scar may cause blindness. In a majority of carefully selected cases, corneal transplants are successful. Eye banks now preserve donor corneas for long periods.

Most of the blood supply to the eye is contained in the pigmented, middle *choroid* layer. Except for its opening in front, which is the *pupil* (seen as the darkest center spot of the eye), the middle choroid layer surrounds the entire eyeball. The choroid layer continues around the pupil as an encircling band, the *iris* (Greek *iris*, rainbow). The iris lends the eye its color. Expanding in front, the choroid is also continuous with the *ciliary body,* which is mostly the *ciliary muscle.* The iris, lying between the cornea and the lens, is attached to the ciliary body. Suspended behind the iris is the crystalline, elastic *lens.* It is attached to the ciliary body by a *suspensory ligament.* The function of the lens is to send light rays to focus an image on the retina. By contracting, the ciliary muscle controls the shape of the lens and helps to adjust the eye to see near objects. Moreover, the iris itself is made up of tiny, exquisitely arranged, radiating and circular muscle fibers. Light waves are collected by the transparent cornea and then pass through the pupil. The muscle fibers controlling the size of the pupil are supplied by the sympathetic and parasympathetic nerve fibers of the autonomic nervous system. By their contraction or dilation, the iris muscle fibers regulate pupil size and, therefore, the amount of light entering the eye (see Figure 7-17).

The innermost layer of the eyeball, the *retina,* is an extension of the optic nerve leading to the brain. It lines the back two-thirds of the choroid of the inner eye chamber. The retina contains a layer of specialized visual receptor cells called *rods* and *cones.* These cells (there are ten layers in the retina) convert light rays into nerve impulses. Tiny nerve fibers, collecting these impulses, combine to form the *optic nerve,* which is the single nerve bundle leaving the orbit for the brain. (The orbit is the bony cavity containing the eyeball.)

The point of exit of the optic nerve from the eyeball is a blind spot, the *optic disc.* The *fovea* of the retina, a tiny pit about one degree wide, and the area surrounding it, the *macular area,* is the region of clearest vision. Using an instrument called an ophthalmoscope (Greek *ophthalmos,* eye + *skopein,* to examine), the physician can examine the retina. A brain tumor, for example, may push the optic disc into the eyeball or, from injury or inflammation, the retina may become detached. A variety of conditions, such as diabetes and arteriosclerosis, are reflected by retinal changes.

Disorders of vision

GLAUCOMA   When the canal draining the aqueous fluid is clogged, drainage cannot occur. Pressure within the whole eyeball increases. The delicate nerve cells and fibers are damaged. This condition is *glaucoma.* Chronic infections and poor general health aggravate this disorder. It may be associated with defective circulation. The individual complains of

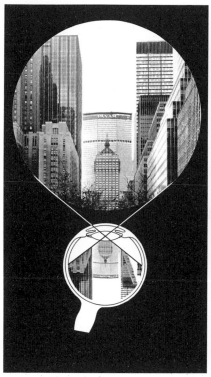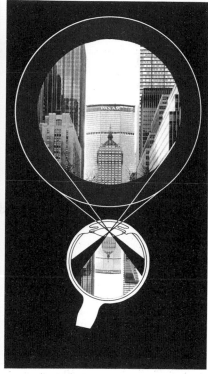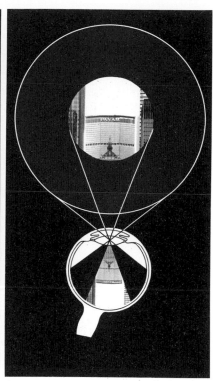

7-18 Glaucoma narrows vision: normal vision (*left*), early glaucoma (*center*), and advanced glaucoma (*right*). Without adequate treatment, the person may eventually lose all sight.

blurred vision, halos, and rainbows around lights. In a darkened room, his eyes may hurt. Frequent changes of glasses do not help. Side vision is the first to go. There is only tunnel vision (see Figure 7-18). Slowly, the nerves of sight are crushed. Delay is disastrous. A painless, quick test measures pressure within the eyeball. With early diagnosis, eye drops usually prevent further blindness. To relieve the pressure, surgery may be necessary.

CATARACT   *Cataract* (Greek *katarregnumi,* to break down) is a cloudiness in the lens. Therefore, light cannot pass through the lens. Cataract can occur at any age. A newborn, infected by the mother's German measles, may be born with cataracts. If no other eye damage is present, surgery is helpful. The cloudy lens is removed and eyeglasses are worn to properly focus images on the retina.

PROBLEMS OF FOCUS   As one ages, the lens dries. It loses elasticity and becomes denser. Its ability to bend light is diminished. Thus images fall in back of the retina. This condition is *farsightedness,* or *hyperopia. Nearsightedness,* or *myopia,* is a disorder in which the images fall in front of the retina. Figure 7-19 illustrates both disorders and also the effect of corrective lenses on each. *Astigmatism* (Figure 7-20) occurs because two adjacent portions of the cornea have different curvatures.

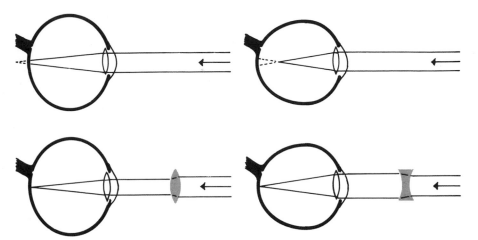

7-19 Farsightedness (*top left*) and its correction with a convex lens (*bottom left*), and nearsightedness (*top right*) and its correction with a concave lens (*bottom right*). In both cases, the corrective lens makes images fall on the retina.

Some light rays focus on the retina, other rays focus in front of it, and still others focus behind it. Part of the image is blurred.[46] A lens that bends only the nonfocusing light rays is corrective.

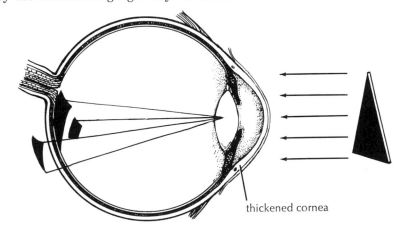

thickened cornea

7-20 Astigmatism. Because two adjacent portions of the cornea have different curvatures, light rays focus improperly.

TWO DISSIMILAR BUT COMMON MINOR EYE PROBLEMS   The *conjunctiva* is the transparent, delicate membrane covering the inside of the eyelid and the exposed surface of the eyeball (see Figure 7-16). Epidemic infection of this membrane (acute bacterial conjunctivitis or "pinkeye") is particularly common in school and preschool children. It is caused by a variety of microorganisms. Eye drops containing an appropriate antibiotic are curative. The surfaces of the conjunctiva are kept lubricated by tear fluid which is continuously secreted by the *lacrimal gland* (see Figure 7-21). Like saliva, tears contain an antibacterial enzyme. Were it not for this constant slight flow of tears the conjunctiva would dry and become inflamed, and vision would be lost.

[46] It was the severe astigmatism of three great Renaissance artists, Holbein, Cranach, and El Greco, that accounts for the distortion of their painted figures. For centures these distortions, in themselves so beautiful and so characteristic of the artists' respective styles, have been widely and rightly admired. (O. Ahlstrom, cited in "Case Study: Vincent Van Gogh," *What's New*, No. 228 [Summer 1962], p. 2.)

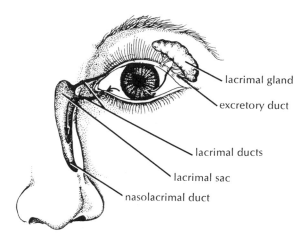

lacrimal gland

excretory duct

lacrimal ducts

lacrimal sac

nasolacrimal duct

7-21 The tear apparatus. Secreted by the lacrimal glands and spread by the blinking eyelids, tears reach the inner corner of each eye. Here they are collected by tiny holes at the inner end of each lid. Each hole leads to a lacrimal sac by way of a minute canal. From the sac, tears reach the nose via a nasolacrimal duct. Hairs in the nose move the tears back to be swallowed. With excessive tearing, the lacrimal apparatus is overwhelmed and tears spill down on the cheek.

Color blindness is an inherited condition due to the mutation of a gene involving color vision in an X-chromosome. Since males possess but one X-chromosome in their body cells, color blindness is more common among them (8 percent of the population) than it is among females (0.4 percent), who have two X-chromosomes. The genes for color blindness are recessive (a recessive gene will usually produce an effect only when it is transmitted by both parents). For a female to be color blind, therefore, the genes of both X-chromosomes must be affected. Most color-blind people are unable to fully see either red or green.

The apparatus for hearing was described in Chapter 4 and diagramed in Figure 4-5 (page 99). Its consummate workmanship, its very fragility, requires its deep encasement in protective bone. Before he sees danger, man usually hears it. Deafness, like blindness, is a cruel handicap. Yet, millions in this nation are chronically deaf to some degree. In older age groups, hearing defects occur in astronomical numbers.

Conductive deafness involves interference of sound transmission through the outer or middle ear. As simple a matter as excessive ear wax may cause deafness. Its removal by a physician is curative. Its removal by an amateur with a hairpin, or some other dangerous instrument, may lead to a pierced eardrum. "He has not so much brain as earwax," wrote Shakespeare in *Troilus and Cressida* (V.i.58). This description might be applied to one who, in this manner, senselessly risks deafness. *Infection* of the middle ear, which sometimes accompanies or follows a childhood communicable disease, is a frequent cause of conductive deafness.

Hearing loss by way of the *Eustachian tube* is not uncommon. As was mentioned earlier (page 99), the Eustachian tube is open only during

Hearing: a special sense— disorders

THE NERVOUS SYSTEM: EASE AND DISEASE **235**

swallowing. In this way an equal pressure on both sides of the eardrum is maintained. During an airplane descent, the passenger should repeatedly swallow. Otherwise, the high-altitude air pressure, trapped in the middle ear, will fail to correspond to the increasing atmospheric pressure on the outside of the eardrum. The eardrum may then rupture. An *upper respiratory infection* may, moreover, cause swelling around the opening and within the Eustachian tube. Sometimes, this causes a mild deafness. An attempt to open the tube by vigorously blowing the nose may force infectious material into the middle ear. Children are more prone to middle ear infection than adults because infection travels more easily via their shorter, straighter Eustachian tubes. Indiscriminate use of nose drops or nasal sprays may promote such infection. The consequences may be serious and chronic.

Sometimes infection will cause stiffening of the joints between the three little bones in the middle ear. The bones become rigid. Their normal ability to vibrate is limited. Sound waves cannot be transmitted through them to the fluid of the inner ear. Hearing is diminished, even lost. But sound waves can be transmitted through the skull to the fluid, and it is on this principle that the hearing aid works.

However, the hearing aid does not help with *nerve deafness*. Here, the problem is in the cochlea of the inner ear, the auditory nerve, or even in the cerebral cortex. For a variety of reasons, many children are born deaf. Such deafness may occur when a pregnant woman's infection with German measles virus also infects her unborn child. A vaccine against German measles is now available (pages 162 and 164). Children born deaf will not speak unless taught through some pathway other than the ear. A deaf child need not be a dumb child. Schools for the deaf are an important societal service.

By injuring the nerve cells of the inner ear, excessive noise can cause deafness, as was discussed in Chapter 4. This deafness may be permanent but is preventable. Individuals working in hazardous areas should wear protective devices such as ear plugs or helmets.

The exocrine and endocrine glands

Their pervasive role in body government

The secretions of some glands are carried through outlet tubes or ducts. These glands secrete externally or into hollow organs. Among these are the breasts or mammary glands (page 464) and the sweat, tear, and salivary glands (pages 234 and 239). These are *exocrine* glands (Greek *exo*, outside + *krinein*, to separate).

Unlike these, the *endocrine* glands are ductless (see body chart 15 in the color section and Table 7-2). *Endocrine* is Greek for "I separate within." From the many chemicals carried in the blood of the arteries, the endocrine glands manufacture their own potent secretions or *hormones* (Greek "I arouse" or "I stimulate"). Releasing their finished hormonal products into the veins over a long time and in perfectly accurate doses, the

the human body

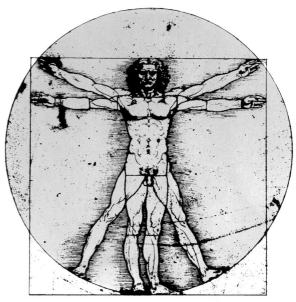

"*Study in the proportions of the human body, based on Vitruvius*" *(1492) by Leonardo da Vinci (1452-1519).*

GUIDE TO CONTENTS

The numbers are the numbers of the body charts.

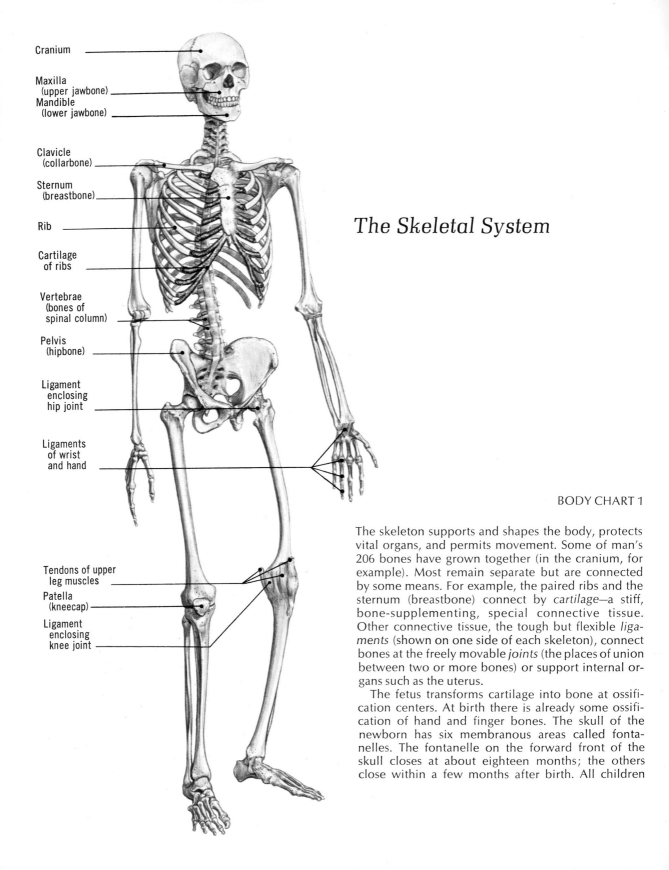

Cranium

Maxilla
(upper jawbone)
Mandible
(lower jawbone)

Clavicle
(collarbone)

Sternum
(breastbone)

Rib

Cartilage
of ribs

Vertebrae
(bones of
spinal column)

Pelvis
(hipbone)

Ligament
enclosing
hip joint

Ligaments
of wrist
and hand

Tendons of upper
leg muscles

Patella
(kneecap)

Ligament
enclosing
knee joint

The Skeletal System

BODY CHART 1

The skeleton supports and shapes the body, protects vital organs, and permits movement. Some of man's 206 bones have grown together (in the cranium, for example). Most remain separate but are connected by some means. For example, the paired ribs and the sternum (breastbone) connect by *cartilage*—a stiff, bone-supplementing, special connective tissue. Other connective tissue, the tough but flexible *ligaments* (shown on one side of each skeleton), connect bones at the freely movable *joints* (the places of union between two or more bones) or support internal organs such as the uterus.

The fetus transforms cartilage into bone at ossification centers. At birth there is already some ossification of hand and finger bones. The skull of the newborn has six membranous areas called fontanelles. The fontanelle on the forward front of the skull closes at about eighteen months; the others close within a few months after birth. All children

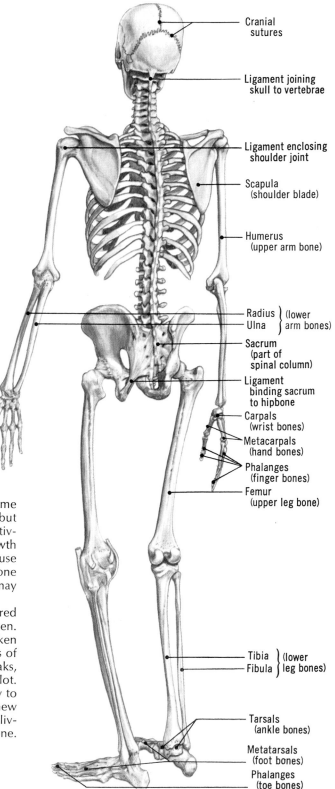

Cranial
sutures

Ligament joining
skull to vertebrae

Ligament enclosing
shoulder joint

Scapula
(shoulder blade)

Humerus
(upper arm bone)

Radius } (lower
Ulna } arm bones)

Sacrum
(part of
spinal column)

Ligament
binding sacrum
to hipbone

Carpals
(wrist bones)

Metacarpals
(hand bones)

Phalanges
(finger bones)

Femur
(upper leg bone)

Tibia } (lower
Fibula } leg bones)

Tarsals
(ankle bones)

Metatarsals
(foot bones)

Phalanges
(toe bones)

BODY CHART 2

ossify bones in the same order but not at the same
rate. Order and rate are genetically established, but
rate is influenced by nutrition, endocrine gland activity, and disease. Adverse effects on cartilage growth
from pituitary or thyroid gland disease can cause
dwarfism. Insufficient vitamin D may retard bone
formation and development in children and may
promote rickets.

Before bone structure appears in the fetus, red
blood cells are formed mostly in the liver and spleen.
As bone develops, red blood cell formation is taken
over by marrow, the soft tissue filling the cavities of
the bones (see body chart 6). When a bone breaks,
the gap between the fragments fills with a blood clot.
From unimpaired blood vessels, new vessels grow to
bring the clot food. From surrounding tissue, new
cells invade the clot. The nonliving clot becomes living tissue and the groundwork for repair of the bone.

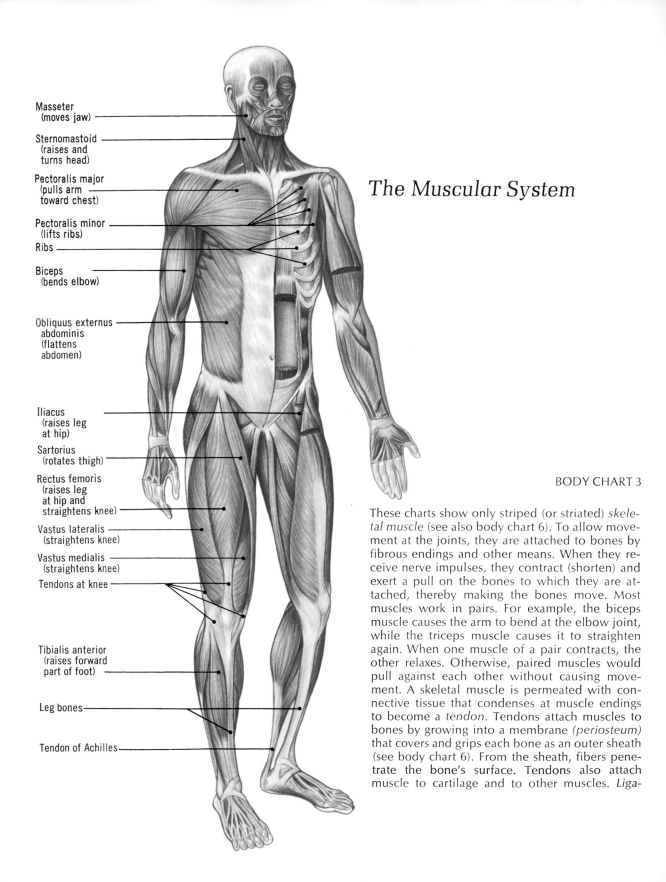

The Muscular System

Masseter
(moves jaw)

Sternomastoid
(raises and
turns head)

Pectoralis major
(pulls arm
toward chest)

Pectoralis minor
(lifts ribs)

Ribs

Biceps
(bends elbow)

Obliquus externus
abdominis
(flattens
abdomen)

Iliacus
(raises leg
at hip)

Sartorius
(rotates thigh)

Rectus femoris
(raises leg
at hip and
straightens knee)

Vastus lateralis
(straightens knee)

Vastus medialis
(straightens knee)

Tendons at knee

Tibialis anterior
(raises forward
part of foot)

Leg bones

Tendon of Achilles

BODY CHART 3

These charts show only striped (or striated) *skeletal muscle* (see also body chart 6). To allow movement at the joints, they are attached to bones by fibrous endings and other means. When they receive nerve impulses, they contract (shorten) and exert a pull on the bones to which they are attached, thereby making the bones move. Most muscles work in pairs. For example, the biceps muscle causes the arm to bend at the elbow joint, while the triceps muscle causes it to straighten again. When one muscle of a pair contracts, the other relaxes. Otherwise, paired muscles would pull against each other without causing movement. A skeletal muscle is permeated with connective tissue that condenses at muscle endings to become a *tendon*. Tendons attach muscles to bones by growing into a membrane *(periosteum)* that covers and grips each bone as an outer sheath (see body chart 6). From the sheath, fibers penetrate the bone's surface. Tendons also attach muscle to cartilage and to other muscles. *Liga-*

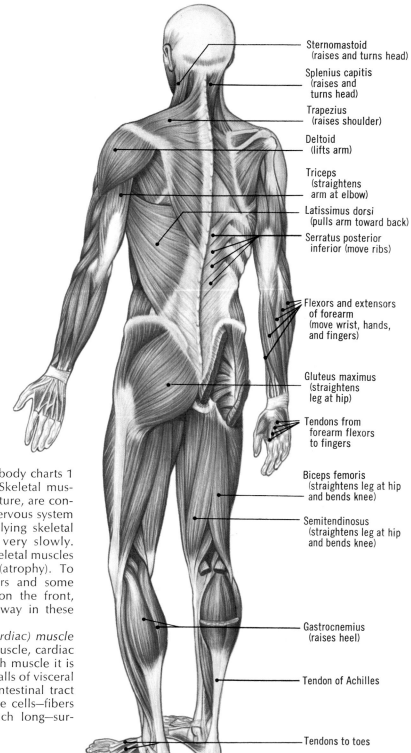

Sternomastoid
(raises and turns head)

Splenius capitis
(raises and
turns head)

Trapezius
(raises shoulder)

Deltoid
(lifts arm)

Triceps
(straightens
arm at elbow)

Latissimus dorsi
(pulls arm toward back)

Serratus posterior
inferior (move ribs)

Flexors and extensors
of forearm
(move wrist, hands,
and fingers)

Gluteus maximus
(straightens
leg at hip)

Tendons from
forearm flexors
to fingers

Biceps femoris
(straightens leg at hip
and bends knee)

Semitendinosus
(straightens leg at hip
and bends knee)

Gastrocnemius
(raises heel)

Tendon of Achilles

Tendons to toes

BODY CHART 4

ments connect bones at joints (see body charts 1 and 2) or support internal organs. Skeletal muscles, the bulk of the body's musculature, are controlled by the will. Unlike central nervous system fibers, peripheral nerve fibers supplying skeletal muscles tend to regenerate—but very slowly. Without adequate physiotherapy, skeletal muscles awaiting nerve repair will waste (atrophy). To show deeper skeletal muscle layers and some bone attachments, some muscles on the front, back, and one side are stripped away in these charts.

Not illustrated here are *heart (cardiac) muscle* and *smooth muscle*. Like smooth muscle, cardiac muscle is involuntary; unlike smooth muscle it is striped. Smooth muscle forms the walls of visceral organs such as those in the gastrointestinal tract and urinary bladder. Smooth muscle cells—fibers less than one-thousandth of an inch long—surround capillaries.

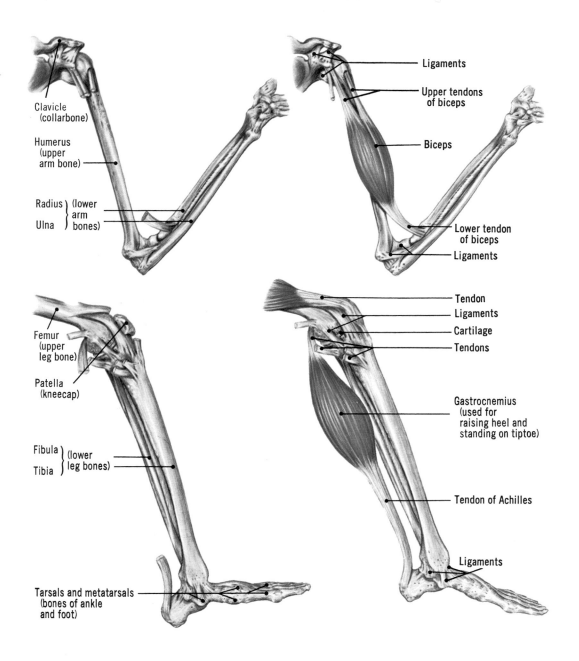

Clavicle
(collarbone)

Humerus
(upper
arm bone)

Radius } (lower
arm
Ulna } bones)

Ligaments

Upper tendons
of biceps

Biceps

Lower tendon
of biceps

Ligaments

Femur
(upper
leg bone)

Patella
(kneecap)

Fibula } (lower
leg bones)
Tibia }

Tarsals and metatarsals
(bones of ankle
and foot)

Tendon
Ligaments
Cartilage
Tendons

Gastrocnemius
(used for
raising heel and
standing on tiptoe)

Tendon of Achilles

Ligaments

The Bone-Muscle Relationship

The structure of an arm and leg clarifies the bone-muscle relationship. Muscles bending a limb at a joint (elbow, knee) are called *flexor* muscles; those that straighten the limb are *extensor* muscles. For movement to occur, bones must be joined at joints, and muscles must pull upon bones by contracting (shortening). Furthermore, the tendons at the oppo-site ends of each muscle must be attached to different bones. For example, the lower tendon of the biceps is attached to a bone of the forearm. Since the elbow is a freely movable joint, contraction of the biceps will cause the arm to bend. (Muscle fibers of the biceps are six to seven inches long and are among the body's longest cells.)

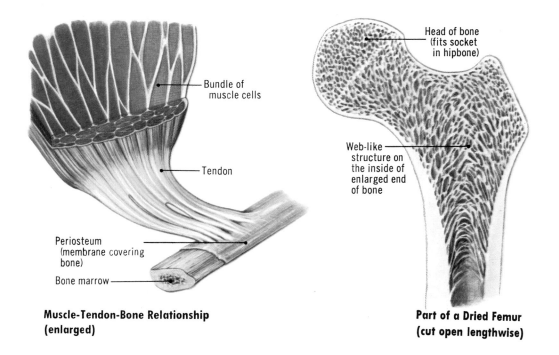

Muscle-Tendon-Bone Relationship (enlarged)

Bundle of muscle cells

Tendon

Periosteum (membrane covering bone)

Bone marrow

Head of bone (fits socket in hipbone)

Web-like structure on the inside of enlarged end of bone

Part of a Dried Femur (cut open lengthwise)

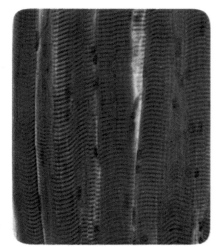

Small Parts of Several Stained Skeletal Muscle Cells (as seen under the microscope)

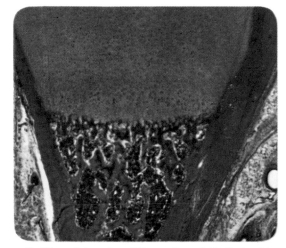

Cartilage (above) and Young Bone Cells (below) in Stained Fresh Bone (as seen under the microscope)

BODY CHART 6

The most versatile joint is that of the shoulder; it has the greatest range of movement. The knee is both the largest and and weakest joint of the body. When a tendon rides over a bony surface, a small sac (a bursa) containing fluid protects it. These bursae are found at such places as about the elbow and knee joints and at the back of the heel. Between the kneecap (patella) and the skin is a bursa. Like other bursae, it may become inflamed (bursitis).

The muscles of adult men are stronger than those of women both because the muscles are larger and because men have a higher oxygen consumption per pound of body weight than do women.

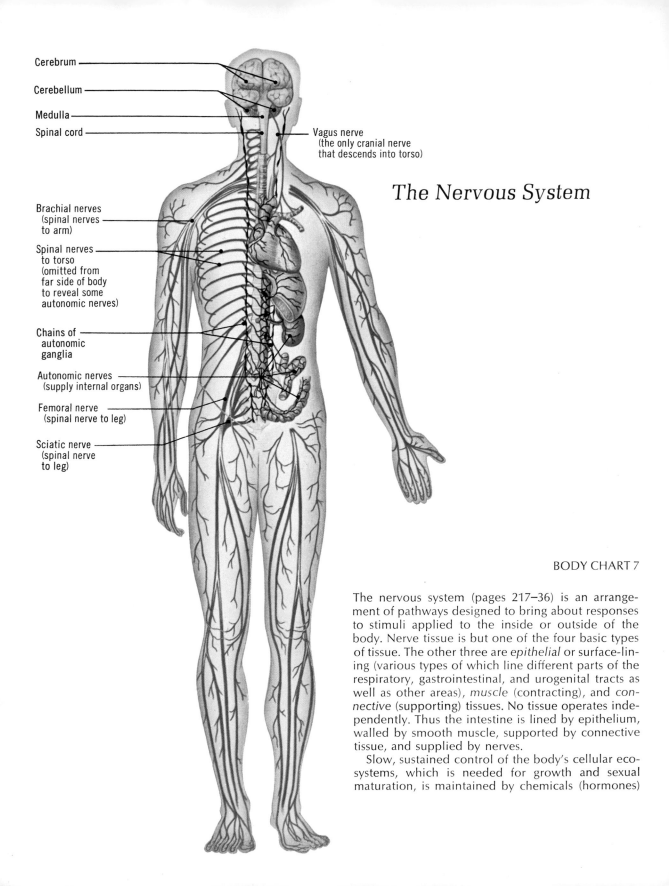

Cerebrum

Cerebellum

Medulla

Spinal cord

Vagus nerve
(the only cranial nerve
that descends into torso)

The Nervous System

Brachial nerves
(spinal nerves
to arm)

Spinal nerves
to torso
(omitted from
far side of body
to reveal some
autonomic nerves)

Chains of
autonomic
ganglia

Autonomic nerves
(supply internal organs)

Femoral nerve
(spinal nerve to leg)

Sciatic nerve
(spinal nerve
to leg)

BODY CHART 7

The nervous system (pages 217–36) is an arrangement of pathways designed to bring about responses
to stimuli applied to the inside or outside of the
body. Nerve tissue is but one of the four basic types
of tissue. The other three are *epithelial* or surface-lin-
ing (various types of which line different parts of the
respiratory, gastrointestinal, and urogenital tracts as
well as other areas), *muscle* (contracting), and *connective* (supporting) tissues. No tissue operates independently. Thus the intestine is lined by epithelium,
walled by smooth muscle, supported by connective
tissue, and supplied by nerves.

Slow, sustained control of the body's cellular ecosystems, which is needed for growth and sexual
maturation, is maintained by chemicals (hormones)

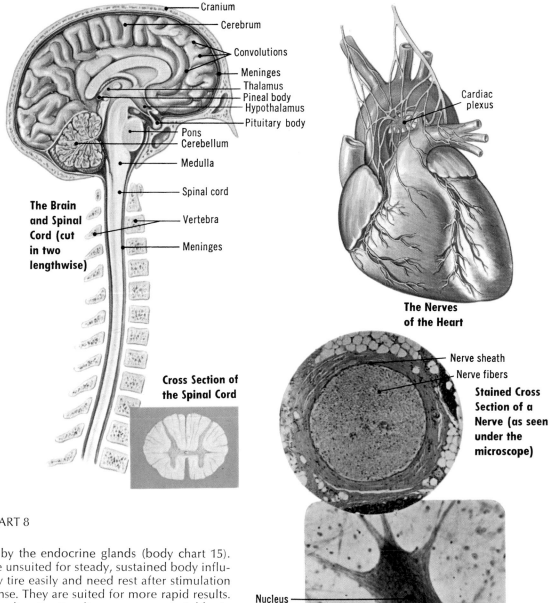

Cranium
Cerebrum
Convolutions
Meninges
Thalamus
Pineal body
Hypothalamus
Pituitary body
Pons
Cerebellum
Medulla
Spinal cord
Vertebra
Meninges

The Brain and Spinal Cord (cut in two lengthwise)

Cross Section of the Spinal Cord

Cardiac plexus

The Nerves of the Heart

Nerve sheath
Nerve fibers

Stained Cross Section of a Nerve (as seen under the microscope)

Nucleus
Cytoplasm

Stained Cell Body of an Efferent (Motor) Neuron (as seen under the microscope)

BODY CHART 8

produced by the endocrine glands (body chart 15). Nerves are unsuited for steady, sustained body influence. They tire easily and need rest after stimulation and response. They are suited for more rapid results.

In responding to stimuli, neurons are *irritable*; in transmitting impulses, they are *conductive*. These two properties combine with their ability to *correlate* and *evaluate* on the basis of memory to make nerve tissue the most specialized of the four basic tissue types. It has been written that the hand without a thumb is but a hook, for it can no longer grasp. But a hand that loses its nerve function loses more than its ability to participate in creation; it loses the more primitive ability to warn its owner of surrounding dangers.

The Circulatory System

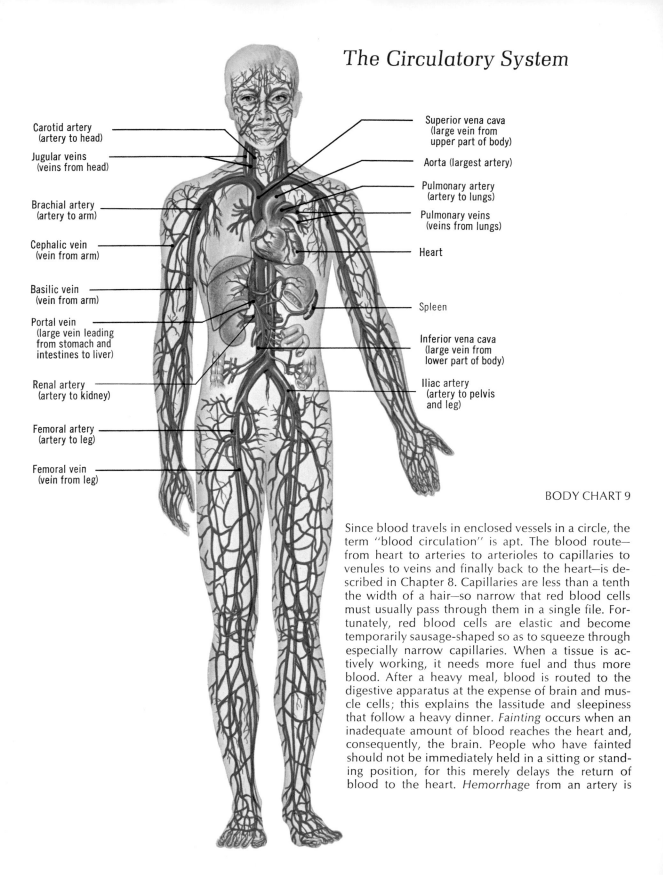

Carotid artery
(artery to head)

Jugular veins
(veins from head)

Brachial artery
(artery to arm)

Cephalic vein
(vein from arm)

Basilic vein
(vein from arm)

Portal vein
(large vein leading
from stomach and
intestines to liver)

Renal artery
(artery to kidney)

Femoral artery
(artery to leg)

Femoral vein
(vein from leg)

Superior vena cava
(large vein from
upper part of body)

Aorta (largest artery)

Pulmonary artery
(artery to lungs)

Pulmonary veins
(veins from lungs)

Heart

Spleen

Inferior vena cava
(large vein from
lower part of body)

Iliac artery
(artery to pelvis
and leg)

BODY CHART 9

Since blood travels in enclosed vessels in a circle, the term "blood circulation" is apt. The blood route—from heart to arteries to arterioles to capillaries to venules to veins and finally back to the heart—is described in Chapter 8. Capillaries are less than a tenth the width of a hair—so narrow that red blood cells must usually pass through them in a single file. Fortunately, red blood cells are elastic and become temporarily sausage-shaped so as to squeeze through especially narrow capillaries. When a tissue is actively working, it needs more fuel and thus more blood. After a heavy meal, blood is routed to the digestive apparatus at the expense of brain and muscle cells; this explains the lassitude and sleepiness that follow a heavy dinner. *Fainting* occurs when an inadequate amount of blood reaches the heart and, consequently, the brain. People who have fainted should not be immediately held in a sitting or standing position, for this merely delays the return of blood to the heart. *Hemorrhage* from an artery is

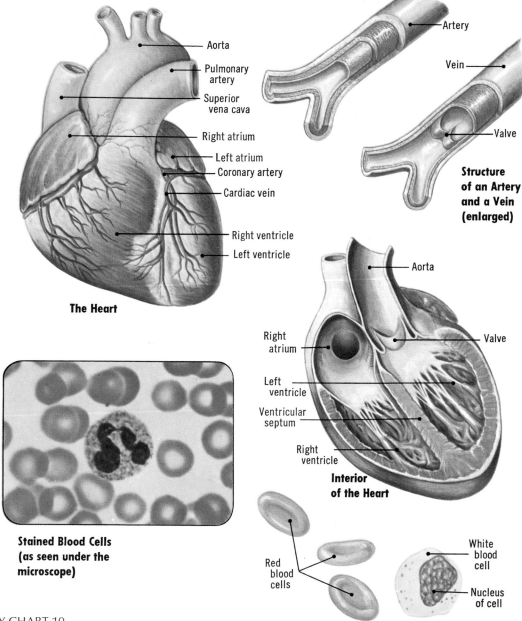

Aorta

Pulmonary artery

Superior vena cava

Right atrium

Left atrium

Coronary artery

Cardiac vein

Right ventricle

Left ventricle

The Heart

Artery

Vein

Valve

Structure of an Artery and a Vein (enlarged)

Aorta

Valve

Right atrium

Left ventricle

Ventricular septum

Right ventricle

Interior of the Heart

Stained Blood Cells (as seen under the microscope)

Red blood cells

White blood cell

Nucleus of cell

Blood Cells (greatly enlarged)

BODY CHART 10

bright red because the blood has been oxygenated. Arterial blood spurts because it escapes under pressure. The spurt may be stopped by the application of pressure between the point of bleeding and the heart. Most venous blood is bluish-red. With hemorrhage, it seeps or wells up into a wound. This bleeding can only be stopped by pressure beyond the bleeding point. Escaping capillary blood merely oozes and clots quickly. When serious hemorrhage occurs, rest is important. Alcohol should not be given. By increasing the force of the heartbeat and raising the blood pressure, both activity and alcohol increase bleeding. Moreover, by dilating the blood vessels, alcohol is certain to facilitate the escape of blood.

The Respiratory System

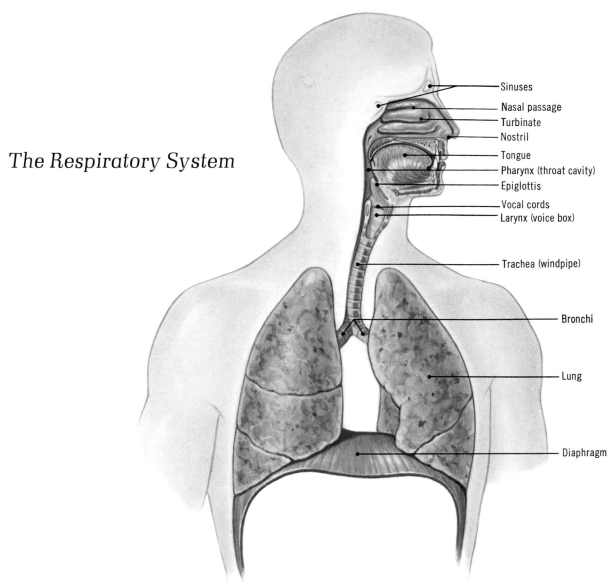

Sinuses
Nasal passage
Turbinate
Nostril
Tongue
Pharynx (throat cavity)
Epiglottis
Vocal cords
Larynx (voice box)
Trachea (windpipe)
Bronchi
Lung
Diaphragm

BODY CHART 11

The nasal cavity extends deep into the skull and is separated into right and left by a septum. Rarely, the septum deviates so much that only surgery permits proper breathing. Each side wall of the nasal cavity supports three shell-like projections called *turbinates,* and the furrowlike *nasal passages* run between these small mounds. The duct carrying tears empties into the lowest of these furrows. Also emptying into the nose are various sinus spaces.

The nose is an efficent filtering and air-conditioning system. Larger particles are trapped by coarse hairs in the nostril. The entire nasal cavity, including

the sinuses, is covered with mucous membrane, which is kept moist by mucus. Mucus also picks up foreign particles and, aided by the sweeping motion of hairlike cilia, moves the particles toward the pharynx to be swallowed. In the upper part of the nasal cavity, the ciliated cells are replaced by specialized receptor nerve cells. This is the olfactory "organ"; bundles of axons run from neurons in this area through the bony roof of the nose and on to the brain. The mucous membrane covering the septum and that of the middle and lower turbinates is thick and full of blood vessels. When inflamed, this mu-

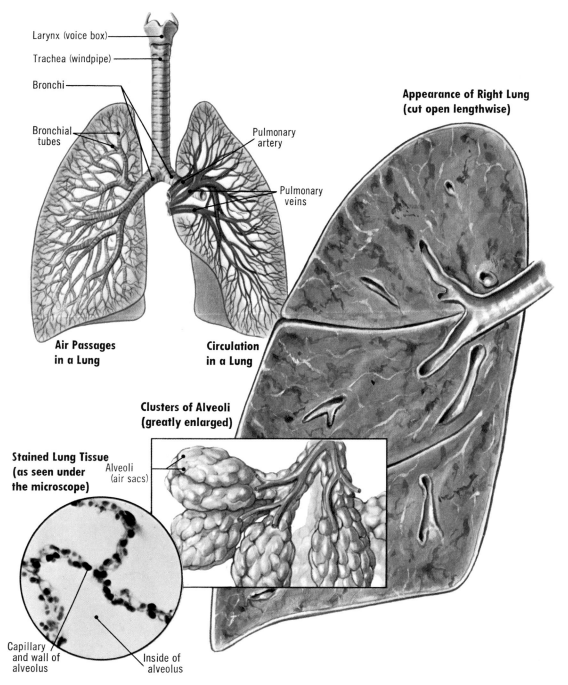

Larynx (voice box)

Trachea (windpipe)

Bronchi

Bronchial tubes

Pulmonary artery

Pulmonary veins

Appearance of Right Lung (cut open lengthwise)

Air Passages in a Lung

Circulation in a Lung

Clusters of Alveoli (greatly enlarged)

Stained Lung Tissue (as seen under the microscope)

Alveoli (air sacs)

Capillary and wall of alveolus

Inside of alveolus

cous membrane swells and blocks the nasal passages. Swollen mucous membrane in the sinuses may also block drainage. The veins in the mucous membrane of the middle and lower turbinates dilate to become venous spaces. With sexual excitement these venous spaces become engorged with blood in much the same way as does erectile tissue of the genital organs. Because of its great vascularity, this area bleeds easily. This very vascularity also makes the nose an excellent ventilating system, for cold air about the capillaries is warmed before entering the lungs. The respiratory tract is further discussed on pages 423–26.

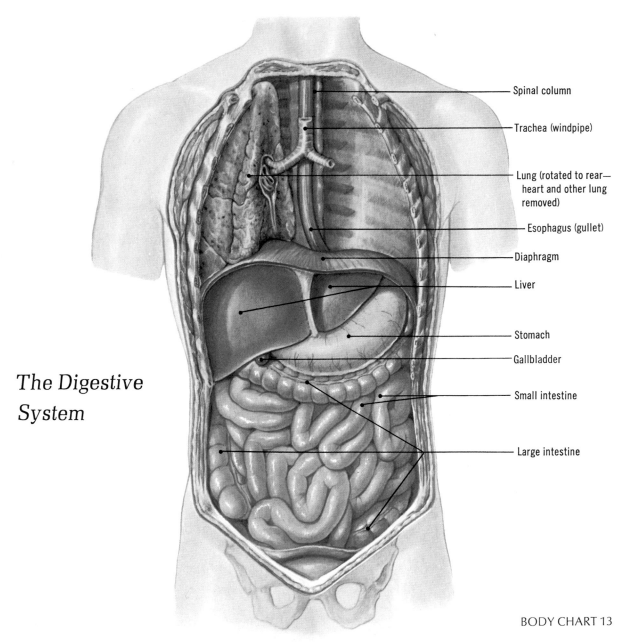

Spinal column

Trachea (windpipe)

Lung (rotated to rear—
heart and other lung
removed)

Esophagus (gullet)

Diaphragm

Liver

Stomach

Gallbladder

Small intestine

Large intestine

The Digestive System

BODY CHART 13

The seventeenth-century English satirist Samuel Butler sardonically described the human body as "a pair of pincers set over a bellows and a stewpan and the whole fixed upon stilts"; he doubtless saw the teeth as pincers and the remaining digestive system as a stewpan. This system is somewhat more comprehensively described in Chapter 9.

From the lips to the anus the adult digestive tract is about 30 to 32 feet long. Two basic kinds of tissue contribute to the wall of the digestive tract from the lower part of the esophagus to the lower end of the small intestine—involuntary *smooth muscle* and the *mucous membrane* lining the muscle. This muscle contracts more slowly than skeletal muscle, and it is able to sustain rhythmic contraction without tiring. The mucosal lining of the digestive tract protects and lubricates. In the small intestine, its absorptive inner surface is unique.

The digestive tract provides the excretory apparatus for food residue; it also excretes other body

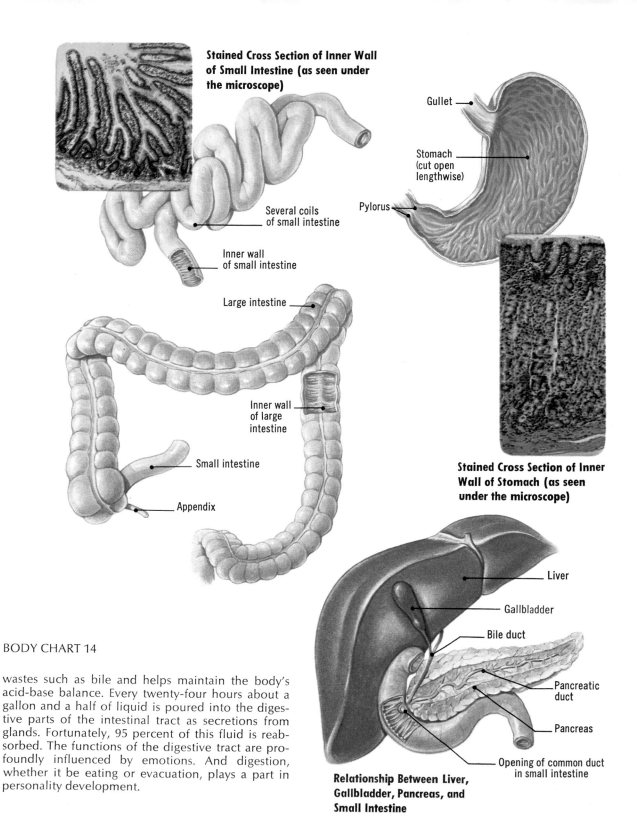

Stained Cross Section of Inner Wall of Small Intestine (as seen under the microscope)

Several coils of small intestine

Inner wall of small intestine

Gullet

Stomach (cut open lengthwise)

Pylorus

Stained Cross Section of Inner Wall of Stomach (as seen under the microscope)

Large intestine

Inner wall of large intestine

Small intestine

Appendix

Liver

Gallbladder

Bile duct

Pancreatic duct

Pancreas

Opening of common duct in small intestine

Relationship Between Liver, Gallbladder, Pancreas, and Small Intestine

BODY CHART 14

wastes such as bile and helps maintain the body's acid-base balance. Every twenty-four hours about a gallon and a half of liquid is poured into the digestive parts of the intestinal tract as secretions from glands. Fortunately, 95 percent of this fluid is reabsorbed. The functions of the digestive tract are profoundly influenced by emotions. And digestion, whether it be eating or evacuation, plays a part in personality development.

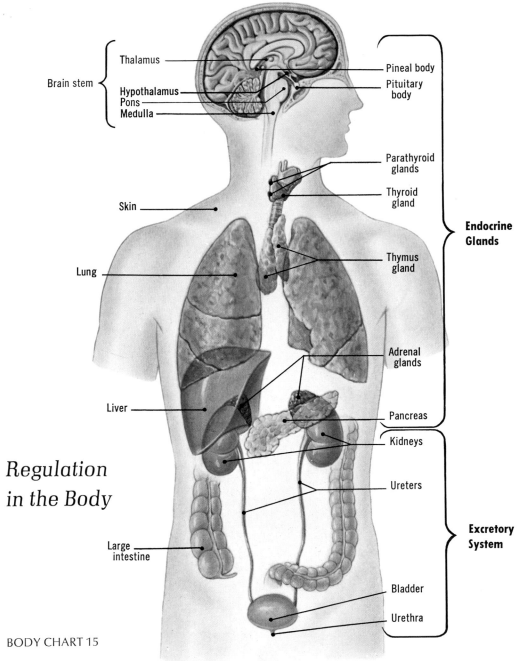

Thalamus

Brain stem

Hypothalamus
Pons
Medulla

Pineal body

Pituitary body

Parathyroid glands

Thyroid gland

Skin

Lung

Thymus gland

Endocrine Glands

Adrenal glands

Regulation in the Body

Liver

Pancreas

Kidneys

Ureters

Excretory System

Large intestine

Bladder

Urethra

BODY CHART 15

"The stability of the interior environment," wrote the nineteenth-century French physiologist Claude Bernard, "is the essential condition of free and independent life...all vital mechanisms, however varied they may be, have only one object: that of preserving constant the conditions of life in the interior environment." This chart illustrates some of the most important body regulators involved in maintaining a harmonious balance among the internal human ecosystems. But one can consider these inner ecosystems of man only as they relate to his outer ecosystems. An unhealthy external environment interferes with the ecological health of the internal environment. Man cannot long safely subject the sensitive organs regulating his "interior environment" to the gross pollutions with which he surrounds himself.

GLAND	ACTIVITIES REGULATED
TABLE 7-2 _Some Typical Functions of the Endocrine Glands_	
Pituitary Anterior	Growth (dwarfism, giantism); as "master gland" influences secretions of thyroid, pancreas, adrenal glands, and gonads.
Posterior	Water metabolism, etc.
Thyroid	Metabolic rate; hence activity and fatigue; body weight.
Thymus	Important in regulation of the lymphoid system, and in the development of immune reactions of the body.
Parathyroid	Calcium metabolism; maintenance of normal excitability of the nervous system.
Pancreas	Via insulin controls sugar metabolism; excess insulin leads to state of shock.
Adrenal Cortex	Secretes life-maintaining regulators; control of salt and carbohydrate metabolism; may be important in mental illness.
Medulla	Active in emotion through the effects of adrenalin and noradrenalin.
Gonads*	Secondary sex characteristics distinguishing the male and female at maturity; maintenance of a functional condition in male and female reproductive apparatuses.

*As glands of internal secretion; to be distinguished from their reproductive functions.

Source: Ernest R. Hilgard and Richard C. Atkinson, _Introduction to Psychology_, 4th ed. (New York, 1967), p. 34.

endocrine system of glands governs various body processes. Among these are the slow, time-consuming growth of bones and the development of the testes and ovaries. Endocrine glands profoundly influence personality. They are supervised by the central nervous system. (There is growing evidence that hormones affect the activity of genes.)

The endocrine glands are the _pituitary, thyroid_ (page 238), _thymus, parathyroid,_ part of the _pancreas_ (page 310), _adrenal,_ and _gonads_ (female ovaries and male testes). Some functions of the endocrine glands are listed in Table 7-2.

The pituitary is attached to the base of the brain. Among the products of its anterior (front) lobe is the growth hormone. If this hormone is produced in excess during the growth period, _gigantism_ may occur (see Figure 7-22); produced in excess in the mature adult, the hormone may cause bone thickening of the face and extremities (_acromegaly_). A genetically based shortage of the hormone is responsible for _dwarfism._ The

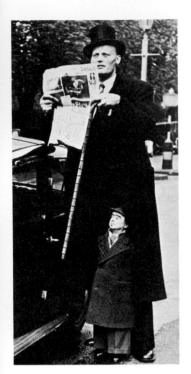

7-22 A giant and a dwarf: the result, respectively, of overactivity and underactivity of the growth hormone of the anterior lobe of the pituitary gland.

anterior lobe of the pituitary also produces hormones that stimulate the gonads (sex glands) and play a major role in reproduction (see Chapter 13). The posterior (back) lobe produces no hormones; it stores and releases hormones produced by brain cells. Thus, it is not true endocrine gland tissue. From it are extracted hormones that affect blood pressure, contract smooth muscle, and inhibit loss of fluid from the kidney.

The thyroid, straddling the trachea (windpipe) and larynx, governs the rate of body metabolism. Infants with severely diminished thyroid function grow poorly and are sexually and mentally retarded (*cretinism,* page 544). Lack of adult thyroid function causes *myxedema,* characterized by diminished physical and mental vigor, hair loss, weight increase, and a thickening of the skin. *Hyperthyroidism,* resulting from an overactive thyroid, produces severe nervousness, weight loss, and protruding eyeballs. Surgical removal of part of the thyroid gland often corrects this condition. *Goiter,* an enlargement of the thyroid, is discussed in footnote 23, page 282.

The *medulla* (central portion) of the adrenal gland secretes both adrenalin and noradrenalin. In concert with the sympathetic nervous system, adrenalin produces the rapid heart rate, increased blood pressure (from constriction of the arteries), and increased blood sugar associated with stress. There is evidence that chronic excitement can cause adrenal damage.

The adrenal *cortex* (outer portion) is essential to life. It provides chemicals called *steroids,* which regulate sugar and salt metabolism. Steroids, such as *cortisone,* are sometimes useful in treating severe asthma and arthritis.

Three groups of steroid hormones are produced by the adrenal cortex. *Hydrocortisone* aids in forming sugar from protein. It also has a widespread anti-inflammatory action throughout the body. It is, moreover, called forth in times of stress such as emotion (anger, fear), excessive muscular exercise, severe infection or trauma, and extreme heat and cold. There is a pituitary-adrenal axis in the sense that the pituitary gland releases a special hormone stimulating the adrenal cortex to make and release enough hydrocortisone in the blood. By its direct action on the kidneys, a second steroid hormone, *aldosterone,* maintains the sodium-potassium balance in the body. The third of the steroid hormones is a group called the *androgens.* In the male most of the androgen is produced by the testes. Only a small amount is normally produced by the adrenal cortex. Rarely, a tumor of the adrenal cortex will produce excess androgen. This can cause serious masculinizing effects even of the female. A normal amount of adrenal androgen in the female does not make her masculine and is, indeed, necessary for her health.

Some glandular dysfunctions

Cystic fibrosis: an exocrine dysfunction

A generation ago *cystic fibrosis* had not yet been classified as a separate disease. Today, this inherited childhood ailment is known as this country's greatest genetic killer of white children. About one of a thousand new-borns has the disease. Cystic fibrosis seems nonexistent in Oriental children and rare in blacks.

Affected are the sweat glands and those ductal glands emptying into organs leading to the outside of the body. Either or both may be involved. The clear, usable fluid usually produced by these glands is replaced, in cystic fibrosis, with a sticky, thick material. There is widespread clogging of the ducts. Complicating these secretory impediments is an excessive salt secretion by the sweat, salivary, and tear glands. On hot summer days, the excessive salt loss of heavy perspiring can lead to serious heat exhaustion.

Not all afflicted children have all or even the same symptoms. Clogging of the pancreatic duct deprives the child of digestive enzymes. The hungry child eats well yet loses weight. His bulky stools are fatty and foul-smelling. The chronic plugging of the air passages leads to a nagging cough. The breathing is labored. The child tires easily.

The future of these little patients depends on constant attention to lung infection. Extra salt and a low-fat diet (supplemented with pancreatic enzymes) also help. As yet, death rates remain high. This afflication needs and is getting much investigation.

Diabetes mellitus: an endocrine dysfunction

Madhumeha, "urine of honey," is the Indian name for diabetes. Fifteen centuries ago the Indian Susruta had noted the sweet taste of diabetic urine.[47] But diabetes has been known even longer—for thirty-five centuries. That oldest of all medical texts, the Ebers Papyrus (1500 B.C.), mentions a treatment for one of its prominent symptoms—frequent urination. To trace the disease to the pancreas required millennia.

Pancreatic tissue is both exocrine and endocrine. By way of a duct, enzymatic digestive juice is delivered to the small intestine. Ductlessly, its insulin, produced by certain of the specialized pancreatic cells in the *islets of Langerhans,*[48] is released directly into the blood. When there is a degeneration of these specialized cells (usually hereditary), insulin is not produced and diabetes mellitus results. How?

By combining carbohydrates and oxygen, cells produce life-sustaining heat and energy. Without insulin from the pancreas, this cannot happen. Insulin controls the entry of carbohydrate (glucose) into the cell. Without insulin very little glucose can enter the cell. Cellular (and body) use of glucose is slowed. Production of energy by the cell is slowed. The inability to use enough glucose for energy is a basic abnormality of diabetes mellitus. Unused, sugar (glucose) collects uselessly in the blood. It spills over into the urine. In the midst of plenty, the cells starve.

The body has no alternative but to seek other sources of heat and energy. Proteins and fats are other sources. But the over-utilization of

[47] N. S. Papaspyros, *The History of Diabetes Mellitus* (Stuttgart, Ger., 1964), pp. 4–5.
[48] Discovered in 1869 by Paul Langerhans, then a University of Berlin medical student.

protein results in a shortage of amino acids for tissue-building. For these reasons, the diabetic grows poorly, infects easily, and heals slowly. Fats, called upon to perform an unexpected duty, are also used to excess so they respond by producing an excess of "ketone bodies." Should the concentration of these "keto acids" rise to a high enough level within and between the cells, cells will be poisoned. The diabetic will sink into a coma and die. A multitude of signs and symptoms besets the diabetic. Because of the excess use of fat and protein, he loses weight, yet he eats voraciously to relieve his constant hunger. Because of the excess glucose in his urine, he loses vast amounts of water via the kidney. He tries to slake his thirst by drinking equally great quantities of water. Fatigue, weakness, blurring of the vision—all these, and more, plague him. What is even worse, prolonged, untreated diabetes promotes atherosclerosis (pages 257–60), and with it a host of circulatory disorders varying from heart disease to stroke. Without insulin the diabetic is doomed. But insulin is available.

It has been almost half a century since two Canadian doctors, Frederick G. Banting and Charles H. Best, quietly announced their epochal discovery (in 1922).[49] It was this: purified animal insulin could replace the natural insulin lacking in the human diabetic. Their finding brought a normal life span to millions. That year, world attention focused on a justifiably proud Canada.

To this day, natural animal insulin has always been used. True, many diabetics do very well with an oral medicine that stimulates a flagging pancreas to yield more insulin. Other chemical products relieve diabetes differently, but their mechanism is unknown. Ordinary insulin and diet are usually satisfactory for a great number of diabetics. But scientists know that the laboratory synthesis of the hormone will advance the understanding of both diabetes and hormones in general. This achievement may have been recently realized by mainland Chinese scientists of Peking and Shanghai universities. Among them are several who were trained in the Western world. One of the reports from China reads, in part:

> Holding aloft the great red banner of Chairman Mao Tse-tung's thinking and manifesting the superiority of the socialist system, we have achieved, under the correct leadership of our party, the total synthesis of bovine insulin.[50]

Banting and Best presented their report of the discovery of insulin somewhat differently. They described the use of pancreatic extracts with seven patients. The first of these was L.T., fourteen years old. He had

> severe juvenile diabetes . . . by January 11 his clinical condition made it evident he was becoming definitely worse . . . The extracts

---

[49] Banting and John James Macleod, a Scottish physiologist, shared the 1923 Nobel Prize for medicine and physiology. Macleod was also associated with the discovery. Best did not receive the Nobel Prize.
[50] "Total Synthesis of Insulin in Red China," *Science*, Vol. 153, No. 3733 (July 15, 1966), p. 282.

given on January 11 were not as concentrated as those used at a later date . . . Daily injections of the extract were made from January 23 to February 4 . . . This resulted in immediate improvement . . . The boy became brighter, more active, looked better and said he felt stronger . . . it justifies . . . hope.[51]

Nowhere in their paper did Banting and Best mention the Canadian Prime Minister. In the pancreas they found not politics, but insulin. It was enough.

[51] F. G. Banting, C. H. Best, J. B. Collip, W. R. Campbell, and A. A. Fletcher, "Pancreatic Extracts in the Treatment of Diabetes Mellitus," *Canadian Medical Association Journal,* Vol. 22, No. 3 (March 1922), pp. 141–46.

8

Of structure, function, and chronic impairments thereto: part II

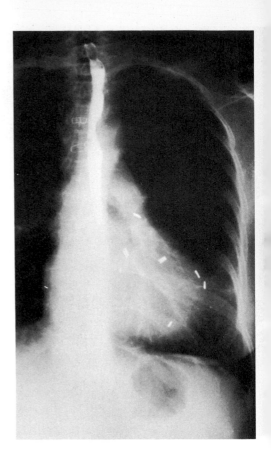

The circulation: structure, functions, and dysfunctions

On a cold January day in 1924, between 11:10 A.M. and 3:50 P.M., in Gorki, near Moscow, an autopsy was carried out. The subject was Lenin, once master of Russia, now dead of his third stroke. Ten doctors signed the final report. Attending, if not mourning, was Josef Stalin.

It was noted that the left side of Lenin's brain was utterly destroyed. The reason was apparent. A main brain artery was blocked. "The surgical instruments sounded as though they were cutting stone,"[1] remarked Health Commissioner Nikolai Alexandrovich Semashko. His comment echoed a long-forgotten report of yet another autopsy, performed by

[1] Stefan T. Possony, *Lenin, The Compulsory Revolutionary* (London, 1966), p. 413.

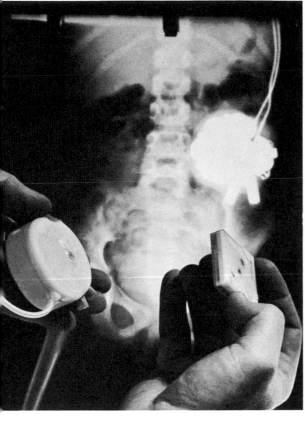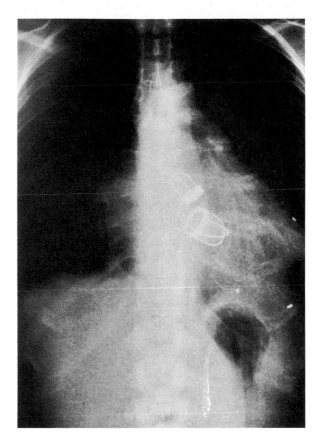

Technology aids the human heart. *Left:* The small white objects on the upper right side in this X-ray are metal clips sewn to the outside surface of a patient's heart during surgery. They allow measurement of changes in the heart's size and movement after the operation. *Center:* Artificial pacemakers (see page 247 and Figure 8-2). The X-ray shows the round one implanted. *Right:* X-ray of a patient's heart in which two artificial ball valves were implanted.

Edward Jenner[2] a century and a half before. Jenner's friend Caleb Parry recorded his words:

> *I was making a . . . section of the heart . . . when my knife struck something so hard and gritty, as to notch it. I well remember looking up to the ceiling, which was old and crumbling, conceiving that some plaster had fallen down. But on a further scrutiny the real cause appeared: the coronaries [the blood vessels supplying the heart] were become bony canals.*[3]

[2] Jenner's smallpox vaccine was to earn him perpetual gratitude.
[3] Caleb Hillier Parry, *An Inquiry Into the Symptoms and Causes of the Syncope Angiosa, Commonly called Angina Pectoris,* quoted in Henry J. Speedby, *The 20th Century and Your Heart* (London, 1960), p. 84.

Both Lenin and the man Jenner examined had succumbed because of a degenerative process of the circulatory system that kills more people in this country today than any other condition—*atherosclerosis*. To understand this and other circulatory problems, one must know something about the circulatory system and how it functions.

The circulatory system

In its broadest meaning, the *circulatory system* refers to the channels through which flow the nutrient and other vital need of the body. As will be seen below, this is a more inclusive term than the word *cardiovascular*, which pertains only to that part of the body's circulatory system composed of the heart and blood vessels. In this section, the heart and blood vessels, as well as the blood within them, will first be discussed. Following the consideration of this cardiovascular apparatus, the discussion of the circulation will be expanded to include "the trade routes of the blood." In tracing these routes of the circulatory system, it will become apparent how the necessities of life are brought to each waiting cell, and how that cell is relieved of its wastes so that it can remain vital. Then will follow a brief description of a circulation not of blood, but of another body fluid called *lymph*. This *lymphatic system* will be seen to be composed not only of vessels in which the lymph flows but also of specialized *lymphoid tissue* or *nodes*. The vessels of the lymphatic circulation are closely related to the blood vessels, but they never connect with them except when they finally empty, via two large *lymphatic ducts,* into the junction of two great veins in the neck.

The cardiovascular apparatus

The cardiovascular apparatus is the body's inner transportation system. By means of the circulation of blood within it, (1) oxygen, nutrients, hormones, and other vital materials are delivered to cells of all the body tissues and organs, and (2) wastes (carbon dioxide and other products) are transported from these cells to points of elimination such as the kidneys or liver. The circulating blood is also involved in (3) fighting infection, and the blood vessels help in (4) regulating body temperature. When skin blood vessels are dilated (widened), body heat is dissipated; when they are constricted (narrowed), heat is conserved.

The heart of a sprightly gentleman

England has had few monarchs so graceful as the ill-starred Charles I (he was executed in 1649). Devoted to ceremony (Charles was the only European monarch of his time who was served on bended knee), he loved good living. But he also appreciated science. This led him to permit his friend and family physician, William Harvey, to dissect deer in the royal park. Such royal empathy helped Harvey to discover the circulation of the blood.

When King Charles heard of the astonishing case of the young Irish Viscount Montgomery, he dispatched Harvey to investigate. As a child, the Viscount had endured an accidental chest wound, leaving in Harvey's words, "a vast hole in his breast, into which I could easily put my three Fore-fingers and my Thumb: . . . I perceived a certain fleshy part sticking out, which was driven in and out by a reciprocal motion, whereupon I gently handled it in my hand." The wound had "miraculously healed and skinned over with a membrane on the Inside, and guarded with flesh all about the brimmes." The Viscount's man servant daily cleansed the wound. Harvey brought "the young and sprightly gentleman" to the king. Thus, more than three hundred years ago, patron king and physican friend together felt the pulsing heart and, through the wound, noted also the "motion of his Heart; . . . in . . . Diastole it was drawn in and retracted, and in the Systole came forth, and was thrust out."[4]

Such dynamic observations helped to make modern heart surgery possible.

The heart as a double pump

The adult heart (Figure 8-2) is a fist-sized, 12½-ounce muscular organ located beneath the breastbone, in the left center of the chest (see body chart 9 in the color section). It is above the diaphragm and between the lungs and is enveloped and suspended in a loose *pericardial* sac containing lubricating (pericardial) fluid.

Each of the two sides of the heart has an upper chamber, the *atrium* (Latin for hall), and a lower chamber, the *ventricle* (Latin for belly, so named because ventricles are the large cavities of the heart). The two sides of the heart are separated by a wall, or *septum*, in which there is normally no opening. Each atrium is a very temporary storage chamber, holding the blood for less than a second. And each atrium is separated from the ventricle below it by a valve. To permit blood to flow through it, the valve opens. To prevent blood from flowing backwards, it closes. The valve between the right atrium and the right ventricle is called the *tricuspid valve* (Latin *tricuspis*, having three flaps or cusps). The two-pointed or *biscuspid valve*, between the left atrium and left ventricle, is also called the *mitral valve*. It is shaped somewhat like a bishop's mitre (see Figure 8-2).

Although the heart is a single organ, it circulates blood in two separate circuits. For each circuit the heart has a separate pump. In the smaller *pulmonary circuit* (Latin *pulmo*, lung), blood is pumped by the right ventricle to the lungs (via the pulmonary artery) and returns to the left atrium (via the pulmonary veins). In passing through the lungs, the blood has given up carbon dioxide and has taken on oxygen (see Figure 8-3). The pump of the larger *systemic circuit* is the left ventricle, which sends blood, via the *aorta*, to the rest of the body. The superior vena cava and the inferior vena cava return the venous blood from the body to the right atrium.

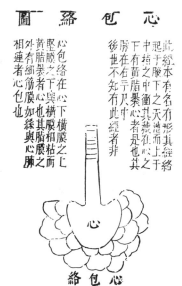

8-1 The heart, from an early 17th-century Chinese book.

[4]From *Anatomical Exercitations*, quoted in George Keynes, *The Life of William Harvey* (Oxford, 1966), p. 156. *Systole* (the contraction of the heart) and *diastole* (the dilatation and relaxation of the heart) are discussed on page 248.

From the pacemaker—the sinoatrial (S-A) node—rhythmic impulses fan out over the atria. The atria then contract. The impulses then continue to the atrioventricular (A-V) node, where specialized fibers begin—the atrioventricular bundle of His. This conducts impulses to right and left atrioventricular bundles, which go on to Purkinje fibers. These distribute impulses to the ventricles and the papillary muscles.

As the ventricles contract, the papillary muscles stabilize the tricuspid and bicuspid valves via their fine tendinous cords (*chordae tendineae*).

8-2 The heart: general anatomy *(bottom)* and electrical pathways *(top)*.

The heart as an electrical mechanism

The sheer labor of the human heart is wondrous. In a seventy-year lifetime, it will beat two and one-half billion times and pump some 600,000 tons of blood. Every minute every drop of blood travels the distance from the heart to the tissues and back again. What keeps the heart beating rhythmically? Specialized cells in the heart known as the *conducting system* are responsible. Within the right atrial wall is one group of such

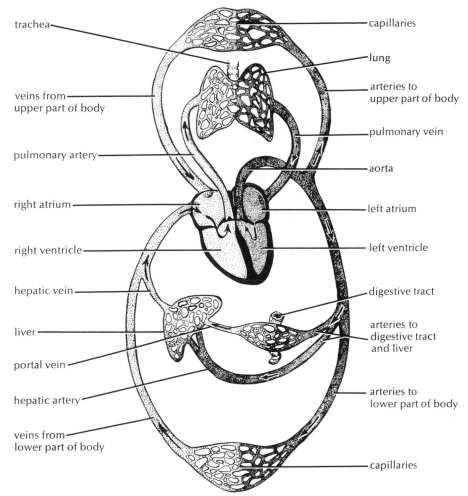

trachea

capillaries

lung

veins from upper part of body

arteries to upper part of body

pulmonary vein

pulmonary artery

aorta

right atrium

left atrium

right ventricle

left ventricle

hepatic vein

digestive tract

liver

arteries to digestive tract and liver

portal vein

hepatic artery

arteries to lower part of body

veins from lower part of body

capillaries

8-3 The two circuits of blood circulation: the *pulmonary,* in which blood is pumped by the right ventricle to the lungs and back to the left atrium, and the *systemic,* in which blood is pumped by the left ventricle to the rest of the body. Oxygenated blood is shown here in darker gray.

cells called the *pacemaker,* located in the *sinus node* (Figure 8-2). Located in the septal wall dividing the atria is another group of specialized cells. This second group of conducting cells is the *atrioventricular node.* Inherent within the pacemaker is the remarkable ability to emit rhythmic bursts of electrical impulses. The pacemaker discharges its impulses and then recharges itself about seventy times a minute. With each electrical impulse, both atria are directly stimulated to contract almost simultaneously. The stimulus then quickly spreads to the atrioventricular node. This node then sends stimuli to the ventricles. The ventricles also contract almost simultaneously. The contraction phase, during which blood is squeezed out of the heart into the systemic and pulmonary circulation, is called *systole.* Between beats the heart rests. This period is *diastole.* During diastole the chambers of the heart fill with blood entering from the veins.

THE CIRCULATION: STRUCTURE, FUNCTIONS, AND DYSFUNCTIONS **247**

In addition to the intrinsic electrical cardiac mechanism described above, the heart can also be greatly influenced by sympathetic nerves, which increase its action, and by parasympathetic nerves, which act oppositely to decrease its activity. Thus, parasympathetic nerves affect the heart during rest. During stress, such as exercise and heat, sympathetic nerves increase the heart rate (see page 225).

The blood vessels

ARTERIES AND VEINS   Blood is carried from the heart to the tissues by a closed system of *arteries;* it is carried from the tissues to the heart by a closed system of *veins.* Within these veins, one-way valves prevent the back-flow (see body chart 10 in the color section). The thick elastic walls of the arteries serve to withstand the heart's pumping pressure of blood. Vein walls are thin. In veins, the blood flows under less pressure, although this flow may be speeded by body muscle contraction.

ARTERIOLES, CAPILLARIES, AND VENULES   Between the arterial and venous circulations are microscopic canals called *capillaries.* They are so narrow that, in some, red blood cells can only pass through in single file. So numerous are the capillaries that, in volume, they make up most of the circulatory system.

The smallest *endings* of the arteries, the *arterioles,* end in the capillaries. The smallest *beginnings* of the veins, the *venules,* begin from capillaries (see Figure 8-4).

THE CORONARY CIRCULATION   How does the heart itself receive its blood supply? From seepage of blood that constantly courses through it? No. The heart has its own blood supply. Like all other organs, arteries lead to it, and veins lead away from it. But the heart receives first choice of the blood that, fresh from the lungs, is newly oxygenated (see Figure 8-3). Even before the great aorta branches off to carry blood to the head, trunk, or limbs, it gives off two crucial branches, the *coronary arteries.* Like an inverted crown or corona, these embrace the heart. After supplying the heart muscle with blood, the coronary arteries eventually terminate in a capillary bed, which empties into veins ultimately discharging venous blood into the right atrium.

Like capillaries elsewhere in the body, the capillaries of the heart have an important characteristic. Unless they are needed because of unusual activity, many lie empty and unused. There is no nerve control of capillaries to make them dilate. Carbon dioxide accumulation in tissue, as well as nerve controls, causes dilation of arterioles. The capillaries respond passively to the arteriolar dilation, thus regulating the volume and flow of blood within them. If a segment of the heart has been damaged, the capillary reserve in heart muscle tissue can be lifesaving.

Now follows a discussion of the blood "that swift as quicksilver . . . courses through the natural gates and alleys of the body."[5]

[5]William Shakespeare, *Hamlet,* I.v.66–67.

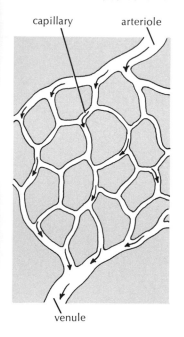

8-4 The relationship of arterioles, capillaries, and venules.

capillary   arteriole

venule

The blood: fluid tissue of transport

The nine liquid pints of blood in the body of the average human being teem with floating, suspended cells. The liquid, called *plasma*, is largely (80 percent) sea water. Man's evolution from sea life involved taking the sea water characteristic of that geological time with him. Sea water and plasma share the same salts but in different concentrations. The precise concentration of the plasma salts must be maintained within narrow limits. Otherwise cells die. With excess sweating, for example, body fluid and salt (sodium chloride) are lost. In some circumstances, the family physician might suggest salt tablets to prevent the salt concentration in the plasma from falling below the proper level.

The cells suspended in the blood plasma are as follows:

1. *Erythrocytes* (Greek *erythros*, red + *kytos*, hollow vessel). In the blood of the average adult male are some twenty-five trillion (one trillion is a million million) red cells. The average adult female's blood contains a somewhat smaller number—seventeen trillion. These comprise 99.9 percent of the total blood cells. They have no nuclei. The average red blood cell circulates about 120 days before it disintegrates and is replaced. Other red blood cells are constantly being manufactured in the bone marrow. For this manufacture, vitamin B_{12} and folic acid are essential.

A complex protein called *hemoglobin* is formed in the cytoplasm of the red blood cells. The iron it contains gives the hemoglobin molecule the ability to combine with and release both oxygen and carbon dioxide. A diet deficient in iron leads to *anemia* (Greek *an*, negative + *haima*, blood + *ia*). Normally, there is a balance between the number of red blood cells produced and the number lost. Health depends upon this ecological balance in the blood's ecosystem. When this equilibrium is disturbed, the concentration of red blood cells in the blood is diminished and anemia results.[6] Added to iron deficiency as a cause of anemia is blood loss. This may be gradual or sudden. Sometimes red blood cells are destroyed, as occurs in *erythroblastosis fetalis*, which is due to problems involving the Rh blood factor (see page 546). Inadequate production of red blood cells can result in *pernicious anemia*; this occurs because of a vitamin B_{12} deficiency. Rarer causes of anemia are poisons or excessive ionizing radiation.

Symptoms of anemia can vary from the mild but extremely distressing headache, weakness, and shortness of breath occurring with moderate iron deficiencies, to the far more serious consequences of severe hemorrhage. With anemia the blood cannot carry enough oxygen to the cells. Oxygen starvation ensues. Also, the heart tries to compensate for a decreased number of red blood cells bringing an inadequate amount of oxygen to the tissues. It works harder, trying to increase the speed of the circulating blood. In doing this, the heart is overworked. In severe and prolonged anemia the heart may enlarge and even fail.

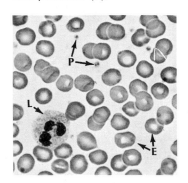

8-5 Human blood cells: erythrocytes (E), leukocytes (L), and platelets (P).

[6]Rarely, an excess number of red blood cells is produced in the marrow, and this may lead to illness.

2. *Leukocytes* (Greek *leukos,* white + *kytos*). Since leukocytes contain no hemoglobin to color them, they are also called *white blood cells.* About seventy-five billion of them defend the body against such stresses as infection. With most bacterial infections, leukocytes increase from a normal quantity of about seven thousand per cubic millimeter of blood to twelve thousand, twenty-five thousand, or even more. This increase is called *leukocytosis.* Pus is partly made of dead and dying leukocytes. Leukocytes consume bacteria by *phagocytosis* (see page 156). Most leukocytes are manufactured in the bone marrow; some (lymphocytes and monocytes) are produced in lymphoid tissue, such as the lymph nodes, instead.

With cancer of leukocyte-producing tissue, white cells are overproduced. Moreover, they are usually abnormal cell types and, unlike normal leukocytes, fight infection poorly. This is *leukemia* (see page 204). The number of leukocytes per cubic millimeter of blood may increase to a quarter of a million. This enormous overproduction interferes with erythrocyte manufacture. Anemia results. The invading white blood cells of leukemia overwhelm other tissues, interfering with their normal functions.

3. The third type of blood cells produced in the bone marrow are the *platelets.* By their involvement in clotting, they help to stop bleeding. Also important to clotting is a protein called *fibrinogen* (Figure 8-6). Plasma from which fibrinogen has been separated in the process of clotting is *serum.*

ABOUT A QUEEN'S GENES   A rare but deservedly famous disease, in which blood clots slowly or not at all, is *hemophilia.* It is hereditary and sex-linked. Like color blindness, the gene for hemophilia is recessive and is carried on the X-chromosome. Since males have only one X-chromosome they are more likely to be bleeders than females, who must have two X-chromosomes carrying the hemophilia gene in order to be bleeders. Bleeder fathers transmit the defective gene not to their sons (since a male child does not receive an X-chromosome from his father) but to their daughters. Unless the daughter has also received an X-chromosome carrying the hemophilia gene from her mother, she will not be a bleeder, but she may transmit the disease to her children. (Female hemophiliacs do not live to maturity, since the onset of menstruation is fatal.)

The family tree of Queen Victoria was riddled with hemophilia (see Figure 8-7). The son of the last Tsar of Russia was a bleeder. This led to the reliance by the royal family on the corrupt quack Rasputin and hastened the decline of the Russian court. The last Tsar of Russia shared this tragic situation with the last King of Spain, who also sired a bleeder. Both had married granddaughters of Victoria. "Thus two of the greatest dynasties of European history, the Spanish in the west and the Russian in the east, ended with uncrowned successors who were bleeders."[7]

BLOOD GROUPS   Before the turn of this century, transfusion was often followed by severe reactions and even death. It was discovered that

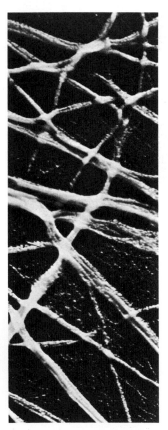

8-6   Fibrin strands (×29,250).

[7]Fritz Kahn, *Man in Structure and Function,* Vol. I, tr. and ed. by George Rosen (New York, 1960), p. 215.

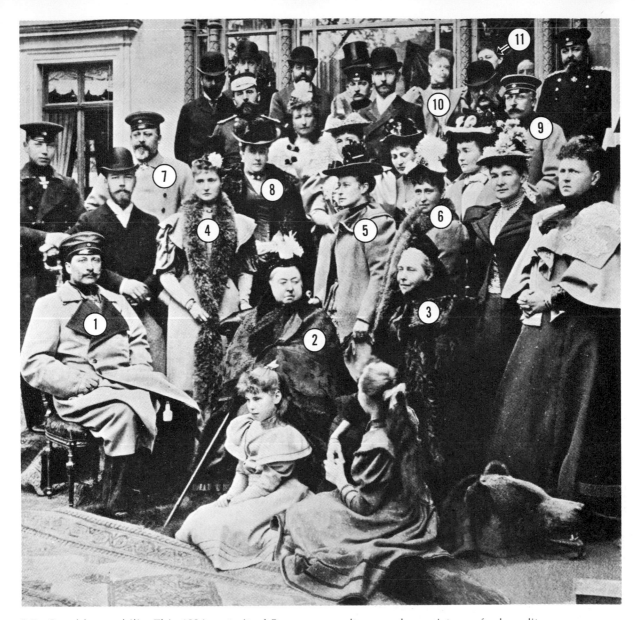

8-7 Royal hemophilia. This 1894 portrait of European royalty was also a picture of a hereditary dynastic misfortune, for Queen Victoria of England *(No. 2)* carried the sex-linked, mutant gene for hemophilia. One of her four sons, Leopold, had the disease; two of her five daughters, Alice (not present here) and Beatrice *(No. 8)*, were known carriers of the gene. Beatrice's daughter, also a carrier, married Alfonso XIII, the last King of Spain; their eldest son was a hemophiliac. Alice's daughter Alexandra *(No. 4)* was, like her mother, a carrier. She married the last Tsar of Russia, Nicholas II (the bearded man standing to her right), and their son was a hemophiliac. The fourth known carrier in this photograph was another daughter of Alice, Irene *(No. 6)*. She married Prince Henry of Prussia and had two hemophiliac sons. The other blood relatives of Victoria shown here are her sons Edward *(No. 7)*, future King of England, and Arthur *(No. 9)*; her daughter Victoria *(No. 3)*, Empress of Germany, a possible carrier; and her grandchildren Kaiser Wilhelm II of Germany *(No. 1)*, Victoria *(No. 5)*, Marie *(No. 10)*, and Elizabeth *(No. 11)*.

TABLE 8-1 *Blood Groups*		
BLOOD GROUP	ANTIGENS (AGGLUTINOGENS) IN THE RED CELLS	ANTIBODIES (AGGLUTININS) IN THE SERUM
O	None	Anti-A and anti-B
A	A	Anti-B
B	B	Anti-A
AB	A and B	None

this occurred because a donor's blood was often incompatible with that of the needy recipient. This meant that the recipient was immune to certain proteins in the donor's blood cells. As a result, the antibodies in the recipient's serum caused clumping and disintegration of the donor's red blood cells. Thus, incompatibility depends on the absence or the presence of antigens in the red blood cells and of antibodies in the serum. A person's red blood cells could contain A or B antigens, both, or neither. His serum could contain anti-A or anti-B antibodies, both, or neither. When a donor's blood, containing one or more antigens, is transfused into a recipient's blood containing incompatible antibodies, the clumping of the recipient's red blood cells that occurs is called *agglutination*. The antigens are called *agglutinogens* and the antibodies, *agglutinins*. Four main blood groups are differentiated (see Table 8-1).

A *universal donor* is a person with group O blood. Since group O red blood cells contain no A or B antigen, group O blood can usually be used for anyone. It is sometimes used in great emergencies when blood-typing of a needy recipient would be too time-consuming. People with group AB blood are *universal recipients*. Since their blood contain no anti-A or anti-B antibody, they can usually receive any blood with relative safety.

THE TRADE ROUTES OF THE BLOOD   To trace the *human blood circulation* one may begin at the tissue-cell–capillary level (see Figure 8-8). These billions of body depots are basic chemical communities. Within them occurs an alchemy of exchange. Tissue cells are wet. They are surrounded by sealike salt water, and the water is within them too.

Through this bathing wetness, the oxygen diffuses into the hungry tissue cell. And, through this same wetness, the tissue cell rids itself of its waste gas—carbon dioxide. Then this waste gas seeps through the capillary wall. Some of it attaches itself to a red blood cell. The rest of it is dissolved in the plasma. At its capillary level each tissue cell breathes. What has occurred? An exchange of gases. And, as a gas, the carbon dioxide waste is eventually capable of being vaporized through the distant lung capillaries.

But much more than an exchange of oxygen and carbon dioxide gas occurs at the tissue-cell–capillary level. Also transferred from capillary blood to the tissue cell are nutrients and hormones, as well as other vital

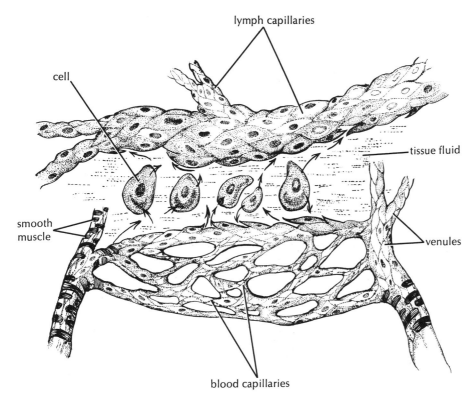

lymph capillaries

cell

tissue fluid

smooth muscle

venules

blood capillaries

8-8 Oxygen, nutrients, and other vital substances in the blood seep through the blood capillary walls into the fluid space surrounding the tissue cell. If there is then a higher concentration of a needed substance outside the cell than inside it, the cell membrane will admit it. Similarly, wastes traverse the cell membrane and reach the fluid spaces between the cells. The wastes may then be carried off with lymph (page 255) to eventually enter the venous blood, or they enter venous blood by seeping directly into a blood capillary. The kidneys, liver, and lungs clear wastes from venous blood.

materials. Fluid from the plasma, not red cells, carries these necessities of life to the tissue cell. To survive, the tissue cell utilizes them. But, just as the tissue cell produced carbon dioxide from the use of oxygen, it produces additional wastes from the use of these other materials. Unlike carbon dioxide, this second type of waste is not gaseous. It cannot be vaporized through the lungs. Only with the help of the kidney and liver can it leave the body. Whether or not arterial blood reaching capillaries contains these wastes depends on whether or not the blood has yet passed through the liver and kidneys.

The blood, having provided the cells with their needs, and loaded with carbon dioxide and nonvaporescent wastes, continues along its route. It leaves the capillaries for the venules. Propelled by the contraction of muscles through which the veins course, the waste-laden blood proceeds toward the right heart. On the way it picks up blood from the liver, via the *portal vein* (see Figure 8-3), which contains nutrients that had been acted upon by this great gland. Now containing nonvaporescent wastes, carbon dioxide, and food for the cells, the "mixed" blood reaches the right heart. It cannot reverse its flow because of the one-way valves of the veins. By way of two great veins—the *superior vena cava* (draining the upper body) and the *inferior vena cava* (draining the lower body)—the blood enters the heart's right atrium (see Figure 8-2).

THE CIRCULATION: STRUCTURE, FUNCTIONS, AND DYSFUNCTIONS   **253**

As soon as the right atrium is filled with mixed blood, it contracts. The tricuspid valve is forced open. Blood pours into the right ventricle. The moment the right ventricle is filled, the tricuspid valve closes (thus blood cannot seep back into the atrium). Immediately the filled right ventricle contracts. Blood enters the pulmonary artery and is propelled to the lungs. It continues on into branching, spreading arteries of diminishing size (arterioles) until it reaches the maze of lung capillaries. Single file, the red blood cells course through the capillaries, ridding themselves of poisonous carbon dioxide and of water vapor (but not of other wastes), while taking on life-giving oxygen. From the lung's capillaries, newly oxygenated blood, still containing nonvaporescent wastes and nutrients, continues on into tiny lung veins (venules) and then to increasingly larger veins until the four large pulmonary veins are reached. These enter the heart's left atrium.

The blood that enters the left atrium contains life-giving oxygen and nutrients and some potentially death-dealing wastes. The first two must be delivered to the waiting cells. The wastes must be eliminated by the kidneys and the liver. How?

When the left atrium is filled, it contracts. The bicuspid (mitral) valve is forced open. Blood pours into the left ventricle. As soon as the left ventricle is filled, the mitral valve closes to prevent back-flow. At once the left ventricle contracts. (Its muscle is thicker than that of the right ventricle because its circuit is longer. The right ventricle needs to pump blood only through the pulmonary circuit. The left ventricle must pump blood a much greater distance.) It pumps blood into that greatest of all arteries, the *aorta*. From the aorta, large arteries carry cellular wastes as well as oxygen and cellular nourishment to the liver and the kidneys. It is the liver and the kidneys that will finally rid the body of all the remaining cellular wastes. As with all other body cells, nourishing food and oxygen are brought to the liver and kidney cells. The liver and kidneys, then, must deal with two different wastes. One is produced by their own cells. The other is the remaining waste not vaporized in the lung. Both kinds of nonvaporescent wastes ultimately end in the urine and the bile, to be eliminated via the kidney and intestine, respectively. Blood, rid of wastes, continues on through progressively larger veins. Eventually, the right heart is reached. After circulating through the lung and left heart, cleansed, newly oxygenated blood is ready for distribution to the cells.

The circle is complete.

The lymphatic system   Like the blood capillaries, the terminal vessels of the lymphatic system begin at the cellular level (see Figure 8-8). (Figure 9-7, page 313, shows the lymphatic blood vessels in the villi of the small intestine.) Unlike the blood capillaries, the lymphatic capillaries do not act as tiny connecting canals between two larger vessels. Originating as blind-ended, microscopic vessels, the lymphatic capillaries, moreover, do not communicate with the blood capillaries, although they may intermingle with them. At

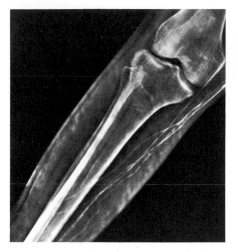

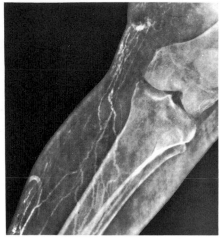

8-9 Lymphangiograms—X-ray photographs of lymphatic vessels, which are made visible by injecting a radiopaque dye into them. In the normal leg *(left)*, the lymphatics appear as thin, straight vessels. In the swollen leg *(right)*, the lymphatics are both more numerous and widely distributed; they are also tortuous, beaded, and dilated. An obstruction to the lymph flow in the groin caused this condition.

the level of the cells, the fluid within the lymphatic capillaries is exactly like the fluid in the extracellular spaces. Within the lymphatic system, that fluid is called *lymph* (Latin *lympha*, water). The lymphatic capillaries coalesce, blending to form larger vessels and these, in turn, coalesce to form even larger vessels. An accessory circulatory system containing lymph is thus formed (see Figure 8-10). In their course the vessels of the lymphatic system never connect with the blood vessels until they finally empty, as two large lymphatic trunks, into veins in the neck. By the lymphatic channels, large protein molecules, which had originally left the blood plasma to seep through blood capillaries into the extracellular spaces, are returned to the blood, and so a critical factor in the body's ecosystem is kept in balance. But lymph also contains white cells loaded with cellular debris, toxins, and other wastes (even bacteria) that must be kept out of the blood. This service is provided by the *lymph nodes.* Lymphatic vessels lead to these discrete organizations of specialized lymphoid tissue. Lymph nodes are not "lymph glands," for they do not secrete anything. Before lymph reaches the circulation, it is filtered in the lymph nodes. By special cells within the nodes, cellular debris and other wastes are digested and rendered harmless. It is in the lymph nodes that lymphocytes are manufactured and plasma cells make antibodies. In some parts of the body, lymph node tissue groups to form organs. The best known are the *tonsils* and *adenoids.* They can become diseased and may require surgical removal.[8] The largest lymphoid organ, the fist-sized *spleen* (see Figure 9-6), is situated in front of the left kidney and to the left of the stomach. It manufactures lymphocytes and antibodies and helps remove used blood cells. The spleen also filters some lymph and blood. It is, moreover, a major site for the manufacture of a protein-clotting factor that prevents normal people from having hemophilia (see page 250). Many

[8]Infection can acutely inflame the lymphatics, causing *lymphangitis.* When this occurs a red line can often be observed extending from the source of infection to enlarged and tender local lymph nodes.

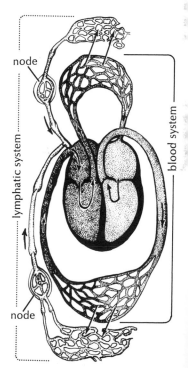

node

lymphatic system

blood system

node

8-10 A schematic diagram of the blood and lymphatic circulatory systems. Oxygenated blood is shown here in lighter gray.

TABLE 8-2 Deaths in the United States Due to Major Cardiovascular Diseases, 1968*

CAUSE OF DEATH		NUMBER	RATE (per 100,000 population)
DISEASES OF THE HEART	Active rheumatic fever and chronic rheumatic heart disease	16,440	8.2
	Hypertensive heart disease	10,000	5.0
	Hypertensive heart and renal disease	7,600	3.8
	Ischemic heart disease		
	Acute myocardial infarction	368,340	184.3
	Other acute and subacute forms of ischemic heart disease	4,960	2.5
	Chronic ischemic heart disease	303,810	152.0
	Angina pectoris and asymptomatic ischemic heart disease	150	0.1
	Total: Ischemic heart disease	677,260	338.9
	Chronic disease of the endocardium and other myocardial insufficiency	7,630	3.8
	All other forms of heart disease	26,430	13.2
	Total: Diseases of the heart	745,360	372.9
HYPERTENSION		8,980	4.5
CEREBROVASCULAR DISEASE	Cerebral hemorrhage	46,200	23.1
	Cerebral thrombosis	61,070	30.6
	Cerebral embolism	1,040	0.5
	Other cerebrovascular diseases	101,110	50.6
	Total: Cerebrovascular disease	209,420	104.8
ARTERIOSCLEROSIS		33,350	16.7
OTHER DISEASES OF ARTERIES, ARTERIOLES, AND CAPILLARIES		24,270	12.1
TOTAL: Deaths due to major cardiovascular diseases		1,021,380	511.0

*Total deaths in the United States, from all causes, were 1,923,000; the overall death rate was 962.2 per 100,000 population.

Source: National Center for Health Statistics, *Monthly Vital Statistics Report*, Provisional Statistics, Annual Summary for the United States, 1968.

of its functions are not clearly delineated. Its removal, a common operation, is not met by serious problems.

Terms describing impediments to the flow of the vital stream

The circulating blood is life's vital stream. And as all parts of the system in which the blood circulates are connected, so are the disorders that affect these parts related. A clot that plugs an artery deprives a portion of the cerebrum of nourishing blood. This condition is called *cerebral ischemia* (Greek *ischein,* to suppress + *haima,* blood), pronounced is-keé-me-ah. Cerebral ischemia can also occur from prolonged spasm of a cerebral artery. Portentous symptoms, such as dizziness and unsteady gait, may occur. The term covering the ailments that result from an inadequate blood circulation in the cerebrum is *cerebrovascular disease.*[9] When a coronary artery leading to the heart is obstructed, the resulting condition is *heart* or *cardiac ischemia* (see page 260). With severe ischemic heart disease, a portion of the heart muscle dies from lack of blood. Since the heart muscle is also known as the *myocardium* and the dead tissue is called an *infarct,* the term for a sudden heart attack is *acute myocardial infarction.* This condition, often called, simply, "heart attack," is a major and epidemic cause of death in this country (see Table 8-2). Another example of the interrelatedness of circulatory disease can be found in the instance of an increased blood pressure in the arteries. Such *hypertension* (see page 266) may result in heart disease. This is because the heart is forced to pump against the increased pressure. The heart may enlarge, even fail. Hence the term *hypertensive heart disease* (see page 266). Sometimes disease of the arteries leading to the kidneys (the *renal* arteries) decreases their lumen. Less blood flows through them. The *ischemic kidneys,* inadequately nourished, respond by producing a general hypertension—and *hypertensive heart disease.* Or, hypertension from other (sometimes unknown) causes can secondarily affect the kidneys. How? The kidney arterioles narrow. Kidney tissue is starved for blood. It deteriorates. This, in turn, promotes hypertension. The afflicted individual is caught in a destructive cycle of disease. Table 8-2 presents the 1968 picture of these diseases in this country.

Atherosclerosis

Now consider *atherosclerosis,* a destructive process of the major and minor arteries of the cardiovascular system. As a degenerative condition of these arteries, atherosclerosis affects them in such a way as to impede the flow of blood within them. It can be so widespread in the body, is so common, and causes so much sickness and death that it will be dealt with as a separate subject. However, atherosclerosis is not a disease but a disease process primarily causing many ailments of the circulatory system but secondarily affecting the organs dependent upon that system. Thus, one cannot, for example, consider atherosclerosis without being

---

[9]The word "vascular" can refer to a vessel or mean "full of vessels." The above context refers to the former. Cerebrovascular diseases cause signs and symptoms referable to the central nervous system, such as paralysis and the inability to speak. For that reason they are discussed in the section dealing with the nervous system (see page 226).

concerned about its effect on the heart or brain or legs. Moreover, the circulatory system may be affected by adversities other than atherosclerosis. Hence, following the discussion of atherosclerosis of the coronary arteries supplying the heart (and leading to heart disease) will be a consideration of other afflictions causing heart disease—such as infections. Atherosclerosis may also result in the already mentioned hypertension, but much hypertension is apparently unrelated to arterial degeneration. And so, although atherosclerosis as a disease process will predominate in this consideration of the ailments of the blood's circulatory system, some of the other problems of that system will also be discussed.

International cooperation with a major health problem

On a summer day in 1965, Adlai E. Stevenson, twice the Democratic candidate for President, fell dead on a London street of a heart attack. His coronary arteries were too clogged to permit blood to enter his heart. As the leading U.S. representative to the United Nations, Stevenson knew international confrontation. But among the most original investigators of the disease that killed him were men of countries whose leaders had caused him his most anxious moments. And among these pioneer investigators were countrymen of Lenin, whose fatal stroke had been caused by the same degenerative condition of the arteries.

Two centuries ago a Frenchman, Pouletier de la Salle, isolated a waxy substance in the bile (a fluid secreted by the liver and poured into the intestine). Fifty years later, another Frenchman, Chevreul, named it *cholesterol* (Greek *chole,* bile + *stereos,* solid). A German, in 1847, noted its presence in lesions (or plaques[10]) of certain arteries. And another German, the great Rudolf Virchow, noting the changing consistency of the lesions, named them *atherosclerosis* (Greek *athero,* soft, gruel + *skleros,* hard.)[11] So atherosclerosis is a lesion primarily in larger and middle arteries, with deposits of yellow plaques containing cholesterol and fatty substances. The plaque itself or a loose, broken-off piece of a plaque or a clot forming around a plaque can occlude an artery and impede the flow of blood. In 1909, a Russian medical officer, A. Ignatowski, observed that army officers had more heart attacks than the lowly mushik (peasant). Could the difference be dietary? The officers could afford meat. Peasants had to be satisfied with vegetables. Ignatowski then produced arterial disease in rabbits by feeding them animal products. Another Russian, N. Anitschkow, fed egg yolk to rabbits. This high-cholesterol diet produced atherosclerosis.

So Russian, German, and French scientists were united in seeking truths for all men. Like pieces of a jigsaw, accumulated evidence fit together to make a picture: atherosclerosis was associated with high-fat, high-cholesterol diets.

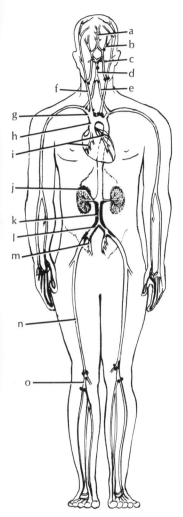

8-11 Common arterial sites of atherosclerosis: cerebral (a–c), basilar (d), vertebral (e), common carotid (f), innominate (g), aorta (h), coronary (i), renal (j), abdominal aorta (k), iliac (l, m), femoral (n), popliteal (o).

[10] A *plaque* is a patch or flat area.
[11] *Arteriosclerosis* is a more inclusive term referring to loss of elasticity, thickening, and hardening of the arteries from any cause.

During the semistarvation years of the German occupation, the Danes experienced less atherosclerosis and heart attacks than in later years, when food became plentiful. Relatively rich countries, such as the United States, West Germany, and Australia, have reported more atherosclerosis and heart attacks than poor countries, such as India and Korea. And in the blood of the inhabitants of India and Korea were low levels of cholesterol and fat. The Bantu of South Africa were studied. They had little atherosclerosis or heart disease. Only 17 percent of their calories came from fats. White South Africans were less fortunate. Over one-third (37 percent) of their total calories came from fats (mostly animal). They were plagued by atherosclerotic heart ailments.[12] An association between dietary animal fat and atherosclerosis is apparent.

How atherosclerosis begins and progresses

That modern magnifier, the electron microscope, combined with other tools, has added much to the knowledge of the atherosclerotic process. The very beginnings of a chronic problem may be observed. The early invasion of the inner arterial lining by fatty substances can now be seen. Small amounts of cholesterol are also detectable. Fatty red streaks and spots, ominous precursors of atherosclerotic lesions, may be stained so as to become visible to the naked eye.

How does atherosclerosis begin and progress? Intestinal absorption first feeds fat molecules into the blood of the arteries.[13] It is now thought that enzymes within the artery break down some of the fat. Then cholesterol and fatty acids are liberated. These irritate the artery wall. Inflammation mars the artery. Next, tiny capillaries grow into the lesion. They rupture. The lesion bleeds, worsens. It ulcerates, then heals. Eventually, it scars. Calcium is deposited. The artery stiffens, hardens, is occluded. When such an artery is cut at autopsy, an inexperienced surgeon might be forgiven for sharing Jenner's impression of falling plaster. An experienced autopsy surgeon may have a fleeting feeling of cutting stone, the sensation experienced by the doctor who performed the autopsy on Lenin.

The arteries of some body sites are particularly prone to atherosclerosis. The atherosclerotic process tends to begin at a point where an artery branches. Figure 8-11 is a simplified diagram showing some locations of arterial branching that are common sites of atherosclerosis. For example: note that the popliteal artery is a continuation of the femoral artery. But then the popliteal artery divides into branches. At the point of division, or branching, atherosclerosis may occur and impede blood circulation to the leg. Complete obstruction would lead to *gangrene*.

Is atherosclerosis a condition only of the aged? Has it now come to

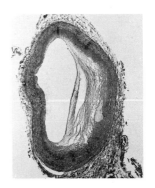

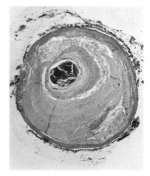

8-12 A normal artery *(top),* an artery with atherosclerotic deposits in the inner lining *(center),* and an artery narrowed by atherosclerotic deposits and now blocked by a blood clot, the dark inner circle *(bottom).*

---

[12] Alton L. Blakeslee and Jeremiah Stamler, *Your Heart Has Nine Lives* (Englewood Cliffs, N.J., 1963), pp. 42–48.

[13] Blood cholesterol levels are increased not only by diet but by several other factors. Among these are cigarette smoking, stress, and lack of exercise.

prominence only because more people live to be old? Decidedly not. Infant autopsies reveal atherosclerosis shortly after birth. Its telltale fatty streaks have been plainly visible in three-year-old arteries. An astonishing majority of autopsied U.S. soldiers killed in Korea (at an average age of twenty-three) revealed atherosclerotic plaques.[14] In many thirty-five-year-old males, other studies[15] show far advanced atherosclerosis, with as much as 50 percent arterial narrowing.

So when the average middle-aged man has a heart attack or a stroke, it has been a long time coming. His symptoms may be agonizingly acute. But for a long time his disease has been brewing within him. Few diseases have so prolonged an incubation period—so long a period between the first body changes and the onset of symptoms.

The four basic ways in which heart disease is manifested

The four basic ways in which heart disease is manifested are:

1. *Inability of a coronary artery to deliver enough nourishing blood to the heart* (*cardiac ischemia*). As a result of this first manifestation four conditions may occur:

a. A *coronary occlusion* takes place when the artery is suddenly closed off by a clot forming at the site of an atherosclerotic plaque or by a plaque swollen by a hemorrhage within it. A *thrombus* (Greek *thrombos,* clot) may be the plug (*coronary thrombosis*). At times, a piece of a clot, an *embolus* (Greek *emballo,* to throw in), may break off and occlude a smaller coronary artery. Although that part of the heart bereft of blood dies, the patient may survive. In that fortunate event, a circuitous blood supply develops around the dead heart tissue. The dead heart tissue is a *myocardial infarct.* So susceptible to occlusion is that part of the coronary artery supplying the front of the heart that it is called "the artery of sudden death."

b. The basic symptom of *angina pectoris* (Latin, a choking in the chest) may vary from a mild sense of pressure to a crushing, viselike chest pain. Often it heralds an occlusion. For an individual with diseased coronary arteries, excitement, exertion, or excessive eating may precipitate an attack of angina pectoris. Often the pain radiates up into the neck or down the left arm, usually into the fourth and little fingers.

c. *Rhythm disturbances* often result from myocardial damage. The infarct may include the conduction pathways from the specialized pacemaking cells responsible for a regular heartbeat. This infarction interrupts the normal pathways of conduction. Many varying disturbances of heart rate and rhythm may result. Should the ventricles twitch (fibrillate), blood cannot reach the body. Death occurs.

For those with faulty pacemakers, implantation of artificial pacemakers is lifesaving. The dramatic inadequacy of several such instruments was recently illustrated. A woman "became pulseless in her automobile while

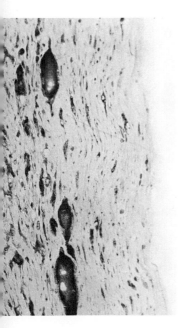

8-13 Lipids (fatty substances) in a coronary artery. The lipids were stained and appear black in this photograph.

[14]William F. Enos *et al.,* "Coronary Disease Among U.S. Soldiers in Korea Killed in Action," *Journal of the American Medical Association,* Vol. 152, No. 12 (July 18, 1953), p. 109.
[15]David M. Spain, "Atherosclerosis," *Scientific American,* Vol. 215, No. 2 (August 1966), p. 49.

the motor was running." Her pacemaker had failed. It was found that "the car's ignition system . . . producing broad-band radio frequency signals, also inhibited five additional pacemakers of the same model up to distances of 15 feet."[16]

There is, then, this added but rare risk of modern living.

d. When *congestive heart failure* has occurred the heart has been considerably weakened by disease. This type of heart failure may occur immediately following a severe heart attack, or it may happen years after damage to the heart muscle. Coronary artery disease is but one of the heart ailments that can result in this condition. It is, therefore, discussed separately (see page 262).

2. With improper development of the embryo heart, inborn or *congenital defects* occur. Every year some forty thousand babies in this country (less than one percent) are born with such a malformation. The heart of such a child cannot pump sufficient blood to the lungs for oxygenation. Some of these affected children have a bluish discoloration of skin and mucous membrane. This is called *cyanosis* (Greek *kyaneos*, dark blue) and is responsible for the term "blue baby."

Inborn heart defects vary in severity. A defect may remain unnoticed until late in life or may not be noticed at all. With mild cases, cyanosis might occur only upon exertion and then is noticeable on the lips and fingertips. In some instances cyanosis does not occur. In many cases, growth is slowed. The child is handicapped. With exceedingly severe heart defects, death may occur soon after birth.

The cause of most inborn heart defects is unknown. A small percentage are due to German measles or other viral infections of the pregnant woman (see below). Many of the more than thirty-five kinds of inborn heart defects are amenable to surgery. The heart-lung machine has been a surgical boon. By shunting the blood from the heart, it temporarily takes over the heart's blood-circulating function as well as the function of the lung in ridding the blood of carbon dioxide and taking on oxygen. The heart is thus "dry." While the machine substitutes for the heart and lungs, the heart can be operated upon.

3. *Infection* can harm the heart at any time, even before birth. Should a woman develop German measles (rubella) in the first three months of pregnancy, she has a twenty percent chance of having a child with the *congenital rubella syndrome* (see page 545). Such children commonly have heart malformations and other defects. Only a small percentage of congenital heart defects, however, are due to German measles. Surgery has dramatically improved the outlook for many of these small patients.

Rheumatic heart disease is no longer the scourge of childhood. This disease is a secondary reaction to a particular streptococcus. Why do some persons develop rheumatic fever after streptococcal infection, while others escape the disease? This is not known. Most often the streptococcal

---

[16]"Convention Report, American Heart Association," *Modern Medicine*, Vol. 35, No. 19 (November 6, 1967), p. 24.

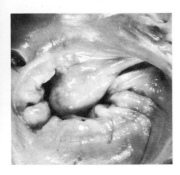

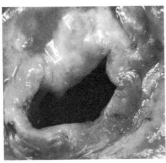

8-14 Normal mitral valve, left atrial side *(top)* and a mitral valve thickened and scarred as a result of rheumatic fever *(bottom)*. The scarred valve cannot open or close completely.

infection is of the throat, nose, and tonsil. The child may have a sore throat or joint pains. He may just feel unwell. Diagnosis is not easy. A good physician may need to watch the child carefully for some time. He is only too aware that, should disease involve the heart valves, eventual healing will result in valve scarring and distortion (see Figure 8-14). In consequence of such scars and distortion, the leaflets of the affected heart valves fail to appose one another properly. The valves try to close tightly but cannot. Blood leaks. Or a valve may fail to open completely. Blood flow is impeded. The physician will hear significant heart murmurs. (Not all murmurs, however, signify disease. Some are quite normal.)

Penicillin and other antibiotics can usually prevent rheumatic fever. One attack of rheumatic fever predisposes a child to another. For a child with a previous attack, penicillin pills are usually given daily until well into adulthood. In this way subsequent attacks are prevented. Surgical repair and replacement of valves scarred by rheumatic disease are now almost commonplace.

Medical advice for children with previous rheumatic fever is to be carefully followed. But the child should not be smothered with over-attention. "The living of strictly by Rule," wrote the seventeenth-century observer La Rochefoucauld, "for the preservation of *Health* is one of the most troublesome Diseases that can be."[17]

4. *Metabolic and endocrine disorders* may adversely affect the heart. An overactive thyroid gland (see page 238) may add to the stress of the heart muscle, as does the excess adrenalin produced by a tumor of the adrenal gland (see page 238), albeit by a different mechanism.

About congestive heart failure

Any illness causing impairment of the heart's action as a pump can result in congestive heart failure. (*Congestion* refers to the abnormal accumulation of blood in a body part.) Normal effectiveness may be seriously reduced by the valvular scarring and distortion of rheumatic fever. A long-standing hypertension may, at last, by its excessive work demands, seriously weaken the heart muscle. A heart frittering away its energy in the wild muscular twitchings caused by a damaged conducting system will result in congestive failure. Or the heart, long ago having endured damage from a coronary thrombosis, at last fails. An acute myocardial infarction may precipitate cardiac muscle incompetence. So congestive heart failure is not itself a disease. It is a complex of signs and symptoms that may result from various types of heart disease.

Either or both of the two heart pumps may fail. If the left heart pump fails, the fluid of the blood backs up into the lungs. There is a "rattling" in the patient's chest. His congestion causes him to cough and to be grievously short of breath. Sitting up relieves him a little. He seeks comfort

[17]From George F. Powell, ed., *The Moral Maxims and Reflections of the Duke de La Rochefoucauld* (New York, n.d.), p. 86.

from the support of several pillows as a back rest. Should the right pump fail, fluid backs up into the abdomen and legs. *Edema* (Greek *oidos,* swelling) results. Press a finger into the leg edema. For a while, the pressure point remains depressed. If both pumps fail, edema may be quite generalized. The kidneys cannot help. The weakened heart muscle cannot pump enough blood to the kidney. Salt that would ordinarily be excreted with the urine is reabsorbed by the kidney. Water is retained with the salt in the body's tissue spaces. Fluid collects. The treatment may include a sodium-restricted diet and the use of *diuretics* (Greek *diouretkios,* promoting urine). Diuretics remove sodium, and thus water, from the body. The patient must restrict his intake of salt.

But it is the flowering *foxglove* plant that provides the classic medicine for congestive heart failure. When its flowers die, its dull green leaves are finger-shaped. So the Scots call the foxglove "bloody fingers," and Welshmen call it "elf's gloves." A sixteenth-century German botanist named the plant *digitalis,* which is Latin for "like a finger." For centuries the practical peasant women of Shropshire, England, had been preparing a foxglove powder with which to treat dropsy. In 1776, Dr. William Withering tried a recipe of herbals he had heard "had long been kept a secret by an old woman in Shropshire."[18] The patient was a lady "nearly in a state of suffocation . . . her breath very short . . . her countenance sunk . . . She could not lye down in bed . . . her stomach, legs, and thighs were greatly swollen; her urine very small in quantity, not more than a spoonful at a time, and that very seldom." His fears of censure by fellow medical men unacquainted with digitalis "soon gave way to desire of preserving the life of this valuable woman . . . five . . . draughts . . . acted very powerfully upon the kidneys, for within the first twenty-four hours she made upward of eight quarts of water . . . our patient being thus snatched from impending destruction."[19] Withering's *An Account of the Foxglove and Some of Its Medical Uses* (1785) is a treasured medical classic.

Plan to live: know the coronary profile

One need not be an early victim of coronary atherosclerosis. Although there is an association between a high-fat, high-cholesterol diet and atherosclerosis, diet is not the only culprit. Kidney disease, high blood pressure, heredity, excessive smoking, diabetes, thyroid insufficiency, physical inactivity, obesity, even previous arterial damage—all these may well be involved. In some cases, several factors in combination may contribute to a heart attack.

However, there are patterns of prevention. Who is most liable to have a heart attack? What elements compound the risk? There is not complete agreement on the answers to these questions. However, some of the most seriously associated factors are these:

[18] William Withering, *An Account of the Foxglove and Some of Its Medical Uses* (London, 1785), p. 3.
[19] *Ibid.,* pp. 13–14.

1. A familial history of coronary heart disease; *the presence of diabetes mellitus, hypertension, obesity, and certain personality characteristics.*

2. Sex and age. *Men are generally more susceptible than women and both become increasingly susceptible with advancing years.*

3. Environmental factors *such as a diet rich in saturated fat and cholesterol, cigarette smoking, and habitual physical inactivity.*[20]

One of the most significant investigations[21] of the causes of heart attacks was conducted in the Framingham, Massachusetts, area. Five thousand men and women, free of overt coronary disease at the beginning of the study, were carefully studied over a period of time. Among these people, heart attack rates rose along with rising blood pressure, weight, and cholesterol levels. Heart attacks were much more common among smokers than nonsmokers. Also, those people who did not exercise not only had heart attacks more often than people who were active, they also died from them more often.

There is a familial tendency to heart attacks. So long as other risks are reduced to a minimum, this hereditary factor need not be alarming. True, the risk of heart attacks is statistically greater among short men with a heavy, rectangularly outlined, hard physique. Height, body build, and, indeed, tendencies to gout and diabetes are genetically influenced. But they do not, as factors, exist alone. A personal preventive program will add the normal years to the life span. Like health, disease exists in an ecosystem. Heart ailments have many causes. To sensibly exercise, to avoid smoking, and to control one's weight, profoundly reduce the risk.

Diet and disorder of circulation

Diet is an important factor in heart disease. Obesity materially increases the risk (see page 268). And those who are overweight for their body build should, with the aid of their physician, lose weight. The type of food is also involved. Many students in this area believe fats to be the food villain in heart disease.

Saturated ("Hard") *fats* usually solidify at room temperature. As a rule, they come from animals. Foods high in saturated (but low in unsaturated) fats include cheeses, butter, cream, lard, and meats, particularly pork, beef, and lamb. "Marbled" meats may be as streaked with fat as an atherosclerotic artery. Pretenderized meat is as tasty, less expensive, and more healthful.

---

[20]American Heart Association, *Diet and Disease* (October 1968), p. 6.
    Recent studies have indicated an increase in coronary heart disease in U.S. and Canadian soft-water areas as compared to hard-water areas. As early as 1957, Japanese scientists linked some quality of drinking water with cerebral hemorrhage—the number one cause of death in Japan. What the relationship (if any) is between water softness and coronary heart disease is now being investigated. ("Soft Water and Heart Disease," *Science News*, Vol. 95, No. 20 [May 17, 1969], p. 471.)
[21]American Heart Association, *Cardiovascular Disease in the U.S., Facts and Figures* (February 1965), p. 24.

Polyunsaturated fats usually remain liquid at room temperature and, generally, come from vegetable or fish oil. Safflower and peanut oil are high in polyunsaturated and low in saturated fats.[22]

Other fatty materials, in addition to cholesterol, are involved in the problem of atherosclerosis. Fat molecules containing phosphoric acid and organic chemicals (*phospholipids*), and *triglycerides* (glycerine combined with three fatty acids) surely participate in the problem. But, for many people, it remains basically true that the intake of saturated fats and high-cholesterol foods should be reduced.

In October 1968, experts of the American Heart Association stated that "in general, a diet designed to decrease the risk of coronary heart disease involves the following three recommendations:

1. A caloric intake adjusted to achieve and maintain proper weight . . .

2. A decrease in the intake of saturated fats, and an increase in the intake of polyunsaturated fats . . . *an intake of less than 40% of calories from fat is considered desirable. Of this total, polyunsaturated fats should probably comprise twice the quantity of saturated fats . . . margarines that are high in polyunsaturates usually can be identified by the listing of "liquid oil" first among the ingredients . . .*

3. A substantial reduction of cholesterol in the diet . . . *Careful planning is necessary to lower the intake of cholesterol without impairing the intake of foods high in proteins.*[23]

These recommendations should not be followed without the family physician's advice. But to restrict one's diet is often not easy.

"The world's most difficult undertakings," wrote Lao Tzu (b. 604 B.C.?) in the *Teh Ching* (Classic of Virtue), "necessarily originate while easy . . . Treat things before they exist. Regulate things before disorder begins . . . Only by becoming sick of sickness can we be without sickness."[24]

In 1867, Walt Whitman wrote:

About a poet's woeful physiology

> *Of physiology from top to toe I sing . . .*
> *Of Life immense in passion, pulse, and power,*
> *Cheerful-for freest action form'd.*[25]

[22]Fats are carbohydrates; that is, they are made up of only three chemical elements—carbon, hydrogen, and oxygen. Saturated fats have the maximum possible number of hydrogen atoms attached to the chains of carbon atoms in their chemical structures. Unsaturated fats have fewer hydrogen atoms in proportion to carbon atoms.

[23]American Heart Association, *Diet and Heart Disease* (October 1968), 4 pages.

[24]Quoted in Paul Carus, *The Canon of Reason and Virtue: Being Lao Tzu's Tao Teh Ching* (Chicago, 1913), pp. 118–19, 124.

[25]Walt Whitman, "One's Self I Sing," in Mark Van Doren, ed., *Walt Whitman* (New York, 1945), p. 311.

On the morning of January 24, 1873, he awoke to find his left arm and leg paralyzed. He had suffered a stroke. Later he wrote such lines as these:

> A batter'd, wreck'd old man . . .
> I am too full of woe!
> Haply I may not live another day;
> I cannot rest O God, I cannot eat or drink or sleep . . .
> My hands, my limbs grow nerveless,
> My brain feels rack'd, bewildered.[26]

For almost twenty years Whitman was ill. His seventh stroke was his last. What manner of disease destroyed him?

Normal pressures of blood

Turn on a water faucet. For water to flow, a steady water pressure must be maintained within, and thus against, the water pipes. A second propulsive pressure, augmenting the first maintenance pressure, must keep the water flowing. In a similar fashion, the heart maintains blood pressure. But healthy arteries are muscular and elastic, not rigid like pipes. They are well able to adjust to the pulsating flow of blood, which may constantly vary in velocity, volume, and pressure. The propulsive pressure of the blood in the arteries is the *systolic pressure*. The *diastolic pressure* is the maintenance pressure.

Abnormal blood pressure (arterial hypertension)

With abnormal narrowing of the terminal twigs of the arteries (the arterioles), blood cannot easily pass through them to the capillaries. The pressure within the arteries increases. This excessive pressure within the arteries is *hypertension*. To overcome it, the heart must work harder. A vicious cycle begins. Artery walls toughen and lose elasticity. To compensate, the heart muscle (the myocardium) thickens. This is particularly true of the wall of the left ventricle. *Hypertensive heart disease* develops. Increased pressure of long duration may damage the kidney and other vital organs. Occasionally, a hardened, weakened, small artery in the brain, under prolonged tension, ruptures. A small amount of blood escapes. The individual thus experiences a "little stroke"—a minor, transient paralysis (see page 227). It is a warning. Treatment and rest may delay a more severe hemorrhage for many years, and it may never occur. Sometimes, fortunately rarely, a more severe hemorrhage does happen. Paralysis, as occurred after the First World War in the case of Woodrow Wilson, may result. A massive cerebral hemorrhage, as in the case of Franklin D. Roosevelt, kills.

[26]Walt Whitman, "Prayer of Columbus," in Hugh I'Ansom Faussett, ed., *Walt Whitman, Poet of Democracy* (New Haven, Conn., 1942), pp. 248–49.

The resting heart rates of warm-blooded animals vary. The mouse heart flutters about five hundred times a minute. A man's heart beats seventy times a minute; an elephant's thirty-five. But for both man and elephant, the blood pressure is about the same. For a twenty-year-old human, the average systolic pressure is about 115 to 120 millimeters of mercury. The average diastolic pressure is about 75. Normal blood pressures vary greatly. For days, even weeks, many individuals have an elevated blood pressure without harm. Exercise, tension, and excitement raise the blood pressure. So does age. At sixty-five, a blood pressure of 135 systolic and 85 diastolic would hardly be considered abnormal. Only when the blood pressure is unduly high, over a prolonged period of time, is disease likely. Many physicians consider a consistent systolic pressure of 150 questionable, and a diastolic of over 90 high. Of the two, the diastolic signifies the lowest constant blood pressure in the arteries. It, therefore, means more.

Partial blocking of a main kidney artery may cause hypertension. Sometimes, kidney inflammation (*nephritis*) or other kidney damage may result in high blood pressure; the exact mechanisms are unknown. By liberating adrenalin, adrenal tumors may raise the blood pressure. This is rare. But most hypertension is unrelated to any other disease, nor is the cause for it known. This type is called *essential hypertension,* not, however, because it is necessary. "Essential," in this context, means "self-existing" or "having no obvious, external cause."

The headache, dizziness, even the shortness of breath of some hypertension may occur with many other impairments. Treatment of hypertension includes drugs, diet, and surgery. Side effects from drugs have, in recent years, been greatly reduced. Diets designed to reduce weight may be helpful. Restriction of sodium (which is most commonly found in table salt) sometimes helps to lower the blood pressure. For hypertensives smoking is especially harmful since it further constricts the arteries. The unduly distressed may be helped by psychotherapy. Of most importance is moderation in all things. By attention to rest and weight and by avoidance of tensions, years of useful living can be added to the life of the hypertensive individual. Today, a case such as Whitman's can be extraordinary. Recent years have seen a distinct drop in death rates from this too common circulatory ailment.

Population patterns of circulatory disability

In terms of human life what is the annual cost of cardiovascular disease in the United States? What is the relationship of age, obesity, and sex to circulatory disability? Every year about one percent of the population of this country dies. In 1968, more than half of these deaths were caused by the major cardiovascular diseases. By a wide margin, heart disease alone leads every other single cause of death, accounting for over 745,000 of the more than 1,923,000 deaths in 1968 (see Table 8-2). Although the death rates from all circulatory disease, as a group, have declined in recent years, mortality from heart disease has increased. Most of these fatalities resulted from atherosclerosis.

CAUSE OF DEATH	TOTAL Number Percent	UNDER 45 Number Percent	46 TO 65 Number Percent	65 AND OVER Number Percent
Diseases of the heart	721,268 100	21,670 3.0	177,733 24.6	521,865 72.4
Stroke	202,184 100	5,682 2.8	31,079 15.4	165,423 81.8
Total deaths (from all causes)	1,851,323 100	255,958 13.8	459,203 24.8	1,136,162 61.4

TABLE 8-3 *Deaths in the United States Due to Diseases of the Heart and Stroke, 1967*

(according to age)

Source: National Center for Health Statistics, *Monthly Vital Statistics Report*, Advance Report, Final Mortality Statistics, 1967.

The effect of age

Among the young, circulatory disease is not a major cause of death. It rarely kills babies; indeed of those who die of heart disease only three percent are under forty-five. Between the ages of forty-five and sixty-five the percentage climbs rapidly to almost twenty-five. In 1967, almost three-quarters (72.4 percent) of those who died of heart disease were over sixty-five years old. Stroke is even more an elderly person's nemesis. In 1967, more than four out of five people who died of stroke were over sixty-five (see Table 8-3). (See page 260 for a relationship between athero-sclerosis and younger age groups.)

Obesity

Obesity increases the risk of circulatory disease. "Mortality from circulatory conditions among males 20 percent overweight is 25 percent higher and for those 30 percent overweight 42 percent higher than for those with normal weight. For women 20 percent overweight, the mortality is 21 percent higher, and for those 30 percent overweight 30 percent higher."[27]

Differences between the sexes

The fragility of the male is discussed in Chapter 16. In no part of his body does the male more abundantly demonstrate that he is the weaker sex than in his cardiovascular apparatus. Table 8-4 merely begins to demonstrate this.

The table does not tell the whole story. The internal lining of a baby boy's coronary arteries is thicker than a girl's. In this respect the baby

[27] Louis I. Dublin, *Factbook on Man from Birth to Death* (New York, 1965), p. 177.

CAUSE OF DEATH	TOTAL Number	TOTAL Percent	MALE Number	MALE Percent	FEMALE Number	FEMALE Percent
TABLE 8-4 *Deaths in the United States Due to Diseases of the Heart and Stroke, 1967* (according to sex)						
Diseases of the heart	721,268	100	415,851	57.7	305,417	42.3
Coronary heart disease	573,153	100	345,154	60.2	227,999	39.8
Hypertension with heart disease	49,975	100	21,542	43.1	28,433	56.9
Rheumatic heart disease	14,176	100	5,988	42.2	8,188	57.8
Stroke	202,184	100	93,071	46.0	109,113	54.0
Total deaths (from all causes)	1,851,323	100	1,045,945	56.5	805,378	43.5

Source: National Center for Health Statistics, *Monthly Vital Statistics Report*, Advance Report, Final Mortality Statistics, 1967.

male gets a relatively poor start. His already narrower coronary passage is more susceptible to occlusion. "Up to the age of 40, twenty-four men to one woman will experience a heart attack."[28] Not until age fifty is the ratio reduced to fifteen to one. At sixty years it is eight to one. By age seventy, the ratio is equal.

Those seeking evidence of male equality will not find it in his coronary arteries. Since the ratios lessen as the woman ages, the female hormone has been tried as a treatment of male coronary heart disease. Its feminizing action has made it an unpopular therapy. This is just as well. It has not proven particularly effective.

The body's filtering system

Every twenty minutes all the body's blood filters through the kidneys. They are not alone in clearing the body of wastes. But the liver, lungs, and skin, important to excretion as they are, do not compare to the excretory activity of the kidney.

The kidneys lie at the back of the abdomen at the level of the lower ribs. A large branch of the great aorta enters each kidney as the *renal*

Kidney structure and function

[28] *Ibid.*, pp. 94–95.

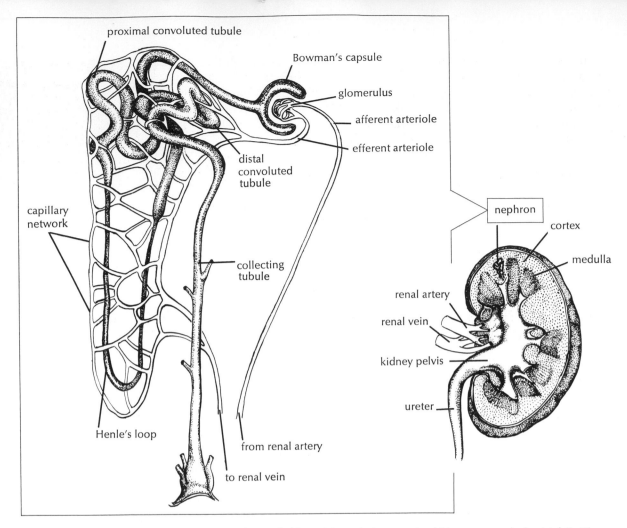

8-15 A nephron *(left)* and its relation to the kidney as a whole *(right)*. The nephron in the illustration of the kidney has been drawn disproportionately large so as to be visible.

artery. Like all other arteries, it progressively divides to become arterioles. But these arterioles (the *afferent arterioles*) do not, like all others, immediately end in capillaries, which, in turn, end in venules. Instead, each afferent arteriole first leads into a tiny tuft of daintily coiled capillaries, a *glomerulus* (see Figures 8-15 and 8-16). Each tubule (Figure 8-15) in the kidney is associated with such a glomerulus. A tiny vessel (an *efferent arteriole*) leads away from each glomerulus to drain it and then branches into a unique second capillary network around the tubule. Other branches of this efferent arteriole end in capillaries that, after feeding the kidney tissue itself, become larger veins leading to the heart.

The capillary tuft fits into the hollow of a *Bowman's capsule*, which is at one end of the tubule (see Figure 8-15). In this way the cavity of Bowman's capsule surrounds the glomerulus. The epithelium of the inner wall of Bowman's capsule that covers the capillaries of the glomerulus is made of specialized cells. These cells have tiny structures (visible only under the electron microscope) resting directly on the capillaries of the glomerulus. These structures can take up material from the blood in the capillaries, and they control not only the amount of fluid leaving the glomerulus, but also the content of that fluid.[29]

Each tubule plus its capillaries is called a *nephron* (Figure 8-15). This is the unit of excretion. As the heart pressures blood into the renal arteries, fluid and salt pass through the glomerulus into the hollow tubule. The fluid traverses the entire length of the tubule—down the proximal convoluted tubule, around Henle's loop, up the distal convoluted tubule, and out the collecting tubule. It then drips into the kidney pelvis (see Figure 8-15). There are some two million nephrons in each kidney; each nephron has its own glomerulus and tubule. So fluid from some two million collecting tubules drips into each kidney's pelvis.

But the fluid that drips into the kidney pelvis is a mere one percent of the fluid that passed into the beginning of the tubule. The other ninety-nine percent is reabsorbed along the way by the capillary net surrounding the tubule. It thus seeps back into the circulation.

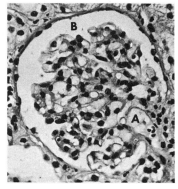

8-16 A glomerulus (× 215). Blood enters and leaves at A. After filtering through the glomerular capillaries, fluid enters Bowman's space (B), which drains into the convoluted tubule.

Kidney dysfunction

Kidney disease costs this country 100,000 lives a year. It is estimated that over 3,300,000 people in the United States have undiagnosed kidney disease. Some kidney diseases give immediate warning. Others do not. Once kidney disease has developed, its progression must be stubbornly resisted.

Pyelonephritis is inflammation of the kidney and its pelvis. At all ages, it is the most common kidney disease. In its early stages, it need not interfere with kidney function. As a chronic disease, pyelonephritis plays havoc with kidney function.

The *nephrotic syndrome* (*nephrosis*) is not an inflammatory disease of the kidney. In this ailment, large amounts of protein molecules escape from the blood into the urine. Body water accumulates (edema). The disease usually affects children. The cause is unknown, yet there is adequate treatment. In most cases, the drug cortisone is helpful.

Acute glomerulonephritis is a noninfectious, rarely fatal inflammation of both kidneys. It usually follows a streptococcal infection. (It will be recalled that rheumatic heart disease is also associated with a streptococcal infection.) During episodes of acute glomerulonephritis many nephrons may be destroyed. Kidney function is diminished. A prominent sign may be blood in the urine. In a few weeks the patient usually recovers from the acute attack. However, repeated attacks of acute glomerulonephritis will destroy an increasing number of nephrons. *Chronic glomerulonephritis* may result from repeated attacks of acute glomerulonephritis. How-

[29]Two common chemicals, caffeine (in coffee) and theophylline (in tea), cause dilatation of the afferent arterioles. This results in an increased pressure in the glomerulus. The rate of its filtration increases and, therefore, so does the urine output.

ever, many people with chronic glomerulonephritis give no history of such previous repeated episodes. Chronic glomerulonephritis results in progressive damage to the glomeruli; uremia (see below) is inevitable. There is no cure. However, much can be done to delay the ravages of the illness.

Polycystic kidneys occur as a result of improper embryological development of the nephron. This condition may be diagnosed at birth. The kidneys may be filled with fluid-filled cysts or cavities of varying size. When there are too many large cysts, the kidney will not function properly. Fortunately, most people with polycystic kidneys have the condition only mildly. They lead normal lives.

Unchecked chronic kidney disease results in a wide variety of symptoms. There may be a burning sensation upon urination, or the affected person may have to urinate frequently. The urine may turn a dark coffee color or appear bloody. In severe cases, widespread swelling of body tissues occurs. Thus the feet, legs, face, or abdomen may swell. Failure of the kidney to excrete waste results in a virtual accumulation of such waste in the blood. This is *uremia* (Greek *ouron,* urine + *haima,* blood), a most serious condition.

Modern miracles have prolonged the life of many kidney disease sufferers. Antibiotics fight infection. *Diuretic* drugs (page 263) help the kidney eliminate salt and water, thus relieving edema. As already noted, *cortisone* is helpful in the treatment of nephrosis; as yet, nobody knows why. *Artificial kidneys* are wonderfully complex mechanical devices that purify polluted uremic blood by filtration. Tragically, the procedure, which is painless, is very expensive, and there are today only about eighteen hundred artificial kidney machines attended by trained personnel, not nearly enough to keep alive all those who could benefit from the treatment. A new, smaller, and less expensive artificial kidney has been developed and is being tested. *Kidney transplants* are today quite common. Over twelve hundred such transplants have been performed on otherwise hopeless cases. A transplant from a living donor is possible because a person can function with just one kidney. A recipient's body is much less likely to reject a transplanted kidney donated by a blood relative than one donated by a nonrelative; the former has a seventy-five percent chance of surviving for a year or more in the recipient's body; the latter has but a twenty-five to forty percent chance. Failure of a kidney transplant need not be mortal. Second and third transplants have been successful. The transplant procedure is the result of long years of scientific labor.

Kidney quacks   The kidney rivals the intestine for the number of quacks who have exploited it. If not an actual kidney quack, Ann Moore, the "Fasting Woman of Tutburg," certainly gave the phonies of her time something to think about. She solemnly swore, in 1809, to have neither eaten nor drunk a thing for five years. Many a credulous Englishman believed her. A doubting Dr. Alexander Henderson revealed the fraud when he noted her sweating skin. Nor did he help Ann Moore's claim when "chance contact of his foot with an earthenware vessel hidden under the bed left him in no doubt that her kidneys were functioning very much as other people's."[30]

Quacks used to diagnose illness, not by examining the patient but merely by inspecting the urine. "What says the doctor to my water?" asks Sir John Falstaff in Shakespeare's *The Second Part of King Henry the Fourth*. His page answers: "He said, sir, the water itself was a good healthy water, but for the party that owned it, he might have moe diseases than he knew for" (I.ii.1–5).

The seventeenth-century English enriched several quacks who claimed to know the secret of turning urine to gold. Today, the injection of a woman's urine into an immature rabbit provides a valuable pregnancy test. A character in a seventeenth-century English play obtains this diagnosis without a rabbit: "I was once sicke and I tooke my water . . . to a doctors . . . The doctor told me I was with child."[31]

Modern quacks have been no less imaginative than their predecessors. But the kidneys are a grim choice for quackery. Chronic kidney disease affects the entire body. Heart disease and hypertension often accompany the kidney's inefficiencies. "Bones can break, muscles can atrophy, glands can loaf, even the brain can go to sleep, without immediately endangering our survival; but should the kidneys fail to manufacture the proper kind of blood, neither bone, muscle, gland nor brain could carry on."[32]

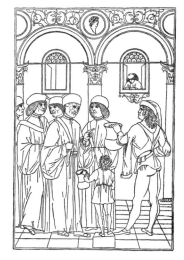

8-17 A 15th-century doctor examining a urine specimen.

[30] Alexander Henderson, *An Examination of the Imposture of Ann Moore,* quoted in J. C. Drummond and Anne Wilbraham, *The Englishman's Food* (London, 1939), pp. 343–44.
[31] Thomas Dekker, *North-ward Hoe,* quoted in Herbert Silvette, *The Doctor on the Stage* (Knoxville, Tenn., 1967), p. 22.
[32] Homer W. Smith, *From Fish to Philosopher* (Boston, 1953), p. 4.

9

Nourishment

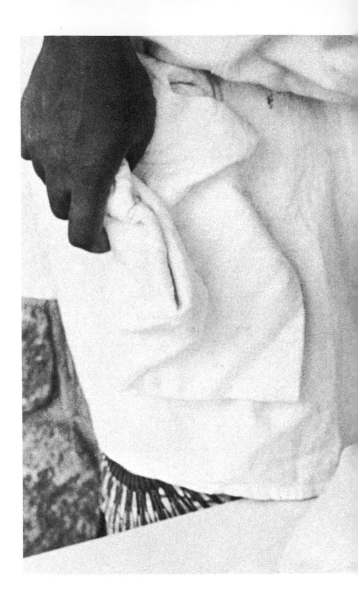

Taste, for which there is some accounting

In that year, 1959, a lot of the citizens of Peoria, Illinois, were shocked, even revolted by the deed. To make matters worse, it had been perpetrated by an officer of the U.S. Army. What had Lieutenant Andrew O'Meara done to so arouse his community?

To demonstrate a means of military survival to some friends, he had killed and skinned a stray dog, and then put it on a spit. The lieutenant

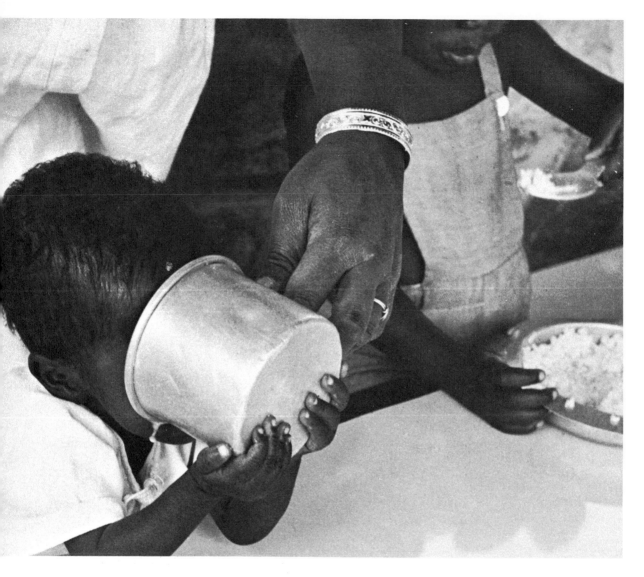

A hungry Biafran child.

was prosecuted, and a judge—under considerable public pressure—fined him the maximum $200 for cruelty to animals. The animal had been killed, not cruelly, but by a sudden blow. The lieutenant could have pleaded innocent, but the furor resulting from his demonstration that dogmeat could prevent starvation was too intense. He did not contest the case.[1]

[1] *Wisconsin State Journal* (August 11, 1959), cited in Frederick J. Simoons, *Eat Not This Flesh* (Madison, Wis., 1961), p. 91.

Food taboos have a long history. Hebrew Biblical instruction forbidding swine, for example, is specific. "Of their flesh shall ye not eat, and their carcase shall ye not touch: they are unclean to you" (Leviticus 11:8).[2] And, more generally, they were told, "Thou shalt not eat any abominable thing" (Deuteronomy 14:3). It was doubtless man's affectionate domestication of the dog that led to strong feelings against consuming the meat of the family pet. Members of Judeo-Christian cultures have had over twenty centuries to learn to abominate dogmeat. The ancient Zoroastrians of Iran considered dogs holy and the eating of them a sin. Moslems also reject dogmeat. But in some cultures puppyhams are a delicacy. Those who consider eating "man's best friend" a savage act should know that, until recently, dogflesh was relished among the Chinese, and their great culture extends over fifty centuries. (Dog breeding for human feeding was urged by one Man Lan-Chun, in an advertisement published in the July 19, 1962, edition of a Peking newspaper. It brought forth little enthusiasm. It seems there was a dog shortage.)[3]

Some religions have banned meat-eating altogether on certain days. On March 18, 1552, the Lord Mayor of London sentenced "a wyfe of Hammersmith . . . and a simple carpenter to public disgrace" for eating meat on "fysshe days." They were forced to "ryde on 2 horses with panelles of strawe about the markettes of the Citie, having eche of them a garland on theyr heades of pyges . . . toes, and a pygge hanging on . . . theyr breastes."[4] Charles IX of France (1550–74) ran no such risks. His marriage to Elizabeth of Austria fell on a meatless Friday. His guests were fed two barrels of oysters, fifty pounds of whale meat, two hundred crawfish, four hundred herring, and eleven hundred pairs of frog's legs.[5]

Food choices have not only been influenced by religion but have also been peppered with politics. Over two hundred years ago, John Adams tartly observed that the English ("absurd masters") had taught the colonists to dislike Parisian cookery.[6] Nevertheless, Thomas Jefferson brought a French cook to the White House. Patrick Henry bitterly attacked Jefferson's affection for French foods.[7]

Even the painfully hungry often reject food to which they are unaccustomed. The Arctic explorer Vilhjalmur Stefansson related that the Eskimos ate berries and strawberries only when on the verge of starvation, before eating their dogs, and finally, one another.[8] Yet many Eskimos are

---

[2] This may have been due to the infestation of pork meat with a parasite that still causes a disease called *trichinosis*. In its early stages the disease is manifested by nausea, diarrhea, and fever; in its later stages, by swelling and pain of the muscles. It is produced by eating undercooked pork containing the parasite.

[3] Jacques Marcuse, *The Peking Papers* (New York, 1967), pp. 60–62.

[4] *A Chronicle of Engleand, 1485–1559*, Vol. II, cited in J. C. Drummond and Anne Wilbraham, *The Englishman's Food* (London, 1939), p. 63.

[5] William Harlan Hale and the editors of *Horizon* magazine, *The Horizon Cookbook and Illustrated History of Eating and Drinking Through the Ages* (Garden City, N.Y., 1968) pp. 126–27.

[6] Charles Francis Adams, ed., *Familiar Letters of John Adams and His Wife, Abigail Adams*, cited in Richard Osborn Cummings, *The American and His Food* (Chicago, 1941), p. 30.

[7] James Schouler, *Americans of 1776*, cited in Richard Osborn Cummings, *The American and His Food*, p. 22.

[8] *World Health*, Vol. 15, No. 5 (September–October 1962), p. 10.

fond of raw birds (bones, feathers, intestines—everything but the bills and feet);[9] they also enjoy caribou dung and the stomach contents of various animals.

During the Second World War the people of the Mediterranean island of Malta were starving. Despite this, rather than eat powdered eggs they threw them into the streets. A century before, the hungry Irish responded similarly. With their potato crop blighted during the famines of 1845, 1846, and 1848, they refused the maize sent to them from the United States. In modern Asia many rice-eaters refuse to eat donated wheat and mullet.[10] Today, in this country, thousands of blacks who have migrated from the South suffer malnutrition compounded by poor food habits and the unavailability, in the new environment, of preferred foods.[11]

Poorly prepared foods are long remembered. The British Tommy of the First World War often referred to his canned meat as "Sweet Fanny Adams." Such sentimental remembrance honored the gentle Fanny, murdered in 1867 and hacked into small (presumably inedible) bits.[12] A century and a half before, the students at Harvard had been no less direct. Spoiled food provoked the Harvard Butter Rebellion of 1766 and the students wrote a Biblical parody, which read in part:

> *And it came to pass in the ninth month of the 23rd day of the Month, that the Sons of Harvard murmured and said*
> *Behold! Bad and unwholesome butter is served out unto us daily; now therefore let us depute Asa the Scribe, to go out unto our Rulers and seek redress*
> *Then arose Asa, the Scribe, and went unto Belcher, the Ruler and said behold our butter stinketh and we cannot eat thereof; now give us, we pray thee, butter that stinketh not.*[13]

But no matter how fresh the food is, many inhabitants of developing countries reject food because of taboos. The weaning of a child in Uganda is hastened if the mother is pregnant. The unborn child is jealous, it is believed, and will poison the mother's milk.[14] In Sierra Leone, eggs are withheld from children under five because eggs are believed to cause them to steal.[15] The Hindu will not eat beef, since the cow is sacred to him. To the Moslem the pig is unclean. He refuses pork.[16] Milk is the favorite

[9] Meyer Klatsky, "Studies in the Dietaries of Contemporary Primitive Peoples," *Journal of the American Dental Association*, Vol. 36, Nos. 4 and 5 (April–May 1948), pp. 385–91.

[10] *World Health*, Vol. 16, No. 2 (March 1963), p. 14.

[11] Jean Mayer, "Food Habits and Nutritional Status of American Negroes," *Postgraduate Medicine*, Vol. 37, No. 1 (January 1965), p. A-113.

[12] *The Mariner's Mirror* (1937), cited in J. C. Drummond and Anne Wilbraham, *The Englishman's Food*, p. 322.

[13] Quoted in C. A. Wagner, *Harvard—Four Centuries and Freedoms*, cited in Adelia M. Beeuwkes, E. Neige Todhunter, and Emma Seifert Weigley, eds., *Essays on History of Nutrition and Dietetics* (Chicago, 1967), p. 154.

[14] Anne Burgess and R. F. Dean, eds., *Malnutrition and Food Habits* (New York, 1963), p. 25.

[15] "Malnutrition in Early Childhood: The Newer Insights," *Clinical Pediatrics*, Vol. 6, No. 8 (August 1967), p. 493.

[16] W. R. Aykroyd, *Food for Man* (New York, 1964), p. 51.

food of men in the U.S. Army.[17] To the Dravidians of Southern India it is a nauseating excrement.[18]

So a multitude of factors—rooted in fear, poverty, religion, and habit—decide a person's food choices. Nobody decides his diet alone. Influencing cultural dietary patterns, moreover, are individual emotions. Few people realize the degree to which food intakes are responses to emotional stresses. Ice cream may be associated with parental reward, spinach with rebellion over parental punishment or authority, coffee with growing up, milk with mother and security. Some people may eat rattlesnake to gain attention. A single food may evoke different responses at various times. Milk, for example, may be both a "reward" and a "security" food.

Mingled with the vast array of cultural and individual emotional factors deciding food tastes are the endlessly subtle sensory perceptions of food. Man smacks his lips over coffee with "body." It provides a pleasurable resistance in the mouth. He also relishes color. Hence, the sprig of green parsley on the plate. Food without salt is deplored by Job. "Can that which is unsavory be eaten without salt?" (Job 6:6). Creamy substances mixed with air are smoothly delicious. A "rough" chocolate insults exquisitely sensitive mucous membranes. Crisp biscuits are tastier than tough meat. Good bread pleases the palate. There is more to food than eating.

The digestive process is often described in terms of combustion machines and hydraulic pressures. As book illustrations, these are useful. But digestion is profoundly influenced by the mind. Hunger is not the same as appetite. And food can cause physiological effects totally unrelated to either hunger or appetite. "Mine eyes smell onions," old Lafeu remarks in Shakespeare's *All's Well That Ends Well* (V.iii.325). Centuries before Pavlov's drooling dogs, the playwright, in four short words, thus defined the conditioned reflex. Yet he well understood the effect of the mind on digestion. "Unquiet meals make ill digestions," says the Abbess in *The Comedy of Errors* (V.i.74). The bard clearly saw the difference between mere hunger and appetite. Macbeth speaks: "Now good digestion wait on appetite, / And health on both!" (III.iv.38–39).

Appetite is a human quality. Animals enjoy food but do not savor sharing meals. "The infant cannot be fed by food alone," writes Dorothy V. Whipple, "he needs to dine . . . He cannot eat until the conditions of dining have been met . . . the infant relaxes and is eager to eat when picked up by gentle, warm, comfortable arms."[19] These are the observations of a pediatrician, but the emotional needs of dining have also been recorded by those who treat the aged—the geriatricians. The aged person who forgets to eat because he is alone is all too common. From the first infant intimacy of mother's warmth to the last suppers of the aged, humans learn this: man eats alone, but dines with others.

[17]Charlotte M. Young, "Food Habits and Faddism," in Abraham E. Nizel, ed., *The Science of Nutrition and Its Application to Clinical Dentistry*, 2nd ed. (Philadelphia, 1966), p. 224.

[18]H. D. Renner, *The Origin of Food Habits* (London, 1944), p. 73.

[19]Dorothy V. Whipple, *Dynamics of Development: Euthenic Pediatrics* (New York, 1966), pp. 368–69.

The basic constituents of foods

The basic constituents of foods are six—*carbohydrates, fats, proteins, vitamins, minerals,* and *water.* In health, all work together. A healthy body is a delicately balanced ecosystem, and a balanced diet helps to maintain that balance. The major nutritional uses and sources of the most important nutrients are outlined in Table 9-1.

All food is made by green plants. From the air, plants take carbon dioxide, which is carbon and oxygen. From the soil, plants take water, which is hydrogen and oxygen. From the sun, they get energy. Chlorophyll in the leaves of green plants uses carbon dioxide, water, and the energy from the sun to form formaldehyde and its related acids. (These acids account for the sour taste of unripe fruit.) With continued synthesis, with ripening, acids become sweet sugars. These, in turn, combine into starches. Then starches combine to form cellulose. These three—sugars, starches, and cellulose—are the most important forms of food *carbohydrates.* Cellulose and maple sugar are found in the leaves, wood, and bark of trees; grains contain starch, cellulose, and some sugars; fruits and vegetables contain all three carbohydrates.

"All flesh is grass" (Isaiah 40:6)— carbohydrates, fats, proteins

But not all carbon dioxide and water in plants becomes carbohydrate. Some combine to form complex acids, the *fatty acids.* These are the chief constituents of *fats.*[20] Unlike carbohydrates and fats, *proteins* contain nitrogen. The nitrogen originally comes from air, which is essentially a mixture of oxygen, nitrogen, a small amount of carbon dioxide, and some rare gases. Twenty-three nitrogen-bearing acids, the *amino acids,* are the constituents of body proteins. According to DNA instructions (Chapter 16), hundreds to thousands of these twenty-three known amino acids are arranged in various ways to become the thousands of body proteins. Of these twenty-three, ten cannot be synthesized in the human body. Since they must be provided in the diet so that the body can make the proteins essential to life, these ten are called the *essential amino acids.* From these ten the body is able to build the remaining thirteen. As sources of the ten essential amino acids, a variety of animal proteins are generally superior to the vegetable proteins.

Carbohydrates, fats, proteins—the three basic food constituents—are, then, all synthesized by green plants. Normally, when consumed, carbohydrates and fats combine with body oxygen (oxidation) to produce life-supporting energy. With a diet deficient in these, the body must resort to using proteins for energy instead of using them for body growth and maintenance. Growth—indeed, basic health—is then impeded. Present in adequate amounts, carbohydrates and fats free the proteins from energy-producing duty and save them for body-building.

---

[20] *Cholesterol,* which is involved in fat digestion, is thought to be related to certain artery and heart diseases, as was noted in Chapter 8.

Before an animal can begin to use the carbohydrate, fat, or protein of another plant or animal, it must break it down or *digest* it. Why? For two reasons. First, ingested food must be reduced to a size small enough to enter body cells. Second, within the far-flung billions of cell factories, the raw material must be reconstructed to resemble more closely the tissues to be rebuilt.

And so the processes of nutrition can become quite complex. However, one fact remains simple: all flesh is grass.

The vital amines

"My company," wrote Sir Richard Hawkins almost four centuries ago, "began to fall sick, of a disease which Sea-men are wont to call the Scurvy . . . The cause . . . some attribute to sloth; some to conceit . . . That which I have seen most fruitful for this sickness is sour Oranges and Lemons."[21] In *scurvy,* a disease of dietary deficiency, there is excessive bleeding. There is bleeding of the gums as well as under the skin surfaces and into the exquisitely tender joints. Observations such as Hawkins' led to a requirement that British sailors drink lemon and lime juices. Hence their nickname "limeys." Prevention and treatment of scurvy are accomplished by the use of vitamin C (ascorbic acid). Unlike the dog, man cannot make his own vitamin C. He must consume it. The commonly used fruits and vegetables are rich in this vitamin. The West Indian cherry of Puerto Rico has the highest known content of vitamin C. Only recently has it become a popular food in that country. If a mother's intake of vitamin C is inadequate, her milk will be poor in the substance. Among infants, scurvy is manifested early by poor growth or brittle bones that fracture easily. Symptoms of mild vitamin C deficiency in babies are frequently reported. However, they also occur in adults.

Vitamin C is unstable, easily destroyed (see Table 9-1). To prevent its being destroyed in the cooking process, a person cooking vegetables should drop the vegetables (undamaged) into a minimum amount of already boiling water. So that air will be kept out (and oxidation reduced), he should immediately cover the pot with a lid. Since even slight alkalinity destroys vitamin C, soda should not be added to food that is being cooked. Modern food canning and freezing procedures retain most of the vitamin C. Contrary to a popular notion, vitamin C is of no proven value in the prevention or treatment of colds.[22] However, some physicians believe that during and following infections there is an increased demand for vitamin C. This may be due to rapid destruction of the vitamin or an increased need. A regular dietary intake of the vitamin is, therefore, recommended by them.

In the 1870's, a disaster struck the newly created Japanese Navy. Almost half the sailors suffered a painful and crippling disease that paralyzed their legs, affected their hearts, and was accompanied by marked mani-

[21] Sir Richard Hawkins, *Observations in His Voyage to the South Seas* (1593), quoted in F. E. Shideman, ed., *Take as diRected* (Cleveland, 1967), p. 36.
[22] Georgina H. Walker, M. L. Bynoe, and D. A. J. Tyrrell, "Trial of Ascorbic Acid in Prevention of Colds," *British Medical Journal,* Vol. 1, No. 5540 (March 11, 1967), pp. 603–06.

festations of impaired digestive function, such as loss of appetite and severe constipation. Kanehiro Takaki, a surgeon in the Japanese Navy, related the disease, *beriberi* (from the Singhakese, "I cannot"), to the sailor's diet of polished rice. Less rice but more wheat, meat, and vegetables were made available. The result: in 1886, there were only three cases of beriberi; in 1879, there had been 1,789. But Takaki erred in attributing the disease to protein deficiency. At the turn of the century, two Dutch doctors stationed in Java noted a curious coincidence in a prison yard. Prisoners and some hens in the prison yard shared both a diet of milled rice and beriberi. A series of classic experiments proved that the "rice polishings," the germ and outer layer of rice, removed by milling, prevented the disease. It is now known that the outer husky portion of the rice grain contains B vitamins, particularly thiamine (vitamin B_1). Infantile beriberi is so rapidly fatal that an afflicted child may die only a few hours after being seemingly well. Even today beriberi is common among breast-fed children in Thailand, Malaysia, and Vietnam. When the mother is given thiamine, recovery is dramatic.

As dietary deficiency diseases, scurvy and beriberi are hardly alone. The first few decades of this century saw science illuminate more old dietary mysteries. The softening of children's bones from *rickets* had long been noted. The relationship of the illness to inadequate sunlight and its cure by cod-liver oil therapy was established many years before 1918, when an antirickets vitamin was first described. It required more years to prove that this vitamin—vitamin D—is manufactured in the skin that is exposed to *sunlight* and that vitamin D promotes the absorption, from the gastrointestinal tract, of calcium and phosphate—two minerals essential to bone formation.

But research into dietary disease was gaining increasing attention. In 1914, an American, Joseph Goldberger, turned his attention to *pellagra* (Italian *pelle*, skin + *agra*, rough). He proved that this disease, which was debilitating many people in the southern United States, is due to the deficiency in the diet of a factor later named *niacin*. Opponents of Goldberger's dietary concept of pellagra insisted that the disease was infectious. In a series of human experiments begun on April 25, 1916, twenty men and two women swallowed capsules of infectious concoctions of blood, feces, and urine of pellagra patients. Dr. and Mrs. Goldberger were among them. None of the human volunteers developed pellagra. By 1912, however, the Polish biochemist Casimir Funk had already summed up what was known at that time. There were four substances containing nitrogen, *amines*, that were vital to life, he postulated. These vital amines he called *vitamines*. Each specifically prevented beriberi, scurvy, rickets, or pellagra. He was right, as far as he went. Now it is known that there are more than four such vital substances. Since new factors have been discovered, the "e" has been dropped in "vitamines."

Each vitamin is either water- or fat-soluble. The water-soluble vitamins are the B complex vitamins and vitamin C (ascorbic acid). The fat-soluble vitamins are A, D, E, and K. Two of them (A and D) are presented in Table 9-1. Although vitamin E deficiency causes male sterility and interferes with the female reproductive ability in some lower animals, its function in people remains unclear. Nor has vitamin E deficiency been demonstrated in human beings. Vitamin K is essential for the manufacture of substances necessary for normal blood clotting. Much of it is made by bacteria in the large intestine, and it is then absorbed into the circulation. When oral antibiotics are ingested, the intestinal ecosystem of these vitamin K–producing bacteria changes, so they may not survive. The termination of the beneficial action of these bacteria in the human intestine can result in vitamin K deficiency—still another potent argument against self-medication.

Vitamin pills never make up for an inadequate diet. Furthermore, their indiscriminate use can be harmful. Folic acid (one of the B vitamins) and vitamin B_{12} are both needed by the bone marrow to make red blood cells. Used in high doses, folic acid relieves some of the symptoms of pernicious anemia. But folic acid does not halt the progressive deterioration of the nervous system caused by pernicious anemia. For a while, a self-medicating individual with the disease may feel better. But he has been lulled into a false sense of security. By the time he seeks medical care it may be too late to correct the error. The toxicity of excessive doses of vitamin D provides still another example of the hazards of self-medication. A host of disagreeable symptoms, including nausea, vomiting, and diarrhea, may occur. Too much intake of vitamin A may cause serious toxic signs and symptoms, including loss of appetite, irritability, abnormal skin pigmentation, dry skin, loss of hair, and bone and joint pains. It is the family physician who should decide about the use of vitamin pills.

Minerals

Disintegrating rocks provide minerals for soil. From soil, growing plants take needed minerals. Man obtains minerals from plants, from animals consuming plants, and from such animal products as milk and eggs. There are nine principal minerals in the human body: calcium, phosphorus, chlorine, potassium, sodium, sulfur, iodine,[23] iron, and magnesium. Some other elements are present in much lesser amounts. These are copper, manganese, cobalt, zinc, fluorine,[24] molybdenum, selenium, and chromium. The amount that is needed of each of them varies. An average-sized man has about two and three-fourths pounds of calcium in his body but just a trace amount of iron. Both are equally essential. Only four percent of body tissue is composed of minerals.

Unlike proteins, fats, and carbohydrates, but like water and vitamins, minerals are not acted upon by digestive juices. Freed from foods by

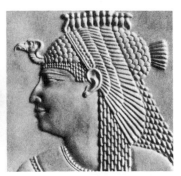

9-1 Cleopatra, Queen of the Nile, and her goiter.

[23] Iodine is essential for the adequate production of thyroxine and triiodothyronine, hormones manufactured by the thyroid gland. With reduced thyroid hormones in the serum, the pituitary gland causes the thyroid to produce more cells to manufacture hormone. This abnormal enlargement of the thyroid is *goiter*. Common goiter is primarily an iodine-deficiency disease.
[24] Fluorine is a gaseous element, and although it has not been proven essential to life, fluorides are important to prevention of cavities (see pages 305–06).

digestion, they are absorbed, used in body building and regulation, and then excreted. To make up for their constant loss, they must, therefore, be regularly supplied in the diet.

It is in calcium and iron that the diet of this nation's people is often poor. Foods with enough protein and calcium usually contain adequate phosphates too. Some foods (milk, for example) contain more calcium than others (such as eggs); some (milk again) contain calcium that is more readily absorbed than the calcium in other foods (such as spinach).

Women need more iron than men. Periodic blood loss and the needs of a baby during pregnancy account for greater iron requirements of women. Iron deficiency among women is common. An adequate diet is necessary. However, iron can be given as a supplement.

Water

Man can live for weeks without food but only for days without water. The water within man is but the earliest sea water that collected on earth. Man did not leave the sea behind. He took it with him, encasing it within his body. Slightly more than half of the adult body weight is water. It is the medium in which all chemical reactions of the body take place. As the most important of all solvents, water brings enzymes (see page 298) into the digestive tract. As a carrier, water is essential to digestion, circulation, absorption, and excretion. Cells waiting to receive food are bathed in water. Two-thirds of body water is inside the cells, and one-third is outside. Nutrients are brought to the cells by the blood, which is about 80 percent water. After food has been used by the cells, there are waste products. These are transferred through watery solutions to the blood and excreted via the kidney in the urine, which is about 97 percent water. In the discussion of water pollution (in Chapter 3), it was pointed out that man is now recycling waste water and using it again after making it pure. The normal kidney has always done this efficiently. Large volumes of water carry waste to the kidney, but in passing through the kidney most of the water is reabsorbed and reused. The urine that is excreted is a concentrated watery solution of the body's waste products (see pages 269–71). Water has even more functions. In its involvement with the movements of the internal organs of the abdomen, and in the lubrication of the joints, water is essential to body mechanics. Too, water helps regulate body temperature.

Some measures of nutrition

Calories

In 1794, the elegant aristocrat and great scientist Antoine Laurent Lavoisier was ordered guillotined by a judge of the French Revolution. Begged to spare his valuable head, the judge curtly answered, "The Republic has no need of scientists." After the execution, Lagrange, an old friend of Lavoisier, whispered wiser words. "It took but a second to cut off his head; a hundred years will not suffice to produce one like it."[25] One of Lavoisier's contributions was to point out that ingested food is burned in a chemical reaction (oxidation) to yield heat and energy. From this "body fuel" concept comes the idea of the *calorie*.

A calorie is the amount of heat required to raise the temperature of one gram of water one degree Centigrade. This is truly a tiny unit of heat. What nutritionists really use is the large kilocalorie, which is a thousand times greater. The term "calorie" is now so commonly used, however, that the "kilo" is dropped in ordinary usage.

Caloric contents of food vary enormously. A given weight of fat contains over twice as many calories as an equal weight of carbohydrates or proteins. Proteins and carbohydrates each have four calories per gram. In a gram of fat there are nine calories.

What is adequate nutrition for the normal, nondieting person? One may rely on the food groups. Table 9-2 provides caloric values in single servings of representative samples of the basic four—the milk, meat, vegetable-fruit, and bread-cereal groups. It also includes representative fats and sweets.

With activity, calorie requirements increase (Tables 9-4 and 9-5). But age, sex, body size, and climate also influence the number of calories a person uses. Because of growth requirements, adolescents need relatively more calories than adults. The aged need fewer calories than the young. Women, who are generally smaller than men, usually need fewer calories. Pregnancy and lactation increase caloric demands. A hot day, mostly because it decreases activity, decreases caloric needs.

Nutritive values of foods, moreover, depend in part on the way the foods are prepared. Fried potatoes, for example, contain much more fat than baked potatoes. In addition, some sick people are unable to digest some foods. Fats are poorly digested by some people with disease of the pancreas (see page 310). Fatigue also impedes the labor of digestion, as do tension and rapid eating. That is why, insofar as possible, one should rest before and after dinner. Thus, the number of calories on a calorie chart is not always the number of calories eventually used by the eater.

Weights and measures

Formerly "ideal weight" was based on average weights according to age, sex, and height. With such an inadequate measure, the ideal weight of an average woman could be considerably more at fifty than at twenty years of age. But it has since been found that people who are of average or slightly less than average weight at twenty-five are healthier and live longer if they maintain that weight for the rest of their lives. In addition, after one's maximum height is achieved, there is no need to gain more weight. Such "ideal weight" tables were especially inaccurate for still another reason. Fat, muscles, organs, bones, and fluid all contribute to weight. Thus, a muscular athlete may weigh more than is recommended

[25] Quoted in Graham Lusk, *Nutrition* (New York, 1964), p. 63.

because of the weight of his larger muscles. He is heavy but his problem is not excessive fat. Although modern charts attempt to correct this by adding body build to weight charts (Table 9-7), the best way to determine actual body fatness is by measuring skinfold thickness with *calipers* (see Figure 9-2). Norms for this measurement have yet to be completely established and agreed upon.

What is meant by overweight? The term does not directly connote excessive fat. A better term might be over-heaviness. However, many nutritionists would agree that someone who weighs 10 to 20 percent over the desirable body weight is overweight. Obesity refers to a generalized bodily condition in which there is excessive storage of fat. The term is commonly used to denote 20 percent or more above the desirable weight.

Harvard nutritionist Jean Mayer describes some "unscientific" yet worthwhile methods of assessing fatness. "If you *look* fat," he writes, in suggesting the *mirror test,* "you probably *are* fat," The *pinch test* involves lifting free a fold of skin and its underlying fat from various body areas such as the back of the upper arm or the abdomen. If the fold is markedly greater than one inch, excessive body fat is indicated. (If the fold is thinner than one-half inch, the individual is probably too thin.) When the *ruler test* is used, the individual lies flat on his back. "If he or she is not too fat, the surface of the abdomen between the flare of the ribs and the front of the pelvis is normally flat or slightly concave and a ruler placed on the abdomen along the midline of the body should touch both the ribs and the pelvic area." In the *belt-line test,* Mayer points out that a man has too much abdominal fat if the circumference of the abdomen at the navel exceeds the circumference of the chest at the nipples. Ordinarily the circumference of the chest exceeds that of the abdomen.[26]

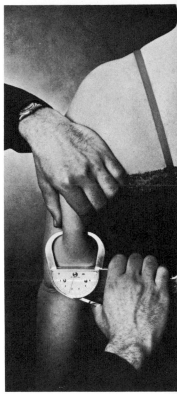

9-2 Skinfold calipers for measuring body fat.

Weighing too much

A relatively small number of people are obese because of an endocrine gland (see page 237) disturbance. Such obesity may be genetically transmitted.[27] (Specific tests help make such a diagnosis.) Most obesity is due to overeating and lack of exercise. Caloric intake simply exceeds energy need. Excess energy is stored as fat and excess fat is detrimental to health. Laborsaving devices have eased life, but the food intake of the U.S. citizen has not decreased with his energy needs. Nothing has added more to the weight problems of the people of this nation than the "snack." Not enough people realize that an average chocolate-covered bar provides more calories than a three-ounce serving of pot roast, that an eight-ounce ginger ale highball has as many calories as two medium-sized white potatoes, that concealed in that tempting cream puff are al-

Why do people weigh too much?

---

[26] Jean Mayer, *Overweight* (Englewood Cliffs, N.J., 1968), pp. 29–30.
[27] Edgar S. Gordon, "Obesity: Gluttony or Genes?" *Postgraduate Medicine,* Vol. 45, No. 2 (June 1969), pp. 95–100.

TABLE 9-1 *A Dozen Leading Nutrients*

NAME	IMPORTANT FOOD SOURCES	WHY NEEDED
CARBOHYDRATES (Sugars and starches)	Breads and cereals Potatoes and corn Bananas Dried fruits and sweet-ened fruits Sugar, sirup, jelly, honey	To supply energy. To carry other nutrients present in the food.
FATS	Butter and cream Salad oils and dressings Cooking fats Fat meats	To supply a large amount of energy in a small amount of food. To help keep skin smooth and healthy by supplying "essential fatty acids."
PROTEINS	Meat, fish, poultry, eggs All kinds of cheese Milk Breads and cereals Dried beans and peas Peanut butter and nuts	To build and repair all tissues in the body. Cellular proteins provide most of the cell's structure and are the enzymes controlling the cell's chemical reactions. To help form antibodies in the blood for fighting infection. To supply energy.

NAME	IMPORTANT FOOD SOURCES	WHY NEEDED	STABILITY TO HANDLING
VITAMINS Vitamin A	Yellow fruits and dark green and yellow vegetables Butter, whole milk, cream, Cheddar-type cheese, ice cream Liver	To help keep skin smooth and soft. To help keep mucous membranes firm and resistant to infection. To protect against night-blindness.	Stable to ordinary cooking temperatures. Unstable to long exposure in warm air. Not dissolved in cooking water.
Vitamin B_1 (Thiamine)	Meat, fish, poultry, eggs (pork supplies about three times as much as other meats) Enriched and whole grain breads, cereals Milk White potatoes	To keep appetite and digestion normal. To keep nervous system healthy. To help prevent irritability. To help body release energy from food.	Unstable to heat, especially in alkaline solutions (soda). Dissolved in cooking water.
Vitamin B_2 (Riboflavin)	Milk All kinds of cheese Ice cream Meat, fish, poultry, eggs	To help cells use oxygen. To help keep vision clear. To help prevent cracking at the corners of the mouth. To help keep skin and tongue smooth. To help prevent scaly, greasy skin around mouth and nose.	Fairly stable to ordinary cooking temperatures, especially in acid solutions. Unstable to ultraviolet light (direct sunlight). Dissolved in cooking water.

Table 9-1 (continued)

NAME	IMPORTANT FOOD SOURCES	WHY NEEDED	STABILITY TO HANDLING
Vitamin C (Ascorbic acid)	Citrus fruits—lemon, orange, grapefruit, lime Strawberries and cantaloupe Tomatoes Green peppers and broccoli Raw greens and cabbage White potatoes	To make cementing materials that hold body cells together. To make walls of blood vessels firm. To help resist infection. To help prevent fatigue. To help in healing wounds and broken bones.	Stable in acid. Unstable: destroyed by oxidation, which is hastened by warm temperature, long, slow cooking, exposure to alkali and copper. Dissolved in cooking water.
Vitamin D	Vitamin D milk Butter Fish liver oil (Also reaches man in sunshine)	To help the body absorb calcium from digestive tract. To help build calcium and phosphorus into bones.	Stable to heating, aging, and storage. Destroyed by excess ultraviolet light.

NAME	IMPORTANT FOOD SOURCES	WHY NEEDED	
MINERALS Calcium	Milk Cheese, especially Cheddar-type Ice cream Turnip and mustard greens Collards and kale	To help build bones and teeth. To help make blood clot. To help muscles react normally. To delay fatigue and help tired muscles recover.	
Iron	Liver Meat and eggs Green leafy vegetables Raisins and dried apricots	To combine with protein to make hemoglobin, the red substance in the blood that carries oxygen to the cells. About two-thirds of the body's iron is in the hemoglobin of the blood. (The minerals copper and cobalt also affect the red blood cell formation.)	
Copper	Essentially the same foods that provide iron	To act in the process by which iron is used in the synthesis of hemoglobin. Also, an essential constituent of many enzymes that function in tissue metabolism.	
Iodine	Iodized salt Salt-water fishes Foods grown in iodine-rich soil Water in nongoiterous regions	To enable the thyroid gland to produce enough of its hormones (thyroxine and triiodothyronine).	

Sources: Adapted from Ruth M. Leverton, *A Girl and Her Figure*, National Dairy Council (Chicago, 1955), and Ethel A. Martin, *Nutrition in Action*, 2nd ed. (New York, 1965), pp. 116, 164–65.

TABLE 9-2 *Caloric Values for Representative Foods, Classified by Food Groups*

FOOD*	WEIGHT OR APPROX. MEASURE	CALORIES	FOOD*	WEIGHT OR APPROX. MEASURE	CALORIES
MILK GROUP			Squash, winter	½ cup	50
Cheese, Cheddar	1⅛ in. cube	115	Sweet potato	1 medium	155
Cheese, cottage, creamed	¼ cup	60	Tomato juice, canned	½ cup (small glass)	25
Cream	1 tbsp.	35	FRUIT GROUP		
Milk, fluid, skim			Apple, raw	1 medium	70
(buttermilk)	1 cup	90	Apricots, dried, cooked	½ cup	135
Milk, fluid, whole	1 cup	165	Banana, raw	1 small	85
			Cantaloupe	½ melon	40
MEAT GROUP			Grapefruit	½ medium	50
Beans, dry, canned	¾ cup	250	Orange	1 medium	70
Beef, pot roast	3 oz.	245	Orange juice, fresh	½ cup (small glass)	60
Chicken	¼ small broiler	185	Peaches, canned	2 halves with juice	90
Egg	1 medium	80	Pineapple juice, canned	½ cup (small glass)	60
Frankfurter	1 medium	155	Prunes, dried, cooked	5 with juice	160
Haddock	1 fillet	135	Strawberries, raw	½ cup	30
Ham, luncheon meat	2 oz.	170	BREAD-CEREAL GROUP		
Liver, beef	2 oz.	120	Bread, white, enriched	1 slice	60
Peanut butter	1 tbsp.	90	Cornflakes, fortified	1⅓ cup	110
Pork chop	1 chop	260	Macaroni, enriched,		
Salmon, canned	½ cup	120	cooked	¾ cup	115
Sausage, salami	1 slice	135	Oatmeal, cooked	⅔ cup	100
			Rice, cooked	¾ cup	150
VEGETABLE GROUP			FATS GROUP		
Beans, snap, green	½ cup	15	Bacon, crisp	2 strips	95
Broccoli	½ cup	20	Butter or		
Cabbage, shredded, raw	½ cup	10	fortified margarine	1 tbsp.	100
Carrots, diced	½ cup	20	Oils, salad or cooking	1 tbsp.	125
Corn, canned	½ cup	85	SWEETS GROUP		
Lettuce leaves	2 large or 4 small	5	Beverages, cola type	6 oz.	80
Peas, green	½ cup	55	Sugar, granulated	1 tbsp.	50
Potato, white	1 medium	90			
Spinach	½ cup	20			

*Foods on this list are in forms ready to eat. All meats and vegetables are cooked unless otherwise indicated.

Source: Adapted from Ethel A. Martin, *Nutrition in Action*, 2nd ed. (New York, 1965), p. 61.

TABLE 9-3 *Caloric Values for Common Snacks*

FOOD	AMOUNT OR AVERAGE SERVING	CALO-RIES	FOOD	AMOUNT OR AVERAGE SERVING	CALO-RIES
"JUST A LITTLE SANDWICH"			CANDIES		
Hamburger on bun	3-in. patty	330	Chocolate bars:		
Peanut butter	1 tbsp. p. b.	330	Plain, sweet milk	1 bar (1 oz.)	155
Cheese	1-oz. cheese	280	With almonds	1 bar (1 oz.)	140
Ham	1-oz. ham	320	Chocolate-covered		
Pizza, cheese	⅛ pie	180	bar	1 bar	270
BEVERAGES			Chocolate cream,		
Carbonated drinks,			bonbon, fudge	1 piece 1-in. sq.	90–120
soda, root beer,			Caramels, plain	2 medium	85
etc.	6-oz. glass	80	Hard candies,		
Pepsi-Cola	12-oz. glass	150	Lifesaver type	1 roll	95
Club soda	8-oz. glass	5	Peanut brittle	1 piece 2½ ×	
Chocolate malted				2½ × ⅜ in.	110
milk	10-oz. glass	500	DESSERTS		
Ginger ale	6-oz. glass	60	Pie:		
Tea or coffee,			Fruit	⅙ pie	375
straight	1 cup	0	Custard	⅙ pie	265
Tea or coffee, with			Mince	⅙ pie	400
2 tbsp. cream and			Pumpkin with		
2 t. sugar	1 cup	90	whipped cream	⅙ pie	460
ALCOHOLIC DRINKS			Cake:		
Ale	8-oz. glass	155	Chocolate layer	3-in. section	350
Beer	8-oz. glass	110	Doughnut, sugared	1 average	150
Highball (with			SWEETS		
ginger ale)	8-oz. glass	185	Ice cream:		
Manhattan	average	165	Plain vanilla	⅙ qt.	200
Martini	average	140	Chocolate and		
Wine, muscatel			other flavors	⅙ qt.	260
or port	2-oz. glass	95	Orange sherbet	½ cup	120
Sherry	2-oz. glass	75	Sundaes, small choco-		
Scotch, bourbon,			late nut with		
rye	1½-oz. jigger	130	whipped cream	average	400
FRUITS			Ice-cream sodas,		
Apple	1 medium	70	chocolate	10-oz. glass	270
Banana	1 small	85	MIDNIGHT SNACKS FOR		
Grapes	30 medium	75	ICEBOX RAIDERS		
Orange	1 medium	70	Cold potato	½ medium	65
Pear	1	65	Chicken leg	1 average	88
SALTED NUTS AND			Milk	7-oz. glass	140
POTATO CHIPS			Roast beef	½ in. × 2 in. ×	
Almonds, filberts,				3 in. piece	130
hazelnuts	12–15	95	Cheese	¼ in. × 2 in. ×	
Cashews	6–8	90		3 in. piece	120
Peanuts	15–17	85	Leftover beans	½ cup	105
Pecans, walnuts	10–15 halves	100	Brownie	¾ in. × 1¾ in.	
Potato chips	1 serving	108		× 2¼ in.	140
			Cream puff	4-in. diam.	450

Source: Adapted from Helen S. Mitchell *et al.*, *Cooper's Nutrition in Health and Disease*, 15th ed. (Philadelphia, 1968), pp. 282–83. Data provided by Smith, Kline, and French Laboratories.

TABLE 9-4 Energy Equivalents of Food Calories Expressed in Minutes of Activity

FOOD	CALORIES	WALKING[1]	RIDING BICYCLE[2]	SWIMMING[3]	RUNNING[4]	RECLINING[5]
Apple, large	101	19	12	9	5	78
Bacon, 2 strips	96	18	12	9	5	74
Banana, small	88	17	11	8	4	68
Beans, green, 1 cup	27	5	3	2	1	21
Beer, 1 glass	114	22	14	10	6	88
Bread and butter	78	15	10	7	4	60
Cake, 2-layer, 1/12	356	68	43	32	18	274
Carbonated beverage, 1 glass	106	20	13	9	5	82
Carrot, raw	42	8	5	4	2	32
Cereal, dry, 1/2 cup with milk, sugar	200	38	24	18	10	154
Cheese, cottage, 1 tbsp.	27	5	3	2	1	21
Cheese, Cheddar, 1 oz.	111	21	14	10	6	85
Chicken, fried, 1/2 breast	232	45	28	21	12	178
Chicken, TV dinner	542	104	66	48	28	417
Cookie, plain	15	3	2	1	1	12
Cookie, chocolate chip	51	10	6	5	3	39
Doughnut	151	29	18	13	8	116
Egg, fried	110	21	13	10	6	85
Egg, boiled	77	15	9	7	4	59
French dressing, 1 tbsp.	59	11	7	5	3	45
Halibut steak, 1/4 lb.	205	39	25	18	11	158
Ham, 2 slices	167	32	20	15	9	128
Ice cream, 1/6 qt.	193	37	24	17	10	148
Ice cream soda	255	49	31	23	13	196
Ice milk, 1/6 qt.	144	28	18	13	7	111
Gelatin, with cream	117	23	14	10	6	90
Malted milk shake	502	97	61	45	26	386
Mayonnaise, 1 tbsp.	92	18	11	8	5	71
Milk, 1 glass	166	32	20	15	9	128
Milk, skim, 1 glass	81	16	10	7	4	62
Milk shake	421	81	51	38	22	324
Orange, medium	68	13	8	6	4	52
Orange juice, 1 glass	120	23	15	11	6	92
Pancake with syrup	124	24	15	11	6	95
Peach, medium	46	9	6	4	2	35
Peas, green, 1/2 cup	56	11	7	5	3	43
Pie, apple, 1/6	377	73	46	34	19	290
Pie, raisin, 1/6	437	84	53	39	23	336
Pizza, cheese, 1/8	180	35	22	16	9	138
Pork chop, loin	314	60	38	28	16	242
Potato chips, 1 serving	108	21	13	10	6	83
Sandwiches:						
Club	590	113	72	53	30	454
Hamburger	350	67	43	31	18	269
Roast beef with gravy	430	83	52	38	22	331
Tuna fish salad	278	53	34	25	14	214
Sherbet, 1/6 qt.	177	34	22	16	9	136
Shrimp, French fried	180	35	22	16	9	138
Spaghetti, 1 serving	396	76	48	35	20	305
Steak, T-bone	235	45	29	21	12	181
Strawberry shortcake	400	77	49	36	21	308

[1] Energy cost of walking for 150-lb. individual = 5.2 calories per minute at 3.5 m.p.h.
[2] Energy cost of riding bicycle = 8.2 calories per minute.
[3] Energy cost of swimming = 11.2 calories per minute.
[4] Energy cost of running = 19.4 calories per minute.
[5] Energy cost of reclining = 1.3 calories per minute.

Source: From F. Konishi, "Food Energy Equivalents of Various Activities," *Journal of the American Dietetic Association*, Vol. 46 (1965), p. 186.

TABLE 9-5 *Energy Expenditures for Various Everyday Activities*

ACTIVITY	CALORIES PER POUND PER HOUR	ACTIVITY	CALORIES PER POUND PER HOUR
Asleep	.4	Playing ping-pong	2.7
Bicycling, moderate speed	1.7	Reading aloud	.7
Cello playing	1.1	Running	4.0
Dancing, mildly active	2.2	Sewing, on a machine or by hand	.7
Dishwashing	1.0	Sitting quietly, watching TV	.6
Dressing and undressing	.9	Skating	2.2
Driving a car	1.0	Standing	.8
Eating a meal	.7	Sweeping, vacuum cleaner	1.9
Horseback riding, trot	2.6	Swimming (2 m.p.h.)	4.5
Ironing	1.0	Tailoring	1.0
Laundry, light	1.1	Typing rapidly	1.0
Lying still, awake	.5	Walking, 3 m.p.h.	1.5
Painting furniture	1.3	Walking, 4 m.p.h.	2.2
Piano playing, moderate	1.2	Writing	.7

Source: Adapted from C. M. Taylor, Grace MacLeod, and M. D. S. Rose, *Foundations of Nutrition*, 5th ed. (New York, 1956).

TABLE 9-6 *A Typical Female College Student's Activities for One Day*

ACTIVITY	HOURS SPENT IN ACTIVITY	CALORIES PER POUND PER HOUR	TOTAL CALORIES PER POUND (Calories × Hours)
Asleep	8	.4	3.2
Lying still, awake	1	.5	.5
Dressing and, undressing	1	.9	.9
Sitting in class, eating, studying, talking	8	.7	5.6
Walking	1	1.5	1.5
Standing	1	.8	.8
Driving a car	1	1.0	1.0
Running	1/2	4.0	2.0
Playing ping-pong	1/2	2.7	1.3
Writing	2	.7	1.4
Total	24		18.2

Total calories used per pound   18.2
Weight in pounds   ×115.0
Total calories expended for the day   2,093

Source: Adapted from Helen S. Mitchell *et al.*, *Cooper's Nutrition in Health and Disease*, 15th ed. (Philadelphia, 1968), pp. 50–51.

TABLE 9-7 Desirable Weights in Pounds for People Twenty-five or Over*

	MEN				WOMEN		
HEIGHT† Ft. In.	SMALL FRAME	MEDIUM FRAME	LARGE FRAME	HEIGHT† Ft. In.	SMALL FRAME	MEDIUM FRAME	LARGE FRAME
5 2	112–120	118–129	126–141	4 10	92– 98	96–107	104–119
5 3	115–123	121–133	129–144	4 11	94–101	98–110	106–122
5 4	118–126	124–136	132–148	5 0	96–104	101–113	109–125
5 5	121–129	127–139	135–152	5 1	99–107	104–116	112–128
5 6	124–133	130–143	138–156	5 2	102–110	107–119	115–131
5 7	128–137	134–147	142–161	5 3	105–113	110–122	118–134
5 8	132–141	138–152	147–166	5 4	108–116	113–126	121–138
5 9	136–145	142–156	151–170	5 5	111–119	116–130	125–142
5 10	140–150	146–160	155–174	5 6	114–123	120–135	129–146
5 11	144–154	150–165	159–179	5 7	118–127	124–139	133–150
6 0	148–158	154–170	164–184	5 8	122–131	128–143	137–154
6 1	152–162	158–175	168–189	5 9	126–135	132–147	141–158
6 2	156–167	162–180	173–194	5 10	130–140	136–151	145–163
6 3	160–171	167–185	178–199	5 11	134–144	140–155	149–168
6 4	164–175	172–190	182–204	6 0	138–148	144–159	153–173

*These figures are based on the person's wearing indoor clothing. For nude weight, women should subtract two to four pounds; men, five to seven pounds. Girls between the ages of eighteen and twenty-five should subtract one pound for each year under twenty-five.

† Height is measured with shoes on: one-inch heels for men, two-inch heels for women.

Source: Metropolitan Life Insurance Company. Derived primarily from data of the Build and Blood Pressure Study, Society of Actuaries, 1959.

TABLE 9-8 Overweight and Excess Mortality

OVERWEIGHT (Percent)	EXCESS MORTALITY* (Percent)	
	MEN	WOMEN
10	13	9
20	25	21
30	42	30

*Compared with mortality of standard risks (mortality ratio of standard risks equals 100 percent).

Source: Metropolitan Life Insurance Company. Derived from data of the Build and Blood Pressure Study, Society of Actuaries, 1959.

TABLE 9-9 Overweight and Excess Mortality from Some Major Diseases

DISEASE	EXCESS MORTALITY* (Percent)	
	MEN	WOMEN
Heart disease	43	51
Cerebral hemorrhage	53	29
Malignant cancers	16	13
Diabetes	133	83
Digestive system diseases (gallstones, cirrhosis, etc.)	68	39

*Compared with mortality of standard risks (mortality ratio of standard risks equals 100 percent). These data apply to people about 20 percent or more overweight.

Source: Metropolitan Life Insurance Company. Derived from data of the Build and Blood Pressure Study, Society of Actuaries, 1959.

most as many calories as will be found in a half-dozen eggs (see Tables 9-2 and 9-3).

Sheer boredom often accounts for overeating. For some people there seems to be little to do but eat and watch old movies on television. Emotional problems are often associated with this cause of overeating. These may originate in the mother who compensates for her rejection of a child by lavishing him with food and other physical comforts. The mother may compound the problem by restricting the child's physical activity so that he will not hurt himself. The child learns that eating earns approval and brings affection. Years later, when feeling disapproval or lack of love, he eats excessively. And his basic training in inactivity does not help him burn up excess calories.

Doubtless this is one reason why obesity tends to be familial. But there are other reasons. There are mothers who have large gastrointestinal tracts and who like to eat. They therefore like to cook. The novelist Thomas Wolfe described a family breakfast menu this way:

> In the morning they rose in a house pungent with breakfast cookery, and they sat at a smoking table loaded with brains and eggs, ham, hot biscuit, fried apples seething in their gummed syrups, honey, golden butter, fried steak, scalding coffee. Or there were stacked batter-cakes, rum-colored molasses, fragrant brown sausages, a bowl of wet cherries, plums, fat juicy bacon, jam. At the mid-day meal they ate heavily.[28]

Lunch and dinner are described no less ecstatically. As one might guess, Wolfe was a large man.

Such a gastronomic family atmosphere may be a symbol of wealth. Time was when the size of the meal and the circumference of the paunch were measures of success. Queen Victoria was once served a dinner of seventy dishes, including four soups, four fish, a haunch of venison, and six roasts.[29] Unlike her husband, she ate sparingly. He had a huge paunch. Perhaps not coincidentally, she lived almost twice as long as he.

Today, obesity caused by overeating is intemperance. A vegetarian, the dramatist George Bernard Shaw was tall and thin. Greeting him on a London street one day, the short and stout English writer G. K. Chesterton said, "From the looks of you, George, one would think there was a famine in England."

"And from the looks of you," replied Shaw, "one would think you had caused it."

Intemperance is often concealable. One can, for example, get drunk, sober up, and (at least for a while) no one will be the wiser. But the obese who eat too much carry their mark of intemperance with them constantly. So it was with Chesterton.

Obesity: a heavy load for mind and body

[28] Thomas Wolfe, *Look Homeward, Angel* (New York, 1929), p. 68.
[29] John Burnett, *Plenty and Want* (London, 1966), p. 68.

The neurotic behavior of the obese is manifested in overeating and in distortions of body image. This latter refers to the idea one has of oneself as an independent object in space. Such distortion can take the form of an overwhelming concern with obesity. For those with this problem, fat is all that matters. People are not better or worse; they are thinner or fatter. Importantly, body image disturbances occur almost exclusively among persons who were obese during adolescence. (If the onset of obesity occurs later in life, body image distortions are rare.) Derogation by parents of obese children later results in body image distortion problems.[30]

To the emotional stress of the obese, one must add physical hazards. Fat people are more susceptible than the thin to sickness and death from heart disease, stroke, nephritis, diabetes, cancers, and various diseases of the digestive system such as gallstones and a variety of liver conditions. And fat people do not live as long as the lean (see Tables 9-8 and 9-9).

How to reduce weight problems

Exercise

The child's training in weight control begins with his mother and may continue at school. School people do well to realize the importance of an overall program of physical activity. Winning football teams are fun but take little weight off the whole student body. People settling into the routines of the late twenties and early thirties soon find themselves fitting tightly into their clothes. It is then that fewer calories are needed to maintain usual weight. Exercise should have been woven into the lifetime pattern long before this. It is never too late to begin walking to the drug store and taking the steps instead of the elevator.

Moderate exercise *over a prolonged period* is an excellent reducer. Half an hour a day of vigorous handball or squash burns up, in a year, the equivalent of sixteen pounds of fat. (Table 9-5 provides the caloric loss per hour resulting from various common activities.)

Sadly, those needing exercise most may get it least. Yet, does this not suggest the role of inactivity in obesity? In one study of normal and obese girls engaged in playing volleyball, it was found that "normal weight girls were motionless, on the average, 50 percent of the time, obese girls 85 percent . . . in tennis normal girls were motionless 15 percent of the time, obese girls, 60."[31]

Dieting

The would-be dieter should seek the help of the family physician. Reliance on quacks, diet fads, and self-medication may all end disastrously. Calorie counting ought to be a way of life. Nothing is more discouraging than repeated weight losses followed by repeated gains. Normal

---

[30] "Disturbances in Body Image of Some Obese Persons" and "Obesity and the Body Image," cited in Albert J. Stunkard, "Body Image Disturbance in Obesity," *Feelings and Their Medical Significance*, Vol. 10, No. 1 (January–February 1968), pp. 1–4.

[31] Jean Mayer, quoted in Herbert L. Jones, Margaret B. Schutt, and Ann L. Shelton, eds., *Science and Theory of Health* (Dubuque, Iowa, 1966), p. 185.

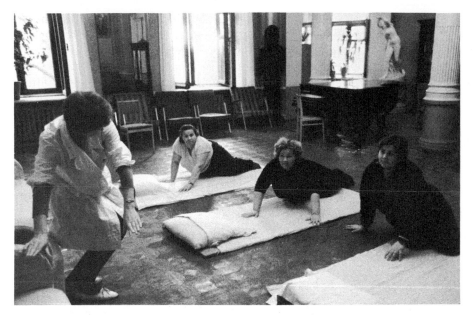

water retention prior to menstruation makes daily weighing meaningless for some women. In other people, early weight loss is loss of fluid, not fat. Weight checks once weekly are quite enough. A varied, tastefully prepared diet is essential to morale. A snack an hour before a meal may be helpful to the dieter in reducing his appetite for the large meal. But snacks and nibbles are calories, and calories do count. A lot of energy is required to use up relatively few calories (see Tables 9-4 and 9-5). For the dieter, exercise is essential. Moderation in both dieting and exercise is basic. A pound of body fat equals 3,500 calories. On a 1,200-calorie-a-day diet, the average woman will lose slightly more than a pound a week. The average male dieter is wiser to consume more—about 1,500 calories daily. Nobody should embark on a strict diet without first consulting a physician. Without his close supervision, losing two pounds a week may be hazardous. Patients on diets of less than 1,000 calories are usually admitted into a hospital for supervision of their diet.

Weighing too little

Justified concern with obesity has made the social life of the underweight individual much more pleasant than it was in former days. Poorly eating infants often suffer from their tense response to an unhappy mother. When an adult is more than 10 percent underweight, particularly if he is in his twenties, a physician's advice is indicated. By increasing their attention to some details, moderately underweight people usually gain weight. Among these details are elimination of infections, particularly of the appendix, teeth, and tonsils. Overactivity of the thyroid gland may need correction. Increased rest or a job change involving less tension may be indicated. Appetite-dulling tobacco is contraindicated. Frequent, extra-high-caloric snacks are better than overeating at mealtimes. Malted milks and milk shakes, cream with cereals, milk instead of soft drinks, extra butter, rich desserts, eggs, and meat—all these increase caloric intake. Vitamin supplements, especially thiamine, stimulate the appetite and improve digestion. In this country, severe malnutrition (as differentiated from a moderate underweight problem) is much less common a problem than obesity.

The hurt of hunger

Retardation—whether physical, mental, or both—has multiple causes varying from hazards within the uterus to those within the slums. The brain weight of a three-year-old is 80 percent of what it will weigh when he reaches adulthood. At that time the body weight is 20 percent that of maturity. It is postulated that during the early years of life malnourishment can do its greatest irrevocable damage.[32] If the malnutrition of poverty can be one of the causes of childhood retardation, the tragedy is double, for the retarded child is unequipped to someday better his circumstances. Adult malnutrition results in inefficiency but is not thought to cause mental retardation.

A study in Mexico indicated that "retardation in physical growth was found to depend upon family dietary practices, and on the occurrence of infectious disease," and in a Guatemala study the same investigators further found "that retardation in height for age relative to other children in the village was accompanied by poorer performance on psychological tests."[33] These studies have shown that episodes of infectious diseases, such as regular measles and chickenpox, may precipitate protein deficiency in children of borderline nutritional status. Such infections diminish appetite and intake of nutrients.

At the second Western Hemisphere Nutrition Congress, evidence was presented to show that "brain growth of infants subject to severe protein malnutrition from the first months of life is markedly impaired."[34] Still another writer says that "apathy typical of chronic protein deficiency, an apathy which translates into diminished learning potential, is estimated to affect 350 million children, 7 out of every 10 children under the age of 6 in the entire world."[35]

Are children in this country affected? Early in 1969, the U.S. Senate Select Committee on Nutrition and Related Human Needs heard a startling

[32] Philip H. Abelson, "Malnutrition, Learning, and Behavior," *Science*, Vol. 164, No. 3875 (April 4, 1969), p. 17.

[33] Nevin S. Scrimshaw, "Infant Malnutrition and Adult Learning," *Saturday Review*, March 16, 1968, p. 84.

[34] "Malnutrition and Innate Capacity," an editorial in *Hospital Tribune* (May 5, 1969), p. 11.

[35] Francis Keppel, "Food for Thought," in Nevin S. Scrimshaw and John E. Gordon, eds., *Malnutrition, Learning, and Behavior* (Cambridge, Mass., 1968), p. 6.

report. Preliminary findings of the first federal nutrition survey in the United States "clearly indicates an alarming prevalence of those characteristics that are associated with undernourished groups." Indeed, 10 to 15 percent of all the children examined showed retarded growth levels and were "therefore, a high risk in retardation of mental and physical performance."[36]

Less than 6 million of the 29 million U.S. poor participate in government food programs. Only one-third of poverty-stricken children attending public school participate in school lunch programs. In the sixties, malnutrition among the poor rose sharply, while, from 1963 to 1969, participation in food programs fell. There are various programs designed to help. But by 1969 over three hundred of the poorest counties had no program because local authorities had not requested them. During harvest time some counties actually discontinue food programs to assure cheap labor. Other programs demand some financial participation by the poor that they cannot afford. Consumer education programs are sadly lacking. A poor man who does not know how to get the most from his scanty food dollars is indeed disadvantaged. Inadequate distribution techniques are among the other failings of food programs.[37]

This richest nation, which finds the means to war and explore, can no longer run the risk of permitting millions of its children to be permanently crippled by malnutrition and hunger.

The process of nourishment

Nourishment depends on an intricate interplay of many organs and body chemicals. A special area in the hypothalamus of the brain tells a person whether he is hungry or full (see body chart 8 in the color section). Destroy the satiety center in an animal, and it will gorge itself to obesity; damage the area signaling hunger, and the affected animal will die of starvation. However, the functions of nutrition begin even before food is ingested. It is now known, for example, that hunger is rarely the stimulus causing an ordinarily obese person to eat. It is his "hungry eye or nose."

Once food is ingested it enters the *digestive system*,[38] so the mouth and its associated structures contribute to the *digestive process*. Digestion is carried out by mechanical and chemical means. For the moment, skip the first part of the digestive system and consider food in the small intestine. Nerves stimulate the contraction of the outer layers of muscle of the small intestine. This *mechanical* process propels the food within it and breaks

[36] "Malnutrition and Innate Capacity," p. 11.
[37] Jean Mayer, "Clinical Nutrition, a Social Pharmacopeia for Nutrition," *Postgraduate Medicine,* Vol. 45, No. 3 (March 1969), pp. 268–69.
[38] The *digestive system* includes the mouth and its associated structures, the pharynx, the components of the digestive tube, and the organs and glands associated with digestion. The *alimentary tract* or *canal* is that part of the digestive tract formed by the esophagus, stomach, and small and large intestines. The *gastrointestinal tract* includes the stomach and intestines. *Gastric* pertains only to the stomach.

it up into finer particles. Stimulated by nerves and hormones, intestinal glands in the lining of the inside of the small intestine produce *enzymes.*[39] The enzymes attack the food, breaking it down into even finer particles. This is a *chemical* reaction. So *digestion* is both a mechanical and chemical process by which nutrients are broken down into smaller units. The digestive process (which began in the mouth) makes possible the transfer of nutrients primarily from the small intestine into the blood and lymph channels. This transfer is called *absorption* and, like digestion, it is part of the nourishment process. After absorption, nutrients must be *transported* by the blood to the tissue cells. By means of a complex activity within the tissue cells called *metabolism,* nutrients are converted into energy and are used to create new molecules for tissue. But not all nutrients are immediately used. Some, such as fat and vitamin A, are *stored* within specific cells. Other nutrients (proteins) are held in *reserve.* The difference between reserve and storage is that reserves are body-wide. Some ingested nutrients are never used; they are evacuated as feces or excreted with the urine.

Digestive activity in the mouth   Even during the first day after birth, the newborn drinks sugar water or his mother's early milk, making good use of his lips. Composed of muscle fibers, the lips are surrounded by a circular band of still more muscle, the *orbicularis oris.* The "little circle around the mouth" (translated from the Latin) curls the lips snugly about the nipple, sealing off air, making sucking possible. The *orbicularis oris* is a sphincter muscle. "Sphincter" is Greek for "that which binds tight." Body sphincters do just that. By constricting a passage, the sphincter keeps it closed. It relaxes temporarily to permit some material to continue through the passage. For example, a constricted sphincter prevents food from prematurely leaving the stomach for the small intestine. When the sphincter relaxes, it helps to govern the amount of food that goes from one part of the passage to the next.

One cannot help but admire the constant labor of the heart. Consider, however, the *mouth.* It is used in talking, breathing, chewing, singing, whistling, coughing, vomiting, laughing, kissing, yawning, spitting, and other activities. But, through it all, one function is constant. The adult human mouth is not diverted from being the receptacle for a daily total of about two pints of saliva.

Food is taken into the mouth, passing under the nostrils. Then taste begins. Taste is partly smell. Eliminate vision and smell and one cannot differentiate between wine and lemonade or between apples and potatoes.

The muscular *tongue* is covered with a great many fine, wartlike *papillae.* Within the walls of the papillae are the *taste buds.* The buds at the back of the tongue are sensitive to bitter. The tip tastes sweet; the sides,

[39] All plants and animals produce thousands of *enzymes.* They are proteins that increase the rate of a reaction without becoming a part of the products of the reaction. Since they are used up in the body's chemical processes, enzymes are continuously produced by the living cell.

sour. In the tongue's center, the "zone of silence," there is no taste. Man makes much of his cultivated taste. Yet, compared to the cow's 35,000 taste buds, his 3,000 buds are few. Nevertheless, the tastes of man (including intermingled smell) are refined enough to recognize the finest size of grains, the subtlest body of liquids, the most piquant wines.

Skillfully guided by the muscular, shoveling, kneading tongue, the incisors cut, the canine teeth tear, and the molars masticate (chew) the solid food (see Figure 9-5). In this maceration and fragmentation, the *salivary glands* (see Figure 9-6) have already begun to help. The mere thought of tasty food set the brain to instruct the salivary glands to increase secretory activity. There are many salivary glands about the lips, cheeks, and tongue. Three pairs of them have been named: the largest of these are the *parotid glands* (in front of and below the ears); the others are the *sublingual glands* (in the floor of the mouth, beneath the tongue) and the *submaxillary glands* (under the jaw). (See Figure 9-6.) All their ducts empty into the mouth.

Since fish eat moist food, they neither have nor need salivary glands. But in one day, a drooling cow, confronted with a dry feed, can muster two hundred quarts of softening saliva. For dry toast man needs, and so produces, more saliva than for milk. In the human, to replace swallowed saliva, and thus to keep the mouth moist, salivary secretion is continuous. In one ordinary lifetime, the specialized microscopic salivary cells secrete over fifty thousand pints of saliva—more than enough to fill two large swimming pools. This secretory activity, like all other body activities, requires energy available only through food.

Glands throughout the entire lining of the gastrointestinal tract secrete a slimy substance called *mucus*. (Its chief chemical constituent is called *mucin*.) Mucus lubricates the lining of the gastrointestinal tract in order to facilitate the passage of its contents. In so doing it protects the inner lining of the tract from damage. Moreover, it can neutralize both acids and bases. Its value, for example, in protecting the stomach from the erosive action of the hydrochloric acid liberated there is obvious. About half of the saliva is mucus, and its mucin makes it sticky. The lubricative action of salivary mucus makes possible the swallowing of food. The other half of the saliva is a solution of a protein enzyme, *ptyalin*. This enzyme breaks down starch into simple sugars (maltose and dextrins). Thus does digestion begin in the mouth. It is in the mouth that food is rendered into a liquid or semiliquid.

The mouth is an anatomic exception. All other body structures or cavities are lined with an unbroken layer of skin or mucous membrane. But in the mouth that protective mucosal layer is penetrated by the erupted teeth. Also, nowhere else but in the mouth are there such singular anatomic connections as there are between tooth and soft tissue or between tooth and bone. Nor does the oral ecosystem promote tooth health. Swarming with microorganisms, often containing a bewildering variety of food chemicals, tolerating wildly fluctuating temperatures ranging from hot soup to frozen ice cream, containing gold, silver, cements, and plastics, enduring endless pollution and even small electric currents between dissimilar metals in the electricity-conducting saliva, the oral ecosystem is a challenge to dental survival. The teeth profoundly affect nourishment and health, and they merit discussion.

The teeth and gums *An old problem*

> *For there was never yet philosopher*
> *That could endure the toothache patiently.*[40]

At twenty-four, George Washington had his first tooth extracted; at fifty-seven, he lost his last tooth. Today, in the country Washington fathered, half of all persons over fifty have lost their natural teeth. For all ages, the ratio is one of eight. The Colonial General would feel at home with this: "For every 100 inductees entering the military service today there are needed 20 dentures, 25 bridges, 80 extractions"[41] and 450 fillings. These figures describe not the soldiers of Washington's day but those of today.

Washington's dental sufferance included more than concern for his speech, chewing, and swallowing. A year before his death, he wrote his dentist of needed "alterations" to his false teeth so they would not "have the effect of forcing the lip out just under the nose."[42]

It was said that Washington suffered more from his "patent masticators" than from the winter at Valley Forge.[43] Less forbearing than Washington was Elizabeth I, the virgin Queen, who also had tooth troubles. When, in 1578, her tooth caused "those in her vicinity no small tribulation,"[44] the old bishop (Aylmer) of London bore pain for peace. To prove extraction bearable, he had one of his last remaining teeth removed in the Queen's presence. Thus reassured, the Queen submitted to the operation.

The "cures" for aching teeth have sometimes been no less dreadful than the aches. Suggested treatments have included biting off the head of a live mouse,[45] filling the tooth hollow with raven dung,[46] and touching the dental organ with the hand of a corpse.[47] The Slovenes wryly advise filling the mouth with cold water and sitting on a hot stove. As the water boils, the tooth is forgotten.[48]

Some people have purposely parted with healthy teeth. In 1862, French soldiers had to bite off the cartridges for their guns. Inadequate dentition

---

[40] William Shakespeare, *Much Ado About Nothing,* V.i.35–36.
[41] John W. Knutson, "Prevention of Dental Disease," in Duncan W. Clark and Brian MacMahon, eds., *Preventive Medicine* (Boston, 1967), p. 229.
[42] Arthur Ward Lufkin, *A History of Dentistry,* 2nd ed. (Philadelphia, 1948), p. 171.
[43] "Reliever of Pain," M.D., *Medical Newsmagazine,* Vol. 12, No. 1 (January 1968), p. 194.
[44] Lilian Lindsay, *A Short History of Dentistry* (London, 1933), p. 37.
[45] Leo Kanner, *Folklore of the Teeth* (New York, 1928), p. 141.
[46] Arthur Ward Lufkin, *A History of Dentistry,* 2nd ed., p. 78.
[47] Leo Kanner, *Folklore of the Teeth,* p. 145.
[48] *Ibid.,* p. 149.

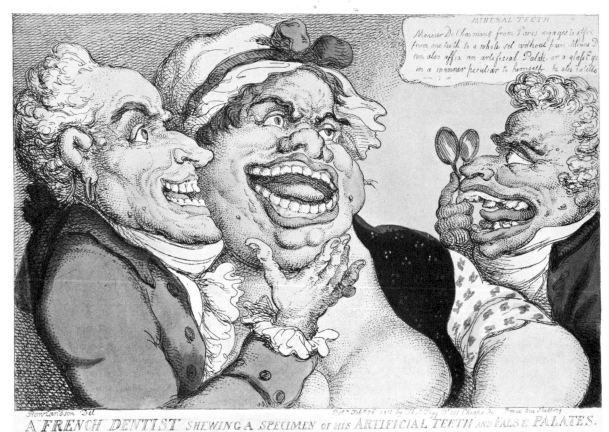

MINERAL TEETH

Monsieur Dellasmont from Paris engages to affix
from one tooth to a whole sett without pain. Means I
can also affix an artificial Palate or a glass Eye
in a manner peculiar to himself. he also instills

Rowlandson Del

A FRENCH DENTIST SHEWING A SPECIMEN OF HIS ARTIFICIAL TEETH AND FALSE PALATES.

9-4 A satire on dentistry and a poke at the French by the English painter and caricaturist Thomas Rowlandson (1756–1827).

meant exemption from military duty. Extracting the teeth became a method of draft evasion.[49] Others sold their teeth. A 1782 advertisement, placed by George Washington's dentist in *Rivington's Royal Gazette,* offered four guineas for each front tooth.[50]

One might conclude this brief historical review of dentistry with some lines published almost a century ago:

> *View this gravestone with all gravity,*
> *Jones is filling his last cavity.*[51]

[49] *Ibid.,* p. 217.

[50] J. A. Taylor, *History of Dentistry* (Philadelphia, 1922), p. 75.
   The seventeenth-century English king James I, on the other hand, paid not for teeth, but for the sheer pleasure of extracting them. Thus did Kunnard the barber earn eighteen shillings for "twa teith drawin furth of his heid by the King." (Quoted in Arthur Ward Lufkin, *A History of Dentistry,* 2nd ed., p. 136.)

[51] "Southern California Practitioner," cited in Henry Harris, *California's Medical Story* (San Francisco, 1932), p. 292.

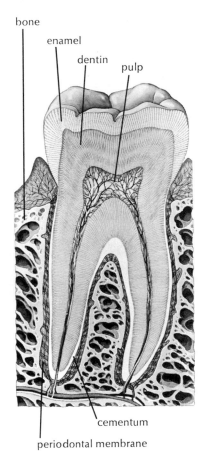

bone
enamel
dentin
pulp

cementum

periodontal membrane

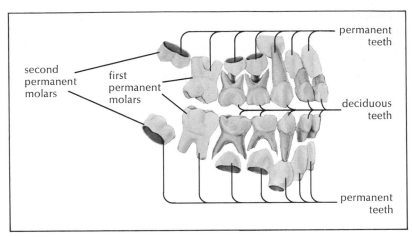

second permanent molars

first permanent molars

permanent teeth

deciduous teeth

permanent teeth

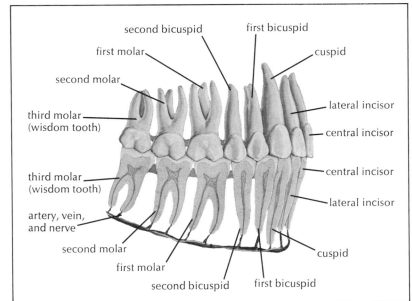

second bicuspid

first molar

second molar

third molar (wisdom tooth)

third molar (wisdom tooth)

artery, vein, and nerve

second molar

first molar

second bicuspid

first bicuspid

first bicuspid

cuspid

lateral incisor

central incisor

central incisor

lateral incisor

cuspid

9-5 Teeth: a longitudinal section of a molar (*above*), the dentition of a six-year-old child (*top right*), and the dentition of an adult (*bottom right*).

Growth and structure

Teeth are almost indestructible. They survive fire and decompose slowly. Ancient skulls are studded with diseased dentition. Not only are teeth resistant, but they are arranged in a highly individual way from person to person. An "oral fingerprint" has been evidence enough to convict more than one murderer who, having set his victim on fire, left nothing behind but a few teeth and, perhaps, a few unincriminating gall-stones.

Anchoring the tooth (see Figure 9-5) in the jawbone is the *root*. The portion of the tooth that one sees in the mouth is the *crown*. Where root and crown meet is the *neck*. Four tissues make up a tooth. The *enamel*, hardest of all body tissues, covers the crown; the bonelike *cementum* covers the root. The ivorylike *dentin*, harder than bone but softer than enamel, forms the body of the tooth. The pulp contains the nerves, blood vessels, and lymphatics. Covering the root of the tooth and extending to line its socket is the *periodontal membrane*. It helps to hold the tooth in place. It is also a shock absorber.

At six weeks, the embryo begins to form tooth buds for the twenty temporary *deciduous teeth*. Shortly thereafter, the buds of the thirty-two *permanent teeth* begin to form. At birth the unerupted deciduous teeth are almost complete. Beneath the deciduous teeth some permanent teeth begin to calcify.

At about six months, the baby shows the first tooth. Before his third birthday, he has a mouthful of deciduous teeth. These will be shed at various times. Neglect of temporary teeth may result in permanent problems. The temporary teeth guide the permanent dentition beneath them. Loss or decay of temporary deciduous teeth may result in crooked permanent teeth, chewing and speech problems, and psychological wounds. Between the age of two and one-half and three years, a child should see the dentist for the first time.

Usually the first or "six-year" molars are the first permanent teeth to erupt (see Figure 9-5). At about this time, the child is losing his front deciduous teeth. The position of the first molars helps determine the position of the other teeth and the shape of the whole lower face. The entire future of the individual's dentition is profoundly influenced by the first molars. "A mouth without grinders," mourned Don Quixote to Sancho, "is like a mill without a stone; and a diamond is not so precious as a tooth."[52] So wrote Cervantes over four centuries ago. Of all the diamonds in the mouth, the most precious is the first molar. As soon as it erupts, this tooth, the "keystone of the dental arch," should be examined by the dentist.

Some major dental problems

Dental cavities (or *caries*) share with the common cold the distinction of being the most common human ailments. How does a cavity form in a tooth? Three things are necessary: a susceptible tooth, sugar, and certain bacteria.

Most teeth are usually covered by a filmy *dental plaque*. This slimy coating collects and holds together an untidy agglomeration of mucus, food debris, and bacteria. The plaque is the same color as the teeth. Some, but not all, of the dental plaque may be temporarily removed by brushing.

[52] Miguel De Cervantes, *Don Quixote De La Mancha,* tr. by Charles Jarvis (London, 1842), p. 188.

But it is the plaque that provides the medium for tooth decay. It is within and around it that the bacteria live and are protected.

From simple sugars formed by the breakdown of food in the mouth, some of these mouth bacteria, the *streptococci,* synthesize complex sugars (polysaccharides) and store them. Between feedings, during food shortages, the streptococci derive energy by converting the stored polysaccharides to destructive acids. How much time do the streptococci need to transform sugar to erosive acid? Within fifteen or twenty minutes most of the damage is done. That is why rinsing or brushing the teeth immediately after eating is so helpful. Emotions may be involved in cavity formation. The rate of salivary flow is influenced by suggestion. A diminished rate of salivary flow encourages cavities. Why? The acid concentration in the mouth rises, and this helps to destroy teeth. Even heredity may play a role in the tendency to cavity formation.

If the tooth-bathing saliva has enough buffers to neutralize acids formed by bacteria, tooth decay can be prevented. If not, the chemical process of decalcification begins. The acid in the saliva, formed by bacterial action on sugar, first destroys the tooth enamel. At this stage there is usually no warning pain. Only later, when destruction has reached the dentin, is there toothache. An unchecked cavity may get to the pulp. Infection sometimes travels from the pulp towards the tissues surrounding the root. Abscess formation may occur. Pus may spread through the blood vessels, causing a swelling of the adjacent soft tissues.

What can be done?

PERSONAL CARE   1. If at all possible, teeth should be brushed after each meal. Even rinsing with a warm drink helps remove food particles. Mouthwashes are not substitutes for brushing. Many dentists recommend water-under-pressure equipment to be used after (but not instead of) brushing. Except for the handicapped, electric toothbrushes are not more effective than the manual.

2. To arrest the progress of cavities, prompt and continuous dental care is essential.

3. During the intrauterine period and first eight years of life, nutrition is critically important. The mother's diet provides minerals for the developing teeth of the child within her. Should her diet be lacking, the child obtains minerals not from the mother's teeth but from her bones. It is after birth that permanent teeth are calcified. So the child's diet should include foods rich in calcium and phosphorus as well as vitamins A, C, and D (see pages 280–82). Moreover, all living tissue needs and contains protein. An adequate diet, so essential for general health, is also an absolute necessity for development of normal tooth structure.

Do adult teeth, permanent and calcified, need calcium? No, but the bone, by which teeth are held in place, cannot remain healthy without calcium.

Does adult dental health require an adequate diet? Indeed it does. Without enough protein for tissue replacement, for example, mouth structures would quickly suffer. And the deleterious effect on adult oral health of shortages of vitamin B and C has long been recognized.

4. Since sugar adheres to the plaque, its intake should be controlled. It is not the amount, but rather the frequency and time-exposure to sugar that is most important. A piece of chocolate cake is not as harmful as an all-day sucker.

5. Foods that stick to the teeth, such as dates or figs, should be avoided. Raw carrots and apples help clean the teeth.

Cavities are not as common in poor countries as in the more affluent. India, for example, endures an agony of chronic undernourishment. Yet the cavity rate of her people is enviably low. This is because food shortages decrease the ingestion of refined sweets. The acid level in the Indian mouth remains low. Moreover, the inadequate diet of many Indians is high in *fluoride*. They profit from this natural cavity preventive.

FLUORIDE   "It is wholly a question of amount whether the influence of fluorine is good or bad."[53] This sums up a remarkable and prolonged scientific adventure that began over sixty years ago. In 1908, "Colorado brown stain" was noted to be prevalent in the teeth of residents in and around Colorado Springs. Not until twenty-three years later was it known, however, that this *mottled enamel* was caused by fluoride in the drinking water. So, too much fluoride causes a condition called *dental fluorosis*. In the intervening years, however, the relationship between mottled enamel and the relative absence of dental cavities had been noted repeatedly. Would fluoride, in lesser amounts, reduce the incidence of dental cavities and still not cause mottled enamel?

For over thirty years the effect of fluoride on human health in general, and dental health in particular, has been carefully investigated. Beginning in the 1930's massive studies have been carried out in communities over the entire North American continent. The answer is summarized here:

> *All studies made prior to 1945, when the first controlled water fluoridation projects were instituted, as well as studies conducted since that time, have added support to the conclusion that optimally fluoridated drinking water in a range of 0.7 to 1.3 parts per million is a safe, relatively simple, and practical health measure that effects a two-thirds reduction in the incidence of tooth decay, with a concomitant and significant reduction in the loss of teeth from dental caries.*[54]

Today, in this country, some four thousand communities, populated by

[53] F. S. McKay, "Fluorine and Mottled Enamel: Historical Survey," cited in David B. Ast, "Dental Public Health," in Philip E. Sartwell, ed., *Preventive Medicine and Public Health,* 9th ed. (New York, 1965), p. 565.

[54] John W. Knutson, "Prevention of Dental Disease," in Philip E. Sartwell, ed., *Preventive Medicine,* p. 236.

some eighty-three million people, have fluoride fed into water supplies. Two-thirds of the major cities in the United States, including New York, Chicago, Philadelphia, and Detroit, have adopted controlled fluoridation. In some cities a vocal minority has succeeded in confusing enough people to delay fluoridation of the water supply. By their misguided action, they condemn millions to needless pain, expense, and disability. Fluoride *solutions* applied to the teeth of children have resulted in a reduction of from 45 to 70 percent of dental cavities. These treatments are more expensive and time-consuming than water fluoridation. They must be regularly repeated. Fluoride *tablets* taken during the early years of life may be ingested only if prescribed. The beneficial results of tablet-taking are comparable to those obtained from water fluoridation. However, a regimen involving the ingestion of fluoride tablets does not provide a reliable method of cavity prevention. Few people can be expected to cooperate on such a long-term basis.[55] Stannous fluoride dentifrices may help.

Periodontal diseases

Disorders of the tissues surrounding and holding the teeth in their sockets are called *periodontal diseases*. For people under thirty-five, cavities cause most of the tooth loss. After thirty-five, periodontal disease is the major cause. It can vary from a mild gum inflammation to actual bone destruction.

Periodontal disease can have several manifestations. The initial signs of inflammation of the gums (*gingivitis*), such as redness, swelling, and bleeding, are usually painless. Poor oral hygiene, tartar or calculus accumulation, and malocclusions are common causes. Less ordinary evidences of periodontal disease are systemic conditions such as diabetes, leukemia, and deficiencies of vitamins B and C. *Vincent's angina* ("trench mouth"), caused by two different bacteria, is amenable to penicillin and good dental hygiene. *Periodontitis* (pyorrhea) can be related to the presence of calculus. Calculus appears when bacteria-loaded plaque calcifies and hardens. The subsequent irritation and infection can promote periodontal disease. *Improper alignment* (*malocclusion*) of the teeth, such as occurs when upper and lower teeth fail to meet efficiently, promotes periodontitis. This can be corrected by an orthodontist. Periodontitis may also be initiated by *improper brushing* or by the trauma of *toothpicks*. In the *Babies Book*

[55] In March 1969 the science editor of the *Saturday Review* cited various reports indicating that fluoridated water used in artificial kidneys was causing bone disease. He wondered whether this had "implications for people with kidney ailments who drink flouridated water every day." (John Lear, "New Facts on Fluoridation," *Saturday Review* [March 1, 1969], pp. 51–59.) In his answer, the Surgeon General of the Public Health Service pointed out that the 900 quarts of water used weekly in artificial kidneys was fifty to a hundred times the amount of fluid consumed by an average person, that most water used in kidney machines should be demineralized, and that "the need to process some water supplies before therapeutic use in large quantities in artificial kidneys has no bearing on the ingestion by anyone of optimally fluoridated water from community water supplies." He again unequivocally endorsed fluoridation of community water supplies "as a medically safe procedure for the reduction of dental caries." (William H. Stewart, Surgeon General, Public Health Service, U.S. Department of Health, Education, and Welfare, in an official statement, "Fluoridation and the Use of Fluoridated Water in Artificial Kidneys," March 1969.)

of about 1475, children were enjoined "youre nose, youre teeth, youre naylles from pykynge."[56] That advice is still good today.

Good mouth hygiene is essential in preventing periodontal disease. Proper brushing is helpful. Professional scaling and polishing of the teeth are important.

Research

Modern dental research involves numerous disciplines. For example, in periodontal disease, the normal connective tissue protein (collagen) breaks down. The enzyme collagenase may be involved. It catalyzes the destruction of collagen. In periodontal disorders, the secretion of this enzyme markedly increases. Biochemists are researching this aspect of periodontal disease. Geneticists and microbiologists have found that minor dietary changes make resistant animals more susceptible to cavities. And, if nursed by susceptible foster mothers, resistant-bred animals become susceptible, too. Moreover, streptococci from decayed teeth of laboratory animals will cause decay in teeth of germ-free animals. From the materials experts comes other help. Implanted into a baboon, a plastic tooth has lasted six years. From rocket engineers and metallurgists has come a powerful light steel suitable for tooth bridges and caps. Using one another's knowledge and ability, scientists are together attacking this nation's enormous dental problems.

Swallowing

Having been cut and ground to a pulp by the teeth, moistened by the saliva, and partly digested by salivary enzymes, the soft food mass is ready to be swallowed. *Swallowing,* or *deglutition,* is the last voluntary digestive act. When the food is slid by the tongue into the *pharynx* (see Figure 9-6), digestion becomes involuntary, automatic. The pharynx is in the neck, as is a small portion of its continuation, the muscular *esophagus* (see Figure 9-6). The pharynx is a muscular passageway for both food and air. Above, it opens into the nasal passages; below, into the larynx. During swallowing, both of these openings, above and below, must be shut off. The *soft palate* and *uvula* (Latin, little grape) shut off the upper nasal part of the pharynx. The *epiglottis* covers the larynx. Thus, without being forced back into the nose or into the larynx and bronchi,[57] swallowed food safely reaches the esophagus. This organ also secretes and is protected by mucus.

Even liquid does not swiftly drop down the ten-inch esophagus. The food dilates it, causing muscular contractions, or *peristalsis.* Unless food is too hot or large, it is not felt in the esophagus. The esophagus travels down the chest behind the heart, between the lungs, and through the *diaphragm* into the abdomen, where it empties into the stomach (see Figure 9-6). Normally it takes about seven seconds for food to pass from the mouth through the esophagus and into the stomach.

[56] J. Menzies Campbell, *From a Trade to a Profession: Byways in Dental History* (London, 1958), p. 59.
[57] The *bronchi* are the larger air passages in the lungs and are continuations of the windpipe (Chapter 12).

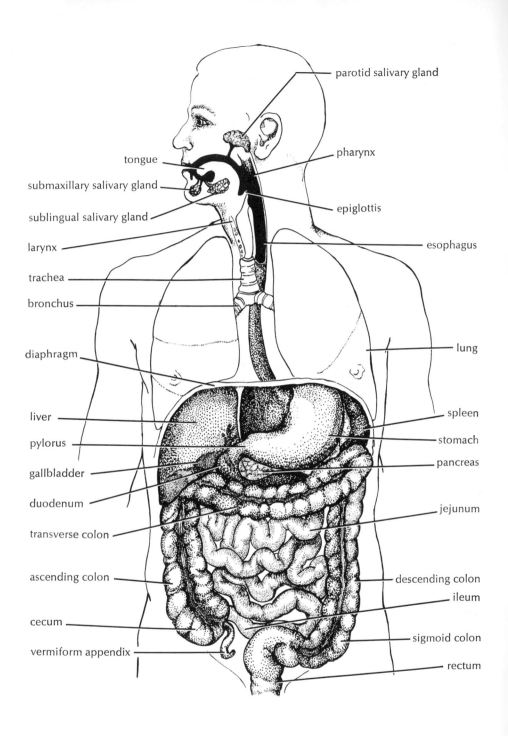

parotid salivary gland

tongue

submaxillary salivary gland

sublingual salivary gland

larynx

trachea

bronchus

diaphragm

liver

pylorus

gallbladder

duodenum

transverse colon

ascending colon

cecum

vermiform appendix

pharynx

epiglottis

esophagus

lung

spleen

stomach

pancreas

jejunum

descending colon

ileum

sigmoid colon

rectum

9-6 The digestive system. Parts of the respiratory system are also labeled here. See also body chart 13 in the color section.

The often abused *stomach* is a muscular, distensable, bottle-shaped tube in the left abdomen (see Figure 9-6). It is separated from the major chest contents (heart and lungs) by the diaphragm. Its usually empty upper portion, the *cardia* (Greek *kardia,* heart), may fill with gas, which can be expelled by belching. The stomach is closed off from the esophagus by the cardiac sphincter and from the small intestine by the pyloric (Greek *pylouros,* gatekeeper) sphincter.

Before leaving the stomach for the small intestine, some food may remain in the stomach for three to four hours. Other foods are fed into the small intestine within a few minutes. What determines this? The nature of the food. In their early digestive stages, meats tarry in the stomach. Soft drinks bubble on into the small intestine. For this reason, meats provide a greater sense of satiety or fullness than do soft drinks.

The inner mucous lining of the stomach contains millions of microscopic *gastric glands.* Their juice contains three enzymes—*rennin, pepsin,* and *lipase.*[58] *Hydrochloric acid*[59] is also a constituent of gastric juice, as is a substance named the *intrinsic factor.* Without this factor, vitamin B_{12} would not be absorbed. This vitamin is necessary for red blood cell formation. (Rennin is found in the human infant, but not the adult.)

The entrance of liquid and semiliquid food from the esophagus (through the open cardiac sphincter) into the stomach is the signal for the gastric glands to produce their juice. This secretion, in turn, stimulates the muscular stomach walls to begin peristaltic waves. Food is then slowly and thoroughly churned with the acid gastric juice. During this process, trapped gas in the stomach may move about, causing the stomach to rumble. (Peristalsis may also occur when the stomach is empty.) Gas pressure against the stomach wall causes "hunger pangs." It is in the stomach that an ironic and paradoxical problem of nature occurs. It is this: how can the stomach secretions carry out their basic function of beginning the digestion of proteins without also digesting the protein stomach lining? The answer lies in the great amount of protective mucus secreted by the stomach. When its production is inadequate to deal with an increase of acid, ulcer soon develops (see below).

So the food is prepared in the stomach for its intermittent entrance into the approximately foot-long *duodenum,* the upper part of the small intestine. The opening of the stomach leading to the duodenum is called the *pylorus.* Only a small amount of food at a time is passed into the duodenal section of the small intestine. Food that is adequately mixed with acid gastric juice causes the pyloric sphincter to open. As soon as food touches the alkaline intestine, the pyloric sphincter closes. Such regulation from acid stomach and alkaline intestine provides for intermittent opening and closing of the pyloric sphincter. Extra mucin made at the top part of the duodenum protects its lining from the acid stomach contents.

[58] Enzymes were defined on page 298.
[59] The normal stomach is insensitive to the acid in the gastric juice. However, the "heart burn" that occurs with regurgitation of hydrochloric acid proves the esophagus to be only too sensitive.

Peptic ulcer

A *gastric ulcer* is an eroded lesion in the stomach lining. A much more common but similar ulcer is found in the duodenum. Both are referred to as *peptic ulcers,* and both are treated similarly. Either ulcer may erode a blood vessel, causing dangerous hemorrhage. Both may penetrate the wall of the involved organ, necessitating emergency surgery. Because gastric ulcers are more likely to be cancers than duodenal ulcers, they can be particularly dangerous.

Peptic ulcers may occur at any age. Usually a peptic ulcer is first noted in the early thirties. Men suffer them four times more frequently than women. However, the increasing number of women exposed to the stresses of the competitive business world is changing this ratio. Although these ulcers do occur in relatively phlegmatic people, they are more common in conflict-ridden, striving individuals. For this reason peptic ulcer is called the "executive's" disease. Stress seems to increase greatly the acid secreted by the lining of the stomach. The stomach and duodenal linings (rarely the lower esophageal) are eroded by the high concentration of acid. Significantly, ulcers occur only in those areas of the digestive tract that come in contact with hydrochloric acid—the stomach, the duodenum, and the lower esophagus. The burning or gnawing abdominal pain of peptic ulcer usually begins two or three hours after meals—between 10 and 11 A.M., at about 2 P.M., and about 9 or 10 P.M., and perhaps again at midnight. Occasionally pain will awaken an individual during the night. Milk, alkali, or food relieves the pain. Several hours after eating there is no food in the stomach to neutralize the excess acid secreted by the mucous membrane of the stomach. The free excess acid acts upon the ulcer, causing the pain. An X-ray usually reveals the ulcer, and laboratory analysis of the gastric juice shows abnormally high levels of acid. A much less stressful environment, frequent feedings of a bland diet emphasizing milk and milk products, and complete abstinence from tobacco, alcohol, and coffee contribute to recovery.

The pancreas   The head of the *pancreas* (Greek *pan,* all + *kreas,* flesh) nestles in the duodenal loop (see Figure 9-6), and its long body lies beneath the stomach, as would a bed. Although it is the second largest body gland, the pancreas weighs only one-twentieth as much as the largest gland, the liver. Along with the duct from the liver, the *pancreatic duct* opens into the duodenal part of the small intestine. Through the pancreatic duct pour the alkaline enzymes produced by the pancreas, *trypsin, amylase,* and *lipase.* Specialized cells of the pancreas also produce a carbohydrate-regulating protein called *insulin* (Latin *insula,* island). These cells are scattered throughout the tail of the pancreas as islands, and they are called the *islets of Langerhans* (see page 239). They do not secrete into the pancreatic duct. Insulin is secreted directly into the blood. Thus, the pancreas is both an *exocrine (ductal)* and an *endocrine* gland (see page 236). Failure of the islets of Langerhans to secrete insulin results in *diabetes mellitus* (see pages 239–41).

The multipurpose human liver fits under the diaphragm and occupies most of the upper abdomen, particularly on the right. It is a veritable chemical factory. Not only does it produce bile, it also chemically treats carbohydrates, proteins, and fats, preparing them for human cellular use. It detoxicates poisons, such as alcohol[60] and caffeine. It destroys bacilli. Like the muscles, it stores glycogen, a sugar. It manufactures carbohydrates from fats. It is also influenced by the emotions. Anger may temporarily stop the flow of bile, robbing one of an essential body juice. Infections, such as *infectious* and *serum hepatitis* (see pages 193–94) may threaten liver function.

The four-lobed liver

A secretion of the liver is yellow, bitter *bile.* "Bile" is a word of uncertain derivation. Another name for it is *gall.* Before reaching the duodenum, bile stops to be stored and concentrated in a two- or three-inch pouch located under the right side of the liver. This is the *gallbladder* (see Figure 9-6). Concentration of bile in the gallbladder is accomplished when part of its water is absorbed by the mucous membrane of the gallbladder and returned to the blood stream.

The sometimes troublesome gallbladder

With entrance of a food morsel into the duodenum, the muscular gallbladder contracts. Bile is then sent to the duodenum via the *bile duct* (see body chart 14 in the color section). Just before the common bile duct enters the duodenum, it is joined by the *pancreatic duct.* Thus one duct carries both bile and pancreatic juice into the duodenum.

Bile contains *bile salts* which hasten fat digestion by helping the moving intestine to break up (emulsify) large fat globules in the duodenum. The smaller, broken-up fat globules have more surface than the large. This increased surface makes the fat more susceptible to the digestive action of the pancreatic enzyme *lipase.* Bile also contains *cholesterol* and a green-pigmented waste product, *bilirubin,* resulting from the destruction of worn-out (and replaced) red blood cells. The normal amount of bile pigment in the blood gives urine its characteristic straw color.

Gallstones

Some animals, such as the horse and the camel, do not have a gallbladder. Many humans have cause to envy them. The normal ability of the mucous membrane of the human gallbladder to absorb water may,

---

[60] An excess of alcohol (or other liver toxin) gradually poisons liver cells. This, combined with poor nutrition, causes the cells to die. They are replaced by fibrous scar tissue. To make up for the loss of liver cells, the remaining liver cells multiply. Finally fibrous scar tissue permeates the liver tissue. Due to local cell multiplication the remainder of the liver becomes knobby. Poor liver function may cause yellow jaundice. The sick liver structure also interferes with the flow of blood from the liver to the heart. It backs up into the veins of the stomach and esophagus. These may rupture and there will be vomiting of blood. With this condition far-advanced, fluid from the blood will leak into body tissues, causing the swelling of *edema.* This liver sickness is *cirrhosis,* or the "hob-nailed" or "gin-drinker's" liver.

in some people, result in *gallstones*. The cholesterol in bile is not very soluble. When the bile becomes concentrated in the gallbladder, the cholesterol may crystallize out of solution and, combining chemically with the bile salts (secreted by the liver) and bile pigment, it will form stones. Often these cause infection and pain and impede bile flow. In the latter case, obstructed bile salts and pigment may then pollute the blood and seep into the skin. The pigments produce *jaundice* (French *jaune,* yellow) and the salts cause intense itching. The stones are removed surgically. Patients are often enchanted by the pretty yellow or green tints of their removed gallstones. Seeing them is more pleasant than feeling them. One may embark on a preventive program to avoid ever feeling or seeing one's gallstones by eating a low-fat diet. A high-fat diet will produce a lot of cholesterol for stone formation. Once stones are formed, however, only surgery helps. Removal of the gallbladder does not interfere greatly with fat digestion because the anatomy and surgery are such that bile continues to be excreted into the intestine.

The tortuously coiled intestine   The *intestine* (see Figure 9-6) is divided into the long, narrow *small intestine* and the shorter, but wider, *large intestine.* Below the point of entrance of the small intestine into the large intestine is the dilated intestinal pouch, the *cecum.* From the cecum projects a narrow tube, the *vermiform appendix.*[61] The entire intestine of a dead human is about twenty-eight feet long. However, the muscle tonus of life shortens the intestine to about ten feet. The large intestine, or *colon,* terminates in the four or five inches of *rectum.*

The small intestine

This is the major digestive organ. Within it, digestion is completed. In its lower portion, absorption of the products of digestion into the blood stream takes place. Encouraged by intestinal peristalsis, food morsels from the duodenum are mixed with pancreatic juice and bile. They are then pushed into the *jejunum* and then to the *ileum,* the final three-fifths of the small intestine.

Covering the inner lining of the small intestine are millions of *villi* (Latin *villus,* tuft of hair). Villi are tiny fingerlike projections extending into the intestinal canal (see Figure 9-7). It has been estimated that the total surface of the villi is about three thousand square feet. Combined with the intestinal folds and coiling, the villi enormously increase the digestive and absorptive surface of the small intestine. But that is not all. The

---

[61] The opening from the cecum to the appendix is usually small. Cecal contents are ejected into the intestine with difficulty. The appendix may become plugged. Then its wall ulcerates. Inflammation (*appendicitis*) progresses. Eventually, the appendix may rupture. If this occurs, its spilled, bacteria-laden contents cause *peritonitis*—inflammation of the peritoneum. (The peritoneum is the membrane lining the walls of the abdomen and pelvis. Peritonitis also occurs with a perforated peptic ulcer.) To prevent all this, it is essential that a diseased appendix be surgically removed (*appendectomy*) as soon as possible. Appendicitis occurs more often in children than in adults, but the disease is more serious in adults.

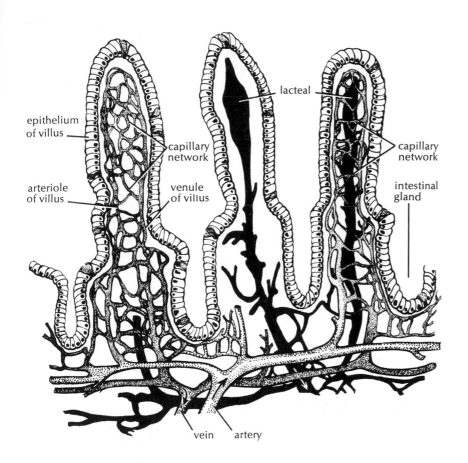

epithelium
of villus

capillary
network

arteriole
of villus

venule
of villus

lacteal

capillary
network

intestinal
gland

vein   artery

9-7 Villi in the small intestine. The villus at the left shows only the blood vessels; the villus in the center, only the lymph vessel (the lacteal); the one at the right is complete, showing both the blood and lymph vessels.

surface of each villus is further increased by *microvilli*, which are visible under the electron microscope. These further increase the effective absorptive surface of the intestine thirty-fold. At the base of each villus, the *intestinal glands* secrete the intestinal juices. Carbohydrate-digesting enzymes, as well as enzymes for fat and protein digestion, are secreted in the small intestine. And along the entire inner surface of the small intestine is secreted a protective film of mucus.

It is from this remarkable inner surface of the small intestine that food is absorbed into the blood and lymph vessels. The ingested food has been broken down. It can now be transported by the blood and lymph to the liver and from there, via the blood, to the body cells to be built up again into the carbohydrates, fats, and proteins of the human type. The products of carbohydrate and protein digestion first go directly to the liver and then to the other body cells. Not all the products of fat digestion follow this route. About sixty percent of the fat is first absorbed into the lymphatic system and then travels on to tissue (see page 254). The rest goes directly to the liver. As droplets, fat may be stored in connective tissue cells. This is called *adipose* tissue.

About twenty million glands in the small intestine secrete an average of a gallon and a half of intestinal juice daily. Every day about ten percent of the body's total water and salt enters the small intestine. Ninety percent of the total secretion is reabsorbed by the body tissues. What is lost is easily replaced. Thus not only digestion and absorption of food take place in the small intestine but also reabsorption of fluid.

In from three to four hours food usually passes through the small intestine into the large intestine.

The large intestine

Entering the *large intestine,* or the *colon* (see Figure 9-6), from the small intestine, through the ileo-colic sphincter, is a semifluid material.[62] Bereft of nutrient, it is waste—largely water. However, salt, bile, and undissolved (even undigested) food are contained in it. Like the esophagus, digestion does not occur in the large intestine. Water absorption in the large intestine causes the contents to solidify and to form *feces* (Latin *faeces,* refuse).

Fecal material should be soft and formed like a column. Consistently fluid adult feces (*diarrhea*) or small pieces expelled with difficulty (*constipation*) merit investigation by the physician. If severe diarrhea occurs, digestive enzymes enter the large intestine. Since they do not normally belong there, they are irritating. Here again the protective mucus secreted by the large intestine is helpful. Feces are expelled from the rectum through the rectal opening, the *anus* (Latin for "ring"). Regulating this final passage of waste material from the body is the anal sphincter.

The human alimentary system has long attracted the special attention of the quack. Although he has not limited himself to this set of organs, his activities have so frequently involved human digestion that he is discussed here.

Fakers and phonies

"For the mind of man is far from the nature of a clear and equal glass, wherein the beams of things should reflect according to their true incidence; nay, it is rather like an enchanted glass, full of superstition and imposture."[63]

Early medicine shows　　Show biz and fake medicine share hardy ancestors. The medieval mountebank would mount a bench and, by act and costume, strive to gain the attention of the market populace. His medicine show drew the gullible crowds, who then bought his phony remedies. Quackery rolled on in

---

[62] A chronic ulceration of the colon (*ulcerative colitis*) occurs in both children and adults. Its cause remains unclear. Many physicians consider it of psychosomatic origin.

[63] Francis Bacon, "Advancement of Learning," Basil Montague, ed., *The Works of Francis Bacon,* Vol. I (Philadelphia, 1844), p. 211.

tandem with performance, and in the eighteenth century, London actor-author David Garrick immortalized the playwright-quack John Hill this way: "For physic and farces, his equal there scarce is / His farce is his physic, his physic a farce is."[64]

In the New World, early California quacks also playacted. During the gold rush days, "they bought diplomas from physicians' widows, thereafter assuming the name of the deceased as a professional alias . . . the tip-off of an abortionist was a medication advertised . . . *not* for pregnant women."[65]

Such widely disparate Americans as "The Hoosier Poet" James Whitcomb Riley and William Avery Rockefeller (the father of the financier) spent years as traveling medicine men. Billed as the "Hoosier Wizard," Riley did everything from playing the violin and drums to giving poetic readings.[66] An engaging entrepreneur, Rockefeller often feigned being deaf and dumb. He attracted crowds by using his talents as a marksman.[67]

Modern showmen of nutrition

P. T. Barnum said, "There's a sucker born every minute." He was not short of followers. Many a modern-day showman has parlayed the digestive system into a successful financial enterprise. Among the most unabashed of these were Bernarr Macfadden and Gaylord Hauser. Both Eleanor Roosevelt and George Bernard Shaw contributed to Macfadden publications. Shaw was a vegetarian. Perhaps he was at home with the Macfadden diets of carrot strips and nuts and fruits. Macfadden had, incidentally, borrowed his philosophy of chewing from a predecessor food fadist, Horace Fletcher. Thirty-two teeth, Fletcher had heard, inhabit the human mouth. It followed that food had to be chewed no fewer than thirty-two times. So he rhymed: "Nature will castigate / Those who don't masticate."[68]

The Duchess of Windsor wrote the introduction to the French edition of a Gaylord Hauser book.[69] What prompted her? Certainly not poverty. Was it the lure of show biz? Did she not, after all, merely join such other luminaries of the day as Greta Garbo and Paulette Goddard? They, too, were Hauser fans.[70] How were they to know the use of blackstrap molasses was nutritional nonsense? And that the M.D. on Hauser's stationery was a mistake:

> Hauser took a degree in naturopathy early in his career; a typographic error that transformed "N.D." into "M.D." on his stationery led to understandable difficulties with the American Medical Association; in recent years he has been careful to disclaim medical

[64] Quoted in C. J. S. Thompson, *The Quacks of Old London* (New York, 1928), p. 325.
[65] George W. Groh, *Gold Fever* (New York, 1966), p. 285.
[66] James Harvey Young, *The Toadstool Millionaires* (Princeton, N.J., 1961), p. 194.
[67] Allan Nevins, *John D. Rockefeller*, Vol. I (New York, 1940), Chapters 2 and 3.
[68] Ronald M. Deutsch, *The Nuts Among the Berries* (New York, 1961), p. 91.
[69] *Ibid.*, p. 163.
[70] *Ibid.*, p. 167.

status and to state that his "wonder foods" are to be regarded only as diet supplements.[71]

Long before Hauser, during the nineteenth century, a stream of medicines had flooded the market, concocted to "open men's purses by opening their bowels."[72] Arnold Ehret, the "professor," claimed that "every disease is constipation." He urged a rigorous regimen of fruits and nuts, fasting, and air bathing. This regimen, he claimed, offered the added dividends of relief from sterility, impotence, masturbation, and prostitution. Women followers were even offered immaculate conception. As Barnum would have predicted, there were plenty of takers.

It was the sheer absorptive qualities of the gut that alcohol peddlers found so useful—that, and human taste. At her death, in 1883, Lydia Pinkham was a respected member of the Woman's Christian Temperance Union. Little, if anything, was said of the 18 percent alcohol content of her "vegetable compound." (Most present-day wines are 13 percent alcohol.) Was it not, after all, "added solely as a solvent and preservative"? The recommended dosage was, nevertheless, more than generous. A full, even overflowing, tablespoon, four times daily, was not too much for "a falling of the womb." For Lydia's devoted customers, prohibition was no hardship. The Pinkham people were part of a pattern. For seventy years, Kansas voted for prohibition, meanwhile merrily tippling such spirited drink as Wild Cherry Tonic and Dr. Worme's Gesundheit Bitters.[73] Another cure-all, called Hostetter's Bitters, originally contained 39 percent alcohol. It was often dispensed in saloons by the shot.[74]

There were quacks who were mechanically inclined and they did not limit their machines to the gut. Perhaps inspired by the Industrial Revolution, many got off to an early start in this country. By the end of the eighteenth century, the Chief Justice of the Supreme Court, numerous legislators, and even George Washington had been hoodwinked. From a Colonial medical humbug, Elisha Perkins, they all bought a pair of brass and iron rods that was supposed to cure all ills. Such wholehearted governmental support helped Perkins become rich.[75] He was but one of the first of a long line. Not long ago, for example, Dinsha P. Ghadiali, the man with "fifteen college degrees," invented the Spectro-Chrome. It was a metal box housing a one-thousand-watt bulb. In front of the bulb, he could slide panes of colored glass. For each disease, he had a different color glass. Ruth Drowns fixed herself the Drowns' Radio Vision Instrument. A drop of blood (any drop would do) was all she needed for a diagnosis. The patient could be miles away. The tragedy of all such fraud remains with the sick. By phony tests and treatment, individuals with

---

[71] *M.D., Medical Newsmagazine*, Vol. 3, No. 5 (May 1959), p. 160.
[72] James Harvey Young, *The Medical Messiahs* (Princeton, N.J., 1967), p. 21.
[73] Gerald Carson, *One for a Man, Two for a Horse* (Garden City, N.Y., 1961), p. 44.
[74] Hostetter V. Sommers, cited in James Harvey Young, *The Toadstool Millionaires*, p. 130.
[75] Morris Fishbein, *Fads and Quackery in Healing* (New York, 1932), p. 12.

early treatable disease, such as operable cancer, may be delayed into a hopeless stage of their disease.

Quacks succeed primarily by exploiting susceptibility and fear of death and disability. Latent in humankind, too is "a primitive craving for the supernatural . . . here primitive medicine and quackery are at one."[76]

Why are quack offerings so successful?

Others who seek quacks do so out of hostile rebellion against the omnipotent parent-physician figure. He is remembered, resented, and cloaked in suspicion. To all this must be added the unfortunate approach of some physicians. Always busy, some are at times unable to take time to listen. A quack always listens.

Particularly vulnerable is the chronically ill person. Some illnesses are characterized by spontaneous episodes of temporary improvement (remission). An individual with multiple sclerosis, for example, may improve for short periods during the progressive downhill course of the disease. Wandering from quack to quack, the patients find renewed but false hope with each new remission, sinking, in the end, into cruel despondency.

One distinguished nutritionist offers these pointers:[77]

How to identify quacks

1. They always have something to sell.

2. They offer quick cures on a money-back basis.

3. They proclaim themselves experts with vastly important "professional" associations.

4. Testimonials and phony case histories, rather than responsible studies published in reputable journals, are their stock in trade.

5. Scientific data are distorted rather than reported.

6. They always condemn one's present way of eating.

7. They claim that such institutions as the American Medical Association and the Food and Drug Administration are "corrupted" by "big business" and conspire to persecute them to hide the "truths" that they alone possess.

How may the quack be defeated? By dispelling the fear on which he breeds. And this can best be accomplished through enlightenment and understanding. In an entirely different context, a distinguished physicist recently quoted still another scientist in a manner singularly appropriate to the present subject. "Maria Sklodowska-Curie said: 'Nothing in life is to be feared—it is only to be understood! Now is the time to understand more—so that we may fear less.'"[78]

How may the quack be defeated?

---

[76]Fielding H. Garrison, "On Quackery as a Reversion to Primitive Medicine," quoted in *Bulletin of the New York Academy of Medicine, 1925–35* (New York, 1966), p. 602.

[77]Frederick J. Stare, *Eating for Good Health* (New York, 1964), pp. 154–55.

[78]Glenn T. Seaborg, "Need We Fear Our Nuclear Future?" *Bulletin of the Atomic Scientists*, Vol. 24, No. 1 (January 1968), p. 42.

10

The emotional life

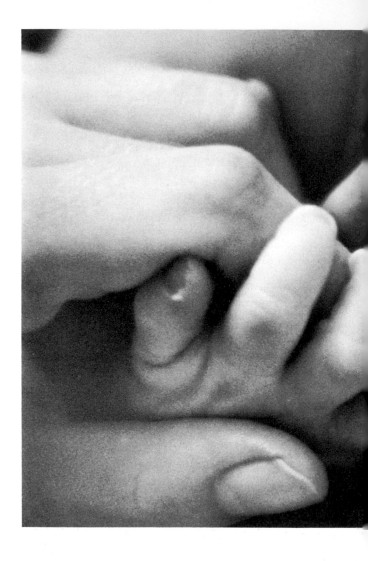

And if the soul
is to know itself
it must look
into a soul:
the stranger and enemy, we've seen him in the mirror. [1]

Personality development

Begin at the beginning. Begin with the birth of the baby. He can suck and he can look, but not at the same time. Through eyes vacant like tiny unwashed windows, he can see only peripherally. He is aware of light

[1]George Seferis, *Collected Poems, 1924–1955* (Princeton, N.J., 1967), p. 9.

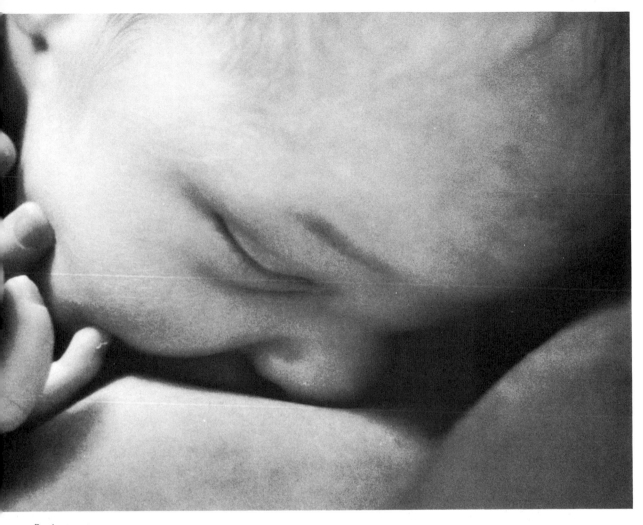

Basic trust.

and dark. He can cry and perhaps raise his head a trifle. Although six months will pass before his teeth can be seen, he has an immediate sweet tooth. He dislikes bitters. He can smell, and even before he was born he could hear. Three to ten minutes after he is born, he will turn his eyes toward a sound. He can feel pressure and warmth and cold. He can cough and sneeze. For a day or two, he will eliminate a blackish-green material called meconium from his rectum. This was formed during intrauterine life, when trial secretions of his digestive glands mixed with swallowed fluid. In a few days he will eat. Most of the time his gut will be able to push the food down. Sometimes he will spit it up. It will be months before he can suck and look at the same time.

During his first day, he will pass between one-half and one and one-half ounces of urine. This amount will increase. His heart beats about 150 times a minute, and he breathes 30 to 50 times a minute. If his head was born first, as is ordinarily the case, he probably breathed before all of him was delivered. Within a week the newborn can smile, not because of a gas pain but from pleasure.[2] Yet there is an old saying that man is expected to grieve. If he does not weep at birth, he is spanked until he does. Be that as it may, the child's first staccato cry heralds the change from aquatic to terrestrial life—an evolutionary change that required millions of years. After his first crying spell, the infant sleeps. When he awakens, he cries again. At this tender age, no other creature can howl so mightily. It is this second episode of weeping that is the concern of this chapter, for it tells that the infant can suffer. And, collecting stress and distress, often he reaches adulthood only to feel like Shakespeare's Antonio in *The Merchant of Venice*:

> In sooth, I know not why I am so sad.
> It wearies me, you say it wearies you;
> But how I caught it, found it, or came by it,
> What stuff 'tis made of, whereof it is born,
> I am to learn.
> And such a want-wit sadness makes of me
> That I have much ado to know myself.[3]

What sadness makes Antonio feel a "want-wit"? What is the root of his anguish? In every time, in every tongue, in every lonely troubled corner on earth, this bewilderment has been uttered. Why is this so? Before the work of Sigmund Freud there were few answers.

Some historical notes The history of the investigation of human emotion may well be divided into before and after Freud. Thirty-four centuries before Freud, in 1550 B.C., the Egyptians wrote, in the *Ebers Papyrus*, that hysteria was caused by a wandering womb. About seventeen hundred years later, the ancient Greek physician Galen, "hoping to lure the vagrant uterus back to its normal position,"[4] recommended actual fumigation of the vagina to cure hysteria. In numerous passages, the Bible mentions madness. Frequently it was considered a punishment from the Lord (Deuteronomy 6:5). In a fit of depression, Saul commits suicide (I Samuel 31:4). The delusion of Nebuchadnezzar, that he was a wolf, is famous.[5] Doubtless such references had a profound effect on later philosophers of religion. The original introspections of St. Augustine (d. 604), the first archbishop of Canterbury, had a penetrating effect on psychology. Spinoza (1632–77), whose philos-

---

[2] *M.D., Medical Newsmagazine*, Vol. 12, No. 3 (March 1968), p. 154.
[3] William Shakespeare, *The Merchant of Venice*, I.i.1–7.
[4] Franz G. Alexander and Sheldon T. Selesnick, *The History of Psychiatry* (New York, 1966), p. 21.
[5] *Ibid.*, p. 23.

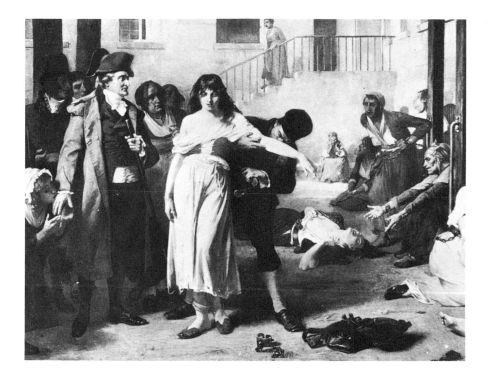

10-1 Philippe Pinel, in 1793, liberating the emotionally ill from their chains.

ophy emphasized insight into oneself as an ethical goal, was an authentic precursor of Freud. "What Freud calls mental health Spinoza calls the freedom of the mind."[6]

In the medieval era the insane of Europe were treated like animals. It remained for the physician-reformer Philippe Pinel to unchain the insane of France (see Figure 10-1). Because of him, many nineteenth-century Europeans were convinced of the need for medical treatment of the emotionally ill.

About the middle of the nineteenth century, the modern era of medicine began. Great discoveries in the natural sciences by Darwin, Pasteur, and others formed the backdrop for the Freudian stage. Freud began his career with significant discoveries about the anatomy of the nervous system. Before his death, in 1939, he had become one of the most influential thinkers in history.

Based on observation, Freud's concepts were ecological. He began by calling attention to the child. Within each child were basic unconscious instinctual drives. Between these drives and the surrounding environment occurred constant and inexorable negotiations. From this interplay human personality resulted. In childhood, basic personality traits were established. With severe emotional trauma and crises, childhood personality development lagged. The resultant adult behaved like a child. The adult person-

[6] *Ibid.*, p. 100.

ality, then, was molded by the stress responses of childhood. "Pubescence," Freud wrote, "is an act of nature; adolescence is an act of man." In this way Freud emphasized the difference between merely growing and growing up. Moreover, Freud taught that the stresses of childhood could be changed. Therefore, patterns of behavior that were based on reactions to stresses could be changed. Early responses to stress, lying deeply buried in the subconscious for long periods of time, often caused eventual emotional problems. If these could be uncovered, confronted, and resolved by an individual who suffered them, cure could result.

Among the most influential of the psychologists who built on Freud's ideas is Erik Erikson. His schema of personality development provides a useful and coherent concept of the flow of psychological happenings through which people must live to grow to emotional maturity. "How does a healthy person grow or, as it were, accrue from the successive stages of increasing capacity to master life's outer and inner tasks and dangers?" [7] This is the basic question that Erikson sets out to answer.

Erikson's eight stages of personality development
For Erikson, every human being's personality develops in eight stages, each of which takes place during a particular age. In each stage the developing individual is faced with a task. If the task is satisfactorily resolved, the individual enters healthily into the next stage. If it is not, the individual is ill-equipped to solve the task of the next stage. Future attempts to solve tasks are hampered by the emotional impedimenta caused by past failures. To heal these wounds to the personality, the individual needs help. Adequate help at critical times stabilizes the individual. Preparation for the next stage and the transition into it are then accomplished with a greater sense of personal competence and security. Better emotional health results. Without help, the person's inadequately resolved tasks turn into cumulative emotional scars—and personality disorders.

Each of Erikson's eight stages is named according to the task that is confronted. The name identifies both the desirable resolution of the task and the contrary development that takes place if the task is not resolved. The desirable resolution of the task of the first of the eight stages is *basic trust.* Its contrary development is *basic mistrust.* Thus the first stage is named *basic trust versus basic mistrust.* But there are no sharp dividing lines between Erikson's stages. During the later stages the resolution (or lack of resolution) of the tasks of earlier stages continues to develop.

As a result of continuous interactions with his environment during these stages, man develops a feeling of self-identity. This feeling, which Erikson calls *ego-identity,* is central to human personality development. Man's ego-identity is his awareness of himself as a distinct person with an influential past, an active present, and a controllable future. What must man live through to achieve this feeling of identity?

[7] Erik H. Erikson, "Growth and Crises of the Healthy Personality," in Clyde Kluckhohn, Henry A. Murray, and David Schneider, eds., *Personality in Nature, Society, and Culture* (New York, 1953), p. 186.

The infant

Basic trust versus basic mistrust is the first stage. In the first year, the infant will make a decision, based on the quality of his maternal care, as to whether the world is dependable and safe or fraught with frustration and fear. It is not a decision reached as the result of one incident or a few. Erikson does not mean that this stage (or any other) is like an obstacle race in which a few missteps forever doom the participant to emotional illness. The infant decision is the product of the ripening relationship between him and his mother. Completely self-centered, yet utterly dependent, he will inevitably be disappointed. No mother can always immediately meet all her baby's needs. And so, as a part of normal development, the child must learn to cope with a degree of frustration. His ability to do this will depend on his overall sense of security or insecurity. If his frustrations are not excessive in amount or in frequency, he will learn that, although things are not always to his liking, most of the time they are fine. A baby can adjust to that. Indeed, this lesson will help him face situations that will arise as he reaches his first year—situations that involve some degree of separation from his mother. If all that has preceded has been characterized by anxiety, he will approach this and future problems with fear and basic mistrust. But if the preponderance of his experience has taught him basic trust, he will have gained a sense of self-esteem that will stand him in good stead.

A CASE OF SEVERE BASIC MISTRUST   What happens to a baby without an opportunity to develop a degree of basic trust? The story of Joey, the "mechanical boy,"[8] provides an instructive, though dramatically extreme, example. "He wanted to be rid of his unbearable humanity," Bettelheim wrote, "to become completely automatic."

> *"I never knew I was pregnant," his mother said, meaning that she had already excluded Joey from her consciousness. His birth, she said, "did not make any difference." Joey's father, a rootless draftee in the wartime civilian army, was equally unready for parenthood. So, of course, are many young couples. Fortunately most such parents lose their indifference upon the baby's birth. But not Joey's parents. "I did not want to see or nurse him," his mother declared. "I had no feeling of actual dislike—I simply didn't want to take care of him." For the first three months of his life Joey "cried most of the time." A colicky baby, he was kept on a rigid four-hour feeding schedule, was not touched unless necessary and was never cuddled or played with. The mother, preoccupied with herself, usually left Joey alone in the crib or playpen during the day. The father discharged his frustrations by punishing Joey when the child cried at night.*

---

[8] The discussion of Joey is drawn from "Joey: A 'Mechanical Boy,'" a classic article by Bruno Bettelheim in *Scientific American*, Vol. 200, No. 3 (March 1959), pp. 117–27.

Joey's existence never registered with his mother . . . When she told us about his birth and infancy, it was as if she were talking about some vague acquaintance.[9]

This parental indifference taught Joey little but basic mistrust. Only mechanical devices could be relied upon to satisfy his greatest needs. Years later Bettelheim described Joey's bizarre behavior:

Entering the dining room, for example, he would string an imaginary wire from his "energy source"—an imaginary electric outlet—to the table. There he "insulated" himself with paper napkins and finally plugged himself in. Only then could Joey eat, for he firmly believed that the "current" ran his ingestive apparatus . . .

Many times a day he would turn himself on and shift noisily through a sequence of higher and higher gears until he "exploded," screaming "Crash, crash!" and hurling items from his ever present apparatus—radio tubes, light bulbs, even motors or, lacking these, any handy breakable object. (Joey had an astonishing knack for snatching bulbs and tubes unobserved.) As soon as the object thrown had shattered, he would cease his screaming and wild jumping and retire to mute, motionless nonexistence.[10]

[9] *Ibid.*, p. 118.
[10] *Ibid.*, p. 117.

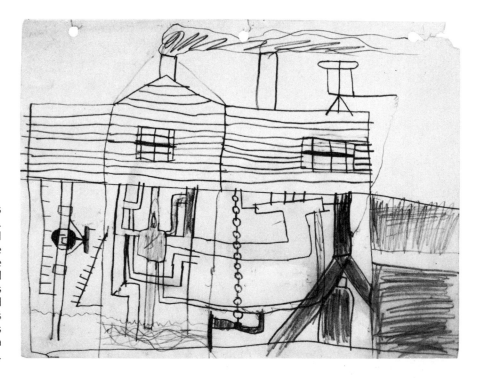

10-2 One of Joey's early drawings. The house is small and simple. The mechanical sewage system is large and complex. Joey's impersonal and rigid toilet training is reflected in his obsessive interest in sewage disposal.

The toddler

Autonomy versus shame and doubt characterize Erikson's second stage of the developing personality. This stage is marked by growing individual muscle controls. As the toddler learns to consciously control his bowel and bladder, he also learns that he can get attention by withholding. If a baby competitor seems to have replaced him, he may use this method of regaining attention. His parents must learn patience. Rigidity and shaming are to be avoided. "From a sense of *self-control without loss of self-esteem* comes a lasting sense of autonomy and pride. From a sense of muscular and anal impotence, of loss of self-control, and of parental over-control comes a lasting sense of doubt and shame."[11]

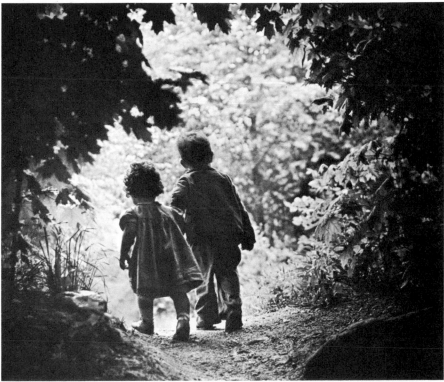

10-3 Early childhood.

At this stage what happened to Joey? He was toilet-trained rigidly. And the rigidity was rooted in indifference, not love:

> *Going to the toilet, like everything else in Joey's life, was surrounded by elaborate preventions. We had to accompany him; he had to take off all his clothes; he could only squat, not sit, on the toilet seat; he had to touch the wall with one hand, in which he also clutched frantically the vacuum tubes that powered his elimination. He was terrified lest his whole body be sucked down.*

[11] Erik H. Erikson, "Growth and Crises of the Healthy Personality," p. 199.

> To counteract this fear we gave him a metal wastebasket in lieu of a toilet. Eventually, when eliminating into the wastebasket, he no longer needed to take off all his clothes, nor to hold on to the wall . . .

> It was not simply that his parents had subjected him to rigid, early training. Many children are so trained. But in most cases the parents have a deep emotional investment in the child's performance. The child's response in turn makes training an occasion for interaction between them and for the building of genuine relationships. Joey's parents had no emotional investment in him. His obedience gave them no satisfaction and won him no affection or approval. As a toilet-trained child he saved his mother labor, just as household machines saved her labor. As a machine he was not loved for his performance, nor could he love himself . . . By treating him mechanically his parents made him a machine. [12]

The preschooler

During the preschool years, the child, armed with the accumulated security of his first stage and the independent body control of the second, seeks to discover more about himself. Erikson calls this stage *initiative versus guilt*.

> Being firmly convinced that he is a person, the child must now find out what *kind* of person he is going to be. And here he hitches his wagon to nothing less than a star: he wants to be like his parents, who to him appear very powerful and very beautiful, although quite unreasonably dangerous. [13]

It is perhaps in this stage that the crushing tragedy of Joey's indifferent parents became most poignantly apparent. For the child, needing love, can endure impatience and even passing anger. He knows that even anger means caring. But indifference is too much to bear.

The preschooler knows his gender and is curious about sex. He examines himself and, when possible, others. He learns that handling his genitals is pleasurable (Freud's "phallic phase"). A shocked, forbidding parent will convince a child that he is basically dirty, unworthy. A relaxed, accepting parent teaches the child that he is worthy and that his worthiness includes the genitalia. Strongly disapproving parents at this phase create guilt and fear of punishment in the child. And untold numbers of children think of the same punishment—that the genitalia will be (with boys) or have been (with girls) cut off. (Figure 10-4 and its accompanying verse illustrate how a closely related fear is manufactured from a normal human activity. Parents need not be concerned about thumb-sucking until the child is about four. Past that age, teeth may be displaced, and the family dentist should be consulted.)

[12]Bruno Bettelheim, "Joey: A 'Mechanical Boy,'" pp. 122, 124.
[13]Erik H. Erikson, "Growth and Crises of the Healthy Personality," p. 205.

10-4 THE STORY OF LITTLE SUCK-A-THUMB

One day, mamma said: "Conrad dear,
I must go out and leave you here.
But mind now, Conrad, what I say,
Don't suck your thumb while I'm away.
The great tall tailor always comes
To little boys that suck their thumbs;
And ere they dream what he's about,
He takes his great sharp scissors out
And cuts their thumbs clean off,—and then,
You know, they never grow again."

Heinrich Hoffman, quoted in Burton Egbert Stevenson, ed., *The Home Book of Verse* (New York, 1922), p. 123.

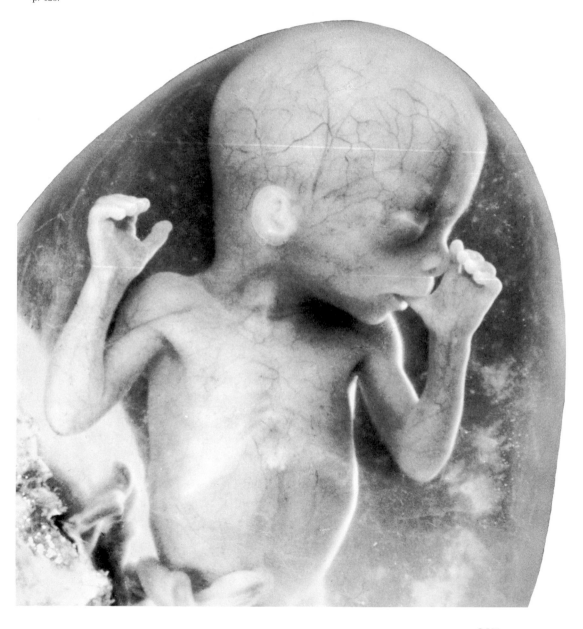

Expressions of the Oedipus[14] complex (which is associated primarily with the work of Freud) are also likely to appear during this stage. With childhood's devastating logic, the four- or five-year-old boy reaches two irreducible conclusions. First, his genitals cannot compare with his fa-

10-5 "Feelings are more important than anything under the sun" (Joey's slogan upon entering the human condition, see footnote 17).

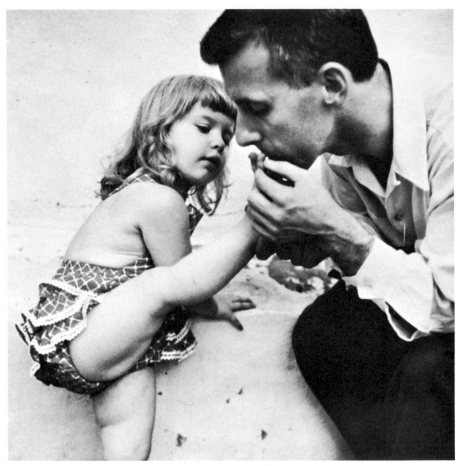

ther's. Second, no matter how much he loves his mother, he cannot replace his father in her affections. Frequently, a male child may express a desire to marry his mother. The little girl may endure a similar experience. Having at first identified with her mother, she now prefers her father. Only he can put her to bed, dress her, and care for her. The mother is rejected. But the girl still needs her mother, just as the boy still needs his father, no matter how much he wishes to be rid of him. It will not be their last entrapment in emotional ambivalence. Three hundred years ago, the philosopher Spinoza clearly defined emotional ambivalence as a "vacillation of the soul."[15]

[14]Oedipus, in the Sophoclean tragedy *Oedipus Rex*, kills his father and marries his mother. Later, upon discovering the true relationship, he blinds himself. See also page 367.
[15]Quoted in Franz G. Alexander and Sheldon T. Selesnick, *The History of Psychiatry*, p. 97.

Parental maturity and skill in handling these emotions, in preventing the humiliation of the searching child, will augment the child's sense of a worthy self. Embarrassing the child will interfere with his ability to conquer future crises.

The school-age child

By the time the child enters school he is in what Freud called the "latency period." His sexual interests have abated. This is the fourth stage of Erikson's schema of personality development, *industry versus inferiority.*

"Personality at the first stage crystallizes around the conviction 'I am what I am given,' and that of the second, 'I am what I will.' The third can be characterized by 'I am what I can imagine I will be . . .' The fourth: 'I am what I learn.' "[16]

No other creature has as long a period of dependency as the human, for no other creature has as much to learn before he can become self-sufficient. The child must learn skills, use tools, and do something he

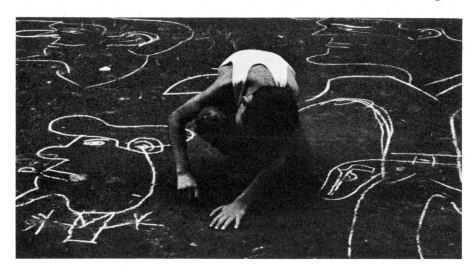

10-6 "Learning is not child's play" (Aristotle).

considers useful. Returning from school to his parents, he will hold out the result of his labor. "Look," he will say hopefully. If he is met with appreciation, he will attempt to do still better. If parental indifference is his lot, a deep sense of inadequacy and inferiority will overwhelm him. But praise must be merited. Should he receive commendation for an effort he knows is inferior, he will lose respect for the person praising him.[17]

[16] Erik H. Erikson, "Growth and Crises of the Healthy Personality," p. 211.

[17] Increasingly sick, Joey spent five years in two schools before coming to treatment by Bettelheim. Three months before, he had attempted suicide. It required almost three years of treatment for the boy to accept his humanness. Bettelheim concludes his description of the case of the "mechanical boy" this way: "When Joey was 12, he made a float for our Memorial Day parade. It carried the slogan: 'Feelings are more important than anything under the sun.' Feelings, Joey had learned, are what make for humanity; their absence, for a mechanical existence. With this knowledge Joey entered the human condition." (Bruno Bettelheim, "Joey: A 'Mechanical Boy,' " p. 127.)

Puberty: the teen-ager

"I felt myself isolated, helpless and always shut up in myself: I do not complain of it, for I believe that my early meditations developed and strengthened my thinking powers."[18] So did that celebrated political magician Talleyrand describe his twelfth year. His was a lonely adolescence. Adolescence generally is. Erikson terms this fifth stage *identity versus self-diffusion.*

10-7 "And the thoughts of youth are long, long thoughts" (Thomas Hood).

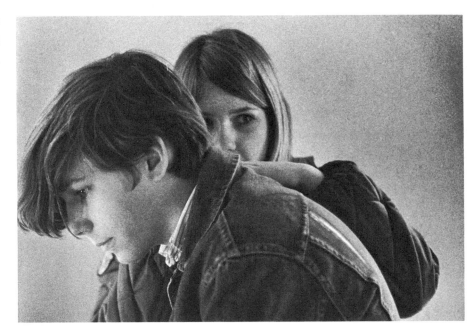

So many changes happen to the adolescent that he needs to become reacquainted with himself. Powerful new sexual urges send him soaring into confused dream worlds. These frighten him and make him feel vaguely guilty. Added to these disturbances are the "inability to settle on an occupational identity" and "the inexorable standardization of American adolescence."[19] Erikson has further described this stage:

> There is a "natural" period of uprootedness in human life: adolescence. Like a trapeze artist, the young person in the middle of vigorous emotion must let go of his safe hold on childhood and reach out for a firm grasp on adulthood, dependent for a breathless interval on his training, his luck, and the reliability of the "receiving and confirming" adults.[20]

[18] From *Memoirs of the Prince of Talleyrand,* quoted in Saul K. Padover, ed., *Confessions and Self-Portraits* (New York, 1957), p. 152.
[19] Erik H. Erikson, "Growth and Crises of the Healthy Personality," p. 218.
[20] Erik H. Erikson, "Identity and Uprootedness in Our Time," in H. M. Ruitenbeek, ed., *Varieties of Modern Social Theory* (New York, 1963), pp. 55–68.

Without reasonably satisfactory resolutions in the previous four stages—without basic trust, for example—adolescence can be a tribulation. Not identity but identity diffusion may result. In this culture this diffusion is common. Temporary identity may be found by some in a gang. With others, self-identity is interminably slow in coming. From his elders, the adolescent hears apprehensive criticism. Parents have been known to say, "Grow up. Stop hanging around the public square and wandering up and down the street. Go to school. Night and day you torture me. Night and day you waste your time having fun."[21] These words are translated from a Sumerian clay tablet 4,000 years old. But the confusion of adolescence is no easier to endure today than it ever was before. Emotional illness still may result.

Adulthood

Henceforth I ask not good-fortune, I myself am good-fortune,
Henceforth I whimper no more, postpone no more, need nothing . . .
Strong and content I travel the open road.[22]

THE FIRST STAGE   Adulthood comprises the next three stages of the Erikson schema of personality development. The first adult stage is *intimacy and distantiation versus self-absorption*. Childhood is over, as is youth. Ostensibly, self-identity is established. Now mature mutual relationships in love, friendship, and work are sought and are possible. The young adult also exhibits what Erikson refers to as "the counterpart of intimacy . . . *distantiation:* the readiness to repudiate, to isolate, and, if necessary, to destroy those forces and people whose essence seems dangerous to one's own." This necessary defensive reaction is not always understood or appreciated by older adults.

THE SECOND STAGE   In this stage, *generativity versus stagnation,* the mature person is prepared to share creatively. He understands that taking can be a way of giving, but that there is a difference between taking and exploiting. Generativity includes a mutual desire for parenthood, for creating the next generation. But it is more than mere reproduction. It is the ability to help another person gain those constructive strengths necessary for effective living.

THE THIRD STAGE: TOWARD THE GREAT EXPERIENCE   This stage is called *integrity versus despair and disgust*. The first Earl of Balfour (1840–1930) was a gentle man and a gentleman. His had been a good and exciting life in the service of his country. His last words were, "This is going to be a great experience."

An originator and leader, he had met life with courage and verve. The last stages of his life were a continuum of doing. He even died with

---

[21] From Samuel Noah Kramer, *Everyday Life in Bible Times,* quoted in Jerome Beatty, Jr., "Trade Winds," *Saturday Review,* (March 16, 1968), p. 18.
[22] Walt Whitman, "Song of the Open Road," lines 4–7.

anticipation. The final stages of his life had given him integrity. His life was a full circle. It excluded despair and disgust.

Thus Erikson unfolds the processes of the development of the human personality. Most people pass through them without too much trouble, gaining the emotional strength to function more effectively. But, at various times during their personality development, some people need help. How much? This may vary from a few quiet conversations with a wise friend to long-term psychotherapy. But help must be available.

Albert Einstein once said that "Every kind of peaceful cooperation among men is primarily based on mutual trust and only secondarily on institutions such as courts of justice and police." Without the basic trust of infancy there cannot be the mutual trust of adulthood.

Personality disorders and emotional problems

Definitions but not human formulae

The emotionally healthy person is able to meet the stresses of life and to choose appropriate methods of solving problems. He has a realistic sense of his own worth and interacts constructively with others. He is able to find satisfaction in efficiently performing his work. Since he adapts well in his environment, and perceives it with minimal distortion, he functions effectively on the health scale.

Emotionally healthy people behave normally; that is, their behavior is, for the most part, culturally acceptable. Behavior is appraised as normal according to degree and in the context of time and place. For an example of degree, consider two women in this culture. One wears a dress that tastefully shows off her feminine attributes; she is normal. The other sheds all her clothes in the street; her exhibitionism is a sign of serious illness. Time is another factor in determining normalcy. The shrieking adolescent girls of seventeenth-century Salem were thought to be possessed by witches. Today, comparable behavior at a rock concert draws little attention. Locale is another context for normalcy. In Java, it is acceptable for two people who are arguing in public to punctuate their epithets with the added insult of shedding their clothes. If this were done on a street in the United States, however, psychiatric investigation might well be suggested. If the concept of normal behavior varies according to degree, time, and place, is there any definition of normalcy? Today, most specialists who diagnose and treat emotional problems accept Freud's concept that the ability to work and to love without undue emotional impedimenta is measure enough of normalcy.

Extent of the problem in the United States

During the Second World War, one of every eight U.S. men examined for the draft was rejected because of emotional problems. On any given day, an estimated two million people are disabled by emotional illness in this country. In this nation's psychiatric hospitals over a million people a year receive treatment for mental illness. From seven to twelve percent of school-age children and youth need professional help for severe emotional problems. It is estimated that about ten percent of the population will, at some point in their lives, suffer serious emotional illness necessitating hospitalization.

It is with reservations that the following limited classification of disorders is introduced. There are many such classifications, and they are convenient for discussing disorders. However, they should not be used to pigeonhole either people or their problems. Indeed, many specialists concerned with emotional health tend to dispense with the labels or classifications altogether, preferring instead to discuss adjustive and maladjustive behavior in broad, uncategorized terms. As Menninger has said:

The limits of labels

> We label mental diseases the way little girls label their dolls. And one little girl's Helen is not like another little girl's Helen. In the same way, Dr. A's "schizophrenia" is different from Dr. B's "schizophrenia." And as long as we think of mental illness as a horrible monster with a name like schizophrenia—we won't be able to prevent it.[23]

A Classification of Personality Disorders

A. *Psychotic disorders*
  1. *Organic causes:* Characterized by lesions[24] in the brain.
  2. *Functional:* There is no demonstrable lesion in the brain.
    a. Schizophrenia
    b. Manic-depressive psychoses
    c. Paranoia
B. *Neurotic disorders*
  1. *Psychoneuroses* (neuroses)
    a. Anxiety states
    b. Phobias
    c. Obsessive-compulsive reactions
    d. Hysterias
    e. Traumatic neuroses
  2. *Psychosomatic disorders:* Peptic ulcer and asthma, for example, may be psychosomatic.
C. *Character disorders:* Examples include drug dependence, alcoholism, and criminal behavior. Some psychologists include sexual deviations, such as homosexuality, in this group. Also included is the psychopathic personality.

Psychotic behavior disorders are more severe than neurotic disorders. The individual displaying psychotic behavior has lost much contact with

[23] "A Conversation with Karl Menninger and Mary Harrington Hall on the Psychology of Vengeance," *Psychology Today,* Vol. 2, No. 9 (February 1969), p. 63.
[24] A lesion refers to any abnormal or harmful change in the structure of a tissue.

reality. However, the psychoneurotic person is still able to view his emotional problems with some degree of objectivity and he attempts to cope with them. Social deviance, rather than emotional symptoms, is the main characteristic of persons with a character disorder. For this reason, they are categorized separately.

Notes on the various disorders

The psychotic disorders

ORGANIC LESIONS   Brain tumors, severe head injuries, and infections such as far-advanced untreated syphilis not uncommonly result in psychoses. The psychotic behavior of *senile dementia* is seen more frequently as greater numbers of people live to be very old. This form of psychosis is due to deterioration of aged brain cells.

FUNCTIONAL DISORDERS   Psychotic behavior is not so easily recognizable as is generally thought. Some people are obviously deranged. Among these are people suffering from the extreme forms of *mania* and the more dramatic types of *schizophrenia*. Many psychotics, however, appear quite normal. Suddenly, without warning or cause, they may go berserk. And just as suddenly, they may return for a time to normal behavior. People suffering manic-depressive states, for example, usually experience a temporary period of lucidity between a "high" jubilant mood and a "low" dejected mood. In this last instance, it is as if the sick individual's moods swing like a pendulum from one extreme to the other, with lucid intervals.

In the United States, *schizophrenia* ("split" or "shattered" mind) is the most common of the psychoses, accounting for about 25 to 30 percent of all first admissions to mental hospitals. About 60 percent of the 500,000 people in mental hospitals suffer from schizophrenia. The term is meant to indicate a split of thought from emotion. Indeed, the patient appears to withdraw from reality and to live in a world of his own. Thus, one of the features of the condition may be consistent behavior utterly inappropriate to the realities of a situation.

Schizophrenia is a good example of the limitation of labels mentioned earlier in this section. It is not a single disease with a known cause and a single treatment. It is, rather, a complex of symptoms of disordered thinking, feeling, and behavior. No known single pattern of interaction between an individual and his environment inevitably leads to schizophrenia. People react to different stresses individually. The time in a person's life that the stress occurs may be as important as the nature of the stress. An emotional experience with which one individual can cope at six years of age may be overwhelming at three.

A great deal of recent research has focused on schizophrenia. The electrical brain waves of the schizophrenic may differ from those of normal people. Certain investigators consider schizophrenia related to an imbalance of body chemistry and function. Proof of this is as yet lacking. Some studies suggest a genetic aspect to schizophrenia, pointing to a

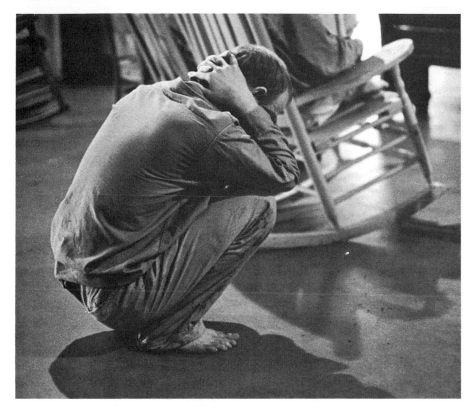

10-8 Assuming the position of a fetus, this catatonic patient has retreated into the womb. Now it is a lonely shelter.

tendency of the condition to occur in families. However, the relative importance of the influence of environment on the incidence of schizophrenia needs study. "The importance of genetic factors . . . has . . . been established . . . although . . . environment too plays its etiologic role."[25]

Because of their predominance in the sixteen to thirty age group, schizophrenias have been called the "psychoses of youth." The very young (six to seven years) and the elderly are not, however, exempt.

A wide variety of symptom combinations are observed in schizophrenia. One schizophrenic individual may either remain utterly motionless for hours (see Figure 10-8) or move about constantly, incoherent and even violent. Another pays no attention whatsoever to his environment. It may even be necessary to feed and dress him. This tragic person seems bereft of the ability to express even basic needs. Still another patient will giggle or babble senselessly. A schizophrenic patient may hear voices or see things that are not really present (hallucinations). He may believe he receives secret messages. One woman accused her dentist of installing a tiny transmitter in the cavity of a molar. By means of this she received constant threatening coded messages, not only from foreign powers, but also from other planets.

[25]Leonard L. Heston, "The Genetics of Schizophrenic and Schizoid Disease," *Science*, Vol. 167, No. 3916 (January 16, 1970), p. 255.

Next to schizophrenia, the *manic-depressive psychoses* are the most common psychoses (afflicting 10 to 15 percent of psychotics). There is, of course, an enormous difference between the occasional "blue mood" to which all normal people are susceptible and this condition. Its onset usually occurs between the ages of thirty and fifty, and women are more commonly afflicted than men. The manic-depressive reaction is manifested by a wild *elation* (*manic phase*) and a deep *despondency* (*depressed phase*). An attack may consist of elation alone or of depression alone, or of alternating elation and depression. A *manic reaction* may be set off by a chance remark or even a mild witticism. There then follows an excessive response with a tendency to irrationality. The *depressive reaction* is marked by retardation of both thought and activity. The patient maintains an air of general hopelessness. Except in exceedingly severe cases, the manic-depressive suffers no intellectual impairment. Even without treatment, recovery is common. The manic phase ordinarily lasts about three months; the depressive phase lasts about three times as long. There is a tendency for the symptoms to recur; about three-fourths of these patients have one or more recurrences.

Paranoia may be manifested by delusions of grandeur or persecution. A paranoid patient might believe himself to be Christ or Mohammed. Persecutions that such individuals feel are generally accompanied by a tendency to seek ulterior motives in the behavior of others. Such was the case of a woman who received the annual prize in law school as the student who had shown the greatest scholastic improvement. Upon graduation, she sued the school for damages. She alleged that the real motive of the faculty, in giving her the prize, was to show the world that in her work was the greatest room for improvement. In this way the faculty was demonstrating that she was not as fit as her associates to be a lawyer. [26]

The neurotic disorders

Every normal individual has his share of neurotic symptoms. These symptoms, resulting from the ordinary stresses and inner conflicts that he has been able to handle, do not interfere with his effective function in society. Thus, a person who has neurotic symptoms does not necessarily have a neurotic *disorder,* or *neurosis.* Whether a neurotic disorder actually exists depends on the degree of involvement of the personality. Neurotic symptoms, arising from an unresolved inner conflict of needs, may take command of the personality for a prolonged time. Effective functioning becomes difficult, even impossible. It is then that a neurotic disorder exists and professional help is indicated. (Those who wonder whether their symptoms are severe enough to merit help should seek such help, if only to remove their doubt.) Unlike most people with psychotic

---

[26] Arthur P. Noyes and Lawrence C. Kolb, *Modern Clinical Psychiatry,* 6th ed. (Philadelphia, 1963), p. 370.

behavior, neurotic individuals do not lose contact with the reality of their environment. Although limited, sometimes severely, the neurotic person is generally able to carry on his usual functions.

PSYCHONEUROSES   Here, briefly described, are the major psychoneuroses.

Anxiety states are one of the most common of psychoneuroses. Everyone shows symptoms of anxiety sometimes, but the neurotic's anxiety is chronic and severe, and he is helpless in handling it. His tension is constant; he feels under severe stress almost all the time. Unbearably acute attacks of anxiety, such as an overwhelming sense of approaching doom, may punctuate his chronic condition. He may suffer a variety of disagreeable physical symptoms such as excessive sweating and heart palpitations. Anxiety states are the most common form of neurosis in young people. Anxiety is so basic to the human experience and so common an emotional problem that it is the subject of the whole of the next chapter.

A *phobia* is a persistent fear of an object or situation that is not really dangerous or that has been blown out of all proportion to the actual danger. Examples are *agoraphobia,* a fear of open spaces; *claustrophobia,* a fear of enclosed places; *acrophobia,* a fear of high places, and *pavor nocturnus,* a fear of the dark, a phobia common to children and some adults.

Obsessive-compulsive reactions are manifested in people who are compelled to think about something that they do not want to think about (obsessive thoughts) or who are compelled to do some act that they do not want to do (compulsive acts). Among the most common compulsive reactions is compulsive hand-washing. For example, an individual who has masturbated may respond with abnormal disgust or a sense of uncleanliness to his action. His excessive thoughts about cleanliness may become obsessive, and he may compulsively wash his hands repeatedly. Such individuals are aware of the absurdity of their thought processes or actions but seem helpless to control them.

There are two types of *hysteria. Conversion hysterias* exhibit the same symptoms as many diseases. They are characterized by body symptoms such as paralysis of the legs, tics, or loss of sensitivity to pain. In *dissociative states,* there is virtual temporary takeover of the individual to the extent that he no longer dictates his own behavior. An example of this is the *multiple personality.* In this instance, two or more different personalities are found in the same person. (The motion picture *The Three Faces of Eve* was based on an actual case of multiple personality.) *Amnesia,* which is "sleepwalking while awake," is another type of dissociative state. This is a hysterical *fugue,* or flight, in which the individual escapes an intolerable situation by totally disassociating himself from it. Thus, he may suddenly appear far from home one day, neither able to identify himself nor to be identified. He may begin an entirely new life. Amnesia of his past is complete. Upon recovering, he will remember absolutely nothing of his fugue.

Traumatic neuroses occur as a result of the distress of extreme stress. A severe automobile crash may, for example, precipitate a severe neurosis. By no means does stress always result in a traumatic neurosis. Some feel that constant activity was responsible for the low incidence of reported neuroses among English, German, and Japanese civilians exposed to bombings. They were too busy to have emotional problems.

Those who study war neuroses usually distinguish between *combat exhaustion* and *combat neuroses*. The neurotic combatant is frequently described as a jumpy, chain-smoking, trembling man. The soldier suffering from combat exhaustion may fall asleep in the middle of a roaring battle. Some soldiers may be more likely to develop chronic war neuroses than others. A soldier who has been raised in a rigid environment, for example, is more inclined to suffer from combat neuroses. The most common feature of the combat neuroses of soldiers of U.S. armies during the Second World War was a deep sense of guilt. (This was not true of soldiers of the First World War.) During the Second World War, these sick men accused themselves of having failed their wounded or dead buddies.

Those with traumatic neuroses may be grievously misjudged. A case in point is the following authentic Second World War story of two heroic pilots. After a long history of bravery in the Pacific, both had been transferred to England. One would walk to his plane but, once there, was unable to board it. His feet turned him around. He would curse himself, swearing to fly on the morrow. But always, just before boarding, his feet would turn him around. His buddy, on the other hand, boarded his plane easily. But as soon as he passed the English side of the channel, he would begin to vomit. Since he had to wear an oxygen mask, he was medically disabled. "The man who could not control his feet was defrocked, demoted, dewinged, and sent to Iceland. The man who could not control his stomach was considered a hero whose stomach just could not take it."[27]

PSYCHOSOMATIC DISORDERS   When the seventeenth-century Englishman John Donne observed that "the body makes the minde," he was not reversing the ancient Roman Ovid (43 B.C.–A.D. 18). "Diseases of the mind impair the powers of the body," wrote the latter. Both poets understood that reciprocal negotiations between mind and body profoundly affect health. "As white as a sheet" or "hot under the collar" takes due note of the skin as a mirror of man's emotions. Whether he blushes or has gooseflesh, his anxiety is being expressed in a physical way. Why? Because the temporary release of tension via a physical reaction is easier to bear than containing the tension.

The term "psychosomatic" originates from the Greek *psychikos,* mind, and *soma,* body. Psychosomatic disorders originate in the mind and are manifested in bodily symptoms. Emotional stimuli are referred by the brain to body organs, resulting in effects ranging from gooseflesh to

[27]Douglas D. Bond, "Management of the Mentally Disabled," in Oliver Schroeder, ed., *The Mind* (Cincinnati, 1962), p. 280.

migraine headaches. Though these symptoms have no actual physical cause, they are nevertheless very real. For example, no condition is seen more frequently by the physician than tension headache. It is caused by sustained muscle contraction about the head and neck. In enduring stress such as cramming for an examination or driving in heavy traffic, the neck muscles contract in positions of maximum alertness. In several patients a physician was able to produce another type of headache, migraine, by discussing with them some of their guilt-producing life situations. Helping these patients understand the reasons for their reactions reduced the number and severity of their headaches.[28] *Asthma* can be precipitated by some substances, such as dust or feathers, to which the individual is sensitive (allergic). But emotional tension may also start an attack. Or both an allergic reaction and emotional tension may be involved and overlap to affect the respiratory system in this manner. The eye is also often involved in anxiety reactions. A case related by Menninger concerns a twenty-four-year-old girl with prolonged disabling eye problems. These had started shortly after the death of her brother in the war. Jealous of him, she had wished him dead. Also, to see if he was really different from her, she had once peeped at him. "The guilt, therefore, was associated not only with the envy of the brother but with the peeping."[29] In such cases psychotherapy can be remarkably helpful.

The effects of the emotions on the body's organs are both numerous and common, and patients with psychosomatic illnesses fill doctors' offices.

Character disorders

The identification of a person as someone who has a character disorder is not a moral judgment. This is a scientific term used to classify some emotionally sick people. The variation in degree of these problems is considerable. One individual may merely be a neurotic nuisance. Another constantly breaks the law. Within this latter group are the *psychopathic personalities*. These individuals are utterly irresponsible. Their sickness is in their lack of conscience. Psychopaths know the difference between right and wrong. However, they are psychologically unable to care about the difference. Preoccupied with the immediate gratification of their own needs, they are oblivious to the needs of others. They lack a sense of guilt and suffer little or no anxiety. Not necessarily lacking intelligence, they are frequently charming. But they feel no love for anyone. Friends, family, minister, and psychiatrist are unable to reach them. Their disorder may result from the lack of an affectionate relationship with an adult during childhood. The antisocial psychopath may reveal bitterness over this deprivation of love.

---

[28] R. M. Marcussen and H. G. Wolff, "A Formulation of the Dynamics of the Migraine Attack," cited in *Harold G. Wolff's Stress and Disease,* rev. and ed. by Stewart Wolf and Helen Goodell, 2nd ed. (Springfield, Ill., 1968), p. 47.
[29] Karl Menninger, *Man Against Himself* (New York, 1938), p. 368.

The criminal Johnny Rocco was not a foundling, but, perhaps worse, he felt like one. These lines from the Anglo-Saxon folk epic poem *Beowulf* can aptly be applied to him:

> *From a friendless foundling, feeble and wretched,*
> *He grew to a terror as time brought change.*

He suffered his way into crime because of a hostile mother. About his mother's reaction to his brother Davie's death he wrote, "When Davie died, she said she wished it was me instead." He adds, pitifully, "Money I stole I would never give to my mother."[30] As a boy, he would only give her money he honestly earned selling the magazine *True Confessions.*

Homosexuality

"There are some persons," wrote Kinsey and his co-workers,

> *whose sexual reactions and socio-sexual activities are directed only toward individuals of their own sex. There are others whose psychosexual reactions and socio-sexual activities are directed, throughout their lives, only toward individuals of the opposite sex. These are the extreme patterns which are labeled homosexuality and heterosexuality. There remain, however, among both females and males, a considerable number of persons who include both homosexual and heterosexual responses and/or activities in their histories. Sometimes their homosexual and heterosexual responses and contacts occur at different periods in their lives; sometimes they occur coincidentally.*[31]

In discussing male homosexuality they wrote further: "Males do not represent two discrete populations, heterosexual and homosexual. The world is not to be divided into sheep and goats . . . nature rarely deals with discrete categories. Only the human mind invents categories and tries to force facts into separated pigeon-holes."[32] Homosexual behavior is not an all-or-none condition, and in evaluating it considerations of time, place, and degree (page 332) are especially important.

HOW MANY INDIVIDUALS PARTICIPATE IN HOMOSEXUAL BEHAVIOR? Possibly millions. Kinsey estimated about four percent of the adult white male population in the United States to be exclusively homosexual after the onset of adolescence. Thirty-seven percent was estimated to have had at least some overt homosexual experience to the point of

---

[30]From Jean Evans, *Three Men,* quoted in Edward A. Strecker and Vincent T. Lathbury, *Their Mothers' Daughters* (Philadelphia, 1956), pp. 179–80.

[31]Alfred C. Kinsey, Wardell B. Pomeroy, Clyde E. Martin, and Paul H. Gebhard, *Sexual Behavior in the Human Female* (Philadelphia, 1953), p. 468.

[32]Alfred C. Kinsey, Wardell B. Pomeroy, and Clyde E. Martin, *Sexual Behavior in the Human Male* (Philadelphia, 1948), p. 639.

orgasm between adolescence and old age.[33] This last figure must be considered in a new light. The present director of the Institute for Sex Research, founded by Kinsey, recently revealed that this estimate is now considered to be high. Since he had ready access to prisoners, Kinsey used them for many of his interviews. He thought that their experience was typical of the lower socioeconomic group. Such is not the case.[34] Indeed, recent revelations of rape of new prisoners by long-term prisoners have shocked the nation. Kinsey's data revealed that female homosexual responses had occurred in about half as many females as males. Homosexual contacts to orgasm had occurred in about a third as many females as males. At any age period, about one-half to one-third as many females as males were primarily or exclusively homosexual.[35] There is much present-day disagreement with Kinsey's estimates of female homosexual behavior. Some research suggests that the number of females participating in homosexual behavior may approximate the number of males.

ROOTS OF HOMOSEXUAL BEHAVIOR   No single series of events or factors can explain homosexual behavior. Several causative factors operating in the individual environment over a prolonged period are usually responsible for it. Neither hormones nor heredity has been proven to be directly related to homosexuality. Furthermore, it is a mistake to associate body types or mannerisms with homosexual behavior. A brawny football player may be exclusively homosexual; a graceful male ballet dancer, heterosexual. Only a small percentage (less than one in five males and one in twenty females) can be identified as homosexual by such attributes as manner or dress.

Every normal person goes through a period of intense interest in the same sex. This is part of normal development and is most pronounced during the period of heightened sexual urges occurring during puberty and early adolescence.

> One therefore finds early adolescents involved in various forms of normal, mutual "homosexual" exploration, including comparing of sexual knowledge, sex talk, and some sex acts. Overt homosexual explorative acts (including mutual masturbation) may also occur and be essentially normal. These acts are no more indicative that such a child will become a homosexual than the sexual exploration at age four means that he (or she) will become sexually promiscuous as an adult. However, the reactions of adults to these acts can have catastrophic results, engendering a sense of guilt which may lead to lasting personality disturbances. [36]

[33] Ibid., pp. 650–51.
[34] "In the News," Medical Aspects of Human Sexuality, Vol. 3, No. 7 (July 1969), p. 104.
[35] Alfred C. Kinsey, Wardell B. Pomeroy, Clyde E. Martin, and Paul H. Gebhard, Sexual Behavior in the Human Female, p. 475.
[36] Marshall Shearer, "Homosexuality and the Pediatrician," Clinical Pediatrics, Vol. 5, No. 8 (August 1966), p. 515.

One recent study of New York adolescent lesbians (female homosexuals) identified disruptive and unstable family background (and not only an unresolved Oedipus complex, see page 328) as a major contributing factor in the homosexual behavior of girls. In these cases a wide variety of emotionally traumatic experiences led to a deep sense of insecurity, which was usually minimally relieved by a woman. This led to the seeking of female relationships.[37] British studies support this view:

> *Children reared in families which are incomplete, disturbed by distortions in personal relationships, or whose sexual attitudes are markedly clouded by repression or ignorance appear to be particularly vulnerable . . . It is particularly important to stress that these homosexual feelings do not inevitably imply homosexuality.*[38]

It should be emphasized that parental attitudes are by no means the only (and frequently not the major) factor in the development of an exclusively homosexual pattern. However, in some instances they can be an important factor. With his son, a father is harsh, unforgiving, punitive. With his daughter, he is gentle, understanding. Will not the son then contemplate the advantages of being a girl? An overbearing, domineering mother constantly ridicules the father. How may the son then perceive the advantages of manhood? So it is, too, with the female homosexual. Possibly the girl's mother gave her reason to fear womanhood.

The wise parent will do more than avoid such pitfalls. Nothing helps a child establish a healthy sexuality more than a discussion of his or her problems with a calm and informed parent. As the child gains the knowledge that homosexual feelings are a normal part of growing up, fears dissipate. More, the parent can show appreciation of the child's budding heterosexual interests. The parent will not encourage these interests by belittling them.

HOMOSEXUAL BEHAVIOR: HUMAN DILEMMA AND HOPE "What is striking about male homosexual alliances, in contrast to both heterosexual and female homosexual alliances, is their fragility, their tendency to be transitory, and the all-pervading promiscuity that characterizes them."[39] Some experts consider this promiscuity to be a consequence of the "disease concept" of homosexuality combined with societal condemnation. To understand the strength of the exclusively homosexual individual's need, one should consider the risk and pains of the average homosexual life. Most people cannot endure prolonged societal condemnation without condemning themselves. Although not universal among homosexuals, self-condemnation and guilt are common among them. The societal reaction to homosexuality doubtless arose from early efforts of Hebrews and Christians to perpetuate and protect the family and the

[37] "Research with Adolescents Sheds New Light on Early Lesbianism," *Science News*, Vol. 96, No. 3 (July 19, 1969), p. 45.
[38] "Female Homosexuality," an editorial in *British Medical Journal*, Vol. 1, No. 5640 (February 8, 1969), p. 331.
[39] Martin Hoffman, "Homosexual," *Psychology Today*, Vol. 3, No. 2 (July 1969), pp. 43–45, 70.

group. In vain does the individual engaged in predominantly homosexual behavior point to the writings of Plato[40] and to the disagreement among many psychologists as to the medical status of homosexuals. In this society the active homosexual (particularly the male) frequently forsakes the comfortable warmth of family and former friends for a life of casual contact. He may endure public contempt and ostracism. And for the male (very rarely for the female) it may be a life of frequent conflict with the law.

No laws of this country expressly prohibit anyone from being a homosexual. Many statutes, however, are directed against various sexual acts, which are grouped in such catch-all phrases as "crimes against nature" or "unnatural" sex behavior. This can confuse some people. "One husband and wife," it has been reported, "turned themselves over to the local police station for punishment when they discovered their specific acts of love subjected them to sixty years of life in prison."[41] The police sergeant was more understanding of them than he might have been if they had been homosexuals. In Western culture, condemnation, not understanding, is the usual lot of the homosexual.

A recent survey showed that, among homosexual women, there is a basic attraction for members of the opposite sex. In this study twenty-four homosexual women were compared to twenty-four nonhomosexual women. Both groups of women were in psychoanalysis. Heterosexual dreams were not significantly fewer in the homosexual group, nor was the desire for pregnancy less prevalent. Even before any psychoanalytic therapy, a majority of the homosexual women (53 percent) had experienced heterosexual activity. Indeed, three-fourths overtly sought social contact with primarily heterosexual men. With adequate treatment, the probability of a change to heterosexuality among the homosexual women was considered to be about 50 percent.[42]

Still another study of 123 lesbians revealed that one in four wished to become exclusively heterosexual.[43] Although the desire to become heterosexual is not always characteristic of those exclusively homosexual, modern therapy does offer hope. In selected cases long-term psychotherapy has been helpful. Group therapy has helped some to change. Homosexuality "is eminently curable—as curable as any other chronic psychologic disorder. Of the people presenting for therapy—and these are the only ones who can be counted legitimately— . . . more than one-third correct their homosexual orientation."[44]

---

[40] It should not be assumed that the entire ancient world was tolerant of homosexuality. Wrote the Roman poet Ovid: "Let youths, got up like women, keep away!" (*Heroides*, 4, 73) and "No bird of air, no thing that breathes, endures female to mate with female" (*Metamorphosis* IX, 731–33).

[41] Robert Veit Sherwin, "Sodomy," in Ralph Slovenko, ed., *Sexual Behavior and the Law* (Springfield, Ill., 1965), p. 428.

[42] H. E. Kaye et al., "Homosexuality in Women," *Archives of General Psychiatry*, Vol. 17, No. 5 (November 1967), pp. 626–34.

[43] F. E. Kenyon in *Journal of Neurology, Neurosurgery, and Psychiatry*, Vol. 31, No. 5 (October 1968), p. 487, and in *British Journal of Psychiatry*, Vol. 114, No. 11 (November 1968), p. 1337 cited in "Female Homosexuality," an editorial in *British Medical Journal*, Vol. 1, No. 5640 (February 8, 1969), p. 330.

[44] Daniel Cappon, "Understanding Homosexuality," *Postgraduate Medicine*, Vol. 42, No. 4 (October 1967), p. A-131.

Wanted: professional help

Who is trained to help?

The treatment of emotional disorders by psychological means is called *psychotherapy*. When other methods, such as drugs, shock treatment, or surgery, are used, the procedure is considered *somatotherapy*. Some physicians use both. Although somatotherapy is generally limited to physicians, psychotherapy is not. The four professional groups involved with psychotherapy are the psychiatrists, psychologists, psychiatric social workers, and psychiatric nurses. Within their various competencies they all contribute to the total treatment available to the patient.

The *psychiatrist* is a doctor of medicine with extensive training in the diagnosis and treatment of emotional problems. All *clinical psychologists,* although they are not M.D.s, have graduate training in their specialty. In addition to diagnosing and treating the emotionally disturbed, psychologists also administer and interpret psychological tests. After earning a master's degree in social work, the *psychiatric social worker* obtains special training in interviewing techniques and psychotherapy. Such training is invaluable in gaining insightful information about a patient's home, work, and community situation. *Psychiatric nurses* are specialists trained to nurse emotionally disturbed people.

Psychoanalysis is a special technique of psychotherapy that uses the basic techniques of Freud. Although clinical psychologists and psychiatric social workers may engage in psychoanalysis, the majority of psychoanalysts are psychiatrists.

In a large *mental hospital,* all four specialists may work together in handling emotional problems. In most *clinics* for the emotionally disturbed, such as child-guidance centers, the psychiatrist, clinical psychologist, and psychiatric social worker are members of a team, each contributing to the patient's recovery. With the exception of psychiatric nurses, these specialists may also be engaged in private practice in the community.[45]

There are only 15,000 psychiatrists in the United States. Added to these are about 18,500 nurses, 7,500 social workers, and 5,200 clinical psychologists working in approximately 600 mental hospitals and 1,800 psychiatric clinics. This means a continuous gross personnel shortage. Twice as many psychiatrists, 10,000 more clinical psychologists, and twice as many social workers are urgently needed. Particularly serious is the shortage of psychiatric nurses. To the approximately one-half million beds presently available for mental patients must be added three hundred thousand more.

[45] Departments of health and mental health (both state and local), local councils of social agencies, and mental health associations are all sources of information regarding local facilities for the treatment of emotional problems. Two national agencies that are especially helpful in providing information about the qualifications of agencies are the National Association for Mental Health, located at 10 Columbus Circle, New York, New York 10019, and the Family Service Association of America, at 44 East 23 Street, New York, New York 10010.

It is understandable that no single technique is used in dealing with complex emotional problems. The *client-centered* technique of psychotherapy directs the patient neither to his problems nor to his early childhood. The therapist makes no effort to suggest either goals or a new way of life. As the patient talks out his problems, the therapist may help to clarify them, but it is assumed that the patient is able to solve his problem. In this atmosphere of patient esteem, the emotionally distressed person comes to realize his worth and his ability to live fruitfully.

Behavior therapy tries to eliminate the behavior pattern that is distressing the patient. Learning techniques are used. One behavior therapist tells of a patient who was unable to have sexual intercourse with his wife

unless he first dressed up as a woman, and he frequently went out on the streets at night dressed in this fashion and wearing a wig. This symptom had become especially uncomfortable to the patient because he feared that his young son, as he grew up, would learn about it. The treatment prescribed was extremely simple. Electrodes were fastened into the woman's clothing that the patient habitually wore; he was encouraged to dress up but warned that at some point he would receive a painful shock or hear a buzzer and that the shock or buzzer would then be repeated at irregular intervals until he had removed the clothing. Each session of therapy included five starts at dressing followed by the shock or buzzer, with a one-minute rest period between each trial. After 400 trials, the treatment was considered ended.[46]

The patient apparently recovered. The aversive conditioning by pain and punishment, rather than by pleasure and reward, has also been used in treating homosexuality and alcoholism.

Toward the end of the last century, Freud and Breuer originated *psychoanalysis*. Severe emotional distress in a hysterical girl had been manifested in deafness and paralysis of an arm. While under hypnosis, she told of many experiences related to her symptoms. Seemingly as a consequence of this, her symptoms disappeared. Psychoanalysis, as a treatment procedure, had begun. Freud discovered that by merely asking patients to relate anything that came to their minds (*free association*), past experiences that had been long repressed in the unconscious and had been causing symptoms eventually came to light. As these unconscious conflicts were revealed to the patient, his symptoms often abated or disappeared. As a result of his earned revelation, the patient developed personality strengths that enabled him to better adjust to his environment. Over the years numerous variations of this procedure have been introduced, but the fundamental approach of psychoanalysis remains unchanged. Dorsey

Some psychological methods used to help emotional problems

[46] C. B. Blakemore *et al.,* "The Application of Faradic Aversion Conditioning in a Case of Transvestism," cited in Jerome Kagan and Ernest Havemann, *Psychology: An Introduction* (New York, 1968), pp. 443–44.

has quoted a little-known poem illustrating what he has called this "growth of self-insight":

> As I walk'd by myself, I talk'd to myself
> And myself replied to me;
> And the questions myself then put to myself
> With their answers I give to thee.[47]

Months or years of from two to five hourly sessions a week may be required for this procedure. The length and intensity of treatment vary with the problem and the patient. Psychoanalysis is work for both analyst and patient. In the very first hours, the analyst seeks to comprehend the patient's problem. He then attempts to sensitively help the patient understand and then deal with the problem. Again, the techniques used depend on the patient. Insight is required of the patient. He must be able to arrive at it, endure it, and use it. Comprehending and confronting his human problems, he will seek ways of resolving them. Not all patients are suitable for psychoanalysis. Among these are those with severely limited intelligence, those who do not come voluntarily, and those who somehow profit financially from their sickness and so remain sick. Persons with severe physical lesions, such as brain tumors, can hardly profit from psychoanalysis. By no means, however, does this exclude all people who are physically ill. Many individuals with physical ailments, such as tuberculosis, may do better under psychoanalysis. A wide variety of emotional problems are amenable to psychoanalysis. Among them are anxieties, psychosomatic problems, and obsessive-compulsive neuroses.

Psychoactive drugs

The use of psychoactive drugs has resulted in a marked drop in the total population of state mental hospitals. Not all of these drugs are new. *Reserpine,* the active principle of the root *Rauwolfia serpentina,* has been used for centuries to treat anxieties and dementias in India, Southeast Asia, and Europe. *Chlorpromazine,* a synthetic drug, shares with reserpine a considerable effectivity in inducing relaxation. Both are particularly useful in treating schizophrenia. The discovery that a certain drug can be used as a tranquilizer for emotionally disturbed people is often incidental. A newly discovered muscle relaxant or antihistamine, for example, may also prove to be an excellent tranquilizer. Why are tranquilizers so often superior to barbiturates? The latter are useful in inducing sleep. With them excitement is reduced, but patients are not able to move about. However, tranquilizers reduce the intensity of the excitement itself. Delusions and hallucinations are reduced without a profound soporific (sleep-inducing) effect. Since tranquilizers do cause some drowsiness, patients so medicated should not drive.

---

[47] Barnard Barton, "Colloquy with Myself," quoted in John M. Dorsey, Preface, in *Illness or Allness* (Detroit, 1965), p. 13.

Lithium carbonate, widely used in Europe, has not yet been licensed in this country, though it is available for research. There is evidence that it may be useful in treating manic and depressed patients.

The very variability and depth of the human mind limits the use of drugs that act on the mind. Research continues into the chemistry of emotional sickness. However, one should not expect the future to yield a drug that will cure schizophrenia just because there is, for example, an antibiotic to cure "simple" pneumonia. Although much has been accomplished with drugs in psychic illness, and there is doubtless more to come, it is well to remember the complexity of human emotions. In psychiatry, drugs do not, as a rule, cure. They merely cause the abatement of gross symptoms so that the patient may be better reached.

Shock therapy

Shock, sometimes through the use of drugs (such as insulin), but usually by electricity, is still extensively employed in therapy by some psychiatrists. This is most effective with depressive states, although its use for other emotional disturbances has met with some success. The trend, however, is away from shock treatment toward the use of tranquilizers. (Some years ago, there was much publicity about a drastic procedure called *prefrontal lobotomy.* In this operation, certain lobes were separated from the rest of the brain. Results were poor. The procedure has now been abandoned.)

Self-help by environmental manipulation

Just as environment may induce stress and anxiety, so may it be manipulated to induce relief. Nobody should try to solve severe emotional problems alone. It is worth reemphasizing that early help can prevent progression of an emotional aberration. Moreover, professional advice is valuable in determining the need for help. However, many people with a mild emotional disturbance can help themselves considerably. Often, the mere presence of an understanding listener helps. Thus, marriage, although no substitute for therapy, may help an anxious individual find relief. For the same reason, friendships may also be effective in relieving anxiety. Unfortunately, some individuals attempt to relieve anxiety by repeated extramarital or premarital affairs. Such affairs may heighten conflict, increase guilt, and leave the sensitive individual more disturbed than before.

Interest in games can be decidedly therapeutic. Anxiety brought on by frustration, is often relieved by appropriate competitive games. Aggressions from frustrations, which otherwise produce anxiety, are thus harmlessly diverted to sports. Spectators at sporting events also achieve this relief. Athletic contests are planned with great skill and forethought. Why are tension-producing favorite teams so avidly supported? People normally enjoy the pleasure from the relief of the deliberately created tensions.

Sublimation of aggressive drives into creative work does not ordinarily resolve conflict. However, sexual and other drives may be sublimated into successful humanitarian efforts.

Noble lives are often led by those who assuage loneliness with humanitarian service. Before he was forty, Albert Schweitzer was world renowned as an outstanding Protestant theologian and as an organ interpreter of Bach. In his middle years, he forsook all the appurtenances of success. He went to medical school, graduated, and became a medical missionary. At lonely Lambaréné, in the African jungle, he built a hospital. "Here at whatever hour you come, you will find light and help and human kindness"[48] is inscribed on a lamp leading to the hospital quay. In the profoundest sense, Schweitzer used his tension to good purpose. If the great man's inner world was loneliness, in work he surely found balm.

What is the best treatment for emotional disorders?

Modern treatment of mental illness has brought emotional strength to countless people who might otherwise have led wasted lives. Today, early diagnosis and treatment offer hope to those who half a century ago would have been forgotten. Nevertheless, therapy for many emotional disorders is still based on empirical methods.

> *Recent studies have indicated that results with different treatments are markedly similar. Most statistical studies show that 65 to 70 percent of neurotic patients and 35 percent of schizophrenic patients improve after treatment regardless of the type of treatment received. Long-term follow-up studies of treated patients have also demonstrated no differences among the various treatments.* [49]

This statement does little to resolve this question: which type of psychotherapy is best suited for the average emotional problem? Because there is no average emotional problem, the answer to that question will probably never be found. Differences in reactions to different stimuli by different people at different times—such variables do not readily lend themselves to measures of psychotherapeutic success. By relatively simple manipulation of his environment, one individual may relieve considerable anxiety-producing stress. At the other extreme, an individual may fail to overcome his emotional hurdles despite intensive appropriate psychotherapeutic treatment. More important than the kind of help received is receiving it from a competent source when it is needed. It is hardly surprising that treatments vary. Considering the complexity of emotions, it is more surprising that they vary so little. That citadel of the mind, the brain, occupies but a third of a cubic foot of space. Under ordinary conditions it uses only ten watts of energy. A single refrigerator light bulb consumes four times that much energy. And yet, assuming that nothing is ever completely forgotten, the average brain is able to store some

[48]Robert Coope, *The Quiet One* (London, 1952), p. 219.
[49]Ari Kiev, ed., *Magic, Faith and Healing* (London, 1964), pp. 4, 5.

280,000,000,000,000,000,000,000,000 "bits" of information. As to the brain's complexity, consider only that part of its structure controlling behavior that is distinctively human—the cerebral cortex (page 222).

> Charles Herrick,[50] the distinguished American neuroanatomist, attempted to get some conception of the number of possible connections among the millions of cortical cells in a single human brain. Based on a series of computations, he inferred that there were $10^{2,783,000}$ such connections. To print this number written out in figures would take about two thousand ordinary book pages.[51]

In the accepting and sorting of numberless human experiences, in its endless relaying of responses, is it to be wondered that the mind falls sick and needs treatment? And that the treatments are so varied?

> Erikson relates the case of a little boy who ate paper. Nobody, however, paid any attention to him. He ate more and more paper. Still nobody cared. So finally he ate the theatre tickets, and then he received treatment.
> One of the ways of looking at symptomatology at any period in any society is: Where is the point where you eat the theatre tickets? We had quite an interesting case brought to the Menninger Clinic of a girl who really didn't need treatment herself, although her parents did. They lived in a house with one bathroom. She used to lock the door and take a three-hour bath. In time, the parents brought her to a psychiatrist, and then she was able to get them treated.[52]

Where is the point where one eats the theatre tickets? Where is the point at which emotional problems must be referred to others for professional diagnosis and treatment? It should be early. A problem that will at first be handled with ease may, if neglected, worsen. To work professionally with emotional problems is difficult. The trained professional understands both his limitations and his potential. He knows how to recognize the need for help in whatever form it appears; he knows when and how to step in and when to leave the disturbed person alone. But most of all, he knows that there are no simple definitions, no easy cures. The mind of man is the most complex and the most autonomous of all created systems. As John Milton wrote in *Paradise Lost* (I.254–55),

> The mind is its own place, and in itself
> Can make a Heaven of Hell, a Hell of Heaven.

[50] Charles J. Herrick, *The Evolution of Human Nature* (Austin, Tex., 1956).
[51] J. Z. Young, *A Model of the Brain*, cited in *Harold G. Wolff's Stress and Disease*, rev. and ed. by Stewart Wolf and Helen Goodell, 2nd ed., p. 172.
[52] Margaret Mead, "The Changing World of Living," *Diseases of the Nervous System*, Vol. 28, No. 7 (July 1967), p. 7.

11

Anxieties
in the 1970s

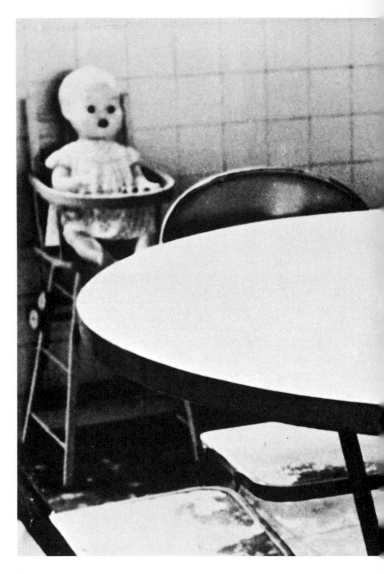

The nature of anxiety

"The problem of anxiety" wrote Freud more than forty years ago, "is a nodal point, linking up all kinds of important questions; a riddle, of which the solution must cast a floodlight upon our whole mental life."[1] What, then, is anxiety? Anxiety is a feeling of foreboding. It is a premonition that something evil is about to happen. As a descriptive term it may be used synonymously with "worry." What is the difference between fear and anxiety? Fear is caused by an immediate experience. One is fearful

[1] Sigmund Freud, *General Introduction to Psychoanalysis*, American ed. (New York, 1920), p. 341.

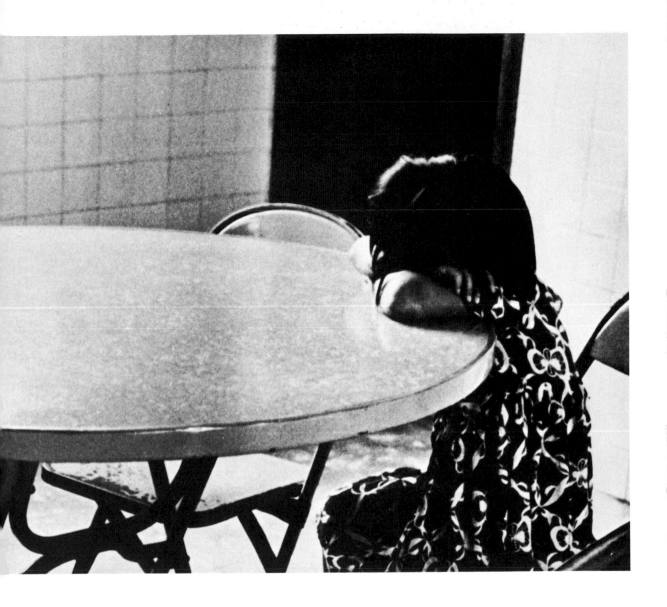

of something or somebody specific and one is afraid now. However, one is anxious about something that may be quite vague. Also, anxiety is always a feeling about the future. The difference between anxiety and fear can be as thin as a hair.

People have a reservoir of anxieties. Most of these anxieties are conquered; others are half-remembered or are deeply buried in the subconscious. The first strange face, the initial separation from the mother, the first day at school—these childhood anxieties are added to the countless anxiety-associated strivings, defeats, and victories that are an inevitable sum of normal living.

THE NATURE OF ANXIETY **351**

The power of anxiety   Of the 6,654 U.S. Army men captured in the three-year Korean war, over 90 percent were taken prisoner during the first twelve months. In those days, enemy treatment of prisoners was atrocious. A ninety-mile death march killed 10 percent of 500 men. Indeed, in the three years of war, 38 percent of the 6,654 U.S. prisoners perished. Of these, over a thousand were victims of atrocities. Even during the beginning weeks of the conflict, the word spread through the U.S. ranks harshly and clearly; capture meant suffering and death. Within him, each man carried this tight knot of anxiety.

For those who were captured, the stresses of war were intensified. Each man had an ancient and crying need to be relieved of his anxieties. Knowing this, their captors did not immediately fulfill the worst expectations of the prisoners. Instead, they fed them and offered them friendship. To agonizingly anxious men, they held out the lure of tranquility. But there was a price: cooperation with the Korean movement for "world peace." Less than two percent of the men collaborated. Doubtless the commitments of most of the men to their own culture induced them to endure. For some, the offer may have even created more tension and anxiety, arising from the conflict between wanting to accept the offer and not wanting to seem cowardly before fellow captives.

So, part of this method of handling prisoners was to offer relief from intolerable anxiety. The plan was intensified by removal of all leaders from their midst. A feeling of abandonment and rejection was cultivated among the prisoners. In a score of ways the men reexperienced a long-forgotten threat of childhood. "If you don't come along, I'll leave you here by yourself!" The unmeant rejections of parents and teachers, the scorn of playmates, the indifference of girls—all these childhood anxieties were consciously or unconsciously renewed, and with their renewal all the old anxious tensions had to be handled again. The newer anxieties were also intensified. Even physical activity of the prisoners was seriously limited—a common source of childhood anxiety. The acute uncertainty of the future, the constant threat of physical and mental harm, the tragic sense of abandonment and rejection, the conflicts and guilts, and the frustration and inactivity of the prison situation—for the prisoners, the cup of anxiety was filled to overflowing.

Some variables of anxiety   The prisoners were in an extreme situation. But few life situations are untouched by anxiety. Anxiety moves the whole of the emotional life. Its more severe manifestations are only too recognizable: the dry throat, the quavering whisper, and, in extremes of anxious terror, the stifled scream. Less dramatic (but just as distressing and more common) manifestations of anxiety are restlessness, cold sweat, palpitating heart, muscular tension in the back of the neck, chest pain, and a hopeless, helpless, sinking sense of impending disaster. However, people differ in their reactions to similar situations. One man's financial ruin does not demoralize him. Expending the energies of his anxiety profitably, he works to recover.

Another is paralyzed by the mere possibility of a relatively minor loss. Still another man is precipitated into mild anxiety by a spot on his clothes. When someone inquired of Einstein why he was so indifferent to his clothes, the great physicist merely answered, "It would be a pity if the wrapping proved better than the meat."

Anxiety: contagion and conscience

Observe a line of small children waiting to be immunized. As one approaches the needle, he begins to tremble, then to cry. One by one, most of the others will lose control and also cry. So it was with the U.S. Army men captured by the Communists, except that most of them thought themselves too old to cry before their buddies. It was no different with the guilt-ridden flagellants of the fourteenth century (Chapter 5), and it is anxiety that dictators have learned to stir in their screaming hordes. Yet, although anxiety can be contagious, to feel it one must have a conscience. A psychopathic criminal does not possess an adequately developed conscience. He suffers no conflict from his actions. He can know no anxiety. In contrast, the anxiety of irreconcilable conflict destroyed the devout minister of W. Somerset Maugham's indestructible story, "Rain." His lust for the prostitute collided with his conscience, sternly forbidding its expression as sinful. From his powerfully conflicting tensions rose guilt and anxiety. He could bear neither and committed suicide.

Anxiety as a motivation

Clearly anxiety is society's tool for maintaining obedience to law and order. But it is more. Because it stimulates man to seek appropriate and constructive solutions to the problems causing it, anxiety may yet save humanity. In this regard, Toynbee[2] drew an illustrative parable. Fishermen, bringing in herring from the North Sea, noticed that the fish in the tanks became sluggish. Because the fish consequently lost some of their freshness, their market value was reduced. By placing catfish into the herring tanks, the fishermen menaced the herring. In the face of this threat, the herring became active, flourished, remained fresh, and retained their market value. Of course, in the end the herrings' "anxiety reaction" did not save them; they were eaten by people. Nonetheless, the threat set in motion constructive defenses against the predatory catfish in their ecosystem. Will human beings turn the tables on anxiety? Will they constructively deal with predators, not only within themselves, but also in their outer ecosystems? A good beginning is to recognize societal threats. Halleck writes:

> The most idealistic, psychologically sound, and committed students have considerable ability to identify themselves with those who are especially oppressed, the persecuted and the poor. In a commonality of brotherhood they feel the oppression of others as if it were their own. This truly Christian, socially responsible attitude

2 Arnold Toynbee, "How to Turn the Tables on Russia," cited in Rollo May, *The Meaning of Anxiety* (New York, 1950), p. 12.

is admittedly only a part of the motivation of activists. Yet at some time or other, for however brief a period, it becomes a powerful factor towards commitment to dissent. Where the attitude of selflessness is persistent, it fosters deep involvement in civil rights work, poverty programs and the Peace Corps.[3]

It is well to remember that the possibility of a destructive reaction to anxiety is in itself cause for anxiety. Fearful, indeed, is "aimless anxiety, which drives us into irrational *action,* irrational *flight*—or, indeed, irrational *denial* of danger."[4]

Escape from anxiety   All human reactions to anxiety are designed to relieve or escape it. Sometimes anxiety may be relieved by a simple expedient, such as changing to a less demanding job. It is more difficult to change a boy friend or girl friend. "I can't afford you anymore," one young woman told a man who had caused her nothing but pain. The normal reaction to anxiety is the realistic appraisal of stress, followed by the taking of appropriate action. Sometimes the reaction to anxiety can be costly. A chronically high anxiety level in college students is related to both lower grades and a higher rate of dropout. Unfortunate as these consequences are, they are certainly remediable. Extreme reactions to anxiety do occur among college students in the form of attempted suicide (see page 378). Such inappropriate reactions to anxiety are manifestations of serious sickness and merit careful medical attention. One preliminary report of a study of suicide among 69 Harvard and Radcliffe students revealed a striking relationship between the suicide attempt and either loss of an intimate person by death and separation or anxiety over academic performance. "Apparently the need to achieve academically and to sustain meaningful relationships are more important to the maintenance of equilibrium in college students than other factors such as extracurricular activities, number of friends, athletic prowess, or physical health."[5] Another study of 1,454 Harvard dropouts showed that psychiatric disorders were four times as high among the dropouts as among the general undergraduate population. A highly encouraging sign of the ability of these young men to handle anxiety was the finding that the "psychiatric dropouts have the same rate of return, attainment of honors and graduation as those who drop out for other reasons."[6]

Anxiety is a paradoxical human experience. An insistent threat to human welfare, it may nonetheless contain the seeds of human salvation.

[3] Seymour L. Halleck, "Why Students Protest: A Psychiatrist's View," *Think,* Vol. 33, No. 6 (November–December 1967), p. 6.

[4] Eric H. Erikson, *Childhood and Society* (New York, 1950), p. 363.

[5] Graham B. Blaine, Jr., and Lida R. Carmen, "Causal Factors in Suicidal Attempts by Male and Female College Students," *American Journal of Psychiatry,* Vol. 125, No. 6 (December 1968), pp. 834–37. For a further discussion of suicide see page 378.

[6] Armand M. Nicholi, Jr., "Harvard Dropouts: Some Psychiatric Findings," *American Journal of Psychiatry,* Vol. 124, No. 5 (November 1967), p. 657

The ability to tolerate and constructively use anxiety may decide more than human health. It may well determine human existence.

For this reason, this chapter is wholly concerned with several anxiety-provoking problems that are central to modern living.

The seventeenth-century French mathematician and philosopher Blaise Pascal wrote:

> *When I consider the short duration of my life, swallowed up in the eternity before and after, the little space which I fill, and even can see, engulfed in the infinite immensity of spaces of which I am ignorant, and which know me not, I am frightened, and am astonished at being here rather than there; for there is no reason why here rather than there, why now rather than then . . . The eternal silence of these infinite spaces frightens me.*[7]

Three centuries later, men ventured out of the world and tentatively explored the moon's ecosystem. During the return trip to earth listeners heard this cosmic conversation:

APOLLO. *So what's new?*
HOUSTON. *Oh, we were wondering what was new with you up there.*
APOLLO. *Oh, very quiet.*
APOLLO (6:21 P.M.). *Nice to sit here and watch the earth getting larger and larger and the moon smaller and smaller.*
HOUSTON (7:35 P.M.). *Hello, Apollo 11. Your white team is now on and we're standing by for an exciting evening of TV and a pre-sleep report.*
            (WILD, HOWLING, SCREAMING NOISES)
HOUSTON. *You're sure you don't have anybody else in there with you?*
APOLLO. *Say again please.*
HOUSTON. *We had some strange noises coming down on the down link and it sounded like you had some friends up there.*[8]

The "wild, howling, screaming noises" were doubtless due to radio interference. If the astronauts were unduly anxious it could not be discerned in their conversation. Such an ability to deal with anxiety under stress is a primary requisite of astronauts. But what of the earthlings to whom they returned? Had the majestic technological triumph nullified some of the anxiety so long ago expressed for them by Pascal? Not for most men. The same anxieties—who am I? what is my relation to other men and to the world outside myself?—remain.

Indeed, modern man's anxieties have increased, partly because of the same technological changes that might have been expected to reassure

[7] Quoted in Theodosius Dobzhansky, *Mankind Evolving* (New Haven, Conn., 1962), p. 346.
[8] Quoted in *The New York Times*, July 23, 1969, p. 26.

him. One must forsake the womb. But is it necessary to get out of the very world? With this added degree of separation, this generation will yet have its anxious rendezvous. Moreover, today the very speed of change troubles people. Impermanence and rootlessness are built into their lives—into their jobs, their automobiles, even into the family unit. Almost a century and a half ago, a French visitor to these shores noted the fever for change:

> *I accost an American sailor and inquire why the ships of his country are built so as to last for only a short time; he answers without hesitation that the art of navigation is every day making such rapid progress that the finest vessel would become almost useless if it lasted beyond a few years.*[9]

If change and rootlessness have grown to be the mark of modern times, anxiety is their common symptom. But it is not quite the same symptom of Pascal nor of those who preceded him. It is compounded. Men now fear that they will be unable to control not only what they know, but also what they are about to know. Destruction by nuclear weapons, dehumanization by computers, devastation by pollution, depersonalization by industry—these threats have not given modern man reason to feel secure with his own technology.

But is it technology itself he fears, or its creators? Man fears man. Why? Because he does not know him. Man's knowledge of himself and his ability to communicate with others has not kept pace with his other discoveries. He has communicated with men on the moon, but not always with men across the table. Man's inner space has not been conquered. Today, the failure to establish human contact disturbs man's relationship with himself, and the group's relationships with other groups. War—the old expression of group conflict—has always been a source of anxiety. Modern war has created the added anxiety of a sense of helplessness. Being able to act positively to reduce one's anxieties—exemplified in the astronauts' cool professional performance—is essential for emotional health. But in the face of Armageddon most people feel powerless.

Global anxieties, then, are assuredly a part of our time. But nearer home, one finds a world of anxieties well worth exploring. What are some of them?

Parental anxiety

A distraught young mother presented her dilemma to her family physician this way:

"It's my fault," she said, her voice trembling. "I should have breast-fed

[9] Alexis de Tocqueville, quoted in Leonard S. Silk, "Business Power, Today and Tomorrow," *Daedalus* (Winter 1969), p. 186.

my baby." Suddenly she was angry. "But I hated it. I couldn't stand it. I never liked it, and I can't hide not having liked it any more. Last month I read an article in this magazine." She held a popular woman's journal. "Is it really that unnatural not to breast-feed the baby? My doctor told me to forget about it. But a friend of mine read that unless you breast-feed your baby, you have lesbian tendencies or something. Is that somebody's idea of a joke?" She wiped her eyes. "I'm beginning to hate this whole thing." She was crying. "I hate it. I hate having a baby. Everybody says something different."

Some women want to breast-feed their babies. They enjoy it, and do it easily. Others, just as normal, do not enjoy breast-feeding. They should not do so. A guilt-ridden mother, resentfully holding her child to her breast, will do that child no good. It is the total experience of dining, of human comfort and tenderness, that is essential to the baby in this, the stage that Erikson calls basic trust versus mistrust.

The young woman described above is still another victim of an endless barrage of conflicting advice. Don't pick up Billie when he screams. Pick up Billie when he screams. Exclude Susie from the bedroom. What if she does feel left out? Don't exclude Susie from the bedroom. She'll feel left out. Never take Willie's hands away from his penis; if you do, he'll masturbate in public. Always divert Willie when he's doing his exploring; if you don't, he'll masturbate in public. And so on, ad infinitum. The result is a confused parent, doubtful of every action, suspicious of his own love, convinced of his inadequacy, and suffering parental guilt.

Parent development

Parents develop too. They pass through stages related to the stages of their child's development (see Table 11-1). Parents and child develop together, experiencing singular, yet interwoven, problems. And, like the child, a parent in the throes of one stage may still be occupied with unsolved problems of a past stage.

It takes time for parents to learn how to interpret the howl of the child. What is the baby trying to tell them? He is dry, fed, fondled. No diaper pin pierces his bottom. Why, then, does he weep? Is it still another gas bubble? Or is it because his bed was accidentally moved six inches from the window and he misses the usual shaft of bright light from an adjacent window?

When the recliner becomes a sitter and suddenly a toddler, he is into everything. Again the parents need time. It is not always easy to wholeheartedly accept a child who seems to be winning an all-day footrace with his mother. No sooner may this acceptance come about than Friedman's third stage of parental development—separation—is reached.

The pain of separation is not limited to children. The child's first day at school, punctuated by the peremptory command, "Mommie, g'wan home," is a trauma that mothers (and grandmothers) are not prone to forget. Nor is the fourth stage, manifested by a child's independence, any easier for the parent. Their child's "declaration of independence" hurts

TABLE 11-1 *Parent and Child Development*

STAGE ONE: Infant	STAGE TWO: Toddler
Parent Development: Learning the *cues*. **Erikson:** Trust. **Spock:** Physically helpless; emotionally agreeable. **Ogden Nash:** *Many an infant that screams like a calliope Could be soothed by a little attention to his diope.*	**Parent Development:** Learning to *accept growth and development*. **Erikson:** Autonomy. **Spock:** A sense of his own individuality and will power; vacillates between dependence and independence. **Ogden Nash:** *The trouble with a kitten is that Eventually it becomes a cat.*
STAGE THREE: Preschooler	STAGE FOUR: School-Ager
Parent Development: Learning to *separate*. **Erikson:** Initiative. **Spock:** Imitation through admiration; learns about friends; preliminary interest in sexuality. **Ogden Nash:** *But joy in heaping measure comes To children whose parents are under their thumbs.*	**Parent Development:** Learning to *accept rejection*—without deserting. **Erikson:** Industry. **Spock:** Fitting into outside group; independence of parents and standards; developing conscience; need to control and make moral judgments. **Ogden Nash:** *Children aren't happy with nothing to ignore And that's what parents were created for.*
STAGE FIVE: Teen-Ager	
Parent Development: Learning to *build a new life,* having been thoroughly discredited by one's teen-ager. **Erikson:** Identity. **Redl:** Conflict to be confined to specific and major issues at hand; peer orientation and fair play. **Ogden Nash:** *O adolescence! I'd like to be present I must confess When thine own adolescents adolesce!*	Source: David Belais Friedman, "Parent Development," *California Medicine*, Vol. 86, No. 1 (January 1957), pp. 25–28.

some parents and angers others. It is almost as difficult for the rejected parent to remember that he is still desperately needed as it is for him to understand the rejection. The fifth stage of parental personality development is marked by an opportunity for the parents to rebuild their lives, not around the child, but with themselves more in mind.

Parental development begins with the parents' own childhood. Parents need help. Almost every parent comes to realize that the child is trying to give that help. This effort, in turn, helps the child to identify with his parents and to grow with them. Their effort is mutually beneficial.

The parent has become the scapegoat of modern times. "Look at how badly you raised me," is the accusation and excuse of many an emotionally distressed young person. The parents' sense of guilt is deep. But "the fact is that children, too, possess freedom of choice. It appears at an early age and develops with the intelligence and other capacities of the youthful personality. Children, then, share the responsibility for their behavior and emerging characters with their parents, relatives, teachers and friends."[10]

And freedom of choice is a durable freedom that may remain when all other freedoms are gone. Frankl writes,

We who lived in concentration camps can remember the men who walked through the huts comforting others, giving away their last piece of bread. They may have been few in number, but they offer sufficient proof that everything can be taken from a man but one thing: the last of the human freedoms—to choose one's attitude in any given circumstances, to choose one's own way.[11]

Undeniably, parents need improving, but the child must share in the responsibility for his own development. It is an opportunity. Again, he can help not only himself but also his parents.

The life of the average mother today is not like her grandmother's used to be. Her grandmother was not isolated with a runabout child in a huge uncaring pile of rock. Her grandmother was not locked up in a carefully measured, stingily allotted, two-room space, a three-dollar telephone call away from her nearest relative. Her grandmother lived among a retinue of relatives and neighbors, all interfering but caring. Her grandmother's time was a time of *kirche, kinder, kochen* (church, children, cooking). Bread was baked at home, not bought practically odorless and neatly sliced. It was a time of the "superhome" not the supermarket. Her grandmother had a single gadget—a music box given her as a wedding present. And when her grandmother bade farewell to her son, who was leaving to be on his own, she had another child at her breast. When her grandmother died that summer at forty-three, and the child died too, it was very sad. Sad, but not unusual. Most grown people died of some infection before they reached the age of fifty; and, in those days, countless babies died of summer diarrhea.

Today's average mother will live well past seventy. She will have borne her children (three) by the age of twenty-seven. She will have raised them before she is fifty. Production of basic services outside the home (education, recreation, food), combined with laborsaving automation, add perhaps as much as ten more years during which child-raising can be a reasonably part-time job. Even a woman who manages to keep busy at home throughout all the childbearing years can count on only about

The child's development: whose responsibility?

The working mother

[10] Corliss Lamont, *Freedom of Choice Affirmed* (New York, 1967), p. 32.
[11] Victor E. Frankl, *Man's Search for Meaning* (New York, 1959), p. 112.

twenty years of complete occupation. These are interim years. They come out of the middle of her life. What is more, some eighty percent of married women become widows—many at a young age. If they hope to remarry, they must become involved in activities outside the home. And they must compete with the growing number of divorcees and other unmarried women.

These potential problems do not contribute to the modern woman's desire to consider domesticity a full-time lifetime occupation. Child-rearing is now a temporary full-time job. Since 1950 the number of married working women in the United States has exceeded the number of single working women. Moreover, the acceptance of women by industry testifies to their success in the business world. Twenty percent of mothers with children under six and over forty percent of mothers with children between six and seventeen work away from home. Millions of these must work because of financial reasons. In the past ten years, however, an increasing number of working mothers have been working because they are unhappy at home. For them, the horizons of home are too limited. They make poor full-time mothers and dull, nagging wives. At work they are happier. But many working mothers are anxious that they are failing their children. They feel guilty. Need they be?

The mother who is content at home need not be defensive about it. A happy full-time mother always will be best for children. But an unhappy mother, resentfully brooding over her missed life outside the home, is best outside that home. An outside job may well improve her performance with her children. And a smaller amount of high-quality mothering is better than a massive amount of poor mothering.

A job, then, may relieve the guilt she feels about being a dissatisfied mother. But what can she do about her new guilt—her feeling that she has deserted the home? She must remember that the home and children remain primarily her responsibility. And, indeed, recent studies have amply indicated that the vast majority of modern young women choose careers that will not lead them into later serious conflicts with their desire to be successful wives and mothers. [12] The greatest problem for the working mother is the care of the infant and preschooler. The care of older children is more easily arranged. People who care for other people's children must have enormous sensitivity, patience, and tenderness. Such people are very hard to find. The degree of the average working mother's guilt will depend in part on her success in meeting the critical problem of substitute care. Also, she must honestly ask herself if she is physically and emotionally able to handle both complex, demanding aspects of her life. The care and feeding of a business executive for eight hours a day, for example, may be just as taxing as caring for any child. (It is possible that experience with one is helpful with the other.) A woman who is exhausted and tense from a high-pressure business or professional life may

[12] Harold L. Wilensky, cited in "Woman's Work Is Never Done: Roundup of Current Research," *Transaction*, Vol. 6, No. 7 (June 1969), p. 8.

find it difficult to be the feminine mother of a child waiting at home. Not only in dress, but also in manner she will need to be a quick-change artist. Children thrive on love, not ticker tape.[13] A child will reject a mother who is masculine in dress or behavior. For this reason and despite "heavy investment in preparing their chosen careers, [she] must impose self-limitations after marriage and children."[14] The guilty working mother who tries to "make it up" to the child for being absent will not mother, but overprotect the child. In the end, the child will fight her off.

What about the father? Without his support, the working mother will fail. If she is prone to constantly remind him of her contribution to the family income, she will receive not support but hate. Work will become for each of them an escape from the other. And the child at home will live on a deserted island threatened by the stormy seas of dissension.

Finally, do not the studies of mother-deprived children provide adequate evidence that a mother's absence deprives and sickens a child? (See the following section.) One must guard against glib conclusions. To begin with, the absent mothers in the studies were usually completely absent. Moreover, maternal deprivation was not the only misfortune of these children. Other factors—such as bitter family dissension, poverty, and racial discrimination—also contributed to the mental sickness of children without mothers. Recent evaluations point to little or no direct correlation between working mothers and childhood instability. Children raised in kibbutzim (the cooperative agricultural communities of Israel) are kept in nurseries. The nursery workers are carefully selected to provide affection and warmth for the children. Every day the children are visited by their own parents. A degree of family life is thus part of each child's day. Some investigators claim that the absence of continual parental attention plus the kibbutz emphasis on the community welfare in ways enhance the child's development.

In summary, many working mothers succeed in raising emotionally healthy children. But they must work at it.

Childhood anxiety

"The relation between infant and mother is a ballet, in which each partner responds to the steps of the other."[15]

Observe a newborn calf. Shakily it struggles to its trembling legs. Still wet, listing, it totters to its mother's teat. Such is its early independence. The dependence of the human newborn, however, is complete. Even the

The need for mothering

[13] "Where I come from," Fiorella La Guardia used to shrewdly say, "we knew the difference between ticker tape and spaghetti." The Little Flower was reflecting even deeper feelings than a social conscience. He was saying: "Society should care like a mother."

[14] Louise Sandler, "Career Wife and Mother," *Archives of Environmental Health,* Vol. 18, No. 2 (February 1969), pp. 154–55.

[15] Jerome Kagan, "The Child: His Struggle for Identity," *Saturday Review* (December 7, 1968), p. 80.

purpose of the breast must be shown him. To completely deprive the human newborn or infant of mothering is catastrophic.

At birth, threats promptly beset the utterly vulnerable human infant. The respiratory center of the brain, the respiratory muscle (diaphragm) separating the chest from the abdomen, the respiratory muscles between the ribs in the newborn—all these need further development. To meet his consequent threat of inadequate respiration, the newborn human must breathe two or three times as fast as the adult. To the respiratory threat is added a gastrointestinal threat. The gut lining is incomplete. For a time, it will function poorly. A third threat is that of an inadequate relationship between the infant and his mother or mother-substitute. And still a fourth threat is that the infant might not be able to satisfy his needs for pleasure, for example, the oral pleasure of enough sucking. For all people, to a varying degree, these threats become realities.

The infant feels hunger. Hunger hurts. He is threatened, anxious. He cries and he is fed. His tension is relieved. But sometimes he cries and the breast (or bottle) does not come. All he can do is cry more. He hurts more. His stress grows. He suffers more anxiety. About six months of a small amount of frustration will teach him how to deal with frustration. Too much frustration, however, will teach him that his most important person cannot be counted upon. He loses his basic trust. At the breast the infant learns, for the first time, love and hate (see page 323).

The effects of prolonged maternal deprivation have long been studied. In 1801, the "wild boy" of Aveyron was found in a French forest. Attempts to help him laid the foundation for present treatment of the mentally retarded. For more than thirty years, reports of children completely deprived of mothering have described their sad expression, pitiable dejection, rigidity, mental and social deterioration, stupor, and even unduly high sickness and death rates.

Animal infants also develop severe emotional problems from maternal deprivation. Laboratory monkeys bred without mothers grieve piteously. At times they clasp their heads in their arms and rock. Some pinch the same patch of skin hundreds of times daily or develop other compulsive mannerisms. Others fail to mate successfully.

One experiment separated young monkeys from their mothers and raised them with mother substitutes constructed of wire. One wire substitute incorporated a bottle containing warm milk from a mother monkey. The other substitute was covered with terry cloth. The young monkeys turned to the bare wire effigy only to feed. Otherwise they clung to the soft terry cloth mother substitute (Figure 11-1). This study indicated "that contact comfort is a variable of overwhelming importance in the development of affectional response, whereas lactation is a variable of negligible importance."[16] Monkeys reared with the never scolding, always warm terry cloth "mother" nevertheless did not mature normally.

[16]Harry F. Harlow, "The Nature of Love," *American Psychologist,* Vol. 13, No. 12 (December 1958), p. 676. Lactation refers to the period of milk secretion.

Observations such as these, combined with highly defensible, if theoretical, schema of normal personality development (see pages 322–32), correctly emphasize the critical importance of the mother to the normal growth of the child. The fact that most psychiatrists vigorously emphasize this has not helped to diminish the widespread sense of guilt and anxiety among many working mothers of young children. And an anxious mother means an anxious child.

Months before birth the first human heart beat pumps not mother's but fetal blood independently produced. Intrauterine life is not mere unremembered slumber. Unborn, the child sucks (often his thumb, see Figure 10-4, page 327), preparing for later oral gratifications of feeding and sex. Within the uterus, jerky movements prelude the initial tottering independence from the mother. Sometime after birth—in body exploration and use, in later creative curiosities at school—the child seeks freedom from dependency. He is dependent, and seeks independence, longer than any other creature. His prolonged dependency gives him the time he needs to learn the behavior expected of him by his culture. But this dependency can also produce frustration, insecurity, hate, guilt, anxiety.

The disciplined, dependent struggle for independence

The childhood struggle for freedom takes place in a milieu of love and hate. He loves the breast that gratifies him; he hates it when it frustrates him. He loves his parents when they comfort him; he hates them when they control him. This love-hate ambivalence is carried into later years. It is a major cause of anxiety. The frustrations of dependency continue, as hostility, into adulthood. The adult loves his child. He hates his child. He loves his mate. He hates his mate. This emotional paradox is not a predicament peculiar to modern man. Twenty centuries ago the Roman lyric poet Catullus wrote these perplexed lines:

> At once I love and hate
> You ask why this should be,
> I know not, 'tis my fate
> A fate of Agony![17]

When the normalcy of this ambivalence is recognized, man will not be so governed by the anxiety it creates. The paths to independence are obstructed by parent-child conflict. But the child will travel those paths nevertheless. The loving parent can help. Should help not come, the child will struggle on alone, unaided. Should the parent impede the child in the normal quest for independence, the child will retaliate with hate, and suffer guilt and anxiety because of it. All normal people have dependent needs. Yet a degree of independence is essential for maturity.

During each stage of personality development, the normal child will collect problems. Usually he learns from them. They do not necessarily become serious impedimenta. Problems vary. Should the heart form im-

[17] Quoted from *Catullus*, tr. into English verse by T. Hart-Davies (London, 1879), p. 122.

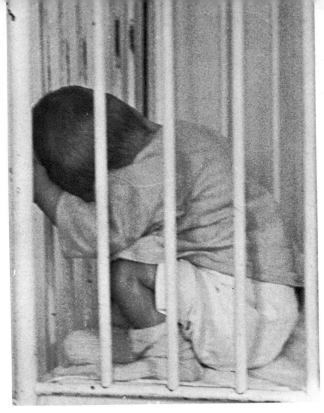

Abandoned and placed in an institution, this Greek child turned his back on the world. Rejected, he rejects. The depression, immobility, and withdrawal of many children suffering maternal and other deprivations may be worsened by insomnia, loss of appetite, loss of weight, and other grave manifestations.

11-1 *Mother love and maternal deprivation*

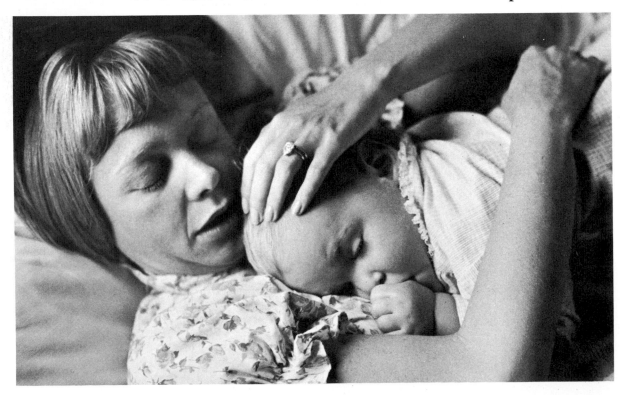

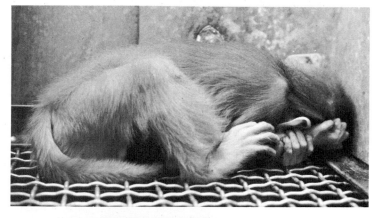

Like the Greek child shown on the opposite page, this baby monkey was denied normal contact with mother and peers. Overwhelmed by his sense of abandonment, the monkey infant, no less than the human, shuts out the world.

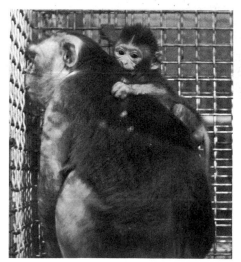

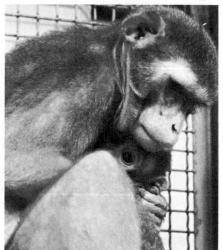

The monkey infant-mother intimacy is a mutual fulfillment (*right*). The mother monkey in the photograph at the left was herself raised with a cloth substitute "mother." She developed abnormally and rejects her infant. Not only food but also cuddling and warmth are the infant's first needs. The normal mother reciprocates by cradling, grooming, caressing, and protecting her baby.

Like the human baby, the infant monkey needs to dine, not just eat. Here, a young monkey clings to the soft terry cloth covered "mother," holding on to it even when feeding from a milk bottle affixed to a plain wire "mother."

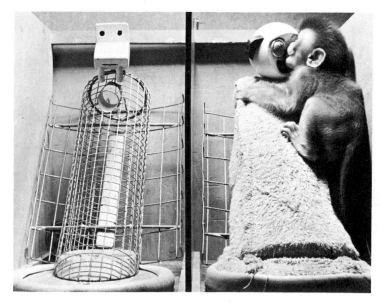

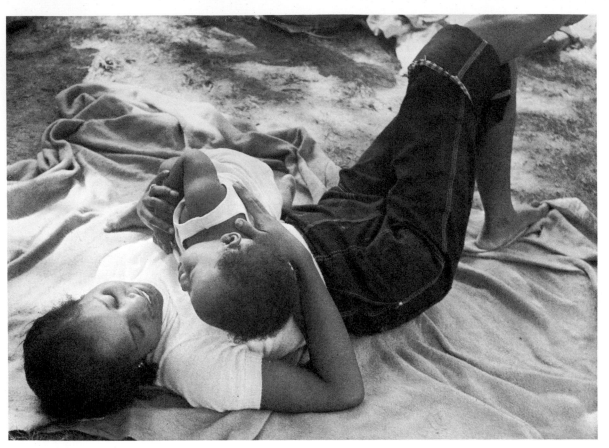

11-2 The nonmysterious parent.

perfectly and leak, it will, nonetheless, beat as long as possible. Should a child's oral needs in the first year be thwarted too often, those needs may well be manifested in later life by constant emotional overeating. But the child will, to repeat, develop nonetheless. Well equipped or not, he will seek independence. This, then, the wise parent will accept.

As he strives for independence, the developing child needs to understand discipline, not continuously suffer from it. The more the child clearly comprehends what his parents expect of him, and why, the less will he need discipline and the less will he suffer when disciplined. The mother who literally screams her emotional responses to a child's behavior is more successful, at least in this respect, than the parent who is sanctimoniously silent and ends by being mysterious. Mysterious parents frighten their children. There may be room for mystery in love of God or love between the sexes. There is no room for it in parent-child love. A child who never really knows how a parent feels has problems with discipline.

One day, the little girl pulls the pots and pans from the cupboard. She is kissed and told she is cute. The next day, repeating the same performance, she turns happily to her mother. But a previous marital tiff has angered the mother. The child is scolded and spanked. The child is hurt, not corrected. One day the father answers his little girl's proposal of marriage with a "sure, honey, aren't you my best girl?" (a lying answer to an honest question). The next week, the little girl repeats her proposal. It is met with cold indifference or even harsh hostility (adding injury to error). Or a little girl, living with her divorced mother, must listen to a constant rehearsal of her father's faults. From her father there is nothing but tenderness. She is confused, then angry. The mother retaliates with discipline. The child retaliates with sullen obedience. Children are not miniature adults. They do not spring into adulthood. They do not develop suddenly after a long quiescence. Neither do their anxieties. They need constancy, not confusion. That is why children love peek-a-boo games. That is why they never tire of hearing the same bedtime story. They know what will happen. They can count on it. Discipline of children works best when it arises from constant love, not intermittent hate.

The Oedipal phase in early childhood development demands the utmost of parental sensitivity. To its subtleties attention is now directed.

Recently, a young man of twenty-two visited a psychiatrist. His chief complaint was that he feared to be alone. Whenever he was by himself, he would become aware of a "creeping" uneasiness. Then slowly terror welled up in him and spread through him "like a stain." He quickly volunteered that he had, for two years, been engaged in homosexual behavior.[18] At present, he was unable to relate well to women. But it was not the sexual orientation that disturbed him. It was the loneliness.

Of Oedipal complexity

Months of psychoanalysis passed. Finally the following story was pieced together. At five, he had worshipped his mother. Now he described her dispassionately. She had been a graceful, beautiful woman, almost childlike. She was fond of picking him up and stroking his hair until he fell asleep. His father was stern and gruff. Sometimes he would grumble, "Be a big boy. Get off your mother's lap." His mother would blush and kiss the child or smooth his hair.

Early one morning his father was ill. The young man remembered every stark detail—the ashen face, the rasping breath, the ambulance, the small clot of onlookers, his own fleeting fright. His mother was inconsolable. All that day she wept. That night he crawled into her bed. "Don't worry, mommie," he said. "I'll be here and keep care of you. He will die. He'll never come back." She slapped him so hard he became confused. She hit him again and again. Then she sent him to his room. In his room he heard her raging at him. Four days later, at his father's funeral, his mother barely spoke to him.

[18]For a further discussion of homosexuality, see p. 340.

From a five-year-old's normal emotion, an abnormal situation had resulted. The child's guilt about wanting to rid himself of his father (a normal desire at that stage) was heightened by both his mother's immature coquetry and his father's disapproval. He was later unable to identify with a father he had never learned to admire. The father's illness intensified the boy's anxiety. But it was the mother's violent renunciation of him that tore him loose from his most urgently needed moorings.

She might have told him the simple truth: she needed both him and his father. Instead, she lost them both. Instead, she sent the boy to a lonely room from which he never emerged.[19]

Masturbation   At about two or three, a normal child explores and stimulates his genitalia. He thereby initiates pleasure in himself and perhaps anxiety in his parents. The parental anxiety originates in conditioning and culture.

The stigma attached to masturbation has ancient beginnings. Early Hebrews and Christians believed children should be seen and sexless. In that period of constant external threat to both groups, it was thought necessary to forbid any practice that might become an internal threat. To strengthen the authority of the family and community, practical controls by adults, including strict sexual repression of the young, were thus deemed essential. One psychiatrist, noting the normal developmental function of male masturbation, nonetheless writes that "We cannot be sure it can be allowed to proceed unchecked. For . . . its inhibition has had a calculable effect on character structure of Western man; and there is no doubt that, in any civilization, the capacity to defer gratification is what distinguishes the healthy person from the impulse-ridden psychopath."[20]

During the Dark Ages, fear of disease was added to sin as a deterrent to masturbation. This medieval attitude died slowly. On August 10, 1897, Michael McCormick of San Francisco was granted patent number 587,994 for a male chastity belt. Fathers were to fit them on their adolescent sons to keep them from masturbating. In Victorian times the young were led to believe that masturbation would visit upon them every malady from sterility to stuttering. Even today, there are unfortunates who believe this. Others, who are fully aware that masturbation does not cause disease, still feel ashamed of masturbating. Thus, an aura of anxiety envelops practically all the males and more than half the females in this culture.

"Don't do that!" This admonition, punctuated with a sharp slap, too often is the two-year-old's introduction to his parent's lack of normal sexual development. The child is taught a crippling lesson: part of him is bad. What is worse, it is a part that feels good. He may never unlearn this. Faced with the catastrophe of losing parental love, he learns early that masturbation is one pleasure that he must enjoy in guilty loneliness.

[19] Problems with parents are by no means the only cause of homosexuality. However, in this authentic case there was a definite relationship.
[20] Milton R. Sapirstein, *Paradoxes of Everyday Life* (New York, 1955), pp. 169–70.

At age two, that is a harsh discovery, especially since he loves his parent with all his dependent heart.

Perhaps he forgets a previous warning. Then he hears: "If you don't stop playing with it, I'll cut it off!" All along the male toddler had fearfully suspected this possibility. Repressed into the unconscious is the child's fear of castration. Years later it will rise, cloaked in anxiety.

The little girl wonders about her absent penis. With a mournful feeling of guilt she remembers her self-manipulation. Did she do something to herself that caused her to lose her penis? Perhaps her parents are punishing her? Unable to dwell on her castration anxiety, she represses it. In the adult woman, this repressed guilt is a common cause of an anxiety neurosis.

The mother who might be aware of these possibilities may become overconscious of them. She is excruciatingly careful not to disturb her child during genital manipulations. There is no reason for this extreme response. A child should be interrupted if his diaper needs changing or for any other sensible reason. Some three- or four-year-olds masturbate publicly. They should be firmly but gently told not to do this. A mother's instruction is better than a stranger's taunt. Ginott writes:

> Parents may exert a mild pressure against self-indulgence, not because it is pathological, but because it is not progressive; it does not result in social relationships or personal growth. The pressure must be mild or it will backfire in wild explosions. The solution lies in so involving the infant with our love, and the child with our affection and interest in the outside world, that self-gratification will not remain his only means of satisfaction. The child's main satisfactions should come from personal relationships and achievements. When this is so, occasional self-gratification is not a problem. It is just an additional solution. [21]

Why is it often more difficult for the normal male adolescent to divert his thoughts from masturbation than it is for the older male or the adolescent female? The aged Sophocles thanked the gods that he was no longer ruled by the tyranny of sexual desire. In our society some believe that the repressed male adolescent lives with that tyranny. They consider it a major cause of his anxiety. As explained in Chapter 13, sex play, kissing, petting—all stimulate sperm production. Pressures are built up. The trapped sperm must be released. Ejaculation occurs. In the normal boy this is a local experience. Without direct stimulation, the adolescent girl does not respond locally to petting. What is a local experience for the boy is a romantic experience for the girl. Ova are not produced in great numbers. Unlike spermatozoa they are not imprisoned to cause pressures that must be released. With the girl there is no ejaculatory reflex stimulation. In the adolescent girl, therefore, sexual stimulation does not neces-

[21] Haim G. Ginott, *Between Parent and Child* (New York, 1965), pp. 161–62.

sarily result in an overpowering desire for release by sexual intercourse. Many students of the subject suggest that, for the adolescent boy, sexual stimulation does have this result.

This difference between the normal adolescent sexes is also manifested by what they want and need to know. Secrecy about sexuality is not conducive to emotional serenity. Many an adolescent girl wants to know about menstruation and pregnancy and delivery, and she wants to know if sexual intercourse hurts. If she sees a magazine double-page spread of children with fins instead of arms, she wants to know all about that, too. She wants to know what kind of sexual activity boys have. And she should know that at least half of all girls masturbate.

Before "wet dreams" happen, the boy should know about these entirely normal nocturnal emissions; he will then realize that they are not dirty. Many authorities suggest that, for the boy, sex and love are quite unrelated. Unlike the girl, he usually does not romanticize his sexual tensions. Almost all normal adolescent boys (over 95 percent) masturbate. The frequency varies from once or twice to several dozen times a month. This the boy needs to know, and he should be told. The realization that virtually all boys masturbate at his age dilutes his sense of guilt.

The senseless guilt and anxiety to which adolescents have been subjected because of masturbation has abated somewhat. There is considerable opinion among psychiatrists that masturbation is a normal and even valuable transition to mature sexual relations. One thing is certain. In this culture, no other activity indulged in by over 95 percent of all males and 50 percent of females is considered abnormal.

The best answer lies in the Greek ideal of moderation. Boys or girls who masturbate privately, moderately, and without guilt or a sense of moral unworthiness will be able to give the best of themselves to a mate. Since they look upon themselves as people of worth, they give something valuable and good.

Those who find in masturbation their only source of gratification and consolation need help. But so does any disturbed person obsessed with one activity to the virtual exclusion of all else in a rich and varied world. From the point of view of body function, however, there is no scientific evidence whatsoever that masturbation can be excessively frequent.

Teen-age anxiety

Each youth sustains within his breast
a vague and infinite unrest.
He goes about in still alarm,
With shrouded future at his arm,
With longings that can find no tongue.
I see him thus, for I am young.[22]

[22] An Oklahoma high school boy, quoted in Evelyn Millis Duvall, *Family Development,* 2nd ed. (Philadelphia, 1962), p. 297.

Today's teen-age culture is a phenomenon of the wealthy society. True, a lot of teen-agers do not have much money. For many, the only source is an impoverished parent. Other teen-agers marry early. A large number must shoulder other responsibilities, possibly prematurely. In the sodden swamps of Asia there are no pampered teen-agers. Nonetheless, a significant share of this nation's economy depends on this powerfully monied leisure class. Without the money the teen-ager spends on movies, records, cosmetics, clothes, cigarettes, and second-hand cars, business would be sorely shaken. Madison Avenue flatters, cajoles, and caters to the teen-ager. Adults criticize him. Along all the remnant Main Streets of the nation, grown-ups at home, school, and church collectively wag a reproving finger at him. This is not a new phenomenon. Consider, for example, this impatient view written some sixteen hundred years ago:

> A youth approached me. He was bearded; his clothes were dirty; he wore a student's cloak and he looked a typical New Cynic of the sort I deplore. I have recently written at considerable length about these vagabonds. In the last few years the philosophy of Crates and Zeno has been taken over by idlers who, though they have no interest in philosophy, deliberately imitate the Cynics in such externals as not cutting their hair or beards, carrying sticks and wallets, and begging. But where the original Cynics despised wealth, sought virtue, questioned all things in order to find what was true, these imitators mock all things, including the true, using the mask of philosophy to disguise license and irresponsibility. Nowadays, any young man who does not choose to study or to work grows a beard, insults the gods, and calls himself Cynic.[23]

How long will it take today's teen-ager to straighten out? the modern elders wonder worriedly. By straighten out, they mean, of course, be more like themselves.

The adult desire for self-perpetuation is natural. The Indian poet-philosopher Tagore wrote that "we must not forget that life is here to express the eternal in us."[24] But if the child is truly to meet the parental need for the eternal, if he is to develop the deepest purpose of their lives, his life must have purpose. In the past, the teen-ager made a definitive financial contribution to the family welfare. This is generally no longer expected of him. It is not completely true that the teen-ager today has a different set of values than adults. His values are just less complex. (Sometimes his elders are tinged with envy at what he can "get away with.") Like his elders he simply buys the pleasures he can afford. And many a teen-ager mimics the adults he knows. He is out for the bigger, the better, and that ultimate measure of having made it—the most.

[23] From the memoirs of the Emperor Julian, Vidal's version, cited in "History Repeats," an editorial in *Perspectives in Biology and Medicine,* Vol. 12, No. 3 (Spring 1969), p. 331.
[24] Rabindranath Tagore, "The World of Personality," in Clark E. Moustakas, ed., *The Self* (New York, 1956), p. 82.

11-3 A fortunate adolescent.

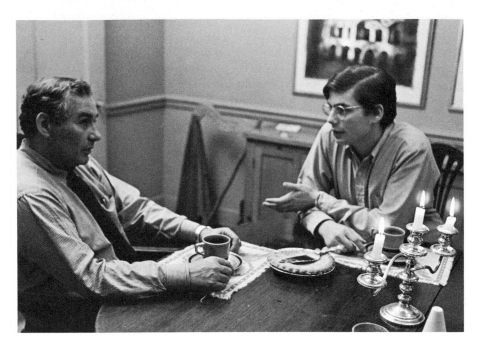

But the same things trouble the teen-ager that used to nag his parents. Who am I? What am I? What will become of me? "Be yourself, Debbie," one kindly parent advised his adolescent. "How can I," came her answer, "until I find out who I am?" And hers is not the best age for waiting. Only too keenly does the teen-ager understand the penetrating cowboy laconism: "I ain't what I ought to be, I ain't what I'm going to be, but I ain't what I was."[25]

Not often does the adolescent of this culture gain confidence from his elders. In France, for example, a young girl is expected to come to her wedding breakfast transformed overnight from innocent ignorance to mature womanhood. In this country, the girl may hear on one day "Stay away from those boys," and on the next day, "Why don't you get married?" Too often there is no apprenticeship to adulthood.

In some cultures, the adolescent is given careful preparation for whatever is expected of him as an adult in the community. The ritualistic puberty rites of many African tribal children marks their initiation into the responsibilities of adulthood.[26] "In view of the sudden switch-over, there is, in practice, no definable period of 'adolescence' in the traditional African culture."[27]

[25] Erik H. Erikson, *Childhood and Society*, p. 219.
[26] After circumcision certain African boys understand they are expected to behave like men. The discontinuance of this rite with some African adolescents is thought, by many natives, to be associated with an increase in antisocial behavior. (Laura Longmore, *The Dispossessed* [London, 1959], p. 182.)
[27] T. A. Lambo, "Adolescents Transplanted from Their Traditional Environment: Problems and Lessons Out of Africa," *Clinical Pediatrics*, Vol. 6, No. 7 (July 1967), p. 439. When the adolescent is transplanted from his rural to an urban environment, however, drug addiction, prostitution, and other delinquency may result.

Frequently, however, the adolescent of this culture must shift for himself. How can he find and identify himself? How can he prevent what Erikson has termed "self-diffusion"?

In the startling changes of his body, there is no remembered and reassuring sameness—only ungovernable, even unsightly change. In his newly overwhelming feelings he finds fatigue and worry. With the sharp and cruel insight of his age, he perceives the frailties of his elders. Must he seek a place in a society in which he has no growing faith? All is anxiety.

The fortunate adolescent will meet an adult who can listen and who faces both adolescent and adult problems squarely. Such an adult will have learned that love means knowing and being known by another person. Such an adult will help prepare the young person for the dignity of adult intimacy. But finding such an adult is not easy.

"Young men mend not their sight by using old men's spectacles; and yet we look upon Nature but with Aristotle's spectacles, and upon the body of man but with Galen's and upon the frame of the world with Ptolemie's spectacles."[28]

Where can a person find a person?

Thus did John Donne, almost three hundred and fifty years ago, criticize his contemporaries for over-reliance upon those who preceded them. His was an ancient concern and it is a modern one too. Today's young person has a problem in communication. He needs to talk to an older person who sees the past, but not through outworn spectacles.

As ever before, an overwhelming welter of rapid changes besets the modern student. And, as John Donne so clearly saw, yesterday's answers do not always fit today's questions. What is right? What is wrong? Tomorrow is unpredictable, uncontrollable, undependable. Why plan? All this and more must be talked over with somebody. Every place is a crowd. Where can a person find a person to talk to? At home? For some, home is too far away. For others, there is nobody home. Still others have no home. In the church? Too often one goes to church out of habit, not because one really wants to go. Teachers? Some teachers look like listeners. But there is a long line there too. The search for a willing adult ear often ends in forlorn failure.

The student turns to his peers. Some of them never ask questions. Within this group are a few moving in an aura of ineffable sadness, theatrical yet strangely mute, involved with nothing but the present tense of themselves. Others, despite a more open, cheerful façade, also ask no questions. They, too, are hard to reach. They, too, are involved with themselves. The members of still another campus group never stop asking questions. Impatient, espousing many causes (some worthy and long overdue for positive action), often as inept when their causes succeed as when they fail, these frequently gifted students have, at many colleges, become campus celebrities. Detracting from the permanence of their con-

[28] John Donne, "Sermon LXXX," in John Hayward, ed., *Complete Poetry and Selected Prose* (London, 1930), p. 672.

tribution is an inability to defer gratification and an insistence on living in the present. Too often they fritter their energies on causes that they have not profoundly examined, but that they know will provoke administrative authority. Deeply suspicious of the past, members of this group fail to hear the centuries-old advice of William Penn to keep their cool: "nothing does reason more right than the coolness of those who offer it. For truth often suffers more by the heat of its defenders than from the arguments of its opposers." [29]

It is to Penn's concept that the average student seems to turn. Never relinquishing his obligation to question or his right to be heard and to listen, he will continue to seek values. He will fall on his face, but only to get up and take a better look. University people are not too late in their efforts to meet student needs. But they need the help of the people. And the people today must hear and heed these words of Socrates: "Citizens of Athens, why is it that you turn and scrape every stone to gather wealth and neglect your children to whom, one day, you must relinquish it all?" If the citizens of Athens heard Socrates, they paid him no mind. Their institutions crumbled. Today's institutions are also shaken. Will they, too, be destroyed in the fires of dispute? Perhaps this next section will suggest some answers. It begins with an extraordinary staff meeting at a famous eastern hospital. [30]

They found a home in the army

That particular meeting would be long remembered. And looking back, it was apparent that even those with the deepest misgivings could not have foretold all that would happen. Present this time had been almost all of the staff of the adolescent ward of Jacobi Hospital in the Bronx. At best their job was never easy: to help some two dozen eight- to eighteen-year-olds with serious emotional problems. Some routine was often a welcome ally. Change was scrutinized. So the abandonment of nurses' and aides' uniforms in favor of street clothes could not have been a casual decision. Almost the whole meeting had been given over to the new proposal. A host of insecurities had surfaced: anxiety about losing status, job identification, lines of authority, controls over patients and one another. At last it had been agreed to try the no-uniform policy for three months.

At a second combined staff-patient meeting the young patients were told of the plan. Like the staff, the children were anxious. But their reasons were different. Impostors would come to care for them. Or nobody would. If the uniforms left, so would the nurses. One small boy, a possible runaway, reasoned worriedly. "The nurses will escape!" he cried. Carefully,

[29] William Penn, *Some Fruits of Solitude*, quoted in Clifton Fadiman, ed., *The American Treasury, 1455–1955* (New York, 1955), p. 691.

[30] The incident at the Adolescent and Latency In-Patient Service of Jacobi Hospital, Bronx, Municipal Hospital Center, New York City, is described in a paper by Donald J. Marcuse, "The 'Army' Incident: The Psychology of Uniforms and Their Abolition on an Adolescent Ward," *Psychiatry: A Journal for the Study of Interpersonal Processes*, Vol. 30 No. 4 (November 1967), pp. 350–75.

gently, the basic reason for the change was explained. The atmosphere would be more relaxed. New patients would perhaps feel more comfortable. Nobody made the mistake of saying that the change would make the hospital more like home. Finally, one adolescent wanted to know why. If street clothes were so much better than uniforms, if they made for such better feelings between everybody, why had the change been so long delayed? Nothing may terminate a coversation between an adult and a child so abruptly as a child's penetrating question. This was no exception. The meeting quickly ended.

As with most carefully planned insurrections there followed a seemingly uneventful period. It lasted six days. Then the adolescent army appeared. It was complete with insignia of rank proclaimed in Magic Marker on pajamas. All was military. An eleven-year-old girl was corps bugler. Around her neck was a carved wooden instrument. Four of the older boys were officers. As allies, they were no longer afraid of one another. There were privates, corporals, and WACs. The disturbed daughter of an army colonel, a pretty and flirtatious girl of sixteen, was the general of the children's army. Accustomed to command, she merely transferred her powers to the military. Armaments (wooden guns) had been manufactured in the occupational therapy shop. The army

> appeared to meet every patient's most acutely felt needs and to solve each one's currently most distressing problems. Depressions lifted. Rivalries waned. Aggression became so bound up in the organization that no one appeared frightened of his own or his fellows' impulses. Individual sexual conflicts were so ingeniously . . . incorporated into the matrix of military roles . . . that they went unnoticed . . . Never were the lines of authority clearer. Never had the dependent and infantile felt better cared for, or the fearful more protected, or the rejected more valued. No one was lonely. Everyone had a vital role and an unmistakable identity. No invading impostors were to be feared. Anyone who craved structure found all he could use. Ambiguities ceased. The vanished uniforms had been restored, as if to demonstrate their value and function to anyone who had not yet gotten the message . . . The only hitch was that this marvel of a device left out the staff.[31]

Nor did the staff accept this lightly.

> Despite its formidable accomplishments the insurgent army was greeted by the now ununiformed staff . . . with distinct displeasure, with dismay and consternation. It was a revolution. The tables were turned . . . Considering how little the army did that was actually disruptive, the near pandemonium that ensued among the staff bears testimony to the extent of their own emotional involvement.[32]

[31] *Ibid.,* p. 362.
[32] *Ibid.,* p. 364.

What had actually happened? To both the sick children and some of the staff members responsible for their care, a change in clothing that was emblematic of their institution, authority, codes, or values was threatening. To some extent, their anxiety depended on whether they saw themselves as the sort of people who control others or who accept controls. In varying degrees, all did both. Both staff and patients needed both. Impressed by reported successes of similar clothing changes elsewhere, the staff had agreed to try to adjust to the change. Too, they, unlike the children, clearly understood that loss of uniforms entailed no real loss of those stable elements in their lives that gave them security. Finally, the staff members were free to leave the ward. Their anxieties could be relieved. The sick children had had no such advantages. Poignantly, they too had sought to adjust. They had met the threat to themselves with a threat to others. A usual reaction. A not unusual result.

The children's army reflected in miniature a well-known human reaction. For whole nations do no less than did these emotionally sick youngsters. Whether the threat is real or imagined matters little. Temporarily, at least, martial law establishes authority, security, purpose, direction. But the formation of the children's army excluded the possibility of treatment and cure. It was the order of the desert, not of hope. This the sick children could not see. And it is this that today's mature young student sees only too well. He needs hope within order. Clearly, he understands that "the art of progress is to preserve order amid change and to preserve change amid order." [33]

But he also sees that, too often, nations are like sick children. Why? Why are nations armed camps? In a biology class he learns that even animals that are instinctively hostile to one another can learn to live peacefully together. In an English class he is told of Stephen Crane, the great war novelist who wrote that "the essence of life is war." Bewildered, searching, he turns to the writings of his father's time. In the lyric prose of Thomas Wolfe, one of the celebrated spokesmen of his parents' generation, he reads this:

> War is not death to young men; war is life. The earth had never worn raiment of such color as it did that year. The war seemed to unearth pockets of ore that had never been known in the nation: there was a vast unfolding and exposure of wealth and power. And somehow—this imperial wealth, this display of power in men and money, was blended into a lyrical music. In Eugene's mind, wealth and love and glory melted into a symphonic noise; the age of myth and miracle had come upon the world again. All things were possible.[34]

And later Wolfe continues:

[33] Alfred North Whitehead, quoted in *Saturday Review* (March 2, 1968), p. 19.
[34] Thomas Wolfe, *Look Homeward, Angel* (New York, 1929), pp. 508–09.

With a tender smile of love for his dear self, he saw himself wear-
ing the eagles of a colonel on his gallant young shoulders . . . For
the first time he saw the romantic charm of mutilation . . . He longed
for that subtle distinction, that air of having lived and suffered that
could only be attained by a wooden leg, a rebuilt nose, or the seared
scar of a bullet across his temple.[35]

The modern student, reading this, begins to reject the past. He feels
a part of a "new race" well described by Emerson a century ago: "There
is a universal resistance to ties and ligaments once supposed essential to
civilized society. The new race is stiff, heady, and rebellious; they are
fanatics in freedom; they hate tolls, taxes, turnpikes, banks, hierarchies,
governors, yea, almost laws."

So some students reject the past. All of it. To them, no past values fit
the present scene. And since the past is gone, there is no future. What
matters is the present. "The most striking change in student value systems
is in the direction of values which lead to immediate gratification."[36]

To treat the severely alienated student, the psychiatrist often must start
by interviewing the parents in the student's presence. One reason for this
is that "the family interview . . . reminds the student that he does have
a past and that the past continues to exert an important influence upon
his present life."[37] At the beginning of therapy such a patient is often
required to "commit himself to a six-month period of therapy. This emphasizes the existence of a future."[38]

Man need not be retarded by the past nor be worshipful of it. But he
does need to understand it. Then he might see, for example, the need for
both peace and national defense. The past helps to teach what is solid
earth and what is shifting sand. As Eiseley has written,

Man's story, in brief, is essentially that of a creature who has
abandoned instinct and replaced it with cultural tradition and the
hardwon increments of contemplative thought. The lessons of the
past have been found to be a reasonably secure instruction for pro-
ceeding against the unknown future. To hurl oneself recklessly,
without method, upon a future that we ourselves have complicated
is a sheer nihilistic rejection of all that history, including the classi-
cal world, can teach us.[39]

[35] *Ibid.,* p. 533.
[36] Seymour L. Halleck, "Why They'd Rather Do Their Own Thing," *Think,* Vol. 34, No. 5 (September–
October 1968), p. 3.

How strikingly similar are the emotional states of such college students to those of some small ghetto
children beginning school. One school superintendent writes: "A victim of his environment, the ghetto
child begins his school career psychologically, socially, and physically disadvantaged. He is oriented
to the present rather than the future, to immediate needs rather than delayed gratification, to the
concrete rather than the abstract." (Carl J. Dolce, "The Inner City—A Superintendent's View," *Saturday
Review* [January 11, 1969], p. 36.)
[37] Seymour L. Halleck, "Psychiatric Treatment of the Alienated College Student," *American Journal of
Psychiatry,* Vol. 125, No. 5 (November 1967), p. 103.
[38] *Ibid.,* p. 102.
[39] Loren Eiseley, *The Unexpected Universe,* quoted in "Activism and the Rejection of History," *Science,*
Vol. 165, No. 3889 (July 11, 1969), p. 129.

So one cannot disregard past institutions, codes, and values. It does not matter whether their symbol is a nurse's uniform, a wedding ring, or a sergeant's stripes. It does matter how a human need for order is met. Institutions, codes, and values need constant, careful reappraisal. Some need changing. Others need to be discarded and, to avoid chaos, replaced by other institutions, codes, and values. In itself, mere rejection of a value is not a value. And mankind cannot do without values.

This much, at least, the emotionally sick children at the Jacobi adolescent ward understood.

Turmoil in a community can arise only from the inner, emotional disorders of its members. The agony of an utter inner chaos, the seemingly total rejection of one's personal worth, provides the subject for the next discussion.

A cry for attention

Tom sulked in a corner and exalted his woes . . . he pictured himself brought home from the river, dead, with his curls all wet and his sore heart at rest. How she would throw herself upon him, and how her tears would fall like rain, and her lips pray God to give her back her boy, and she would never, never abuse him anymore! But he would lie there cold and white and make no sign—a poor little sufferer whose griefs were at an end. [40]

It is interesting to note that Tom Sawyer (Mark Twain's typical American boy) often envisions his own death. [41] The above passage reflects Tom's response to his Aunt Polly's misunderstanding of him. A short while later Tom reflects in this way about the girl he loves: "She would be sorry someday, maybe when it was too late. Ah, if he could only die *temporarily!*" [42] Later still, Tom, hidden under the bed, watches his aunt weep over his supposed death. In a spasm of self-pity, he even weeps with her. And, as this great story of American boyhood reaches its climax, Tom sees his own funeral services: "at last the whole company broke down . . . in a chorus of anguished sobs, the preacher himself giving way to his feelings and crying in the pulpit." [43]

All this in the gentle, happy summer of boyhood. Yet the novel is among the most beloved of all literature. Why? Because Tom Sawyer's emotions are universally understood. By dreaming of dying, perhaps even by his own hand, the child wreaks the sufferings of guilt on the more powerful. Thus, he avenges his helplessness. A Japanese used to accomplish this by committing hari-kari on the doorstep of his tormentor for all the

[40] Mark Twain, *The Adventures of Tom Sawyer,* (New York, 1950), pp. 23–24.
[41] It may be similarly significant that, as a boy, Mark Twain deliberately exposed himself to small pox "to get it over with." He almost perished from the disease.
[42] Mark Twain, *The Adventures of Tom Sawyer,* p. 69.
[43] *Ibid.,* p. 143.

neighbors to see. He differed in method (though not in basic reasons) from many a Western suicide today.

There are no simple reasons for suicide. Sociological, cultural, physical, psychological—these are among the factors involved. Suicide rates among college students, for example, are increasing. For some, adjustment to increased permissiveness combines with an intensely competitive atmosphere and a bewildering loss of individuality to contribute to severe emotional distress. A certain number (perhaps 10 percent) of all suicides are impulsive reactions by the mentally deranged. Other suicides act deliberately, after carefully weighing for themselves the pros and cons of living. A deep hurt or sense of shame precipitates others to suicide. Barbiturate-takers frequently hover on the edge of death and accidentally slip over to be listed as suicides. Though an estimated 20,000 people kill themselves in this country yearly, between 100,000 and 150,000 (again, this is estimated) try unsuccessfully to commit suicide. Why estimated? Because in this culture suicide is taboo and is underreported as a cause of death. First suicide attempts, although of critical importance in predicting the second (and often more successful) attempts, are rarely reported to health departments.

The most common suicide takes place on a Monday in the spring when a single or divorced elderly white male Protestant kills himself. In this country, the annual suicide rate among physicians is triple that of the whole population. Suicide is more frequent in urban than in rural areas, and suicide rates vary too from city to city; in San Francisco, for example, the rate is five times that of New York City. Today, of all cities, West Berlin has the worst suicide rate. Russian-created tensions are not necessarily the cause. Suicide rates in that city were high long before the Second World War. The twentieth century's highest overall suicide rates are in Austria and Switzerland.

Whether attempted or threatened, suicidal behavior is portentous. It urgently merits the professional assistance of a psychiatrist, psychologist, or social work specialist. Such attention may be lifesaving.

An attempt at suicide is a cry for help. In his play *Death of a Salesman*, Arthur Miller put meaningful words into the dialogue of Linda, the wife of the suicidal salesman. To her self-centered sons she speaks of their father:

> *Willy Loman never made a lot of money. His name was never in the paper. He's not the finest character that ever lived. But he's a human being, and a terrible thing is happening to him. So attention must be paid. He's not to be allowed to fall into his grave like an old dog. Attention, attention must be finally paid to such a person . . . A small man can be just as exhausted as a great man.*[44]

But, later, Willy commits suicide.

[44] Arthur Miller, *Death of a Salesman*, (New York, 1949), Act I.

In the great gulf, in the long years, between the normal vengeful dream-ings of Tom Sawyer, the boy, and the despairing agony of Willy Loman, the salesman, much happens. But again and again do people like these, who are as one in their loneliness, cry out for the attentions of help and love. If attention is not paid, an American childhood may become an American tragedy.

Human loneliness has many costs. In the next section still another of its prices is considered.

The loneliest ones

Sitting up straight in her chair, almost primly, a little defiant, tightly clasping ringless fingers, she tells the social worker her name. She is nineteen and came to town eight months ago. It has been five months since she has menstruated. She is not sure who the father is. And then, suddenly, she begins to cry.

"I don't care," she says, "I hate him anyway."

Scenes like this are twice as common in this country today as they were twenty years ago. Over three hundred thousand out-of-wedlock babies were born in the United States in 1969, over nine percent of the total number of births.

What do we know about the unwed mother? Who is she? What are some of her problems?

One anxiety of many an unwed mother is in her sense of being unloved. Yet often she cannot love. She may come from an over-coercive home. Perhaps her parents do not respect the person in the girl. Her individual speed and pattern of doing things are faults to be constantly corrected. She is directed and overdirected. Little do her parents realize the signifi-cance of this poetic advice:

> You may give them your love but not your thoughts,
> For they have their own thoughts.
> You may house their bodies but not their souls,
> For their souls dwell in the house of tomorrow, which
>   you cannot visit, not even in your dreams.
> You may strive to be like them,
>   but seek not to make them like you.[45]

Constant coercion causes anxiety in the child. It is met in various ways. The child may dilly-dally, daydream, and develop a fine "forgettory." Or the anxiety may be manifested by rebelliousness. Any parental advice then becomes a tyranny to be ignored. Moreover, the child feels unworthy. She may think everything she does is wrong. She feels rejected. She is thrown back on herself.[46] She loses the ability to give love to others. How

[45] Kahlil Gibran, *The Prophet* (New York, 1923), p. 18.
[46] Percival M. Symonds, *The Dynamics of Human Adjustment* (New York, 1946), p. 552.

can she again risk giving love when the people who mean the most to her, her parents, think her very existence a wrong? Out of rebellion, out of desire to retaliate, or in a desperate search for appreciation, she has sexual intercourse. But this arises from a feeling of rejection, not love.

Other girls are the victims of the opposite extreme. The parents are oversubmissive and overindulgent. No whim of the child is denied. The child is showered with unneeded gifts in such profusion that their meaning is lost. Such a girl is bored. She need consider nobody but herself. A severe anxiety about her health (hypochondriasis) may develop. As an attention-getting mechanism, it is useful. She may, moreover, fix all her expectations on the all-powerful, always sacrificing, parents. Her ability to love anyone else is diminished. Even the very thought of loving someone else may be threatening. She is without discipline, without the ability to love, for to love requires discipline. Passion requires compassion. Her doting parents have impoverished her with indulgence.

The disadvantages of the unwed mother are considerably more than emotional. Some are socioeconomic. Others are manifested by an increased risk to health, even to life.

Relatively few unwed mothers give birth in private hospitals. Over half of unmarried mothers get late or no prenatal care. Eighty percent of married women, on the other hand, receive prenatal care in the first six months of pregnancy. In the first three months of pregnancy, less than ten percent of unmarried mothers get prenatal care. But almost half of married mothers get this crucial early care in the first three months.

The poorer care of the unwed mother is apparent in the greater threat to the life of both herself and her child. Eclampsia (a toxic condition of pregnancy, once common) and syphilis are both more frequent in unmarried mothers than in married mothers. Unmarried-mother maternal death rates are over three times higher than those of married mothers. The life of the unmarried white mother is at tragic risk. Her pregnancy ends in her death eight times more often than the married white mother. Both black and Puerto Rican unmarried mothers have a better chance of surviving pregnancy than the white unmarried mother. [47]

The reasons for this are cultural. Black and Puerto Rican unmarried mothers are generally more accepted by their families. The white unmarried pregnant girl is cruelly cast out of her milieu. Often she cannot share her great burden with those who brought her into the world. She must skulk on the perimeter of society. Former friends shun her. By delaying prenatal care as long as possible, she risks her life. More often than the unmarried Puerto Rican and black mother, she submits to a dangerous, illegal abortion. And, much more often than they, she is killed by it.

Compared to the baby of the married mother, the baby of the unmarried mother is twice as likely to be premature, is twice as likely to die in the first month, and is twice as likely to be stillborn.

[47] National Council on Illegitimacy, *Illegitimacy: Data and Findings for Prevention, Treatment and Policy Formulation* (October 1965), pp. 34–36.

Maimed by emotional maldevelopment, more than a quarter of a million young girls of this wealthy country every year experience hazards that alienate them still further. They need help. Their help must start with the education of parents.

Moreover, too often only the plight of the unmarried mother has been considered. Whenever possible, the unmarried father should be helped. The popular idea of the elderly, uneducated, totally maladjusted seducer is not accurate. In one study, most unmarried fathers were found to have at least a high school education, were but a few years older than the mother, and functioned quite adequately in school or work. Delinquency patterns were not usual. Nor is the relationship between unmarried parents so casual as has often been assumed. On the other hand both young people may be suffering emotional inadequacies established in childhood. Deferment of personal gratification for the more lasting satisfactions of societal approval is difficult enough for the mature, let alone the immature. Thus "when neither sexual partner possesses any strong identity, and when neither one is strong in the area of responsibility and maturity, each reinforces the other to satisfy personal needs, with little regard for the consequences of the act."[48]

Love versus anxiety

"There is a land of the living and a land of the dead and the bridge is love, the only survival, the only meaning."[49]

Life begins and ends with separation. Both are inevitable. Each has its own poignancy.

There is separation at birth. Filling the gulf is love. Without mothering, without embracing love, the infant suffers. Yet, mothering is not smothering. True mother love teaches further separation. The constancy of a mother's love, even after her child's departure, is mirrored by the child's ability to learn to love others in later life.

As the normally learning child explores his body, he learns the glories of self-love. This self-love is not necessarily selfish. The child was born selfish. He will remain selfish only if he learns to hate himself. But if he learns self-worth, he will love this worthy self. And, by giving of a worthy self, he will be able wholeheartedly to enter into the long learning process of loving others. He must, for example, learn to love his neighbor. Were he born with the ability, he would not have had to be commanded.

But how may the child learn to hate himself? He can be taught that he is evil. He can be told a thousand times that he is naughty, that he is bad, that he should be ashamed of himself. A devaluated child deval-

[48]Reuben Pannor, Fred Massarik, and Byron W. Evans, *The Unmarried Father,* Final Report, Children's Bureau, Welfare Administration, U.S. Department of Health, Education, and Welfare (February 1967), pp. 230–31.
[49]Thornton Wilder, *The Bridge of San Luis Rey* (New York, 1927), p. 235.

uates himself still further. And such a child has been cruelly robbed of life's paramount need—the need to give a worthy love. When it is necessary, a child should be corrected, even punished, briefly and to the point, but never heartlessly. He must never feel unloved.

Love is not lust. Love gives. Lust takes. True, both find expression through coitus. Yet, coitus satiates lust, but continues love. With neither animals nor man is love a prerequisite for coitus. However, the profound need of love is characteristic only of man. Sexual desire may result from loneliness, vanity, a desire to conquer or be conquered, a need for social status, a desire to hurt or destroy someone. Any strong emotion (of which love is but one) can stimulate sexual desire.[50] After that desire is satiated, the individual may experience physiological relief. But the deeply significant mutuality, the need to do for another without direct reward, so characteristic of human love, has evaded him. He has given the least of himself. He has not given tenderness nor given up greed. He remains separate, alone.

In Chapter 15 there is some discussion of the techniques of sexual intercourse. These are important. However, the techniques of sexual intercourse do not replace the art of loving. Both may be learned. But, as food without love leaves the infant emotionally starved, so does sex without love leave the adult still hungering. Only love can solve the anxiety of separation.

Entering adolescence with self-esteem unshaken, convinced of a wholesome personal value, the young person can further develop the vital enrichments of his humanness. Since he has self-respect, he respects. For a few years, a "best friend" occupies the interest, then members of the opposite sex. In these years, slowly, now clearly, then beclouded, but ever recurring, there comes to the youth a new perception. Love is the art of giving. When he has learned to give, the young person is ready for adulthood. Prepared to exchange separation for union, he seeks a mate.

[50] Erich Fromm, *The Art of Loving* (New York, 1951), p. 54.

12

Drug dependence: escape into captivity

CLEOPATRA. . . . *Give me to drink mandragora.*
CHARMIAN. *Why, madam?*
CLEOPATRA. *That I might sleep out this great gap of time*
My Antony is away.[1]

Mandragora, or mandrake, may have lent rest to the Egyptian queen; the plant contains sedative properties. Another plant, the deadly nightshade, produces altogether different effects. A few years ago a Riverside, California, professor brewed some and took a large dose of it. His wife became so alarmed by his droll behavior that she called the family physi-

[1] William Shakespeare, *Antony and Cleopatra*, I.v.4–6.

384

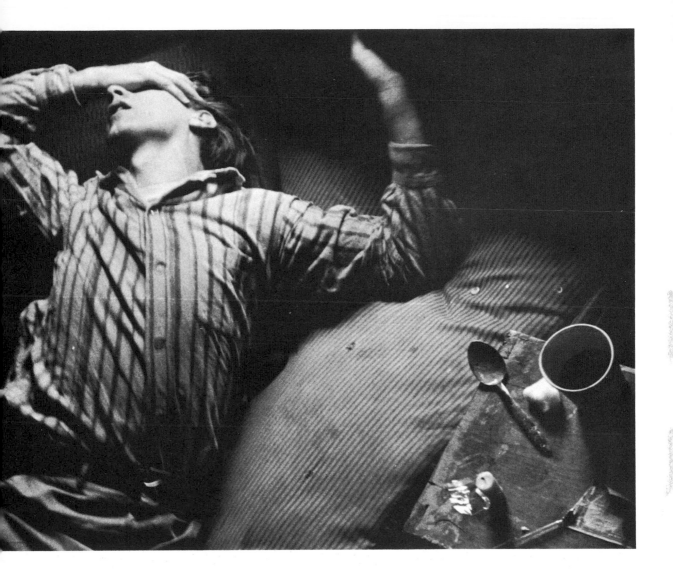

cian. In a nearby hospital, a barred-window cell was found for the befuddled pundit. There he was tied hand and foot, spread-eagle, to the bedposts. From this vantage point he could clearly watch the goings-on in his tiny cell. Part of his published report reads as follows:

> Most rooms usually have shuttered air vents situated either near the ceiling or floor. The vent in my cell was located just above the door. To my amazement it began to fill up like a small football stadium with tiered rows of my former students. They were wearing brightly colored berets and horn rimmed colored glasses. Each had a bottle of coke and a bag of popcorn. They single filed into the bleachers, finally filling it to capacity. Now they sat very rigid

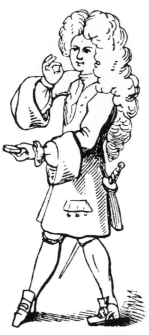

12-1 A snuff-taker.

without appearing to notice my presence. However, when I turned my head as if to look at some other area of the room the scene suddenly became highly animated. As they guzzled their cokes and stuffed popcorn into their mouths they pointed their fingers at me and laughed sardonically. Whenever I focused my eyes on their antics, they suddenly froze and took no notice of me. It is of interest to note that I recognized every face in the group and that I had given each and every one of them the D or F grade in beginning Biology.[2]

"My beloved sweet darling," Sigmund Freud wrote to Martha Bernays almost eighty years ago,

my tiredness is a sort of minor illness; neurasthenia it is called . . . I must aim at being with you . . . for a long time . . . the bit of cocaine I have just taken is making me talkative . . . Here I am making silly confessions to you, my sweet darling, and really without reason unless it is the cocaine.[3]

Mrs. Margaret Thompson took snuff, as did other London ladies of her day. She died on April 2, 1776, but she left a will that has caused her to be long remembered:

I, Margaret Thompson, . . . being in sane mind . . . desire that all my handkerchiefs that I may have unwashed at the time of my decease . . . be put . . . at the bottom of my coffin, which I desire may be large enough for that purpose, together with a quantity of the best Scotch snuff . . . as will cover my deceased body.

According to the will, her bearers were to be the six greatest snuff-takers of the parish of St. James, Westminster. Snuff-colored, not black, hats were to be worn. As they went along, six maidens bearing her pall were to take snuff for refreshment. Her servant was "to walk before the corpse, to distribute . . . snuff to the ground and upon the crowd."[4]

She was not the only one to desire interment with her vice. Some years ago in Camembert, France, a man obeyed his wife. He preserved her in the town's best Calvados brandy cider and so buried her. In her memory, he composed this touching rhyme:

> Here lies my wife. Her dying wish:
> "I think it would be dandy
> To be preserved, when comes the end,
> Like a ripe plum in brandy."[5]

[2]Cecil E. Johnson, "Mystical Force of Nightshade," *International Journal of Neuropsychiatry*, Vol. 3, No. 3 (May–June 1967), p. 274.

[3]Ernest L. Freud, ed., *Letters of Sigmund Freud*, Letter No. 94 (New York, 1960), pp. 201–02. This letter was written from Paris on February 2, 1886. Freud married Martha Bernays in 1884. He died in 1939 at eighty-three. Martha Freud died in 1951 in her ninetieth year.

[4]H. V. Morton, *Ghosts of London* (New York, 1940), pp. 33–34.

[5]Lucia Masson, *La Belle France* (New York, 1964), p. 23.

What is buried in some graves is surprising. What is inscribed on some of the stones marking them is no less startling. Consider this memorial found in a churchyard at Burlington, Massachusetts:

> *Here lies the body of Susan Lowder*
> *Who burst while drinking a*
> *Sedlitz Powder.*
> *Called from this world*
> *to her heavenly rest,*
> *She should have waited till it*
> *effervesced. 1798*[6]

Cleopatra took her drug to ease the pain of separation. The California professor perhaps took his to publish (though he almost perished instead). Freud took cocaine because it stimulated him—maybe to write better love letters. Mrs. Thompson snuffed for sheer pleasure. The French lady willingly left these earthly premises stewing in brandy cider. And poor Susan Lowder probably never revealed why she took a powder.

People have found a variety of purposes for a variety of drugs and have developed profound attachments to some of them. In considering these attachments, the substances producing dependence will be discussed; however, as much interest will be given to those who abuse drugs. Recent years have seen a remarkable increase in the abuse of some drugs in this country. The welter of opinion evaluating this phenomenon has not always been scientifically based. Considerable reliable effort is now being made to rectify this. In appraising the available information, it is well to remember that the effects of a drug may vary from individual to individual, and from time to time with the same individual. (This is particularly true when there is a change in dosage or social setting.)

Terms and classification

"The terms 'habituation' and 'addiction' plagued scientists for years and ultimately came to have a distorted sociological rather than scientific import . . . Fortunately, better perspective has been brought to this complex field by the abandonment of the terms habituation and addiction as having meaningful scientific value."[7] In 1964, the World Health Organization Expert Committee on Addiction-Producing Drugs recommended substitution of the term *drug dependence* for both drug addiction and drug habituation. Agreement in this country was promptly obtained from the Committee on Drug Addiction and Narcotics of the National Academy

---

[6] Ann Parker and Aaron Neal, "What a Way To Go!" *Ciba Journal,* No. 39 (1966), pp. 20–29.
[7] Nathan B. Eddy *et al.,* "Drug Dependence: Its Significance and Characteristics," *Bulletin of the World Health Organization,* Vol. 32, No. 5 (May 1965), p. 721–33.

TABLE 12-1 Some Characteristics of Certain Types of Drugs That Induce Dependence

TYPE OF DRUG DEPENDENCE*	BASIC ACTION	PSYCHOLOGICAL (PSYCHIC) DEPENDENCE	PHYSICAL DEPENDENCE	WITHDRAWAL SYMPTOMS (ABSTINENCE SYNDROME)	DEVELOPMENT OF TOLERANCE
Morphine and morphinelike drugs	Depressant	Yes, strong	Yes, develops early	Severe, but rarely life-threatening	Yes
Barbiturate-alcohol	Depressant	Yes	Yes	Severe, even life-threatening	Yes, but only partial for alcohol
Cocaine	Stimulant	Yes, strong	No	None	No
Cannabis (marihuana)	Stimulant	Yes, moderate to strong	No	None	No
Amphetamine	Stimulant	Yes, variable	No	None	Yes, slowly
Hallucinogen (LSD)	Stimulant	Yes	No	None	Yes, rapid

*Khat is not included here because the chewing of its leaves (producing an amphetaminelike drug effect) is not a problem in this country. Despite a renewed effort to reintroduce cocaine into the United States, its use in this country remains extremely limited.

of Sciences–National Research Council. "Drug dependence is a state of psychic or physical dependence, or both, on a drug, arising in a person following administration of that drug on a periodic or continuous basis."[8] A variety of chemical substances affect man's central nervous system to cause only a psychological (psychic) dependence. However, other drugs also provoke a physical dependence. This latter type of dependence becomes manifested by withdrawal symptoms (the *abstinence syndrome*) when the effects of the drug are interrupted. So a physically dependent drug abuser undergoes withdrawal symptoms when he can no longer obtain the drug, or when he is given another drug that nullifies the effects of the one on which he is dependent. If he has had experience with the more severe evidences of the abstinence syndrome, the drug abuser has reason to fear it. A delirium occurs, which is usually characterized by hearing strange voices and seeing alarming things that are nonexistent (*hallucinations*) as well as by unreasoning, false beliefs (*delusions*). These, combined with body-shaking tremors and other discomforts, cause the individual to suffer intensely. Some investigators suggest that abstinence-syndrome–producing drugs, such as alcohol, the barbiturates, and the opium derivatives, interfere with the "dream-sleep" that is characteristic

[8] *Ibid.*, p. 722.

of the last third of the night and that is associated with rapid eye movements (REMs). Abrupt withdrawal of such drugs, they theorize, results in a sudden, overwhelmingly chaotic resurgence of the dream sleep, which precipitates the delirium of the abstinence syndrome. Many drugs that produce dependence, both psychic and physical, also produce *tolerance;* that is, the drug abuser finds that he must use increasingly larger doses of the drug to achieve the effect obtained with the initial dose. As will be seen below, tolerance to a drug may become so great that doses that would ordinarily be lethal are used without killing the drug abuser. Tolerance to one drug can result in tolerance to a similar one, as in the case of heroin and morphine.

The World Health Organization Expert Committee has described seven different types of drug dependence according to the patterns of their action and the responses they bring about.[9] These are:

1. morphine type
2. barbiturate-alcohol type
3. cocaine type
4. cannabis (marihuana) type
5. amphetamine type
6. khat type
7. hallucinogen (LSD) type

Table 12-1 indicates some of the basic criteria by which part of this classification was made.

Depressants

THE JUNKIES

*When they are
in the street
they pass it
along to each
other but when
they see the
police they would
just stand still
and be beat
so pity ful
that they want
to cry.*

Marie Ford, 12 years old[10]

The morphine type of drug dependence: the opiates

me pharmacologists consider marihuana a depressant, not a stimulant.
, 36 *Children* (New York, 1967), p. 147.

Some historical notes

Greek mythology tells that in the underground kingdom of the dead, ruled by Hades, runs the river Lethe. A drink of its waters produced oblivion. Thus, long ago, the Roman poet Vergil wrote of "poppies steeped in Lethe's slumber" (*Georgicus*, I.78).

Twenty centuries before Vergil, Egyptian mothers used poppy juice to bring slumber to their fretful children. Much later the Chinese used opium dependingly. Not until Ch'ung Ch'en outlawed tobacco smoking in 1641 did they savor the poppy, Centuries before, Chaucer had mentioned "nercotikes[11] and opie" (*The Knight's Tale*, line 1472), and Shakespeare's Othello refers to the poppy and "all the drowsy syrups of the world" (III.iii.331–32). In *Samson Agonistes* (lines 629–30) John Milton, too, wrote of "death's benumbing Opium." Centuries later, in Eugene O'Neill's play *Long Day's Journey into Night*, the tragic Mary refers to symbolic clouds, but means opium, when she says, "It hides you from the world and the world from you . . . No one can find or touch you any more." So, throughout the ages, writers have woven the poppy into their plots. It is a good device. For mankind, the flower has powerful and exotic meanings.

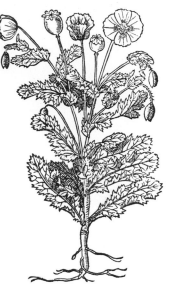

12-2 The delicate opium poppy.

The sleep-producing poppy, *Papaver somniferum* (see Figure 12-2) flowers in beguiling white, red, and purple. A century ago, John Ruskin rhapsodized its beauty as "the most transparent and delicate of all the blossoms of the field . . . the poppy is painted glass . . . always, it is a flame, and warms the wind like a blown ruby."[12]

The poppy's milky juice oozes, not from its delicate petals, however, but from the cut pods. For centuries, its use has released man. Its abuse has imprisoned him. Most of the world's opium is grown in Turkey, Burma, India, Persia, China, Laos, Thailand, and Mexico. Legal opium is auctioned "in such ports as Istanbul and Calcutta by quotas submitted via the Commission on Narcotic Drugs in Geneva and filed with the United Nations Economic and Social Council (handled in the U.S.A. under the Internal Revenue Code)."[13]

The drugs

The risk of dependence on *morphine*, the principal active component of opium, is great, as are its pain-killing properties. Heating morphine with acetic acid (acetylation) synthetically produces the more potent *heroin*. Unlike Britain, the United States has outlawed heroin. Other synthetic opium derivatives are *dilaudid, demerol*, and *methadone*. Because its withdrawal symptoms, described below, are relatively mild, methadone

---

[11] In the broadest meaning, however, any agent producing insensibility or stupor is a narcotic. Medically, in the U.S., the term narcotic is today usually limited to opium, morphine, and heroin. Since morphine is derived from opium, these two terms will be used interchangeably in this section.

[12] John Ruskin, "Love's Meinie" and "Proserpina," in E. T. Cook and Alexander Wedderburn, eds., *The Works of John Ruskin*, Vol. XXV (London, 1906), p. 258.

[13] W. Z. Guggenheim, "Heroin: History and Pharmacology," *International Journal of the Addictions*, Vol. 2, No. 2 (Fall 1967), p. 329.

is used in the withdrawal treatment of chronic opium users. *Codeine,* a derivative of morphine, is commonly used in cough medicines. Many drug abusers start with this substance. *Nalline,* an antagonist of opium, does not produce a euphoria. Injection of nalline will dilate the constricted pupils of the chronic heroin user and will also start withdrawal symptoms within half an hour. The careful use of nalline is helpful in diagnosing heroin dependence.

The action

Opiates are depressants. "The depressant actions include analgesia (relief of pain), sedation (freedom from anxiety, muscular relaxation, decreased motor activity), hypnosis (drowsiness and lethargy), and euphoria (a sense of well-being and contentment)."[14] The chronic opium user, moreover, loses interest in sex. He also becomes severely constipated.

The alchemy of opium chains man in two ways. The first way is by the development of a physical dependence. This can be initiated by repeated small doses of the drug. If he is without the drug for about twelve hours, the dependent opium user gets sick (the withdrawal or abstinence syndrome). The second chain is forged by the body's ability to adapt to the drug (tolerance). Because of tolerance, increasing quantities of drug are required to produce the same effects and to avoid the intense discomforts of withdrawal. Eventually, to experience the original euphoria, the abuser may take doses that ordinarily would be lethal. And, with this increased dosage, the degree of both the dependence on and the tolerance to the drug also increases. This distinguishing characteristic of morphine and morphine-like drugs is the trap of the abuser.

During drug withdrawal the nose runs and the eyes water. The pulse and blood pressure shoot up. Muscles twitch, and vomiting may be uncontrollable. And surrounding the patient is the smell of his vomitus. Restless, sleepless, he hurts everywhere. Worst of all, he has a consuming craving for the drug. Unless he is very old or very ill from other disease, the person undergoing withdrawal will suffer intensely but will not die. Within about twenty-four to forty-eight hours, the abstinence syndrome reaches its peak. Then it spontaneously subsides. Gradually, the physical dependence on the drug abates. But the psychic dependence lingers on for a long time. It may persist for the rest of the individual's life.

Opium dependency can kill. Babies born of opium-dependent mothers may also be dependent on the drug. Unless diagnosed and treated promptly, they perish.[15] An opium abuser thought by the pusher to be a police informant may be deliberately provided with a lethal overdose. How many opium deaths are murders is not known. In the fifteen years

---

[14] David P. Ausubel, *Drug Addiction* (New York, 1958), p. 18.
[15] Jane S. Lin-Fu, *Neonatal Narcotic Addiction,* Children's Bureau, U.S. Department of Health, Education, and Welfare (1967), pp. 1–11.

between 1950 and 1964, the number of opium deaths in New York City rose markedly. Almost half (48 percent) were labeled "acute reaction to dosage or overdosage."

In New York City heroin dependency is the leading cause of death between the ages of fifteen and thirty-five; in 1968 over four hundred heroin-dependent persons died in Manhattan alone. Suicides and homicides are comparatively high among these individuals. So are infections such as serum hepatitis, carried by unclean needles, and tetanus.[16] Moreover, recent research indicates that the severe liver damage seen in heroin-dependent people is due not only to the viral infection of serum hepatitis (see page 194) but also to the toxic damage resulting from long-term drug use.

The people

In December 1964, the Federal Bureau of Narcotics reported 55,899 chronic opium users. Of these, over half were blacks, about 12 percent were Puerto Ricans, and 15 percent were Mexican-Americans. Over 20 percent were "other whites." Among the socioeconomically disadvantaged groups, an increased incidence was apparent. Males predominated by about five to one. Under the age of twenty-one, a shift occurred: almost half (47.6 percent) were white and only 26.6 percent were black. Most opium abusers are between twenty and thirty-five. The trend is to younger users. About 50 percent are unemployed.[17] In 1970, estimates indicated increased heroin abuse (over 100,000) spreading to all socioeconomic levels. The rate of physicians and nurses who become dependent is estimated to be a hundred times that of the general population. Nurses and doctors usually abuse demerol.[18] However, in this country, 90 percent of those who abuse opiates are dependent on heroin.

Where do opium abusers live? In 1962, it was in the large slum areas of the large cities of New York (46.4 percent), California (15.6 percent), Illinois (14.8 percent), and Michigan (3.8 percent). In that year the highest rate of opium dependence (130 per 100,000 population) was in New York City. Washington, D.C., was a close second with a rate of 101.8.[19]

Most people who are dependent on opiates need to commit crimes. It is only through stealing, prostitution, and "pushing" narcotics that they obtain sufficient funds for their drug. Many drug abusers, beset by increasing tolerance, develop a prohibitively expensive problem. Their drug may cost as much as $125 daily. Often, to control this expense, they voluntarily commit themselves, undergo withdrawal, and then promptly return to lesser doses. Every year, in the United States, about 7,000 more people

[16]Michael M. Baden, "Of Drugs and Urine," *Medical Tribune and Medical News,* Vol. 10, No. 84 (October 20, 1969), p. 15.
[17]Jordan Scherer, "Patterns and Profiles of Addiction and Drug Abuse," *International Journal of Addictions,* Vol. 2, No. 2 (Fall 1967), p. 75.
[18]Solomon Garb, "Narcotic Addiction in Nurses and Doctors," *Nursing Outlook* Vol. 13, No. 11 (November 1965), p. 30.
[19]D. M. Wilner and G. G. Kassebaum, eds., *Narcotics* (New York, 1965), pp. 4–55, 85–286.

become dependent on opium. Most do not get their first drug from a "pusher." The quickest way to become a drug abuser is to know one.

Why do some people take these drugs? Few (perhaps 5 percent) become dependent as a result of being medically treated with opiates. Some will begin drug abuse to be an accepted member of the group. Basically, drug abuse is due to psychiatric illness. But grinding poverty also plays a part. Deeply felt insecurities and inadequacies combine with sordid socio-economic deprivation to produce the average opium abuser. The word "narcotic" is derived from the Greek *narkotikos,* meaning benumbing. Emotional numbness is what the drug abuser seeks. Uninvolvement is his goal. Life's problems are not encountered. The drug answers all. Hovering on the border of withdrawn sleep, he is easily awakened. This he calls "being on the nod." For the abuser of opium, however, there is one reality. Somehow, more drug must be gotten. The irony of his situation is complete. He takes the drug to escape. Yet he lives in a constant pressure cooker.

The treatment

The dependent opium user may be treated in several ways: "Cold turkey" refers to the abrupt withdrawal of the drug. As it is a cruel experience, few physicians approve it. Abrupt withdrawal with some supportive therapy is a second method. Withdrawal symptoms are curtailed by the use of other drugs or by electroshock therapy. Still a third method, approved by most physicians in this country as the most humane, is gradual withdrawal with supportive therapy. For a few days the patient may be kept on minimal doses of morphine. Then, for about a week, methadone is substituted. After being given in gradually reduced doses, it is discontinued. Withdrawal must be carried out under hospital conditions. Therapy in a group of peers with similar problems is helpful.

The treatment program at the Rockefeller University Hospital in New York slowly substitutes methadone for heroin. The patient is indefinitely maintained on methadone. A maintenance dose of the drug is taken orally once a day. This eliminates the infecting three to four daily injections with a narcotic needle. Moreover, methadone has a uniform action. Unlike other morphine-like drugs, it induces no high. Thus a reinforcing factor to take heroin is blocked. It then becomes possible to put the mind to constructive use. The tendency to prey on society is diminished. As of January 1, 1968, of the 750 patients who had been accepted into the program (about half were rejected), 282 had remained on it for at least one year. One-third were steadily employed; a second one-third worked intermittently or were students.[20] This treatment is spreading. A more recent study at the New York Correctional Institute for Men appears to confirm that methadone has a "blocking" effect, thus preventing heroin dependence. A constructive rehabilitation program using methadone reduced

[20]Donald B. Louria, *The Drug Scene* (New York, 1968), pp. 179–80.

antisocial behavior. It should be clearly understood, however, that such patients are dependent on methadone. The program is being continuously evaluated.[21] Cyclazocine,[22] an experimental narcotic antagonist, also offers promise, as does a compound with the formidable name of dl-alpha-acetyl-methadone.[23]

It is easier to get a willing patient off drugs than to keep him off. Except for physician-patients, relapse rates are as high as 90 percent. That less than 10 percent of physicians return to drugs indicates the importance of having some life interest apart from drugs—of having "something to go back to."

Federal narcotic treatment centers in this country include the Public Health Service hospitals at Lexington, Kentucky, and Fort Worth, Texas. Despite active therapy, designed to help the patient deal with conflicts between his ego and environment, the follow-up studies of released patients show a disappointingly high rate of return to drug dependence. California also maintains an advanced treatment program. The California State Rehabilitation Center program involves compulsory civil commitment, detoxication, diagnostic study, and transfer to a rehabilitation center for mandatory treatment periods lasting from six to fourteen months. Halfway houses, for those not quite ready for societal onslaughts, are provided.[24]

The prevention of this type of drug dependence can be promoted by intensive social programs aimed at improving the wretched environment that spawns emotional problems. As has been seen, character disorders underlie compulsive drug abuse. These are poorly understood and more research is surely indicated. However, even better knowledge will be to no avail unless the environment of the vulnerable individual is improved.

Some experts laud the British approach to morphine or morphine-like drug dependence. There the physician may legally provide the patient with drugs. Ostensibly, the profit motive is removed. The English narcotic problem is hardly solved, however. In fact, it is presently growing. The tolerance of the drug-dependent individual increases. The profit motive has not entirely disappeared. Some registered drug patients demand more of a drug only to sell it. Some (by no means all) experts in this country feel that policing and penalties were the critical factors in reducing the number of chronic drug abusers from 200,000 to 60,000 between the two world wars.

---

[21] "Methadone Looks Good," *Science News,* Vol. 96, No. 1 (July 5, 1969), p. 2.

[22] Alfred Freedman et al., "Cyclazocine and Methadone in Narcotic Addiction," *Journal of the American Medical Association,* Vol. 202, No. 3 (October 16, 1967), p. 119.

[23] "Methadone Replacement on the Way?" *Journal of the American Medical Association,* Vol. 209, No. 11 (September 15, 1969), p. 1617.

[24] It was in Santa Monica, California, that Synanon, a private foundation, was founded. Today, for some abusers, it offers a haven and a hope. Not all applicants are admitted. Not every resident can obey its rigid rules. It affords harsh reality for a harsh sickness. Synanon has survived because other methods have not. It deserves careful professional evaluation. The two facilities of Daytop Lodge and Village are in Staten Island, New York, and in Sullivan County, New York. Here again, the rules are strict and the program rigid. Narcotics Anonymous and Teen Challenge also work voluntarily to help the individual with a drug problem, as does Exodus House.

Unlike the abstinence syndrome induced by withdrawal of morphine and morphine-like drugs, the abstinence syndrome following discontinuance of both barbiturates and alcohol depends on a prior prolonged and continuous ingestion of relatively high doses. In addition, the signs and symptoms resulting from the prolonged excessive use of alcohol and barbiturates are similar. So are the signs and symptoms ensuing from the withdrawal of either drug. Also, barbiturates will suppress the withdrawal symptoms of the alcoholic and, to some extent, alcohol will suppress withdrawal symptoms for the chronic barbiturate abuser. These are among the reasons for the grouping of these drug dependencies into one type. However, because of psychological and social differences among those who use them, they will be discussed separately in this section.

Sedatives: barbiturates and barbiturate-like drugs

Since they allay excitement, barbiturates are sedatives. Among these are the short-acting *Seconal* and *Nembutal* and the longer-acting *phenobarbital*. Recently, a host of nonbarbiturate sedatives have been developed; two of the better known are *Doriden* and *Dormison*. Tranquilizers, such as *Equanil* and *Miltown* (trade names for the same drug), and *Librium* also have a barbiturate-like action. There is no question that these drugs, and the many others like them, have great medical value. They are generally used to control signs and symptoms resulting from psychic, circulatory, respiratory and gastrointestinal distress. However, all barbiturates and barbiturate-like drugs can be abused. They should never be used without the advice of the family physician. As with all other drugs, constant informational material comes to the physician about both their uses and dangers. He is particularly concerned with the patient who will attempt to conceal a dependence because of shame or the desire to obtain still another prescription. Some patients in large cities go from physician to physician seeking a prescription for the drug upon which they have become dependent. Of all the sedatives, the barbiturates are the most abused.

Every year barbiturates kill more people (over 3,500) in this country than any other drug; many die as suicides. As with the opium derivatives, prolonged and excessive use causes not only profound psychological and physical dependence but also tolerance. The true barbiturate abuser may daily pop between ten and twenty pills or capsules into his mouth. They are not hard to get. Counting refills, about 175 million prescriptions for sedatives and stimulants are filled every year in the nation's drug stores. To this must be added the millions of doses illegally supplied.

Acute barbiturate poisoning may, at first, make an individual seem sociable. This is due to the alcohol-like effect on inhibitions. As has been pointed out, barbiturate and alcohol intoxication are similar. Soon moodiness and depression replace the cheerfulness. The barbiturate abuser slurs his speech, staggers. He seems to suffer an inner agony. Finally, he may sink into a coma. Without attention, he may not waken.

But this is not the only way to die from barbiturates. To avoid a sleepless night, a barbiturate abuser may take one or two pills at bedtime. Within an hour or two, he wakens, his mind a cloud of cotton. Two more pills. Again, he sleeps. A deeply disturbed person may repeatedly waken, each time more confused, each time swallowing more barbiturates. The lethal dose is not much larger than the therapeutic dose. This individual, too, may not awaken. Should he have ingested alcohol before bedtime, he is indeed at grave risk. Both alcohol and barbiturates are depressants. One enhances the action of the other. Together, their effect may be disastrous. People have been found dead with an amount of barbiturate and alcohol in the blood that, if either had been taken without the other, would not have been fatal.

Withdrawal from barbiturates may be hazardous. Symptoms begin within twenty-four hours after the last drug dose. Soon, anxiety, headache, and vomiting give way to grave threats to life. Both delirium and psychoses occur often. A patient undergoing withdrawal may require as long as six weeks or more of scrupulous care. Psychotherapy to examine the cause of the dependence is essential.

Alcohol

"How sweet is everything that is moderate . . . For Mnesitheos says that one should always avoid excesses in everything."[25]

CULTURAL CONCEPTS   The primitive Cocomas Indians of the Amazon Valley grind the bones of their dead to a fine powder that they then gulp down with their beer.[26] Sometimes Jivaro Indians dip enemy shrunken heads in beer before tasting the brew.[27] And so devoted are the primitive Dusun to potent drink that writers have reported entire village populations, including children, quite drunk.[28] Among the primitives, every important event, from birth to marriage to death, was and is celebrated with alcohol.

Where did the word "alcohol" begin? The Arabic *al kohl* originally referred to a fine antimony powder used for staining the eyes. From it was derived the word *alcohol*. Whether this is the origin of the toast "here's mud in your eye" is unknown.

Nor is it known when alcohol was first made. Stone age beer jugs, ten to fifteen thousand years old, have been discovered. Forty centuries ago, the Babylonian Code of Hammurabi provided careful regulations for the sale of beer. In about 1500 B.C., an ancient Egyptian book of etiquette warned: "Make not thyself helpless in drinking in the beer shop . . . Falling

---

[25] Athenaeus (419 B.C.), quoted in Sterling Dow, "Two Families of Athenian Physicians," *Bulletin of the History of Medicine*, Vol. 7, No. 1 (June 1942), p. 18.

[26] Ernest Crawley, *Dress, Drinks, and Drums* (London, 1931), p. 219.

[27] William Curtis Farabee, *Indian Tribes of Eastern Peru, Papers of the Peabody Museum of American Archaeology and Ethnology*, cited in Chandler Washburne, *Primitive Drinking* (New York, 1961), p. 105.

[28] Owen Rutter, *British North Borneo*, cited in Chandler Washburne, *Primitive Drinking*, p. 250.

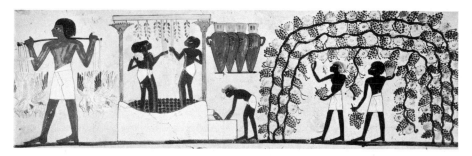

down thy limbs will be broken, and no one will give thee a hand to help thee up, as for thy companions . . . they will say, 'Outside with this drunkard.'"[29] Nor was it without reason that Plato had an Athenian reflect: "Then not only an old man but also a drunkard becomes a second time a child?" Alcohol seems to have been a problem even at ancient Greek athletic events. The Greek stadium at Delphi still has a sign, *circa* 5 B.C., forbidding wine in the stadium. Violators were to be fined five drachmas. Today, the Southern Methodist University stadium boasts a comparable prohibiting sign.[30] One of Harvard College's first projects was a brewery.[31] Nevertheless, a similar regulation now forbids drinking in the Harvard University stadium.[32]

Nor is the Bible short of references to alcohol. As soon as he left the ark, Noah built an altar (Genesis 8:20). But then he planted a vineyard and got drunk (Genesis 9:20, 21). That his inebriety led to poor behavior and a bad example for his sons is, however, made abundantly clear. Use of alcohol was permitted among the Jews—wine "cheereth God and man" (Judges 9:13)—and was even part of religious life. But to be intoxicated was considered an abomination; self-control was the rigid rule. This age-old approach is reflected even today in the drinking habits of Jews.

The early Romans were also abstemious. Nevertheless, the later progressive societal decay, during and following the years of the Punic Wars, saw drunkenness rampantly accompany promiscuity. Both Roman debauchery and Hebrew restraint profoundly influenced the early Christians (see page 470). Those desiring to be known as followers of Christ were instructed, "be not drunk with wine" (Ephesians 5:18). However, the use of wine was not completely forbidden, as Paul's advice to Timothy makes clear: "but use a little wine for thy stomach's sake and thine often infirmities" (I Timothy 5:23). Today, to the Catholic, temperance is an important religious virtue. Although neither Luther nor Calvin was an absolute teetotaler, modern Protestant churches tend strongly to support abstinence.

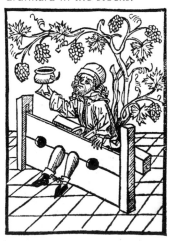

12-4 A 15th-century drunkard in the stocks.

[29] Sir E. A. Wallis Budge, "The Dwellers on the Nile," cited in "Alcoholism as a Disease," *World Health* (January 1966), p. 21.
[30] Arthur P. McKinlay, "Non-Attic Greek States," in Raymond G. McCarthy, ed., *Drinking and Intoxication* (Glencoe, Ill., 1959), p. 51.
[31] J. C. Furnas, *The Life and Times of the Late Demon Rum* (New York, 1965), p. 20.
[32] Arthur P. McKinlay, "Non-Attic Greek States," p. 51.

DEPRESSANTS   **397**

Primitive people drank partly to relieve anxiety. Added to relief from tension were pleasures of the senses, such as taste and smell. Enveloping the pleasant package were companionship and religious meanings. The ancient civilized peoples doubtless had some reasons for drinking that were similar to those of the primitives. But a remark of Sholem Asch might be considered to have a universal application to drinking: "Not the power to remember, but its very opposite, the power to forget, is a necessary condition of our existence."[33] A Guatemalan Indian expressed this even more succinctly: "A man must sometimes take a rest from his memory."[34]

THE FATE OF ALCOHOL IN THE BODY   According to a Japanese proverb,

> *First the man takes a drink,*
> *Then the drink takes a drink,*
> *Then the drink takes the man!*

Swallowed, alcohol stops first at the stomach. This often mistreated organ promptly helps its owner. Its walls allow only twenty percent of the alcohol to be absorbed into the circulation. The rest must await entrance into the small intestine, where complete absorption is quick. But this entrance is delayed, or even temporarily halted (depending on the amount of alcohol taken), by spastic closure of the pyloric valve at the juncture of the stomach and small intestine. The delay prevents a sudden absorption (and a walloping dose) of all the ingested alcohol into the circulation. Absorption is further best retarded by protein foods (eggs, meat) and by dilution (water, milk, or juices). Whether absorbed into the circulation from the stomach or small intestine, alcohol in the blood means its rapid access to its next stop, the liver.

Alcohol is a toxin, or poison. Detoxication is accomplished by oxidation—a chemical process involving body oxygen. During the body detoxication of alcohol, three oxidation processes occur.

1. The first occurs in the liver. The liver receives much more alcohol than it can handle at one time. It oxidizes a tiny amount of its received alcohol into acetaldehyde. (The fate of this irritating substance is detailed in 2 below.) The rest of the alcohol leaves the liver utterly unchanged. It is then carried by the blood to the right side of the heart and then continues on to the lungs. As the blood in the lungs goes through its usual process of exchanging carbon dioxide waste for fresh oxygen, it also rids itself of a very little of its freeloader, alcohol. Thus, a tiny amount of alcohol is evaporated with breathing. This is not the alcohol that can be smelled. But it can be accurately measured. The alcohol that can be smelled is that in the mouth.

From the lung, the alcohol that has not evaporated on the breath (and this is, by far, the greatest part of it) returns, with the newly oxygenated

[33]Sholem Asch, *The Nazarene*, tr. by Maurice Samuels (New York, 1939), p. 3.
[34]Louis Lewin, *Phantastica: Narcotic and Stimulating Drugs*, cited in Norman Taylor, *Flight from Reality* (New York, 1949), p. 17.

blood, to the left heart. Then, not yet detoxicated, still not oxidized, the alcohol is pumped throughout the body.

So, the hitch is in the liver. It cannot oxidize all the alcohol it gets in one fell swoop. The liver works slowly, oxidizing alcohol a little at a time. The rest gets into the circulation via the heart and lungs. The alcohol distributed throughout the body must wait its turn for bit-by-bit detoxication by the liver. It is during that waiting period that the famed reactions to alcohol occur. Thus, alcohol acts with relative rapidity, but it leaves the body slowly.

2. While alcohol travels unchanged over the circulatory route, the liver busily, but slowly, oxidizes a few drops at a time to acetaldehyde. The acetaldehyde is very toxic. Fortunately, it quickly undergoes a second oxidation. This occurs not only in the liver but throughout the body. Acetic acid is formed.

3. A third, and final, oxidation also takes place throughout the body. Acetic acid is oxidized to water, carbon dioxide, and caloric energy.

THE EFFECT OF ALCOHOL   Alcohol is not a stimulant. It is a depressant. But most people who drink spirits moderately do not seem depressed. On the contrary, they are relaxed, even gay. Those drinking too much were described by Benjamin Rush, a Quaker doctor and signer of the Declaration of Independence, as "singing, hallooing, roaring . . . tearing off clothes . . . dancing naked."[35]

Depression only comes later. Why the delay? Alcohol does indeed depress and anesthetize the nervous system. But it also releases inhibitions. Carried by the blood through the brain, it courses through the cerebral cortex. It is in the cortex that the numberless nerve connections of learning are laid. Alcohol numbs them. If one has learned to hold his tongue, for example, alcohol loosens it. If it slips enough, he may halloo.

How do hangovers happen? How does too much drink take the man? The body cells lose fluid. There is thirst. Circulatory changes cause headache. Decreased inhibitions promote overactivity. There is fatigue. The alcohol irritates the stomach. There is nausea. It assaults the nervous system, causing dizziness.

However, in concentrations high enough to cause drunkenness, alcohol does not directly damage the brain. There is "no sound evidence whatsoever that alcohol causes permanent direct damage to the body."[36] Does that mean that alcohol, taken excessively, is harmless?

Hardly.

ALCOHOL AND BODY WEIGHT   Alcohol, in itself, does not cause one to be fat. Its calories (the average ounce of whiskey provides seventy-two) are not stored as fat. They do, however, replace food calories, which are then stored. Unless the drinker cuts down on his food calories to the extent of his alcohol caloric intake, he will fatten.

---

[35] Benjamin Rush, "Inquiry into the Effects of Ardent Spirits upon the Human Body and Mind," reprinted in *Quarterly Journal of Studies in Alcohol*, Vol. 4, No. 2 (September 1943), p. 325.
[36] Morris E. Chaefetz, *Liquor, the Servant of Man* (Boston, 1965), p. 48.

ALCOHOL AND SEX Alcohol releases sexual inhibitions. Confirmed alcoholics, however, lose interest in sex. Shakespeare's porter in *Macbeth* says about alcohol, "it provokes and unprovokes. It provokes the desire, but it takes away the performance" (II.iii. 33–35). Getting drunk, like being promiscuous, is a sign of deep emotional instability. In small amounts, alcohol need not result in immature behavior.

ALCOHOL AND DRIVING There is little question of the relation between drinking and poor driving. In over half the fatal traffic accidents, a driver is involved who has been drinking.[37] Some recommend a reevaluation of the "don't mix drinking and driving" rule.[38] Others, however, point out that "the variable effects of food taken with drink, tiredness, minor illness and remedies taken for it, and other factors including habituation to alcohol, make it impossible to advise any 'safe' upper limit for alcohol consumption before driving."[39] Several chemical tests are available for measuring the alcohol content in the system. The spinal fluid, saliva, blood, urine, and breath all have been accurately tested. Such evidence can, of course, be used in court (as was noted in Chapter 4).

ALCOHOLISM Of the estimated seventy-five million people in the United States who drink, one in fifteen is poisoned. He is an alcoholic. Without treatment he may become human backwash, gutted, guttered.

Why can one person drink alcohol convivially, while another becomes a confirmed alcoholic? There are no simple answers. The causes of alcoholism are many and complex. In some cases the reasons reach into childhood. For example, as a child, an alcoholic may have been grossly overprotected. He comes to need this excess protection. He learns to fear its loss. To keep it, he remains dependent. Then, one day, he is an adult. Suddenly he must compete. He must be independent. He is bereft. He may reach for alcohol, which, he may have learned, will embolden him.

Even before the alcoholic reaches his first phase, he has warnings. His very first drink may be an unexpected delight. He can hardly wait for another. His course begins.

The symptoms of alcoholism (Table 12-2) need not follow in sequence. Some come together. Others may not occur. Throughout the first "blank period or amnesia" the potential alcoholic will act normally. He may be cheering at a football game with friends. On the following day, he remembers nothing. Deep within him is a gnawing uneasiness. Later, this will be a wild fear. What did he do and say? He cannot recall. He drinks more. For many alcoholics the tolerance for the liquid drug increases. For others it seems to decrease. The first phase may last five years—sometimes less.

Item seven, in the second phase, is the milestone in the alcoholic's

---

[37] W. Haddon, Jr., and V. A. Bradess, "Alcohol in the Single Vehicle Fatal Accident: Experience of Westchester County, N.Y.," *Journal of the American Medical Association*, Vol. 169, No. 14 (April 4, 1959). p. 1587.

[38] Robert F. Borkenstein, "A Realistic Approach to Drinking and Driving," *Traffic Safety*, Vol. 67, No. 10 (October 1967), p. 11.

[39] "Drinking Drivers," an editorial in *British Medical Journal*, Vol. 2, No. 5544 (April 8, 1967), p. 67.

TABLE 12-2 *Phases and Symptoms of Alcoholism*

FIRST PHASE

1. First blank period or amnesia.
2. Sneaking drinks.
3. Preoccupation with drinking.
4. Gulping drinks.
5. Becoming evasive about drinking.
6. Second blank period or amnesia.

SECOND (OR CRUCIAL) PHASE

7. Loss of control of drinking.
8. Manufacturing alibis.
9. Extravagant and grandiose behavior.
10. Aggressive behavior.
11. Persistent remorse.
12. Periods of total abstinence ("going on water wagon").
13. Tries changing pattern of drinking.
14. Begins dropping friends.
15. Leaves or loses jobs.
16. Becomes *more* preoccupied with alcohol.
17. Loses outside interests.
18. Indulges in orgies of self-pity.
19. Impulse to escape from environment (actual or contemplated).
20. Experiences unreasonable resentments.
21. Protects his supply of alcohol (hides bottles).
22. Malnutrition (the alcoholic neglects to take food).
23. Hospitalization.
24. Decrease or loss of sexual desire.
25. Alcoholic jealousy.
26. The morning drink (needs a "bracer" to start the day).

THE FINAL (OR CHRONIC) PHASE

27. First prolonged intoxication . . .
28. Ethical deterioration.
29. Impairment of thinking.
30. Drinking with social inferiors.
31. Debasement of taste—if necessary drinks methylated spirit, bay rum, or surgical spirit in toilet preparations.
32. Loss of tolerance for alcohol.
33. Vague, indefinable fears.
34. Presistent tremors.
35. Cannot perform simple muscular tasks without alcohol.
36. Drinking becomes obsessive.
37. Vague religious desires develop.
38. Alibis and rationalizations fail, and the patient admits defeat.

Source: Lincoln Williams, *Tomorrow Will Be Sober* (New York, 1960), p. 34.

journey. Without adequate treatment, it marks a downhill course. In this stage the moral argument concerning alcohol does the alcoholic the greatest disservice. That quarrel helped create the concept of the average alcoholic as a skid-row bum. Less than ten percent of the nation's alcoholics inhabit skid row. The rest live with their families, desperately hanging on to their jobs. It is the skid-row caricature of the alcoholic that his important people—his wife, boss, and even minister—cannot accept of him. He is not really that, they say. He will straighten out.

The alcoholic helps with the delusion. Tomorrow will be sober. Pale, trembling, furtive, he pulls himself together. To those worrying about him, he gives false hope. They vacilate. He is not treated. He rejects such help as Alcoholics Anonymous. Then he is drunk again. His remorse is their despair.

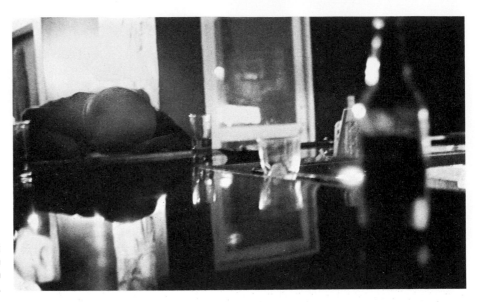

12-5 The alcoholic: this nation's fourth greatest public health problem.

His last stage is a haunting torment that he will run out of alcohol. Hours are spent in searching for and then hiding it. Often he cannot keep the alcohol down. Days are spent on his knees, like an animal, crawling, vomiting, perhaps resting his throbbing head on a toilet bowl.

His body, long resentful, is now an angry protest. He may have already become hoarse from his swollen throat (brandy voice). His bloodshot eyes, pasty skin, red "brandy nose" have become part of him. Poor nutrition wastes him. Vitamin deficiency diseases plague him. Without alcohol he may develop delirium tremens (the abstinence syndrome). Numberless "worms" or "ants" torture him. "Snakes" bite into him. Delirium tremens is a true psychosis. Five percent of alcoholics develop delirium tremens. Without attention, perhaps twenty-five percent of those with delirium tremens die. With care, less than five percent die.

Other signs of vitamin deficiency may occur. Prickly burning of the hands and feet herald the onset of the pain and paralysis of *polyneuritis.* Prompt treatment with vitamin B can prevent permanent disability. *Korsakoff's psychosis* (seen with diseases other than alcoholism) is characterized by periods of amnesia filled in by the patient with all sorts of preposterous tales. Full recovery has not been reported. *Wernicke's syndrome* is the result of impeded brain tissue metabolism. With vitamin B therapy, improvement is likely. *Cirrhosis of the liver,* a destructive infiltration of that organ, first with fibrous tissue and later with fat, has frequently been reported. Like the other complicating conditions of alcoholism, it is probably due to malnutrition.

THE INCIDENCE OF DRINKING   Most people in the United States handle alcohol very well. But the exceptions number into millions. The alcoholic is a major public health problem. His tragedy is incalculable.

The damage to his role as mate, parent, and employee is a grievous price that he and his society pay for alcohol.

Two out of three adults in this country drink some kind of alcoholic beverage. Half of these use distilled spirits. One-fourth of them drink at least three times weekly. Among occasional drinkers, men outnumber women three to two. "The value placed on sexual purity remains potent . . . a general intolerance of drunken women exists at all levels."[40] Three times as many men as women drink regularly. Among the better educated and the more affluent, drinking is more common. City people drink more than rural dwellers. Protestant abstainers outnumber the Jewish three to one, and the Catholic two to one. Blacks drink as commonly as do whites.[41]

With some relatively rare (and highly overpublicized) exceptions the teen-ager does not get drunk. He drinks primarily to taste adulthood. Beer is his favorite beverage. About 60 percent of all high school students take some alcoholic drink before graduating. A Toronto study showed that this rises about 10 percent during the first year of college.[42] U.S. data show similar results. Almost 75 percent of all college students in this country use alcohol to some extent. There are five times as many abstainers among college students from nondrinking families as from families in which one or more parents drank. College students, particularly girls, drink for social reasons. Heavy drinking among college students occurs but is not common.[43]

THE TREATMENT OF ALCOHOLISM   In the treatment of alcoholism, five carefully supervised methods may be used. These are the five A's: *aversion therapy, apomorphine, antabuse, adjustment* (psychological and spiritual), and *Alcoholics Anonymous.* In *aversion therapy* the patient is first given injections of a nauseant drug. He then drinks various whiskeys. He may associate his resultant nausea with the ingested alcohol. For many, this treatment has been successful.

The effectiveness of the drug *apomorphine* is not based on a conditioned reflex. It is used after alcohol has been ingested. Upon injection of apomorphine, nausea and even severe vomiting occur. The alcoholic is too sick to drink more. This treatment is not often used. Another drug, *antabuse,* makes even a small amount of ingested alcohol a dangerous experience—the patient becomes seriously ill. *Alcoholics Anonymous* is a splendid supportive organization offering much psychological and spiritual aid, which may, however, need *professional supplementation.* The best approach is multidisciplinary.[44] Some health departments have embarked on alcoholism prevention and treatment programs.

[40] Harrison M. Trice, *Alcoholism in America* (New York, 1966), p. 20.

[41] *Ibid.,* p. 22.

[42] Milan Korcok and Dianne Jones, "Toronto School Drugs Survey," *Addictions,* Vol. 16, No. 1 (Spring 1969), p. 4.

[43] *Alcohol Statistics,* Report by George Gallup of the American Institute of Public Opinion, "Percentage of Drinking Population to Total Population by Years," p. 2.

[44] Ruth Fox, "A Multidisciplinary Approach to the Treatment of Alcoholism," *International Journal of Psychiatry,* Vol. 5, No. 1 (January 1968), pp. 34–46.

Some minor depressants: sniffing for dreams

Greek mythology refers to the priestess Pythia, seated on the side of the mountain Parnassus. From the earth she inhaled cold vapors that already had convulsed goats and a goatherd. Her vapor-inspired thoughts were carefully interpreted by the priests. Thousands of years later, stylish English gentry of the early nineteenth century used laughing gas to sniff themselves silly at dinner parties. Soon college students in this country were sniffing and laughing too. Ether sniffing became popular both in this country and abroad; one nineteenth-century report states that "the students at Harvard used to inhale sulfuric ether from their handkerchiefs, and it intoxicated them and made them reel and stagger."[45]

Today, a ten-cent tube of glue and a paper bag provide some children and adolescents with their dreams. In the drug culture this is called "snorting." Airplane model glue is most popular. However, plastic cement, antifreeze, paint thinner, cleaning and lighter fluids, gasoline and kerosene—all have their followers. The vapors are central nervous system depressants. With chronic abuse, tolerance has been reported. With discontinuance of the drug, withdrawal symptoms can be severe but are usually mild. Nausea, vomiting, dizziness, and ringing of the ears have all been reported. At first, the sniffer is exhilarated. As he sniffs, euphoria and hallucinations may occur. Occasionally hallucinations persist for several hours. Homicides have been associated with the abuse of the vapors of glue, lacquer thinner, and plastic cement. With the beginnings of the sniffing experience, there is no established evidence that irreversible physical damage results.[46] However, there is considerable clinical opinion that physical damage to both kidney and central nervous system is likely.[47] Persistent glue sniffing can result in severe anemia and bone marrow and liver damage. Chronic gasoline sniffers can develop lead poisoning. By decreasing the supply of oxygen to the lungs the Freon aerosol spray sniffer risks his life.

Several deaths from plastic bag suffocation and accidental ingestion have been reported. But the major problem is the sniffing itself.

Stimulants

The amphetamine type of drug dependence

Differences among the stimulants: speed freaks vs. acid heads

Basically, depressants such as morphine, the barbiturates, and alcohol reduce psychic and motor stimuli. The depressive drug abuser is often psychically and physically incapacitated. His senses are deadened, and he exists on the foggy border between consciousness and unconsciousness. He drifts into a troubled sleep. This loss of consciousness limits the

---

[45] W. T. G. Morton, "A Memoir to the Academy of Sciences at Paris on a New Use of Sulfuric Ether," cited in Sidney Cohen, *The Drug Dilemma* (New York, 1969), p. 99.

[46] Edward Preble and Gabriel V. Laury, "Plastic Cement, The Ten-Cent Hallucinogen," *International Journal of Addictions*, Vol. 2, No. 2 (Fall 1967), p. 275.

[47] John C. Pollard, "Teen-Agers and the Use of Drugs: Reflections on the Emotional Setting," *Clinical Pediatrics*, Vol. 6, No. 11 (November 1967), pp. 618–19.

amount of drug he takes. His antisocial behavior, such as stealing, is rooted in the need to secure more drug. Stimulants, on the other hand, excite psychic and motor activity. Thus, hallucinogens such as LSD and marihuana are included in the stimulant group, along with the amphetamines. Nevertheless, although the amphetamine-type abusers ("speed freaks") and the LSD abusers ("acid heads") both take stimulants, their choice of stimulant is largely determined by their needs and their personalities. And each of these stimulants produces bizarre but different behavior.

The speed freak seeks one result; the acid head, another. The amphetamine-type drug abuser takes the drug primarily to experience a "flash" or "rush." This he describes as a "full body orgasm." The acute anxiety and the hallucinations and paranoia associated with amphetamine abuse are secondary. This psychic storm may combine with an undiminished, even a temporarily increased, physical strength. This mixture of irrationality and strength can suddenly explode with the murderous violence of a hand grenade. The LSD abuser wants a different drug reaction and his secondary behavior is different from the speed freak's. "Rather than seeking a *flash* or a thrill as do the speed freaks, the chronic LSD user develops a complex set of motivations for his drug use, involving self-psychoanalytic, pseudoreligious and creative aspirations." The speed freak is often violent; this the acid head rejects. Thus "speed always drives out acid."[48]

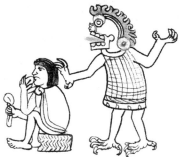

12-6 An Indian eating mind-affecting mushrooms before the god Mictlanteccuhtli, from a 16th-century manuscript.

Amphetamine: the bitter pill

The proprietary names for methamphetamine central nervous system stimulators are methedrine and Desoxyn. For dextroamphetamine, they are Dexedrine or Benzedrine. In street terminology, "speed," "crystal," or "meth" usually refers to an amphetamine.

Amphetamine abusers develop no physical dependence. Withdrawal is, therefore, neither dangerous nor painful. However, psychological dependence is marked. So is tolerance. An abuser may gobble as many as 150 "pep pills" a day to attain the effect first experienced with just one.

Amphetamine drugs are commonly used as an appetite depressant for weight reduction. They have, moreover, been remarkably effective in the treatment of school children's learning disorders.[49] When swallowed, they are tasteless, but they can become a bitter pill. With abuse, the drugs cause sleeplessness, extreme hyperactivity, profound behavior changes, and hallucinations. Even relatively moderate doses may cause such marked psychic changes as to make college attendance, for example, impossible.[50] Chronic amphetamine abuse has led to brain damage.[51]

[48] David E. Smith, "Speed Freaks vs. Acid Heads," *Clinical Pediatrics,* Vol. 8, No. 4 (April 1969), pp. 187, 188.

[49] C. K. Conners, L. Eisenberg, and A. Barcai, "The Effect of Dextroamphetamine on Children with Learning Disabilities and School Behavior Problems," *Archives of General Psychiatry,* Vol. 17, No. 4 (October 1967), pp. 478–85.

[50] Richard M. Steinhilber and Albert B. Hagedorn, "Drug Induced Behavioral Disorders," *GP,* Vol. 35, No. 5 (May 1967), pp. 115–16.

[51] "Drug Dependency," the UCLA Interdepartmental Conference, Anthony Kales, moderator, *Annals of Internal Medicine,* Vol. 70, No. 3 (March 1969), p. 591.

Most people who abuse amphetamines begin by taking these drugs orally, but many individuals now "shoot" the drug by vein. After many injections, scars develop along the veins; these the abuser calls "tracks." A rapid tolerance is developed. Soon the amphetamine abuser gives himself astronomic amounts. With each fresh injection he experiences the "rush." He is then known as a "speed freak." How much does he take? It is impossible to be certain. His drug source is the black-market laboratory. Dosage and content vary widely.

A perilous pattern develops. The drug is injected about every two hours around the clock for three to six days (rarely more). During this period the abuser remains continuously awake. This is called a "run" or "speed binge." The abuser than "falls out." Exhausted, tremulous, disorganized, enduring terrifying visual and auditory hallucinations, and paranoid, he goes to sleep. Once asleep, he cannot be awakened. Following a three- or four-day run, the drug abuser sleeps twelve to eighteen hours. He awakens hungry. His paranoia is largely gone. But now he is plagued by a depression of extraordinary intensity. One seventeen-year-old girl put it this way: "Without speed I feel so lousy that I'd rather shoot speed and live for one week than live for forty years without it."[52] To escape the terrible depression, the abuser must start another run. If the drug is available, he does. If not, the desperate search for it begins.

During a run, appetite disappears. The experienced abuser may force himself to eat. To control the growing anxiety, hallucinations, and paranoia, barbiturates or opiates may be added to the regimen. It is with the first injection that the severe paranoia may appear, though usually it is delayed several days. Everyone is suspect. Friends "bug" the phone. Every car is a police cruiser. Trees are detectives. To track down his enemies one abuser set out with his pet Doberman. Excited, he is liable to become violent. He may hurt or kill somebody. "If the patient is large or violent, the physician may be in some immediate jeopardy."[53] But often the sick and suspicious person will not go to the doctor.

During a run, the "methhead" has purposeless compulsions. One abuser may shine his shoes, again and again, all day long. Another will take a radio or an automobile motor apart. Completely absorbed, he seems untroubled by his lack of coordination and failure to "repair" it.[54] For extended periods he may engage in nonejaculatory intercourse. Eventually this will lead "to the inability to get or maintain an erection at all, and a chemically produced total impotence."[55] With discontinuance of the drug, this disappears. But the psychotic symptoms often persist.

During a period of chronic use, twenty to thirty pounds may be lost. Commonly seen, and in part due to malnutrition, are abscesses, non-healing ulcerations, and brittle fingernails. Among amphetamine abusers,

[52] Quoted in David E. Smith, "Speed Freaks vs. Acid Heads," p. 185.
[53] *Ibid.*, p. 186.
[54] John C. Kramer, V. S. Fischman, and Don C. Littlefield, "Amphetamine Abuse," *Journal of the American Medical Association*, Vol. 201, No. 5 (July 31, 1967), pp. 89–93.
[55] Jordan Scherer, "Patterns and Profiles of Addiction and Drug Abuse," p. 182.

serum hepatitis is common. It is caused by a virus transmitted by dirty needles. The mortality from this liver disease is much higher than that seen with infectious hepatitis (see page 193).

It is estimated that, in the major cities of this nation, thousands of young people take intravenous amphetamines. Those amphetamine abusers who want to stop taking it find that difficult. Why? "Meth" abusers generally live together, communally. They cannot bring themselves to leave their friends.[56] Yet even in this human need for companionship, there is an added and ironic danger. Amphetamine toxicity is augmented in a crowded ecosystem. Aggregation of animals increases the toxicity of amphetamine fourfold. "It has become obvious that taking the drug in a high-density population situation increases its toxicity."[57]

A particularly dangerous complication has developed. LSD is now often contaminated with methamphetamine crystal. "The tachycardia [excessively rapid heart rate], muscle tremor and anxiety produced by 'speed' is often magnified by the LSD-sensitized mind into a panic reaction."[58]

The ability of the amphetamines to induce tolerance is almost unique among stimulants of the central nervous system. So great can the slowly developing tolerance become that an abuser of this group of stimulants is eventually able to withstand a dose several hundred times greater than that ordinarily used by physicians. The drugs causing dependence of the hallucinogen (LSD) type include *LSD, psilocybin* (a drug found in a mushroom), and *mescaline* (found in the buttons of a small cactus— "mescal" or "peyote"—and in the seeds of varieties of the morning glory). In this country, some Indian tribes use the mushrooms, cactus buttons, and morning-glory seeds during their religious rites. Their medicine men and women also use them for treatment. Like the amphetamines, the LSD type of hallucinogens have the capacity to induce tolerance. This, however, is not characteristic of drug dependence of the *Cannabis,* or marihuana, type.

The hallucinogen (LSD) type of drug dependence

LSD

Elephants interest some psychiatrists, too. The adult male elephant periodically goes berserk and, for two weeks, is a menace. To study this cyclically recurring mental derangement, investigators in this country chose Tusko, a 7,000-pound resident of Oklahoma City's Lincoln Park Zoo. LSD was chosen to simulate the madness. Why? Because of "its well-known personality-disrupting effect upon humans and other animals."[59] An elephantine dose killed Tusko in one hour and forty minutes.

[56] David E. Smith and Alan J. Rose, "Observations in the Haight-Ashbury Medical Clinic of San Francisco," *Clinical Pediatrics,* Vol. 7, No. 6 (June 1968), p. 316.
[57] David E. Smith, "Speed Freaks vs. Acid Heads," p. 187.
[58] David E. Smith and Alan J. Rose, "Observations in the Haight-Ashbury Medical Clinic of San Francisco," p. 319.
[59] Louis Jolyon West, Chester M. Pierce, and Warren D. Thomas, "Lysergic Acid Diethylamide: Its Effect on a Male Asiatic Elephant," *Science,* Vol. 138, No. 3545 (December 7, 1962), p. 1101.

Tusko had received 297 milligrams (297,000 micrograms) of LSD. The human dose is but 0.1 to 0.2 milligrams (100 to 200 micrograms). No human death directly attributable to LSD has been reported. The effective dose of LSD is tiny. One ounce would provide 300,000 adult doses. Two pounds, equally distributed, "would mentally dissociate every man, woman, and child in greater New York for an eight-hour period . . . 'an average dose' . . . 100 micrograms . . . can barely be seen with the naked eye."[60] Taken by mouth, LSD does not act for about forty-five minutes. By the time its effect begins, it is gone from the brain. About four hours after consumption, the effects begin to decrease. In six to twelve hours, they are gone. Tolerance to LSD is rapidly developed. Unlike opium tolerance, LSD tolerance may be developed in a few days and is usually lost in two or three days. Over a period of days, therefore, some users build up an LSD tolerance of 1,000 or 2,000 micrograms (sometimes even more). The average dose is but a tenth this size. For the original effect, therefore, massive doses may be taken once a tolerance has been built up. There is no evidence of a physical LSD dependence.

Two major types of reactions are attributed to LSD, one psychic and the other nonpsychic. Each will now be examined.

PSYCHIC EFFECTS   For thirty-five to forty minutes after ingestion of LSD, nothing happens. Then, for a brief period, there is a sense of well-being. This is followed by a feeling of unreality, of depersonalization and loss of body image. In new users this may be terrifying. The following case was reported from Bellevue Hospital in New York:

> A 21-year-old woman was admitted to the hospital along with her lover. He had had a number of LSD experiences and had convinced her to take it to make her less constrained sexually. About half an hour after ingestion of approximately 200 microgm., she noticed that the bricks in the wall began to go in and out and that light affected her strangely. She became frightened when she realized that she was unable to distinguish her body from the chair she was sitting on or from her lover's body. Her fear became more marked after she thought that she would not get back into herself. At the time of admission she was hyperactive and laughed inappropriately. Stream of talk was illogical . . . Two days later, this reaction had ceased. However, she was still afraid of the drug and convinced that she would not take it again because of her frightening experience.[61]

The illusions following LSD ingestion may include an orgy of vividly colored shapes and patterns, some beautiful, others bizarre. These are

[60] Sidney Cohen, *Drugs of Hallucination* (London, 1964), pp. 34–35.
[61] William A. Frosch, Edwin S. Robbins, and Marvin Stern, "Untoward Reactions to Lysergic Acid Diethylamide (LSD) Resulting in Hospitalization," *New England Journal of Medicine*, Vol. 273, No. 23 (December 2, 1965), p. 1236.

called "pseudohallucinations." While knowing that the perception of bizarre designs has no basis in external reality, the individual sees them anyway. True hallucination, in which one perceives something that is not actually there, is not common with LSD abusers. What does occur is a perceptual change. The LSD abuser sees what is in the environment, but for him it has changed markedly in shape or color and in meaning. These are illusions not, strictly, hallucinations. *Synesthesia,* the translation of one type of sensory experience into another, may also occur. Music may be felt as body vibrations. Colors may beat in rhythm with music.[62] (The song "Good Vibrations" refers to synesthesia.) Some individuals seem to recall long-forgotten events. Others claim feelings of transcendence. Smith has described a *psychedelic syndrome.* A belief in nonviolence, a desire to return to nature, a belief in magic, signs, and mental telepathy, and a tendency to live in groups are among its characteristics.[63]

Today, legal use of LSD is limited to research. Its official distribution is by the National Institute of Mental Health. As it is a colorless and tasteless substance, its illegal handling is difficult to detect. A reasonably sophisticated chemist can make it. The chemical search for "soul" has become a spreading cult. What objective data are available regarding the psychic effects of LSD?

> By June, 1967 . . . 21 reports . . . contained the details of . . . adverse reactions to LSD . . . these were 142 cases of prolonged psychotic reactions, 63 nonpsychotic reactions, 11 spontaneous recurrences, 19 attempted suicides, 4 attempted homicides, 11 successful suicides, and 1 successful homicide . . . An additional 9 cases shared possible suicidal intent . . . There were 6 cases of convulsions which may be seen as tic reactions.[64]

Still another question remains to be considered. Were the above adverse reactions reported in the medical literature by June 1967 all that had occurred? By no means. Ungerleider and others surveyed 2,700 psychiatrists, psychiatric residents, general practitioners, and psychologists in the Los Angeles County area. As a result of their studies of returned, carefully prepared questionnaires, they found that more than twenty-three hundred adverse reactions had been noted between July 1, 1966, and January 1, 1968. They consider this figure conservative. What percent of LSD users have adverse reactions? This is unknown because a reasonably accurate estimate of LSD-dependent abusers is not available.[65]

Some individuals who experienced prolonged psychoses after LSD

---

[62]David E. Smith and Alan J. Rose, "The Use and Abuse of LSD in Haight-Ashbury," *Clinical Pediatrics,* Vol. 7, No. 6 (June 1968), p. 318.

[63]David E. Smith, "Speed Freaks vs. Acid Heads," p. 318.

[64]Reginald G. Smart and Karen Bateman, "Unfavorable Reactions to LSD," *Canadian Medical Association Journal,* Vol. 97, No. 20 (November 11, 1967), p. 1214.

[65]J. Thomas Ungerleider et al., "A Statistical Survey of Adverse Reactions to LSD in Los Angeles County," *American Journal of Psychiatry,* Vol. 125, No. 3 (September 1968), pp. 352–56.

ingestions had had no previous psychiatric disturbance.[66] One dose of LSD has, in many cases, produced a psychosis (the duration of the psychoses varies).

There is no explanation for the recurrence phenomenon of an LSD experience weeks or months after the last ingestion of the drug. Despite discontinuance of LSD, one woman had spontaneous recurrences of hallucinations for months. "She . . . has terrifying involuntary illusions of people decomposing in the street in front of her and had nightmares in vivid color. She continued to have these experiences five months after her last drug experience."[67]

So it was with Stevenson's Dr. Jekyll. Without his drug, and while sitting in the park, he "was once more Mr. Hyde."[68] The "reappearance of LSD symptoms a month to over a year after the original use, without reingestion"[69] is ominous indeed.

Some nonpsychotic reactions have been prolonged. Acute panics, confusions, and psychopathic behavior have been reported. Of these, panic reactions are most frequent. Some of these have required long-term psychotherapy.

LSD-associated suicide has occurred. One successful suicide (of the 11 reported) was of a twenty-year-old college student. "A few days prior to his death he discussed plans for the immediate and distant future with friends . . . He took LSD in the company of others . . . and without explanation, while by himself, disrobed and took his life."[70]

DOES LSD HAVE NONPSYCHIC EFFECTS?   Science is seeking the answers to the following questions:

1. Does LSD ingestion damage human chromosomes?

2. Does LSD have a teratogenic effect? (Teratogenesis refers to the production of physical defects in offspring while in the uterus.)

The lymphocyte[71] chromosomes of LSD users have been studied, with inconclusive results. One group found chromosomal aberrations in eighteen patients who had taken different doses of LSD for various lengths of time. But these individuals had taken other drugs too. Also examined were the chromosomes of four children born of three mothers who had taken LSD during pregnancy. Two of these children had a markedly increased frequency of chromosomal breakage. During the first three or four months of pregnancy, their mothers had ingested high doses of LSD.[72]

[66]Medical Society of the County of New York, Public Health Committee, Subcommittee on Narcotics Addiction, cited in Reginald G. Smart and Karen Bateman, "Unfavorable Reactions to LSD," p. 1216.

[67]Saul H. Rosenthal, "Persistent Hallucinosis Following Repeated Administration of Hallucinogenic Drugs," *American Journal of Psychiatry*, Vol. 121, No. 3 (September 1964), pp. 240–41.

[68]Robert Louis Stevenson, "The Strange Case of Dr. Jekyll and Mr. Hyde," in Damon Knight, ed., *A Century of Great Short Science-Fiction Novels* (New York, 1964), p. 59.

[69]"LSD—A Dangerous Drug," an editorial in *New England Journal of Medicine*, Vol. 273, No. 23 (December 2, 1965), p. 1280.

[70]Martin H. Keeler and Clifford B. Reifler, "Suicide During an LSD Reaction," *American Journal of Psychiatry*, Vol. 123, No. 7 (January 1967), p. 885.

[71]A lymphocyte is a variety of white blood corpuscle.

[72]Maimon M. Cohen, Kurt Hirschhorn, and William A. Frosch, "In Vivo and In Vitro Chromosomal Damage Induced by LSD-25," *New England Journal of Medicine*, Vol. 277, No. 20 (November 16, 1967), pp. 1043–49.

Other researchers have verified these findings.[73] Indeed, one such study involved examination of the chromosomes of fifty LSD users and fourteen nonuser controls. The mean chromosome breakage rate of the LSD users was twice that of the nonusers. And three of four children born to mothers who had ingested LSD showed high levels of chromosome breaks.[74]

But some studies show no such evidence. One controlled experiment involving "32 patients before and after they took [LSD and] five black-market LSD users . . . revealed no significant difference between the before- and after-LSD chromosomal aberration rates."[75]

Criticisms have been leveled at both positive and negative results of other human studies. Some are these: the unreliability of dosage information from LSD users; lack of knowledge of other drugs used at the same time (which might also cause chromosomal abnormalities); the lack of information about other illness such as virus infections (rubella, for example) that might cause chromosomal injuries. Indeed, there seems to be incomplete agreement on the normal level of chromosomal abnormalities.

Limited study of the LSD effect on animal sperm has added little that is decisive. On various occasions one researcher injected six mice with LSD and inspected the germ cells for excess chromosome breaks. Increased abnormalities were noted far more often in the LSD-injected mice than in the controls.[76] However, the animal dose was about five hundred times as high as the usual human dose.

LSD has been injected into pregnant mice, rats, and hamsters[77] (see Figure 12-7). When injected early in pregnancy, an increase of congenitally malformed fetuses occurs. In the case of rabbits, however, LSD proved a much milder teratogen than thalidomide.

In various concentrations and for various lengths of time, LSD was added to test tubes containing human leukocytes.[78] Compared to leukocytes not so treated, a marked increase in chromosomal breakage was noted. On the other hand, a careful study of drosophila (fruit fly) cells treated with LSD revealed no increase in chromosomal abnormalities.[79]

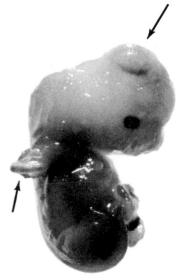

12-7 A hamster fetus with deformed brain and legs (arrows). Its mother had been injected during early pregnancy with a very high dose of LSD.

[73] Samuel Irwin and Jose Egozcue, "Chromosomal Abnormalities in Leukocytes from LSD-25 Users," Science, Vol. 157, No. 3786 (July 21, 1967), pp. 313–14; J. Nielson et al., "Lysergide and Chromosome Abnormalities," British Medical Journal, Vol. 2, No. 29 (June 1968), pp. 801–03.

[74] Jose Egozcue, Samuel Irwin, and C. A. Maruffo, "Chromosomal Damage in LSD Users," Journal of the American Medical Association, Vol. 204, No. 3 (April 15, 1968), pp. 214–18.

[75] Joe-Hin Tjio, Walter N. Pahnke, and Albert A. Kurland, "LSD and Chromosomes," Journal of the American Medical Association, Vol. 210, No. 5 (November 3, 1969), p. 849.

[76] N. E. Skakkebaek, J. Philip, and O. J. Rafaelsen, "LSD in Mice: Abnormalities in Meiotic Chromosomes," Science, Vol. 160 (June 14, 1968), pp. 1246–48.

[77] Reports of such studies include E. R. Auerback and J. A. Rugowski, "Lysergic Acid Diethylamide: Effect on Embryos," Science, Vol. 157, No. 3791 (September 15, 1967), pp. 1325–26; G. J. Alexander et al., "LSD: Injection Early in Pregnancy Produces Abnormalities in Offspring of Rats," Science, Vol. 157, No. 3791 (September 15, 1967), p. 453; W. F. Geber, "Congenital Malformations Induced by Mescaline, Lysergic Acid Diethylamide and Bromolysergic Acid in the Hamster," Science, Vol. 158, No. 3798 (October 13, 1967), p. 265.

[78] Maimon M. Cohen, Michelle J. Marinello, and Nathan Back, "Chromosomal Damage in Human Leukocytes Induced by Lysergic Acid Diethylamide," Science, Vol. 155 (March 17, 1967), pp. 1417–19.

[79] Dale Grace, Elof Axel Carlson, and Philip Goodman, "Drosophila melanogaster Treated with LSD: Absence of Mutation and Chromosome Breakage," Science, Vol. 161 (August 16, 1968), pp. 694–96.

How may these contradictory findings be interpreted?

At present, the case for the chromosomal effects of LSD in human users is not proved, although sufficient evidence exists to justify the expectation that further studies may confirm such an effect.[80]

and

The evidence for a teratogenic effect of LSD is very strong but not unanimous. Certainly, it is strong enough to warrant a great deal of further research on the whole topic.[81]

The seeds of psychoses

As has been pointed out above, other hallucinogens, producing reactions similar to LSD's, include *mescaline, psilocybin,* and *morning-glory seeds.* A suicide following the use of morning-glory seeds has been reported.[82] Another disturbed twenty-four-year-old male "first learned of the hallucinogenic effects of morning-glory seed ingestion through a newspaper article cautioning against the use of the seeds.[83] Before going into shock, he experienced a variety of hallucinations. Four months later hallucinations were occurring at will and against his will.

The "pink wedge"

On November 11, 1967, the "pink wedge" was sold to some young people in San Francisco. It was not much larger than a saccharine tablet. Users thought they were buying LSD. They were. But it was contaminated with STP (named for a motor fuel additive, Scientifically Treated Petroleum). Upon analysis, STP was found to be DOM, an experimental compound developed by the Dow Chemical Company. Somehow, the formula had fallen into illicit hands. It was not long before the Haight-Ashbury Medical Clinic was deluged by young people in a toxic panic. After treatment, many could remember nothing of their experience.[84]

STP has added meanings. A Canadian psychiatrist writes,

The letters stand for Serenity, Tranquility and Peace—and any associations with a tombstone may not be inappropriate in view of the occasional fatal outcome of STP ingestion . . . The actual

[80] Reginald G. Smart and Karen Bateman, "The Chromosomal and Teratogenic Effects of Lysergic Acid Diethylamide: A Review of Current Literature," *Canadian Medical Association Journal,* Vol. 99 (October 26, 1968), p. 809.

[81] *Ibid.,* p. 810.

[82] Sidney Cohen, "Suicide Following Morning-Glory Seed Ingestion," *American Journal of Psychiatry,* Vol. 120, No. 10 (April 1964), pp. 1024–25.

[83] P. J. Fink, M. J. Goldman and I. Lyons, "Morning-Glory Seed Psychoses," *Archives of General Psychiatry,* Vol. 15, No. 2 (August 1966), p. 210. Many experts hold that the wide publicity concerning dangerous drugs has piqued the curiosity of the vulnerable and promoted drug use.

[84] David E. Smith and Alan J. Rose, "The Use and Abuse of LSD in Haight-Ashbury," p. 321.

TABLE 12-3 *Comparative Strengths of LSD and Other Hallucinogens (Approximate)*	
HALLUCINOGEN	COMPARATIVE STRENGTH*
Marihuana (leaves and tops of *Cannabis sativa*, swallowed)	30,000 mg.
Peyote buttons (*Lophophora williamsii*)	30,000 mg.
Nutmeg (*Myristica fragrans*)	20,000 mg.
Hashish (resin of *Cannabis sativa*)	4,000 mg.
Mescaline (3,4,5-trimethoxyphenylethylamine)	400 mg.
Psilocybin (4-phosphoryltryptamine)	12 mg.
STP (2,5-dimethoxy-4-methyl-amphetamine)	5 mg.
LSD (d-lysergic acid diethylamide tartarate)	0.1 mg.

*That is, each of these dosages has an equivalent effect.

Source: Sidney Cohen, "Pot, Acid and Speed," *Medical Science*, Vol. 19, No. 2 (February 1968), p. 31.

psychedelic experience lasts for four to five days, with effects similar to though much more intense than those of LSD. The subject is unable to sleep for the first 20 hours or so, then sleeps for 4 to 10 hours; on awakening he finds himself in an even more intense psychedelic experience than before sleep, and the effects are highest at this time, gradually wearing off in the next few days and leaving the subject exhausted.[85]

Over-the-counter hallucinogens

Not all hallucinogens are illegally sold. A number of intoxications have been reported recently from a considerable diversity of over-the-counter products. They are sold for a variety of symptoms, ranging from diarrhea to constipation. Many, such as cold tablets, cough depressants, and sleep inducers, are intensely advertised. They should be kept "under the counter" and sold only by prescription.

This old Persian tale is still told today in Southwestern Asia:

The cannabis (marihuana) type of drug dependence

Three men arrived at Ispahan at night. The gates of the town were closed. One of the men was an alcoholic, another an opium-addict, and the third took hashish. The alcoholic said: "Let us break down the gate"; the opium smoker suggested: "Let us lie down and sleep until tomorrow"; but the hashish-addict said: "Let us pass through the keyhole."[86]

[85] J. Robertson Unwin, "Illicit Drug Use Among Canadian Youth: Part I," *Canadian Medical Association Journal*, Vol. 98, No. 8 (February 24, 1968), p. 405.

[86] *World Health: The Magazine of the World Health Organization*, Vol. 13, No. 1 (January–February 1960), p. 24.

It is the dried tops, leaves, and flowers from the female form of the plant *Cannabis sativa* that yield marihuana. The longer male plant is used for fiber or hemp. which is probably why marihuana is sometimes called "hemp."[87] Forty-seven centuries ago the Chinese Shen Nung knew of the seductive powers of the resinous flower top. It was called "the Liberator of Sin." The Indians, however, named it "the Heavenly Guide." With them its cultivation became an art. Even today, near Bombay, a pure cannabis product called *ganja* is prepared. The notoriously potent *charas* is rarely used; Indian physicians attribute much insanity to it. *Bhang,* the cheapest cannabis product in India, is the marihuana known in this country. Marihuana is a Mexican term denoting an inferior tobacco. It is Spanish for "Mary Jane." All cannabis products have been called hashish, after a schemer of the eleventh century. To embolden his men to assassinate, he was reputed to have fed them cannabis. The schemer was Jusan-i-Sabbah. The word "assassin" is derived from Hasan's full name: Hashishin. Many experts disagree with the statement that Hashishin used cannabis and suggest the drug was opium. Today, hashish is charas.

In most countries of the world, there is at present no known medical use for marihuana. A few years ago Israeli and U.S. chemists synthesized the active principle of marihuana, making possible its further study.

Marihuana smoking is usually a lonely group affair. To rebreathe one another's smoke, some avid smokers may hole themselves up in a closet. In the past, marihuana has been used in religious customs and ceremonial rites. Mohammedans and Hindus have used it in their religious services, as have the members of the American Indians' Native American Church. In this country today, people at all levels of society smoke marihuana for escape. For many, use of the drug is an expression of inner conflicts. It may be a way of gaining social acceptance, of handling real or imagined rejection, or escaping anxiety or depression.

Great numbers of young people experiment. Of these, the great majority either promptly give up marihuana or become casual users. Most experimental casual users of marihuana, as well as those who become dependent on the drug, do not go on to opiates or other drugs. On the other hand, marihuana has been abused by most abusers of other drugs.

Effects

Marihuana acts on the central nervous system. If smoked (and depending on the amount taken), its effect, which can be felt within a few minutes, may last from four to (rarely) twelve hours. There is no physical dependence on the drug. Therefore, abrupt discontinuance of the drug does not result in withdrawal sickness. It has not yet been demonstrated that marihuana causes permanent mental or physical changes. Psycho-

---

[87] The early settlers in this country planted hemp in the soil of the colonies. They reaped the hemp and made rope from it. During the Second World War, the weed was planted in six Midwestern states. It was feared that the Philippine source of hemp would be lost to the Japanese. The weed was needed not to relieve the stress of war but for rope.

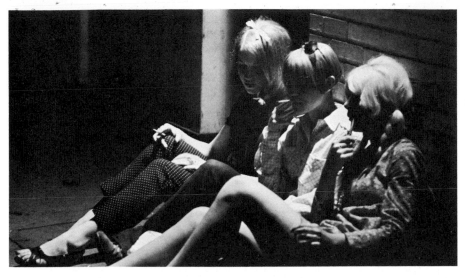

12-8 High school girls sneaking a smoke.

logical dependence does occur. Development of tolerance is slight. There is thus little or no tendency to increase the dose.

Lethargy or hilarity is usual. Time, space, or body image may be distorted. Intensification of visual and auditory stimuli occurs. A user "may meditate on the beauties of art, nature and music or he may inexplicably step out of an eighteenth story window to pick up a butterfly on the lawn below."[88] Depersonalization may occur. "One user relates . . . I float up and up and up until I'm miles above the earth. Then, Baby, I begin to come apart. My fingers leave my hands, my hands leave my wrists, my arms and legs leave my body."[89] To a varying degree, inhibitions are lost. Impairment of judgment and memory, instability, and confusion are common. "Persons high on marihuana have subtle difficulties in speech, primarily in remembering from moment to moment the logical thread of what is being said. Marihuana may interfere with retrieval of information from immediate memory storage in the brain."[90] One young man exemplified this phenomenon in this way:

> *I often drive my automobile when I'm high on marihuana . . . I'll come to a stop light and have a moment of panic because I can't remember whether or not I've just put my foot on the brake. Of course, when I look down, it's there, but in a second or two afterward, I can't remember having done it. In a similar way I can't recall whether I've passed a turn I want to take or whether I've made the turn.*[91]

[88] Edward R. Bloomquist, "Marijuana: Social Benefit or Social Derangement?" *California Medicine*, Vol. 106, No. 5 (May 1967), p. 348.

[89] *Ibid.*, p. 348.

[90] Andrew T. Weil and Norman E. Zinberg, "Acute Effects of Marihuana on Speech," *Nature*, Vol. 222, No. 5192 (May 3, 1969), pp. 434.

[91] *Ibid.*, p. 437.

Marihuana does not arouse the sexual instinct. It influences the sexual response, however, by permitting greater freedom of participation. Because of the time-space distortion, orgasm may seem more prolonged and intense than usual.

Repeated administration or high doses of the drug may result in hallucinations, illusions, and delusions. These predispose the individual to antisocial behavior marked by aggressiveness, intellectual derangement, and insomnia. With some unstable individuals, even a small amount of marihuana may induce a transient psychosis (see below). Usually recovery occurs within a few days. Occasionally a marihuana-triggered psychosis may last for several months.[92] This is very rare.

The increased hunger caused by marihuana is due to the drop in blood sugar. About sixty percent of those who chronically smoke marihuana experience a marked (and sometimes ravenous) increase in appetite. Chronic bronchitis and asthma, engorgement of the lining of the eyes (conjunctivitis) and throat are other common complications.

MARIHUANA-INDUCED PSYCHOSES: A STUDY OF U.S. SOLDIERS IN VIETNAM By 1969, marihuana smoking had become exceedingly common among U.S. troops in Vietnam. Aside from other considerations, a combat soldier under the influence of marihuana is at a gross disadvantage in a war zone. Hallucinating, he can no more be expected to avoid a land mine than some civilians in the same condition can drive an automobile. "The Vietnamese war is surely the first in which the army has been more concerned with marihuana than in the venereal diseases." Recently Talbott and Teague[93] reported twelve cases of acute toxic psychosis occurring among U.S. soldiers (from 1967 to 1968) that were clearly associated with the use of cannabis derivatives. In all but one case, more than one psychiatrist made the diagnosis. Several important factors emphasized by these writers enter into the consideration of this report:

1. The stress of combat in Vietnam is unique. That these cases occurred in that ecosystem is significant. Although their stress is less severe, most marihuana smokers seek to escape tension that, to them, is considerable.

2. An individual, here or in Vietnam, undergoing an adverse marihuana reaction is usually treated with the patience that is accorded a person who has taken too much alcohol. Only when symptoms are severe or persistent is medical help sought.

3. Unless a marihuana cigarette filling is removed or the cigarette is smoked, Vietnamese marihuana is so skillfully disguised in U.S. cigarette packs that it cannot be distinguished from an ordinary cigarette.

4. Vietnamese marihuana has a much higher concentration of active resin than that sold in this country. This may account for the greater number of psychoses associated with its use.

5. Half of all Vietnamese marihuana is polluted with opium.

[92] William H. McGlothin, "Cannabis," in David Solomon, ed., *The Marihuana Papers* (New York, 1966), p. 414.

[93] John A. Talbott and James W. Teague, "Marihuana Psychosis," *Journal of the American Medical Association*, Vol. 210, No. 2 (October 13, 1969), pp. 299–302.

6. In this country, psychotic behavior directly resulting from marihuana smoking is very rarely noted or reported.

With these points in mind consider this case:

CASE 2—*A 19-year-old, single, white soldier, private first class, was referred for examination by another psychiatrist. He was alleged to have shot and killed an individual while on guard duty.*

Sworn statements and a formal judicial investigation revealed that while on guard duty the victim shared a "marihuana cigarette" with the subject, the subject's first. The victim was described as a joker whose humor was sometimes "a little sick and cruel." Shortly after having the cigarette the victim began to pick on some nearby Vietnamese children. He reportedly told them that he was "Ho Chi Minh" and fired his weapon near them. Although the subject questioned if he was Ho Chi Minh, when the victim showed him the name on his shirt, the subject became terrified and fired his rifle. He then left his guard post and entered the base camp in a confused fashion, saying that he had killed Ho Chi Minh. Upon saying this he displayed a T-shirt with that name written on it and urged those around him to accompany him to see the body. On the way, he spoke in a disjointed and confused fashion. Upon arrival at the guard post, actually an observation tower, the bare-chested body of a Negro soldier, with several gunshot wounds on the left anterior [front] portion of the chest, was found. Due to the subject's confused state and his bizarre story, he was taken to the division psychiatrist.

Upon examination the patient was confused and apprehensive, but quite proud, in a patriotic manner, of having killed Ho Chi Minh. When confronted with the fact that the individual killed was an American Negro soldier, the subject held up the bloody, bullet-torn T-shirt, with Ho Chi Minh written across the chest, and stated rather emphatically that he had shot Ho Chi Minh, not an American soldier. He stated that the victim had told him that he was Ho Chi Minh, that the victim was disguised and had infiltrated American lines, and had proved his identity by showing his name written on the shirt. The subject then believed him, became scared, shot him, and took the T-shirt back to camp to prove that he had indeed shot and killed Ho Chi Minh. The psychiatrist's opinion was that the subject was delusional and suffering from an acute toxic psychosis, one of us (J.W.T.) concurred at a later examination.

Further examination revealed no evidence of hallucinations nor any other indication of a thought disorder. The subject was concerned and became increasingly anxious with any mention of the victim being an American soldier. He was apprehensive and unable to understand why no one believed him. He was puzzled at being seen by a psychiatrist rather than being treated as a hero for having killed Ho Chi Minh.

TABLE 12-4 Marihuana Psychoses Among U.S. Soldiers in Vietnam, 1967–68: Twelve Cases

CASE NO.	AGE	FIRST EXPOSURE TO MARIHUANA	PHYSICAL SYMPTOMS	IMPAIRED COGNITIVE FUNCTIONING	MENTAL SYMPTOMS	DELUSIONS	PREMORBID PERSONALITY	DURATION OF SYMPTOMS
1	26	+*	+	+	Paranoid, anxious	+	−	36 hours
2	19	+	+	+	Paranoid	+	−	3 days
3	24	+	+	+	Paranoid, anxious	+	Aggressive	7 days
4	21	+	+	+	Paranoid	+	Psychopathic	2 days
5	20	+	+	+	Paranoid	+	−	2–3 days
6	22	+	+	+	Anxious	−	−	1 day
7	21	+	+	+	Anxious	−	−	2 days
8	21	+	+	+	Paranoid	+	−	3 days
9	22	+	+	+	Suicidal, paranoid	+	−	11 days
10	22	+	+	+	Anxious, paranoid	+	−	2 days
11	19	+	+	+	Anxious, paranoid	+	−	3 days
12	19	+	+	+	Paranoid	+	−	2 days

* + indicated positive; −, negative.

Source: Adapted from John A. Talbott and James W. Teague, "Marihuana Psychosis," *Journal of the American Medical Association*, Vol. 210, No. 2 (October 13, 1969), p. 300.

Following a short period of hospitalization, the subject's condition changed and he evidenced grief and depression about the preceding events.

Contact with this individual continued over the next several months without any further signs of psychotic thinking or behavior. It should be noted that the subject also stated that upon first smoking the cigarette containing cannabis derivatives he experienced a burning-like irritation and an urge to cough. In addition to this he noted some mild sensations of choking and transient tingling in his extremities.[94]

[94] *Ibid.*, pp. 300–01.

The cases of psychoses among soldiers that were due to marihuana consumed in a stress environment are summarized in Table 12-4. Note that these were all first exposures. Only two had previous psychiatric histories (premorbid personalities). Physical symptoms included burning and irritation of the respiratory tract, an urge to cough, irritation of the conjunctivae, and poor coordination. Among the features of the diminished cognition (awareness, understanding, perception) were impairments as to time and place as well as to memory and attention span.

Marihuana and the law

Marihuana is not a narcotic. It does not depress the individual. Nevertheless, its control in this country is under narcotics laws. In California alone, scores of new arrests for marihuana violations are recorded each month. These usually involve persons with no previous record of drug abuse. Considerable and responsible opinion recommends constructive review of some existing drug laws so that they do "not routinely make felons out of students seeking a new thrill."[95] Testifying before the Senate subcommittee to investigate juvenile delinquency, the Director of the National Institute of Mental Health stated that marihuana "should not be associated with narcotics—either medically or legally."[96] One of the indirect effects of marihuana is that the user deals with an illicit segment of society. On the other hand, there is no direct evidence linking marihuana to crime.[97]

ARGUMENTS PRO AND CON   Various arguments are offered in favor of legalizing marihuana. What are they? How do they stand up under examination?

1. *Marihuana is no more harmful than legal alcohol.* This is probably true, although it has not been completely proven. Certainly marihuana and alcohol have comparable effects. However, alcohol is deeply rooted in Western culture. Indeed, for many it is part of a religious sacrament. The societal cost, moreover, of legal alcohol is at least five million emotional and physical cripples. Society seems willing to pay this price. But marihuana is foreign to this culture. Why add millions of possible problems to the society?

2. *Legal tobacco is more harmful than marihuana.* No responsible observer can ignore the tobacco disaster. However, there are considerable differences between the use of marihuana and tobacco. Tobacco can be smoked without danger to others and while the smoker is engaged in other activity. It produces neither erratic nor unproductive behavior. Dependence on others, reduced energy and motivation, decreased participation

[95] Neil L. Chayet, "Law, Medicine and LSD," *New England Journal of Medicine,* Vol. 277, No. 5 (August 3, 1967), p. 254.
[96] "Pinning Down the Weed," *Science News,* Vol. 96, No. 13 (September 27, 1969), p. 263.
[97] Leonard M. Zunin, "Marijuana: The Drug and the Problem," *Military Medicine,* Vol. 134, No. 2 (February 1969), p. 109.

in the societal order—these are characteristic of chronic marihuana, not tobacco, abusers. Tobacco affects primarily the user. Marihuana may harm the abuser's associates. For example: while smoking tobacco one can drive a car; marihuana produces hallucinations,[98] which certainly preclude such activity. Tobacco, moreover, does not lower inhibitions. Marihuana does.

3. *It's nobody else's business!* There is no such thing as a purely private vice. "He who overindulges . . . with respect to drugs . . . alters the lives of others . . . he is unavailable for civic obligation."[99] Society must pay heavily for the cost of individual social derelictions.

4. *People of other countries use marihuana without problems.* This is not true. The use of marihuana is now legally restricted in practically every civilized country in the world. African nations are searching for better methods of control. Indeed, for growing and distributing marihuana in some parts of Africa the death penalty may be incurred. After twenty-five centuries of use, during which cannabis became part of her religious life, India has undertaken a program aimed at the elimination of her "pot skid rows." (Moreover, the United States is a cosigner of the United Nations treaty controlling marihuana. To legalize the drug, this nation would have to abrogate its treaty.)[100]

5. *Since marihuana is cheaper and quicker than alcohol, and does not cause physical dependence, it will drive the alcohol industry out of business.* This argument is invalid. During the years of legally available bhang, India had serious alcohol enforcement problems.

6. *In the doses ordinarily taken in this country, marihuana is harmless.* Here one is faced with the changing meaning of the word "ordinary." Stronger preparations of marihuana are reported to have caused India countless problems varying from indolence to insanity. Is there any guarantee that more potent marihuana preparations will not reach this country? Hardly. The active principle of marihuana is thought to be tetrahydrocannabinol (THC). Tablets alleged to contain this chemical and to be as potent as five marihuana cigarettes are available in Canada.[101]

Marihuana is a problem. In some areas, drugs (especially marihuana) are hardly strangers to the college campus. Despite this, "constructive idealism is the badge of youth. Society renews itself from the oncoming generation. Liberty and order rest more upon the harnessing of adventurous insights than on a mere repetition of ancient patterns."[102] If this society is to solve its drug problems, it will have to look to its young people to participate in that solution.

[98] Martin H. Keeler, "Marihuana Induced Hallucinations," *Diseases of the Nervous System*, Vol. 29, No. 5 (May 1968), pp. 314–15.

[99] Charles E. Wyzanski, Jr., "Marijuana: It's Up to the Young to Solve the Problem," *New Republic*, Vol. 157, No. 17 (October 21, 1967), p. 16.

[100] Sidney Cohen, "Pot, Acid and Speed," *Medical Science*, Vol. 19, No. 2 (February 1968), p. 33.

[101] Lionel P. Solursh and Wilfrid R. Clement, "Hallucinogenic Drug Abuse: Manifestations and Management," *Canadian Medical Association Journal*, Vol. 98, No. 8 (February 24, 1968), p. 409.

[102] Charles E. Wyzanski, Jr., "Marijuana: It's Up to the Young to Solve the Problem," p. 16.

Tobacco: drug dependence in a class by itself

"A filthie noveltie . . . A custome lothsome to the eye, hatefull to the nose, harmefull to the braine, dangerous to the Lungs, and in the black stinking fume thereof, neerest resembling the horrible Stigian smoke of the pit that's bottomlesse." [103]

Some historical notes

There is no evidence of ancient Greek, Roman, or German smoking. In West Indian, Central American, and Mexican antiquity, Mayan Indian relics testify to the use of tobacco. In a report dated 1497, a priest, Romano Pane, first described the habit. The Indians inhaled smoke through a Y-shaped pipe called a "tabaco." The two forks of the Y fitted into their nostrils.

Tobacco was the first commercial export from the New World to the Old. Without it, the colonization of Virginia might have been long delayed. First explored by Sir Walter Raleigh (who enjoyed a pipe of tobacco before going to the scaffold in 1618), the colony was constantly threatened by disease, hunger, and Indian attack. Nevertheless, it prevailed. How? The gallant Captain John Smith made friends with the Indians. And food came from England. Most important, however, John Rolfe, the settler who married the Indian princess Pocahontas, discovered a method of curing tobacco. In England, despite the bitter antagonism of James I, demand for the leaf grew. Still the lonely Virginians were unhappy. Then a major problem was solved. Ninety marriageable girls were sent to them from London. The settlers, mostly young men, paid only traveling expenses. Since tobacco took the place of money, from 120 to 150 pounds of good Virginia leaf were traded for each girl.[104]

James and his supporters persisted in their opposition to tobacco. Darkly, they suggested that it caused impotence:

It dulls the sprite, it dims the sight,
It robs a woman of her right.[105]

In those days, the Russians whipped tobacco smokers or slit their noses. In 1642, a Papal Bull exorcised "infecting the churches with . . . noxious fumes."[106] Excommunication was threatened.

But nothing stopped smoking. Today, the threat of possible death fails to accomplish this.

Why do people smoke?

Curiosity probably prompts the average adolescent to start smoking. To prove his adult status, he continues despite his initial distaste. The young mimic becomes a rebel. Smoking demonstrates resistance to

[103] James I of England, in *A Counterblaste to Tobacco* (1604), cited in E. Corti, *A History of Smoking,* tr. by Paul England (London, 1931), p. 83.
[104] *Ibid.,* p. 92.
[105] C. M. Fletcher *et al., Common Sense About Smoking* (Baltimore, 1963), p. 81.
[106] E. Corti, *A History of Smoking,* p. 129.

parental authority. But no single theory can account for the eventual profound hold of tobacco on the young person. Nor will any single theory of cure help break the habit.

Some aspects of the origins of tobacco dependency merit particular mention.

Emotional roots

Even in the womb's security, an unborn baby may suck his thumb (see Figure 10-4). At birth, and before the cord is cut, the newborn may pop a thumb into his mouth. To eat, healthy babies must suck. Many babies normally continue to suck after their hunger is satiated. Sucking, then, is a basic instinctive need of the infant, a drive associated with the mother's warmth, with food, with security. Some babies are more avid suckers than others, rejecting cup and spoon, weaning late. A child to whom sucking is not so important may be weaned earlier. Others wait three years or longer. A content child, satisfied with his early sucking experience, will usually venture easily into the next phase. An insecure child, not satiated by his sucking experience, perhaps because of a constantly agitated mother, will only reluctantly part with early comforts. Sucking can become excessive. This is seen with older children who continuously suck their thumbs or with chain-smokers.

The infant relieves the pain of hunger by sucking the nipple. The child finds succor with a blanket or thumb. The adult drags on a cigarette or pipe. This can be a continuous behavior pattern, a prolonged emotional shelter.

"Sucking or smoking, therefore, is innately capable of reducing the negative effect of distress and of evoking the positive aspect of enjoyment . . . Many adults experience distress frequently enough every day to seek to reduce this distress by smoking."[107]

Economic aspects of smoking

The tobacco industry employs about 100,000 people, and sales of tobacco and tobacco products amount to several billion dollars a year. These products are a major source of government revenue: in the fiscal year ending June 1965, the federal government collected tobacco taxes totaling more than $2 billion, and the states collected $1.2 billion. For the individual smoker, the habit is expensive indeed, running into many thousands of dollars over a lifetime.

Tobacco advertising constitutes but a small percentage of total advertising in this country. Nevertheless, it involves large sums of money: about $31 million in magazine ads, $26 million in radio ads, and $170 million in TV ads annually. Does advertising induce people to smoke or increase a smoker's consumption of tobacco products? One communications expert

[107] Silvan S. Tomkins, "Psychological Model for Smoking Behavior," *American Journal of Public Health,* Vol. 56, No. 12 (December 1966, supplement), p. 18.

recently wrote that "advertising does not sell many cigarettes."[108] It may be that advertising merely affects the sale of particular brands without increasing the total number of cigarettes bought. Czechoslovakian and Italian experience supports this statement. Despite minimal advertising, cigarette consumption in both countries increased. However, the precise relationship between advertising and smoking is not known. Those people in this country who are pressing for the abolition of all cigarette advertising are particularly concerned about the possible influence of ads on would-be smokers, especially children.

Social aspects of smoking

Some people smoke to feel more intimately a part of a convivial group, to share a relaxing group activity. For others, a cigarette provides a protective smokescreen in an uncomfortable social situation such as a party at which the smoker feels ill at ease. For still others, smoking provides an outlet for the tensions of a busy world. These are but a few of the social aspects of smoking.

What specific human harm comes of tobacco smoking? Before examining the evidence, one must visualize the airway system.

Inhaled air traverses the nasal and (if the mouth is open) oral cavities, passes the *pharynx* to the *larynx,* and reaches the hollow, stiff *respiratory tree* (see Figure 12-9 and body charts 11 and 12 in the color section). This is indeed a tree, but upside down, with its branches spreading out on each side of the chest cavity.

The normal respiratory tree

The main trunk, the four-inch-long *trachea* (windpipe) divides into two main branches, the *bronchi* (singular, *bronchus*). Division and subdivision continue until tiny twigs are reached called the *bronchioles*. These end in thin-walled air sacs, the *alveoli* (see Figures 12-9 and 12-11). There, through the capillary network embedded in the alveolar walls, oxygen is absorbed into the blood and carbon dioxide is eliminated. The oxygen from the inhaled air is carried in the blood from the lungs to the heart through the pulmonary veins, and it reaches the rest of the body via the aorta, the great artery from the heart. The carbon dioxide has been delivered to the alveolar capillary network through the pulmonary arteries, which feed blood to the lungs from the heart. The carbon dioxide is expelled from the alveolar capillaries when breath is exhaled.

The trachea and bronchi are kept rigid and open by regularly spaced, C-shaped rings of hard fibrous tissue called *cartilage*. The bronchioles, however, are not held open by cartilage but by *elastic fibers*. Thus, they get larger with inhaling and smaller with exhalation.

Covering the whole respiratory tract, from nose to bronchioles, is a thin, moving film of mucus. Every day about three ounces of mucus are pro-

[108]Frederic C. Decker, "The Economic Effect of Reduced Cigarette Consumption on Advertising," *American Journal of Public Health,* Vol. 56, No. 12 (December 1966, supplement), p. 30.

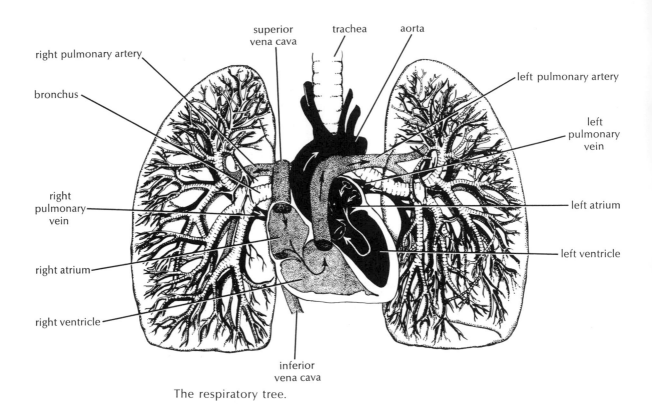

The respiratory tree.

12-9 The respiratory system

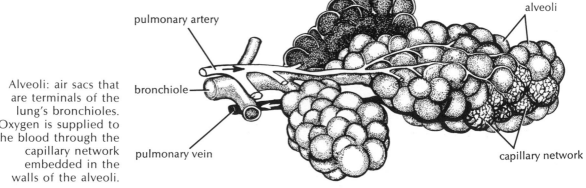

Alveoli: air sacs that are terminals of the lung's bronchioles. Oxygen is supplied to the blood through the capillary network embedded in the walls of the alveoli.

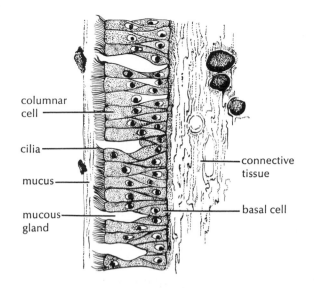

columnar cell

cilia

mucus

mucous gland

connective tissue

basal cell

Respiratory epithelium resting on connective tissue. When the surface layer of epithelial cells is damaged, the damaged cells are cast off and replaced by upgrowing deeper cells, which grow cilia when they reach the surface. Although the epithelial cells lie at different levels, they all reach the underlying connective tissue and are in contact with the nerves in connective tissue, which control the beat of the cilia. The columnar cells reach the connective tissue by narrowing. The cells of this type of respiratory epithelium are found throughout the entire respiratory tract except in the alveoli and in the smallest air passages leading directly to the alveoli. The extremely thin epithelium in the alveoli is unlike the rest of the respiratory epithelium to permit an efficient exchange of oxygen and carbon dioxide gases. In addition, cilia are absent in the passage of the vocal cords. Were they present there, voice production would be hampered. Therefore, this passage is cleared by clearing the throat or by a slight cough.

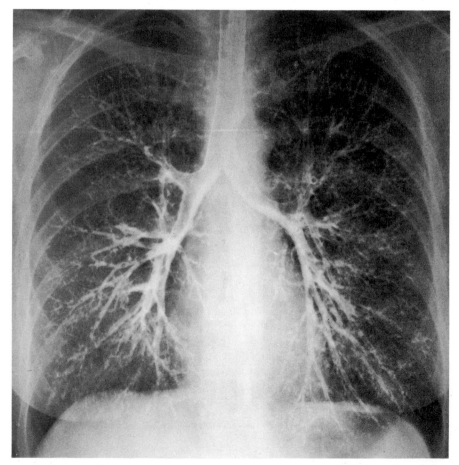

A bronchogram, an X-ray of the lungs taken after instilling an opaque medium in the bronchus.

duced by glands in the lining of the air passages. The mucus is kept moving towards the throat by countless sweeping, hairlike *cilia*. Like millions of tiny brooms, the cilia project from the lining of the bronchial tubes (see Figure 12-9). The moving mucus blanket keeps the air passages moist and protects them. Inhaled dust, germs, and other foreign particles stick to the mucus blanket and are swept away by the ciliary brooms. Anything that interferes with ciliary action interferes with the normal housekeeping of the respiratory system.

Smoking and sickness

On January 11, 1964, *Smoking and Health,* the report of the Advisory Committee to the Surgeon General of the Public Health Service, was released. In 1967, a second report, *The Health Consequences of Smoking,* was made available by the Surgeon General, and supplements to it were issued in 1968 and 1969. The later reports reinforce the first one. What are some of the findings?

1. Because of illness, cigarette smokers spend over a third again as much time away from their jobs as persons who never smoke. Women who smoke are sick in bed 17 percent more than women who never smoke.[109]

2. Total death rates for cigarette smokers are nearly 70 percent higher than for nonsmokers. Heavier smoking means higher death rates. For example, with those smoking forty or more cigarettes daily, the death rate rises to 120 percent more than that of nonsmokers.[110] The ratio of smoker to nonsmoker death rates is greatest in the precious peak years, forty to fifty.[111] Furthermore, "life expectancy among young men is reduced by an average of 8 years in 'heavy' cigarette smokers, those who smoke over two packs a day, and an average of 4 years in 'light' cigarette smokers, those who smoke less than one-half pack per day."[112]

3. The death rates from cancers of the lung, larynx, oral cavity, esophagus, kidney, urinary bladder, and pancreas are all markedly higher with smokers than nonsmokers.[113]

The earlier smoking is started, the sooner death occurs. Children are mimics. The impact of advertising, the example of parents and others important to the child, the child's search for symbols of maturity—all combine to impress the pre–teen-ager with a favorable picture of the smoker.[114] The rapid increase of smoking among high school students has led to recommendations that education against smoking begin no later than the third grade.[115]

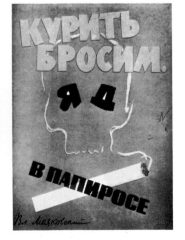

12-10 "Stop smoking. Tobacco is a poison": a Russian poster.

[109] *Smoking and Illness* (1967), prepared by the National Clearinghouse for Smoking and Health, Public Health Service, and based on a report issued by the National Center for Health Statistics, *Cigarette Smoking and Health Characteristics.*
[110] *Smoking and Health* (1964), Report of the Advisory Committee to the Surgeon General of the Public Health Service, "Summary of Research,"
[111] *Ibid.,* "Summary and Conclusions."
[112] *The Health Consequences of Smoking,* 1969 Supplement to the 1967 Public Health Service Review, "Summary of the Report," p. 1.
[113] *The Health Consequences of Smoking,* 1968 Supplement, pp. 94–106.
[114] Charles L. Leedham, "Pre-Teen Smokers," *Clinical Pediatrics,* Vol. 6, No. 3 (March 1967), p. 135.
[115] Eva J. Salber and Theodor Abelin, "Smoking Behavior of Newton School Children," *Pediatrics,* Vol. 30, No. 3 (September 1967), p. 371.

TABLE 12-5 Causes of Death of Current Male Cigarette Smokers

Excess Deaths and Percentage Elevation of Death Rates Compared to Males Who Never Smoked

CAUSE OF DEATH	OBSERVED DEATHS AMONG CURRENT CIGARETTE SMOKERS	EXPECTED DEATHS*	NUMBER OF EXCESS DEATHS (observed minus expected)	PERCENTAGE OF EXCESS DEATHS DUE TO SPECIFIED CAUSE	MORTALITY RATIO (observed divided by expected)	PERCENTAGE ELEVATION OF DEATH RATE COMPARED TO NONSMOKERS (excess divided by expected, multiplied by 100)
Coronary heart diseases	1,380	860.0	520	35.8%	$\frac{1,380}{860.0} = 1.60$	$\frac{520}{860.0} \times 100 = 60\%$
Other heart and circulatory diseases	674	359.7	314	21.6%	$\frac{674}{359.7} = 1.87$	$\frac{314}{359.7} \times 100 = 87\%$
Total: Heart and circulatory diseases	2,054	1,219.7	834	57.4%	$\frac{2,054}{1,219.7} = 1.68$	$\frac{834}{1,219.7} \times 100 = 68\%$
Lung cancer	325	21.8	303	20.9%	$\frac{325}{21.8} = 14.91$	$\frac{303}{21.8} \times 100 = 1,391\%$
Bronchitis and emphysema	115	13.2	102	7.0%	$\frac{115}{13.2} = 8.71$	$\frac{102}{13.2} \times 100 = 771\%$
Total: Major lung diseases	440	35.0	405	27.9%	$\frac{440}{35.0} = 12.57$	$\frac{405}{35.0} \times 100 = 1,157\%$
All other causes	1,659	1,446.1	213	14.7%	$\frac{1,659}{1,446.1} = 1.15$	$\frac{213}{1,446.1} \times 100 = 15\%$
TOTAL: ALL CAUSES	4,153	2,700.8	1,452	100.0%	$\frac{4,153}{2,700.8} = 1.54$	$\frac{1,452}{2,700.8} \times 100 = 54\%$

*Based on the age-specific death rates of men who never smoked.

Source: Adapted from E. W. R. Best *et al.*, "Summary of a Canadian Study of Smoking and Health," *Canadian Medical Association Journal*, Vol. 96 (April 15, 1967), p. 1106.

Table 12-5 presents the results of a Canadian study demonstrating the elevation of death rates from various diseases of smokers as compared to nonsmokers.

Emphysema and chronic bronchitis

The smoke from cigarette combustion produces gases that paralyze cilia. Mucus cannot move. In the bronchioles, a traffic jam is created. How? With inhaling, the bronchioles expand. Air can squeeze in past the unmoving mucus. But as air is exhaled, the bronchioles diminish in size. They clamp down on the trapped, accumulated mucus. Air cannot get out. It stretches the air sacs (alveoli). These balloon. They form large air blisters. Some rupture. Lung tissue is destroyed (see Figure 12-11). Breathing efficiency is diminished. To accommodate the damaged, overstretched lung, the entire bony chest cage enlarges. Then the diaphragm, the breath-

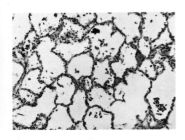

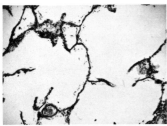

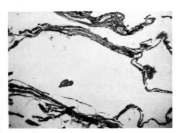

12-11 Normal lung alveoli (*top*), alveoli partly destroyed (*center*), and extensively destroyed alveoli (*bottom*).

ing muscle separating the chest and abdomen, loses efficiency. All this is *emphysema.*

Emphysema is generally seen in conjunction with a *chronic bronchitis.* The accumulation of mucus and the paralysis of cilia combine to prevent the elimination of germs. These, in turn, infect the bronchial tubes.

"Cigarette smoking is the most important cause of chronic bronchitis . . . [and] evidence indicates that cigarette smoking is the most important agent in the development of pulmonary emphysema in man."[116] Moreover, "for chronic bronchitis and emphysema . . . the death rate for cigarette smokers is 500 percent higher than for nonsmokers."[117]

Smoking and cancer

"Carcinoma of the lips occurs most frequently where men indulge in pipe smoking: the lower lip is particularly affected by cancer, when it is compressed between the tobacco pipe and the teeth."[118] This was written one hundred and seventy-five years ago. In our own time, the study of cancer and smoking has taken on new urgency. The following statement was issued by the Public Health Service in July 1969:

> *Additional evidence substantiates the previous findings that cigarette smoking is the main cause of lung cancer in men. Cigarette smoking is causally related to lung cancer in women but accounts for a smaller proportion of cases than in men. Smoking is a significant factor in the causation of cancer of the larynx and in the development of cancer of the oral cavity. Further epidemiological data strengthen the association of cigarette smoking with cancer of the bladder and cancer of the pancreas.*[119]

The relationship between smoking and lung cancer has been intensively studied. These are some of the findings: (1) The average male cigarette smoker has nine to ten times the chance of the nonsmoker of developing lung cancer. For heavy smokers this risk doubles.[120] (2) If smoking is discontinued, the risk of dying from lung cancer sharply decreases.[121] (3) Since 1930, the lung cancer death rate in women has increased over 400 percent. Compared to the increase in the male lung cancer rate, after 1960, there was noted a "greater relative rise in mortality from lung cancer in the female population."[122] This increase continues. (4) Only one of twenty diagnosed lung cancers is now cured.[123] Of all the common malignancies,

[116] *The Health Consequences of Smoking,* 1969 Supplement, "Smoking and Chronic Obstructive Broncho-pulmonary Disease," pp. 1, 3.
[117] *Smoking and Health* (1964), "Summary and Conclusions," p. 29.
[118] S. Th. Sömmering, "De Moribus Vasorum Absorbentium Corporis Humani," 1795, p. 109, tr. in Ernest L. Wynder and Dietrich Hoffman, *Tobacco and Tobacco Smoke* (New York, 1967), p. 1.
[119] *The Health Consequences of Smoking,* 1969 Supplement, "Summary of the Report," p. 2.
[120] *Smoking and Health* (1964), "Summary and Conclusions," p. 31.
[121] *The Health Consequences of Smoking,* 1969 Supplement, "Smoking and Cancer," p. 1.
[122] *The Health Consequences of Smoking,* 1968 Supplement, p. 97.
[123] Alton Blakeslee, *It's Not Too Late to Stop Smoking Cigarettes,* Public Affairs Pamphlet No. 386 (New York, 1966), pp. 10–12.

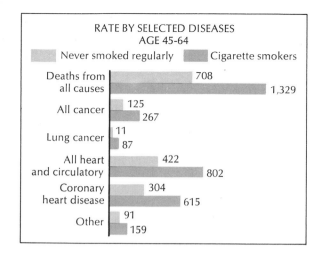

RATE BY SELECTED DISEASES
AGE 45-64

Never smoked regularly · Cigarette smokers

Disease	Never smoked regularly	Cigarette smokers
Deaths from all causes	708	1,329
All cancer	125	267
Lung cancer	11	87
All heart and circulatory	422	802
Coronary heart disease	304	615
Other	91	159

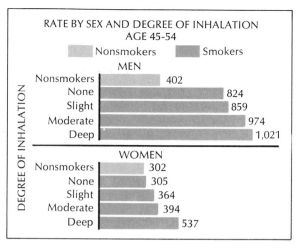

RATE BY SEX AND DEGREE OF INHALATION
AGE 45-54

Nonsmokers · Smokers

DEGREE OF INHALATION

MEN

Nonsmokers	402
None	824
Slight	859
Moderate	974
Deep	1,021

WOMEN

Nonsmokers	302
None	305
Slight	364
Moderate	394
Deep	537

Source: E. C. Hammond, *Smoking in Relation to Death Rates of One Million Men and Women* (1966).

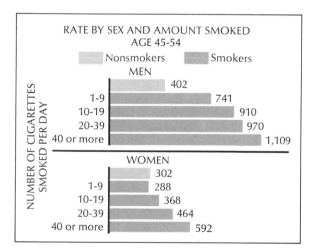

RATE BY SEX AND AMOUNT SMOKED
AGE 45-54

Nonsmokers · Smokers

NUMBER OF CIGARETTES SMOKED PER DAY

MEN

	402
1-9	741
10-19	910
20-39	970
40 or more	1,109

WOMEN

	302
1-9	288
10-19	368
20-39	464
40 or more	592

12-12 Death rates (per 100,000 person-years) of smokers compared to nonsmokers.

lung cancer offers by far the least hope of cure (see page 211). (5) The microscopic appearance of about 100,000 specimens of lung tissue (taken from people who had either died or were undergoing lung surgery) was correlated with smoking history. The results:[124]

Those who had never smoked had normal lung tissue.

"Pre-cancerous lesions" were found in proportion to the amount of cigarette smoking.

The tissue of those who had smoked and stopped showed less lung disease changes. Reversibility is possible when smoking is stopped.

If smoking continues, pre-cancerous cells go on to malignancy. Deeper tissue is invaded. The changes then do not reverse. Man suffers few illnesses so presently incurable as cancer of the lung.

[124] *Ibid.,* p. 10.

Cigarette smoking: the heart and blood vessels[125]

Increasing evidence suggests "that cigarette smoking can contribute to the development of cardiovascular disease and particularly to death from coronary heart disease . . . Some of the harmful cardiovascular effects appear to be reversible after cessation of cigarette smoking."[126] Depending on other risk factors (such as high blood pressure and high serum cholesterol), the death rate of cigarette-smoking males is from 70 to 200 percent higher than that of nonsmoking males. And the tragedy of these figures is deepened by the fact that it is the young smoker who dies more often. "Additional evidence . . . indicates that young smokers between the ages of forty-five and fifty-four have the highest mortality ratios—three times as great for men, and twice as great for women, if they smoke ten or more cigarettes per day, as compared to nonsmokers."[127]

How does tobacco affect the heart? Indications are that nicotine may cause an increased heart muscle need for oxygen. Having created that need, cigarette smoking may nevertheless prevent its being met. By reducing the blood's ability to transfer oxygen to tissues, the carbon dioxide absorbed from smoking may cause a decrease in available oxygen. So cigarette smoking may indeed be a double blow to the heart. It is not surprising that those more susceptible to coronary disease have heart attacks more often if they smoke—and less often recover. For smoking seems to accelerate blood clot formation—a situation hardly beneficial to an individual with coronary artery malfunction. As for atherosclerosis, "autopsy studies suggest that cigarette smoking is associated with a significant increase in atherosclerosis of the aorta and the coronary arteries."[128]

Smoking and tooth loss

Periodontal disease (particularly gum inflammation, bony-tissue destruction, and loss of teeth) is much more common among smokers than nonsmokers. For example, women smokers between twenty and thirty-nine years of age have twice the chance of losing their teeth, even all their teeth, than nonsmoking women in that age group. Among men smokers, the chance of being toothless between thirty and fifty-nine years of age is double that of nonsmokers.[129]

Smoking and pregnancy

Babies born of mothers who smoke weigh, on the average, half a pound

---

[125] The material in this section is drawn from *The Health Consequences of Smoking*, Public Health Service Review, Public Health Service Publication No. 1696 (1967), pp. 25–28, and its 1968 and 1969 Supplements.

[126] *The Health Consequences of Smoking*, 1969 Supplement, "Summary of the Report," pp. 1–2.

[127] E. C. Hammond, "Smoking in Relation to the Death Rates of One Million Men and Women," quoted in *The Health Consequences of Smoking* (1967), p. 25.

[128] *The Health Consequences of Smoking*, 1969 Supplement, "Summary of the Report," p. 3.

[129] Harold A. Solomon et al., "Cigarette Smoking and Periodontal Disease," quoted in *Medical Bulletin on Tobacco*, Vol. 6, No. 4 (December 1968).

less than those born of nonsmokers.[130] For the child, this may be critical. Spontaneous abortions, stillbirths, and premature deliveries occur more frequently with mothers who smoke (see page 553).

More research is needed. One recent study[131] compared urinary excretions of nicotine by cigarette, pipe, and cigar smokers. Cigarette smokers excreted three times as much nicotine as the others. This was thought to be due to the lesser inhalation by pipe and cigar smokers. Moreover, other "evidence indicates that there is little risk of coronary heart disease associated with cigars and/or pipe smoking."[132] In addition, "there is a much smaller increase of the lung cancer death rate associated with pipe and/or cigar smoking than with cigarette smoking."[133]

Are pipes and cigars safer than cigarettes?

Another study, however, is less encouraging. It concludes this way: "heavy cigar and pipe smoking may be more hazardous than previously thought and should not be considered a safe alternative to cigarette smoking."[134] Supporting this opinion is the unduly high incidence of cancer of the lips and larynx among pipe and cigar smokers.[135]

Do filters strain out the cigarette sickness? Research workers report "no." In studying the effects of nine popular filter tip cigarettes in reducing tar and nicotine, they concluded that "cigarette filters did not offer protection against the health hazards of smoking."[136] The best tip, then, is to quit smoking.

The best tip?

The English essayist Charles Lamb rhymed: "For thy sake, tobacco, I / Would do anything but die."[137]

Every year thousands go him one better.

[130]C. S. Russel, R. Taylor, and R. N. Maddison, "Some Effects of Smoking in Pregnancy," *Journal of Obstetrics and Gynecology,* Vol. 73, No. 5 (October 1966), pp. 742–46.
[131]Alfred Kershbaum *et al.,* "Effect of Cigarette, Cigar and Pipe Smoking on Nicotine Excretion," *Archives of Internal Medicine,* Vol. 120, No. 3 (September 1967), p. 314.
[132]*The Health Consequences of Smoking* (1967), p. 25.
[133]*Ibid.,* p. 34.
[134]Theodor Abelin and Otto R. Gsell, "Relative Risk of Pulmonary Cancer in Cigar and Pipe Smokers," *Cancer,* Vol. 20, No. 8 (August 1967), pp. 1295–96.
[135]*The Health Consequences of Smoking,* (1967), p. 35.
[136]Alfred Kershbaum *et al.,* "Regular, Filter Tip and Modified Cigarettes," *Journal of the American Medical Association,* Vol. 201, No. 7 (August 14, 1967), pp. 545–46.
[137]Charles Lamb, "A Farewell to Tobacco," in *Bookman's Pleasure,* comp. by Holbrook Jackson (New York, 1947), p. 164.

13

Human overproduction and reproduction

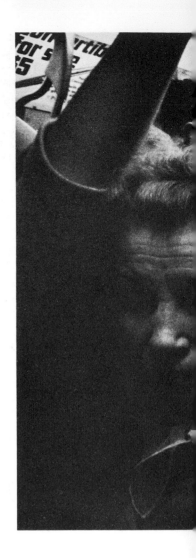

Overproduction

Pushers and peelers

Several years ago the following item appeared in the *New York Times:*

> The Japan National Railways has hired 470 more sturdy "pushers"
> to help cram long-suffering Tokyo commuters into trains already
> crowded far beyond capacity at the height of the winter crush hour.
>   The new "oshiya-san" (honorable pushers), mostly students hired
> on a part-time basis, bring to 2,500 the number stationed at key

432

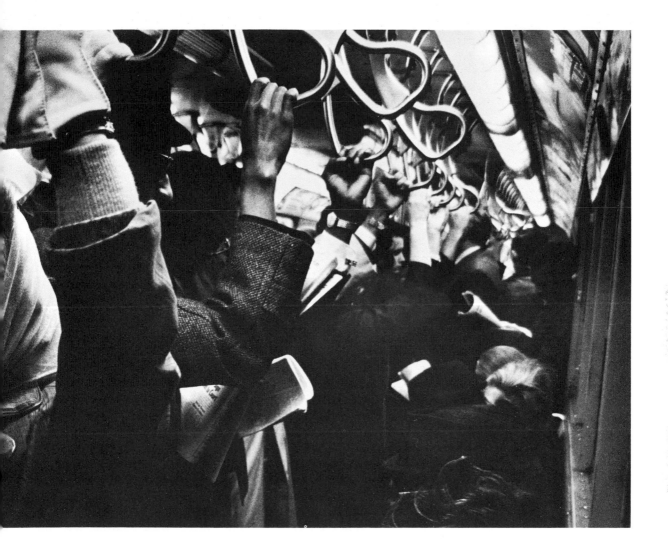

Tokyo rail points to help move an average of nearly four million commuters daily between their homes and places of work . . .

. . . The "oshiya-san" double as "hagitoriya-san"—pullers or peelers—with the frequently vital job of snatching surplus passengers out of the cars to permit the doors to close and the tight two-minute operating schedules to be maintained.[1]

With this quotation, a central problem of this era is approached. Long ago the prophet Isaiah (5:8) warned against overpopulation. Today the "pushers" and "peelers" of the elegant Japanese symbolize a world threat.

[1] *New York Times,* January 16, 1966, Sect. 1, p. 8.

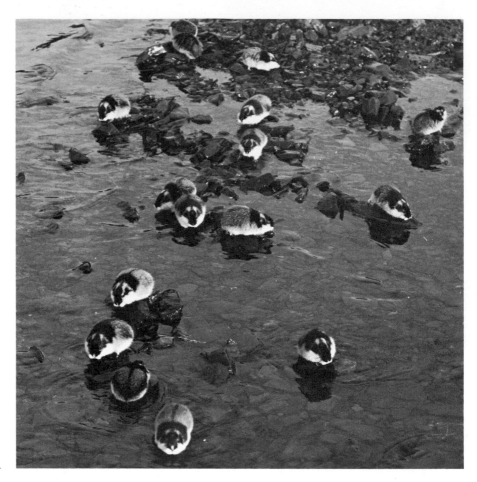

13-1 Excess lemmings.

Why is a book on health concerned with the problem? Better health is one cause of the population explosion. In the past, famine, war, and pestilence winnowed mankind. By these three fertility and mortality ratios were equated. But today communicable disease is under increasing control. The twentieth-century plague in Los Angeles killed fewer than forty people. In the fourteenth century, the same microorganism cost over forty million lives. Famine and war still threaten, but there can be only opinionated meditation about their future effect. Those spared today live to propagate tomorrow. Better health promises too large a population and, ironically, threatens health.

It is in a crowded and threatening ecosystem that man competes with other life. Only to the extent that he can best his competitors in environmental control can man hope to prevail. Man is not lacking in the capacity to reproduce. With all his sophistication, he escapes no biological laws. Nature insures multiplication (and thus survival) of humankind by providing superabundant numbers of reproductive cells. Each human ovary contains about 200,000 primitive, undeveloped eggs (*ova*). Only one is needed for conception. Each ejaculation of human semen contains 250 to 500 million spermatozoa. Only one is needed for fertilization.

In its abundance, human seed is not unique. About every twenty minutes, the bacterium *Escherichia coli* divides in two. Were a hundred percent to survive, one bacillus would, in a day and a half of such increase, film the surface of the earth several times. If unchecked and immortal, a single primitive protozoan, the tiny *Paramecium,* would, in a few quick days, produce protoplasm ten thousand times the volume of the earth. If all the progeny of one April mating of houseflies were to live, they would, by August, cover the entire earth with a layer of houseflies forty-seven feet deep. Ruthlessly nature provides for no such endurance. Why do not bacteria, paramecia, or flies inherit the earth? By limiting space and food, nature prohibits their overmultiplication. And, if these two are not enough to control the *Escherichia coli,* for example, nature sees to it that by its very increase it produces self-destructive poisons. True, resistant strains develop. These may live on to increase. Nonetheless, the wages of overcrowding are death.

More complex species have more complex methods of population limitation. The little lemming has long intrigued zoologists. Every four years, Europeans observe these rodents increase in number and then scurry straight into the ocean (see Figure 13-1). Their mass "suicide" helps limit their number. Populations of Minnesota jack rabbits rise and fall cyclically. After a rise, episodes of mass dying occur. Neither food shortages nor predators account for this. The dead jack rabbits have been examined. Their livers and other glands are diseased. They have signs of high blood pressure. Their arteries are hardened. These result from "stress sickness." Similar tensions of crowding have produced this illness in many other animals.

Human overcrowding is being studied. The pituitary-adrenal system of man responds to stress in the same fashion as that of animals. Exactly how does overcrowding contribute to a human stress syndrome? Does it directly cause sickness and death? These remain incompletely answered questions. That overcrowding contributes to social sickness is, however, undeniable.

Malthus on man

Robert Thomas Malthus was among the first to dramatically portray overpopulation as a social problem. It was an anonymous work that made him famous: *Essay on the Principle of Population as It Affects the Future Improvement of Society, with Remarks on the Speculations of Mr. Godwin, M. Condorcet and Other Writers.* The essay brought bitter attack. A calm, cheerful man, Reverend Malthus was alluded to as a gloomy parson, a prophet of doom. Both Hazlett and Dickens excoriated him. The former called him a slave to sex. The latter gave the name Malthus Gradgrind to an unpleasant character in *Hard Times.* Karl Marx accused Malthus of a plot to prevent the revolution of the masses by diminishing their numbers. As unkind a cut as any was the opprobrium hurled at him: anti-Cupid! "It is an utter misconception of my argument," he wrote mildly in the 1817 edition of his *Essay,* "to infer that I am an enemy of population. I am only an enemy of vice and misery."

The basic thesis of his book was this: human populations, like other species, can increase faster than their means of subsistence.

To support this concept, Malthus postulated that unchecked population growth increases by a geometrical progression, whereas food increases by but an arithmetical progression. In other words, people would increase as do the numbers 1, 2, 4, 8, 16, 32, 64, 128, 256, and so on. Food or subsistence, however, would progressively increase only as the numbers 1, 2, 3, 4, 5, 6, 7, 8, 9, and so on. He theorized that if the population could be assumed to double every twenty-five years, in two centuries the number of people would increase by 256 times, whereas food would increase only 9 times. In three centuries the ratio of population to food increase would be as 4,096 to 13. In time, an astronomical number of people would be fiercely foraging for a dwindling food supply. To forestall this, the Reverend urged late marriage and moral restraint. Malthus was an outspoken foe of contraceptive techniques, labeling them "improper arts to conceal the consequences of irregular connections." Without moral restraint to control population growth, Malthus warned, the miseries of vice, war, and starvation would inevitably ensue.

Many shortcomings weaken the Malthusian theory. For example, he could not recognize the vast untapped resources of the undiscovered agricultural areas of the Americas, Africa, and Oceania. Nor did Malthus consider the possibility of scientific advances increasing food productivity. He failed, moreover, to emphasize that mere reproductive power did not necessarily mean reproduction. Many peoples, including some who do not have access to the modern methods of birth control, successfully limit population.

Nevertheless, Malthus drew serious attention to a spectre.

Mankind's limited land[2]

Everything man uses comes from the land. The total land area of the earth is approximately 58 million square miles. Only 25 percent of the earth's total surface is suitable for farming. Impossible climates or unproductive soil, frequently both, force men to forgo millions of acres of land.

Much high mountain area is uninhabitable. The highest permanent habitations on earth are in Peru (17,100 feet). There, crops are not grown at altitudes over 14,000 feet. People live by grazing sheep, alpacas, and llamas. Some high tropical areas have a friendly climate (Mexico City is over a mile high). However, earth's mountainous land is only about 5 percent arable.

[2]Langdon White, "Geography and the World's Population," in Stuart Mudd, ed., *The Population Crisis and the Use of World Resources* (The Hague, 1964), pp. 16–25.

About 17 percent of the land area of earth is desert. In it lives less than 3 percent of the world's population. Little desert land is now cultivated. Someday, perhaps, desalination and other projects will bend desert areas to man's will. The ingenuity of scientists (such as Israel's Duvdevani) has turned some deserts into gardens. On a more inclusive scale such accomplishment, however, is unlikely. It is estimated that "even when the small 'islands' made productive by irrigation are added, the world's deserts probably have not more than two to five percent of their total areas cultivable."[3]

Cold lands take up about 29 percent of the surface of this planet. Antarctica is almost twice the size of the United States. Not one single human being lives there permanently. Covering millions of square Arctic miles are the frozen, treeless landscapes of the tundras, the world's coldest areas. They offer little hope for food. Seasons without frost are short. The soil is generally infertile. Summer drainage is poor. Russia issues glowing reports of success at the agricultural stations of her tundra, but development of the tundra is still only experimental. Few Russians voluntarily migrate to them. Finland, Sweden, and Greenland have grown food in previously unused Arctic areas. But, on a considerable percentage of the world's icy wastes, the day of good crops is not even in the distant future.

Tropical rain forests are not more hospitable. The huge and almost empty Amazon Basin, for example, provides the population with but a bare subsistence. Disease, poor soil, and dense forests combine with an insufferable climate to discourage investment and migration. Exploitation of these vast areas would require more money than is presently available to any government.

Are there other, better, more distant frontiers?

Is the solution out of this world?

Much "nonsense arithmetic" about expanding population is, unfortunately, not nonsense. This chilling warning is an example:

> The current rate of [population] growth would lead to an eventual limit of some 60 quadrillion people by the year 2864. This would constitute 220 persons for each square meter of the earth's surface; to house them, the planet would be covered with continuous 2000-story buildings over land and sea alike, providing 7.5 square meters of floor space per person in 1000 stories. The other 1000 stories would be for food production and refrigeration machinery needed to pump heat to the solid outer roof skin where it would radiate directly into space. The temperature of this outer skin would rise to 2000°C . . . as regards emigration to other planets, it would be necessary to send 73 million people a year to maintain the present level of population. Even if this were possible, the solar system's presumably habitable planets would soon be filled. Venus is about the earth's size; with

[3] Ibid., p. 20.

population doubling every thirty-seven years, Venus would reach the earth's population density in that time span. Mercury, Mars and the moon together have half the same area; the excess population of earth and Venus would fill them up in another ten years.[4]

Settlement of other worlds is often mentioned as a possible solution for this world's overpopulation. First stop, the moon. Perhaps a scientific laboratory may someday be built there. It may become an interplanetary bus stop. But the recent visits to this cinder revealed little about its ecosystem to seriously invite human colonization.

Mars? Oxygen and water are incredibly rare. After nightfall, it is bitter cold. Venus? Vast clouds apparently cover this unfriendly planet. Temperatures would melt lead (800°F). In this harsh ecosystem, the atmosphere is mainly carbon monoxide. Great fog, dust storms, intense heat, bitter cold, and carbon monoxide make of Venus a huge, tropical, poisonous planet of "smog." Mercury has an impossible climate. Pluto is far and dark. Jupiter, Saturn, Uranus, and Neptune freeze. Many hundreds of millions of miles separate them from enough warmth to keep people alive. Countless other planets whirl outside earth's solar system. Some may be paradise. But, for man, no planet can be anything but a hell without a sun to warm it. The nearest sun to earth's is many millions of miles away. To arrive near it would require more years than one lifetime can afford. And the trip would have been in vain. For man's needs it warms too weakly. One would not even shiver to death, for to shiver one must first be warm. And so, should an excess of the world's population seek a nourishing home outside of this world, they would have to go on and on, careening past endless, lonely emptiness, occasionally passing faintly glimmering suns that would fail to keep any planet decently warm. Sometimes twin suns would be seen. They maintain deadly heat. After over a century of travel, the constellation Alpha Aquilae (about 94 million million miles from earth) might be reached. Maybe it maintains a kindly planet or two for human comfort. Perhaps even a vacation spot. Perhaps not. Nobody knows. But it is quite a long, even tiring, journey, and there is always the return trip to be considered.

No, it is on earth that man must seek solutions to his overpopulation problems. And he must always remain cognizant of his environmental limitations, of the confines of his ecosystem.

---

[4] *M.D., Medical Newsmagazine*, Vol. 10, No. 4 (April 1966), p. 116. A further illustration of this train of thought was provided by Carl E. Taylor: "It is possible to demonstrate mathematically that at present rates of increase we will have standing room only by 2500 A.D. or that in 5,000 years the human race will be expanding so fast that it will form a solid ball of flesh growing out into space at the speed of light." (Quoted in "Crosscurrents of Opinion," *Medical Tribune* [December 18–19, 1965], p. 7.)

But these figures point to the far-distant future. The past is no less instructive. If the current two percent per year rate of increase in the world's population "had existed from the time of Christ to the present time . . . there would be over 20 million individuals in place of each person now alive or 100 persons for each square foot." (C. L. Markert, "Biological Limits on Population Growth," cited in William D. McElroy, "Biomedical Aspects of Population Control," *BioScience*, Vol. 19, No. 1 [January 1969], p. 19.)

		TABLE 13-1 *Estimate of Births*	
		in Three Periods of Human History	
PERIOD	NUMBER OF YEARS IN PERIOD	NUMBER OF BIRTHS IN PERIOD (in billions)	AVERAGE ANNUAL RATE OF INCREASE (per 1,000 population)
600,000 B.C.– 6000 B.C.	594,000	12	0.02
6000 B.C.– A.D. 1650	7,650	42	0.6
A.D. 1650–1962	312	23	4.35

Source: Annabelle Desmond, "How Many People Have Ever Lived on Earth?" from *The Population Crisis and the Use of World Resources* (The Hague, 1964), pp. 45–46.

The arithmetic of population growth

By 1962 about 77 billion people had been born into this world (Table 13-1). By 1975 (barring a catastrophic disaster) about a billion more will have been added. Of the 78 billion people who, by 1975, will have inhabited the earth, over 95 percent will be dead. At the present rate of increase, the 1975 estimated world population will be some 4 billion (see Table 13-2). A medical wag once remarked that statistics are used by some people like a drunk uses a lamp post—more for support than for illumination. So figures must be related to meanings. If the meanings of populations figures signify trouble for mankind, then man must reason a course of action.

The seventy-six centuries from 6000 B.C. to A.D. 1650 (Table 13-1) begin with the New Stone age, sweep through the Bronze and Iron periods, go on past antiquity and the dark medieval ages and on to the Renaissance in the south of Europe and the Reformation in the north. Like a child full of questions, man entered this last age. In seeking and finding answers, he opened a Pandora's box of population problems.

The 23 billion people born during the three centuries following A.D. 1650 are almost half the number born in the seventy-six preceding centuries. In those relatively brief three hundred years, almost twice as many births occurred as in the 5,940 centuries of prehistoric times. The surge in world population of the middle seventeenth century continues today. What happened to start the increase?

Why did people grow in number?

Because man succeeded in better controlling his ecosystems. One of the most significant marks of his environmental triumph was the invention

Some general dimensions of overpopulation

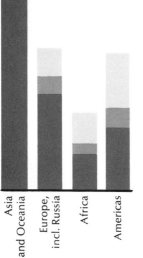

CONTINENT	POPULATION AT GIVEN TIMES (in millions)						
	1000	1600	1800	1900	1960	1975 (est.)	2000 (est.)
Asia and Oceania	165	279	599	921	1,700	2,231	3,900
Europe, including Russia	47	102	192	423	641	751	947
Africa	50	90	90	120	244	303	517
Americas	13	15	25	144	407	543	904
Total	275	486	906	1,608	2,992	3,828*	6,268

TABLE 13-2 *Estimated World Population:* A.D. *1000*–A.D. *2000*

*More recent projections indicate that world population will pass the 4 billion mark by 1975 (Population Reference Bureau press release, April 1969).

Source: Annabelle Desmond, "How Many People Have Ever Lived on Earth?" from *The Population Crisis and the Use of World Resources* (The Hague, 1964), p. 39, abstracted from *The Future Growth of World Populations; Population Studies, No. 28* (New York, 1958), p. 23.

13-2 World population: a graphic view (based on Table 13-2).

of the microscope. For, with its magnifications, man identified some of his most persistent predators. Previously invisible, these competitors of man had been totally elusive. Seen, they could be attacked.

"With the point of a needle," wrote Leeuwenhoek (see Chapter 6),

I took some . . . substance from the teeth of two ladies, who I knew were very punctual in cleaning them every day, and therein I observed . . . these animalcules . . . [In] the same substance taken from the teeth of an old gentleman, who was very careless about keeping them clean, I found an incredible number of living animalcules, swimming about more rapidly than any I had before seen, and in such numbers, that the water which contained them, (though but a small portion of the matter taken from the teeth was mixed in it) seemed to be alive.[5]

This experiment, detailed by the seventeenth-century Dutch lensgrinder, is the kind of observation that quickened a series of epochal revolutions in human history. Men wrought a scientific approach to life—and death. They looked and saw for themselves. Doors were opened to new thought and experiment. Pasteur, Freud, Koch, Ehrlich, Lister, Mendel, Semmelweiss, Einstein—all built the scientific edifice for the twentieth century. From the back of mankind they lifted a load of sickness

[5] Isabel S. Gordon and Sophie Sorkin, eds., *The Armchair Science Reader* (New York, 1959), pp. 188–89.

TABLE 13-3 *Number of Survivors at Various Attained Ages for Eighteenth-Century France, India 1941–50, and Norway 1946–50*

AGE (in years)	NUMBER OF SURVIVORS (per 1,000 births)		
	EIGHTEENTH-CENTURY FRANCE (before demographic revolution)	INDIA 1941–50 (developing)	NORWAY 1946–50 (developed)*
Birth	1,000	1,000	1,000
1	767	818	970
20	502	574	950
40	369	422	916
60	214	216	818
80	35	27	388
85	12	2	214

*These data for modern Norway, which are similar to those of other developed countries, indicate more than the advantages of modern public health programs. They emphasize that success in prolonging life brings about a need for programs for the aged (see page 591).

Source: Alfred Sauvy, *Fertility and Survival* (New York, 1961), p. 40.

and death; by so doing, they also undermined death control. For a high death rate, albeit cruel, is an efficient control of population growth. The absence of both death control and birth control quickly resulted in vast overpopulation.

With *scientific* revolution came *agricultural* change. Plant breeding, crop rotation, cultivation—these improvements wrested more food from the earth. During prehistory, man ate what was available. In the Old Stone age he developed tools to farm. In time, his most powerful tool was his mind.

Scientific, agricultural, and industrial changes brought Europe a better life. On that continent today, infant mortality is one-seventh what it was two centuries ago. In the last two centuries, life expectancy in the Western world has increased from thirty years to more than seventy. What does this mean? When babies do not die and live on to reproductive age, the seed is sown for more population.

Compare the figures for eighteenth-century France with those for modern Norway (Table 13-3). In the past two hundred years the number of survivors at age twenty has almost doubled and, at sixty, has almost quadrupled. Two hundred years ago a French baby had only a 50 percent chance of reaching reproductive adulthood. Today, that figure in Norway (and in other developed countries such as modern France and the United States) is 95 percent. Thus, in industrial nations, almost all children live

TABLE 13-4 · World Population Data for Selected Countries

REGION OR COUNTRY		Population Estimates Mid-1969 (millions)	Birth Rate (per 1,000 population)	Death Rate (per 1,000 population)	Current Rate of Population Growth[a]	Number of Years to Double Population	Infant Mortality Rate (deaths under one year per 1,000 live births)	Population Under 15 years (percent)	Population Projections[b] to 1980 (millions)	Per Capita Gross National Product (US$)[c]
AFRICA	Congo (Dem. Rep.)	17.1	43	20	2.3	31	104	39		60
	Ghana	8.6	47	20	2.5	28	156	45	12.2	230
	Kenya	10.6	50	20	3.0	23	132	46	14.6	90
	Nigeria	53.7	50	25	2.5	28		43		80
	South Africa	19.6	46		2.4	29		40	26.8	550
	Sudan	15.2	52	18-22	3.0	23		47	21.0	100
	UAR	32.5	43	15	2.9	24	120	43	46.7	160
ASIA	Ceylon	12.3	32	8	2.4	29	56	41	16.3	150
	China (Mainland)	740.3[d]	34	11	1.4	50			843.0	
	China (Taiwan)	13.8	29	6	2.6	24	20	44	17.6	230
	India	536.9	43	18	2.5	28	139	41		90
	Indonesia	115.4	43	21	2.4	29	125	42	152.8	100
	Israel	2.8	25	6.6	2.9	24	25	33		1,160
	Japan	102.1	19	6.8	1.1	63	15	25	112.9	860
	Jordan	2.3	47	16	4.1	17		46	3.3	220
	Pakistan	131.6	52	19	3.3	21	142	45	183.0	90
	Philippines	37.1	50	10-15	3.5	20	73	47	55.8	160
	South Korea	31.2	41	10-14	2.8	25		42	43.4	150
	Thailand	34.7	46	13	3.1	23	31	43	47.5	130
	Turkey	34.4	46	18	2.5	28	161	44	48.5	280
AMERICA[e]	Argentina	24.0	23	9	1.5	47	58.0	29	28.2	780
	Brazil	90.6	38	10	2.8	25	79.0	43	124.0	240
	Canada	21.3	18.0	7.3	2.0	35	23.1	33	22.3	2,240
	Chile	9.6	33	10	2.3	31	108.0	40	12.2	510
	Colombia	21.4	45	11	3.4	21	80.0	47	31.4	280
	Cuba	8.2	27	8	2.0	35	40.0	37	10.1	320
	Guatemala	5.0	43	15	2.8	25	92.0	46	6.9	320
	Mexico	49.0	43	9	3.4	21	63.0	46	71.4	470
	Puerto Rico	2.7	26	6	1.1	63	33.0	39	3.1	1,090
	United States	203.1	17.4	9.6	1.0	70	22.1	30	240.1	3,520
EUROPE	Albania	2.1	34.0	8.6	2.7	26	86.8		3.0	300
	Czechoslovakia	14.4	15.1	10.1	0.5	140	23.7	25	15.8	1,010
	East Germany	16.0	14.8	13.2	0.1	700	21.2	22	17.7	1,220
	France	50.0	16.9	10.9	1.0	70	20.6	25	53.8	1,730
	Ireland	2.9	21.1	10.7	0.5	140	24.4	31	3.5	850
	Italy	53.1	18.1	9.7	0.7	100	34.3	24	58.8	1,030
	Poland	32.5	16.3	7.7	0.8	88	38.1	30	36.6	730
	Spain	32.7	21.1	8.7	0.8	88	33.2	27	34.8	640
	Sweden	8.0	15.4	10.1	0.8	88	12.6	21	8.6	2,270
	United Kingdom	55.7	17.5	11.2	0.6	117	18.8	23	60.2	1,620
	West Germany	58.1	17.3	11.2	0.4	175	23.5	23	61.0	1,700
U.S.S.R		241	18	8	1.0	70	26	32	277.8	890
OCEANIA	Australia	12.2	19.4	8.7	1.8	39	18.2	29	15.2	1,840

[a]Latest available year.   [b]Assuming continued growth at current annual rate.

[c]1966 data supplied by the International Bank for Reconstruction and Development.

[d]U.N. estimate. Other estimates range from 800 to 950 million.

[e]Mid-1969 population estimates for the Latin American countries are taken from the latest figures of the Latin American Demographic Center of the United Nations. These figures are more recent than those on which most of the rest of this table is based.

Source: Population Reference Bureau. Data derived primarily from the 1967 U.N. Demographic Yearbook.

to have children of their own. Two centuries ago only half of them survived long enough to accomplish this. What is more, most people in developed countries live through the reproductive age. Not only do they live long enough to begin a family, they stay alive to add to it.

Today, not only are people increasing in number, but the rate of increase is also accelerating. Every year, mankind reproduces a larger percentage of a larger number. It now takes less time to double population than formerly. For world population to reach 3 billion took about 600,000 years. To double that number to 6 billion will take less than 40 years.

Complicating the population dilemma is the uneven multiplication of peoples (see Tables 13-2 and 13-4). In 1960 Asia had 57 percent of the world's peoples. By 1975 that proportion will increase 2 percent. At the present rate of growth, by A.D. 2000 almost two out of every three human beings on earth (62 percent) will be in Asia. Will Asia be ready for them?

Some modern meanings of overpopulation

Population increase without preparation: Ceylon

Since time immemorial, both fly and mosquito buzzed and hummed triumphantly over the prostrate people of Ceylon. Fly-borne diarrhea decimated the child population. Malaria brought tragedy to the daily lives of these gentle people inhabiting the island to India's south.

In 1946 a DDT campaign was introduced. The Western world had two centuries of economic preparation for death control. For Ceylon, the knowledge was immediate. She was caught unprepared.

The insects were destroyed in Ceylon. In one year the death rate was reduced 40 percent. But the birth rate did not fall. From 1950 to 1960 the number of Ceylonese increased by 28.9 percent. At this rate the population of Ceylon will be doubled about every thirty years. Within a limited economy, she now desperately strives to meet her sudden spurt of population.

Other areas of crisis

It is not only in Ceylon that sudden population increases have resulted from failure to bring high birth rates into line with lower death rates. Already, countless people in underdeveloped countries of South America, Asia, and Africa do not have enough to eat. Most of the malnourished preschool children in the world live in these countries. With one hand, progress gives them life. With the other, it takes it away.

Technical knowledge exists to meet the world's food shortage for some years to come. But arable land is unevenly distributed. Asia is in direst straits. "At present, 400 million human beings in the western industrial nations consume as much protein as 1,300 million of their fellowmen in Asia."[6]

---

[6]Robert C. Cook, "Population and Food Supply," in *The Population Crisis and the Use of World Resources* (The Hague, 1964), p. 474.

Man can be no more hopeful of soon meeting the housing shortage. In those countries with the largest populations the worst housing exists. Millions in Africa, Asia, and Latin America live in dwellings of mud, straw, or cardboard. Countless others swarm in the streets of crowded cities. They beg, they prostitute, they hold out a skinny hand to a heedless world. Still others have an address of sorts, but the housing is dilapidated beyond description. Fundamental sanitation is a luxury. In such facilities the population will double in less than a generation.

What are the realistic financial opportunities of these malnourished, inadequately housed peoples of the developing countries? The average per capita income for the modern Asian is about $100 a year. For the Indian and Pakistani it is between $70 and $80 yearly. The average Latin American garners some $300 per year. The future of any nation rests with her children. Excluding mainland China, almost 700 million children under fifteen years of age live in countries with a national per capita income of less than $500 per year; of these, 450 million live in countries where the income is under $100 annually.[7] May one hope to see these incomes rise? A major impediment is the increasing population. In Egypt, for example, the annual population increase (2.7 percent) will negate any economic benefit that might accrue from the completion of the Aswan Dam.

Watch us grow!

The population of the United States is now well over 203 million. After eleven years of steady rise, the U.S. birth rate descended from its historic 1957 peak of 25.3 per 1,000 population. Continuing steadily downward, the 3,520,000 live births registered in 1967 marked the third successive year that the total had fallen below the 4 million mark. By no means should these figures give rise to the belief that the population growth in this nation is under control. In 1968 there were 7 million women between the ages of eighteen and twenty-one. These are the peak marriage years. The products of the post–Second-World-War baby boom, these young women represent a fertility potential never before reached. By 1970 they will be in the midst of determining the future population growth of the United States. The peak child-bearing years are between the ages of twenty and twenty-nine. By 1980 the number of U.S. women of that age will have increased from 14 million (in 1968) to 20 million. In 1995 their number will be about 28 million. At present rates of growth, and if the two-to-four-child family desired by many couples continues to be the rule, the population of the United States will approach 300 million by the year 2000. The pill? It is at best merely delaying population growth. The size of this nation's average family in 1968 was about the same as it was in 1955 and in 1960—long before the pill was so extensively used. Oral contraception

---

[7] United Nations Children's Fund, *Assignment Children*, cited in "The Needs of Children," *Clinical Pediatrics*, Vol. 8, No. 6 (June 1969), p. 6A.

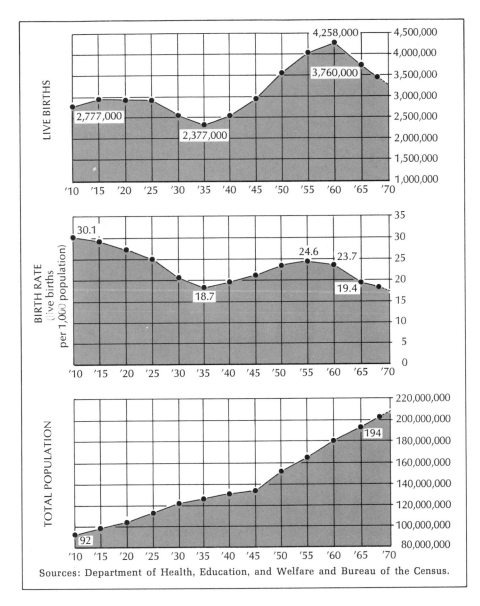

13-3 U.S. live births, birth rates, and total population: 1910–70.

Sources: Department of Health, Education, and Welfare and Bureau of the Census.

has made contraception more pleasant. But to control population people must decide upon smaller families. To maintain the U.S. population at its present level, an average of 2.3 children per family is desirable. Today, it is 3.3. Education is sorely needed.

"Watch Us Grow!" used to be the challenge of little cities to the big. Los Angeles grew. And an astronaut gets around the world in less time than one can travel forty miles of the Los Angeles freeways on a busy afternoon. Manhattan grew. At day's end, people flee the island. Rather than live in cities, commuters have forgone the hard-earned eight-hour

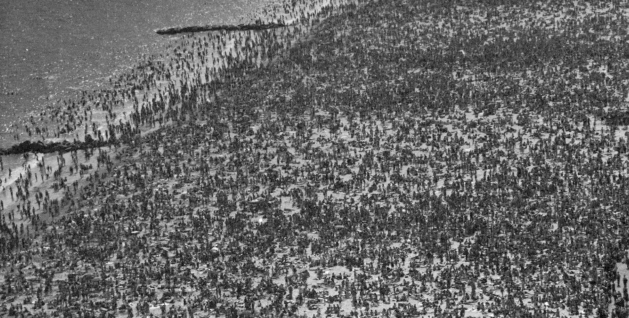

day. By adding three hours a day for travel to and from the job, they have regressed to a working day of eleven hours. This nation is also short of power, which costs more to distribute than to create. Schools are crowded, air is sewage, water is scanty (millions now drink treated sewage), noise is deafening, housing is short.

But perhaps the most subtle and erosive evil of overpopulation is the loss of personal significance. In his marvelous essay "Civil Disobedience," Thoreau tells of his night in jail for failure to pay a poll tax. In prison Thoreau felt free because he felt significant. One cannot but reflect that this lover of solitude found his original significance in a cabin near Walden Pond, today a polluted watery receptacle for various wastes.

George Washington headed a nation of 4 million. Today, the President worries about more than 200 million. By 1975 each Senator will court two and a quarter million people; each Representative about 525,000. As population increases, taxes increase, but representation inexorably lessens.

Where can modern man find a Walden Pond? Every year over three thousand acres of lush countryside are bulldozed. Cities stream noisily into one another. Within a generation, half of this nation's population will concentrate in three megalopolitan areas—along the California coast, on the Eastern seaboard, and around the Great Lakes. A bumper-to-bumper existence in these areas is a valid nightmare.

No, the bumper-to-bumper concept is no exaggeration. By 1975, 120 million vehicles, traveling 1,000 billion miles yearly, will slay over 60,000 people a year. For this purpose, roads will be built at about $3.5 million a mile. For each road mile, about forty acres of agricultural land will be sacrificed. Add to this decrease in agricultural land the amount needed for airfields, cities, reservoirs, flood control, and other similar purposes.

Well, Thoreau, at least, found a quiet spot.

If not war, then what solution?

Is war the inevitable "solution"? In the past it has been suggested that man's proclivity for killing other men has helped limit population. Overpopulation promotes war. This generation finds 740 million restless Chinese seeking more real estate. Will the next generation find more than one billion Chinese less restless? Eighty-five percent of the Chinese are now forced to live on but one-third of their available land (much of China's territory is sacrificed to uninhabitable desert or high mountains). If China's population goes unchecked, where will her people go? Or those of India? Africa? Latin America? Will the human tragedy that is war be used as a solution?

The tragedy of war's waste is heightened by irony. War does not relieve population growth. If anything, it forces improvements in medicine. And, as occurred after the Second World War, it can create an economic boom that stimulates population growth.

Some recommend *abortion* (see pages 569–71). Japan practices it with remarkable success. In 1947 Japan's birth rate was 34.3 percent. Her death rate was 14.6 percent. Her natural increase (the difference between the two) was 19.7 percent. In 1948 a law authorized the individual physician, on his own responsibility, to induce abortion for physical or financial reasons. By 1957, ten years after the abortion law, the birth rate had dropped to 17.2 percent. The death rate was 8.3 percent. The rate of natural increase was less than half of that of 1947, 8.9 percent. Every year about 1,250,000 abortions are performed in Japan. Since these are done only by physicians, no undue mortality is noted from the procedure.[8]

Abortion, however, is not the only cause of the low Japanese birth rate. About 60 percent of the decreased birth rate is due to abortions. Birth control accounts for the rest.

Considerable segments of U.S. citizenry would not accept widespread governmentally approved abortion. (With distaste, many recall the since discontinued "abortariums" that existed in Russia before the Second World War.) Yet, there are as many, if not more, illegal abortions in the United States as there are legal ones in Japan. About 20 percent of pregnancies in this country terminate in criminal abortions. Thousands die. Educated women seek abortions more commonly than those without a college education. Illegal abortions are not largely a problem associated with unmarried pregnant girls. They are sought more often by married women who have been pregnant several times.

An *economic* solution has been recommended. Can greater efficiency in food production resolve the problem? As long as population numbers outstrip ability to meet needs, this concept remains unrealistic. Today, hundreds of millions starve in miserable housing. Despair is their constant companion. What realistic reason is there to think that the next generation will have solved the overwhelming problem of poverty for twice the number of people who live in poverty today? As one distinguished biologist writes:

> Some feel that the battle to feed the world population is now lost, and that it is a foregone conclusion that by 1985 we will have world-wide famines in which hundreds of millions of people will starve to death. I must admit I see no major crash program which would lead me to disagree with this conclusion.[9]

The need for such a program is great and urgent.

An *educational* approach has been suggested. As with other public health programs, it should permeate the birth control effort. Directing such programs to maternity services would seem particularly indicated. Of special importance is the education of the mother who has borne her first child. It is she who has the greatest potential for adding to the population.

[8]Kitaoka Juitso, "How Japan Halved Her Birth Rate in Ten Years," in *The Sixth International Conference on Planned Parenthood* (London, 1959), pp. 27–36.
[9]William D. McElroy, "Biomedical Aspects of Population Control," p. 19.

There is, moreover, expert opinion that instruction in population problems and family planning should begin during the high school grades. Indeed, in Baltimore detailed information on family planning and family growth is given to the high school student. The material, incorporated into the social studies and biology courses, has been found to be valuable to both student and parent. Although obtaining competent teachers in this area is a problem, it too can be solved by intensive education.[10]

The *demographic* solution has been offered. This suggests a reduction of the birth rate to the point where it equals the death rate, so that population growth either slows or stops. Birth control and education are the tools of this solution. Birth control is further discussed in Chapter 16.

So, a major threat to man's survival is overproduction. Yet, it is brought about in the only way he can survive—by reproducing. It is to this—the human miracle—that attention is now turned.

Reproduction

The pituitary: a master gland

The endocrine influence

The pituitary gland is attached to the base of the brain by its own short stem (see body chart 8 in the color section). It is snugly encased in its own bony fortress. The ductless, endocrine pituitary gland weighs no more than two baby-dose aspirins. It is no larger than a cherry. It has a front (anterior) lobe and a back (posterior) lobe. The posterior lobe releases several hormones; one stimulates contraction of the pregnant uterus. From its lordly position, the anterior lobe prepares and dispenses hormones. These both activate and control other endocrine glands—thyroid, adrenals, and ovaries and testes. That is why the pituitary is called the master gland. The present concern is with the effect of the pituitary on the testes and ovary. For the reproductive system, the chain of command is from the main part of the brain (cerebral cortex) to the hypothalamus (part of the brain near the pituitary) to the pituitary to the ovary to the uterus. It is not surprising that psychic or emotional distress can lead to disturbances of reproduction.

Similarities

The reproductive systems

During the first half-dozen weeks of human embryonic life, it is not possible to microscopically differentiate male gonadal tissue from the female cells which are already present. The male gonads (testes) arise from female primordia according to genetic instruction. Not until the third month of life within the uterus are the external sex organs distinguishable as male or female without the microscope (see page 561).

[10]*Ibid.*
[11]A gonad (Greek *gone*, seed) is a gland producing spermatozoa or ova.

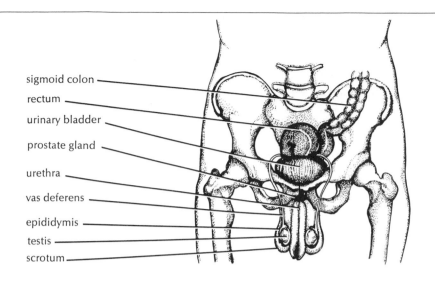

sigmoid colon

rectum

urinary bladder

prostate gland

urethra

vas deferens

epididymis

testis

scrotum

13-4 *The male reproductive system*

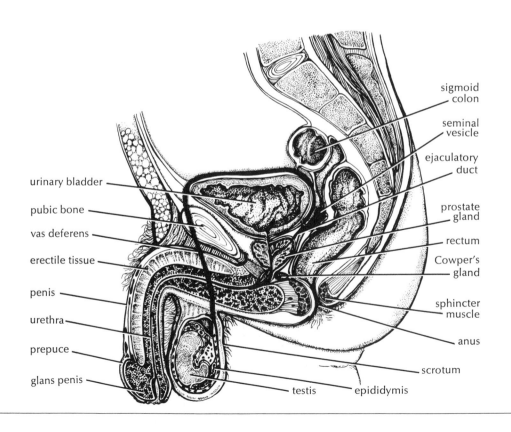

urinary bladder

pubic bone

vas deferens

erectile tissue

penis

urethra

prepuce

glans penis

sigmoid colon

seminal vesicle

ejaculatory duct

prostate gland

rectum

Cowper's gland

sphincter muscle

anus

scrotum

testis

epididymis

The male reproductive system (Figure 13-4)

This system consists of a pair of male gonads (testes) and excretory ducts (the epididymis, vas deferens, and ejaculatory ducts). The accessory structures are the seminal vesicles, prostate gland, Cowper's glands (also called the bulbo-urethral glands), and penis.

THE MALE REPRODUCTIVE ORGANS About two months before birth, the *testes* usually descend from the abdomen into the external sac, the *scrotum*. It is crucial that this occur before adolescence. Only at a temperature cooler than that of the abdominal cavity can the development of spermatozoa in the testes occur. Should both testes fail to descend, sterility results. Should only one testicle reach the scrotum, there would probably be enough normal spermatozoa to insure fertility. In some males only one testicle will descend and years may elapse before the other descends. In many cases, surgery and hormones have been successful in the treatment of undescended testicles.

A basic purpose of the testes is to produce *spermatozoa* (Greek *sperma,* seed). This first function is carried on by germinal cells of the *seminiferous tubules.* These coiled little tubules (straightened out in both testes they would be a mile long) are supported by connective tissue in which special cells carry out the second basic function of the testes—the production of the hormone *testosterone.* The same hormone of the anterior pituitary that maintains the corpus luteum (see page 458) in the female is responsible for the production of testosterone in the male. It is the testosterone that causes the male genitalia to develop, the voice to deepen, the bones to increase in size, the beard to appear, and the psyche to change. The growth of the external genitalia is the first sign of puberty in the boy.[12]

Eventually, the seminiferous tubules unite in a single convoluted tube at the back of each testis called the *epididymis.* Mature spermatozoa leave the seminiferous tubules and are temporarily stored in the epididymis. At maturity, enough spermatozoa have accumulated in the epididymis for ejaculation.

The *vas deferens* (or spermatic cord) is a continuation of the epididymis. It goes upward along the back of the testes and, by way of a canal in the groin, into the abdomen. Eventually the vas deferens joins the duct of the *seminal vesicle* of its side of the body. The two seminal vesicles are

---

[12]*Androgens* are substances capable of producing masculine body characteristics. Thus, *testosterone* is an androgen. Testosterone is the major hormone of male sexual development. By their action on the *sebaceous glands* of the skin, androgens predispose teen-agers to acne. The intense self-concern characteristic of the pubescent person does not make acne easy to bear. This disease of the sebaceous glands in the skin occurs in some 75 percent of children at puberty. Usually it is mild. The normal sebaceous glands produce an oily substance called *sebum.* In acne an abnormal amount of sebum blocks the outlet of the gland. It enlarges. The outer part of the lesion turns black, not from dirt, but because of chemical changes. These are the "blackheads." Infection may occur and spread deep into the skin. Washing several times daily with a disinfectant soap is wise. However, there is no evidence whatsoever that the initial lesion of acne begins because of uncleanliness. Moreover, the prevalent belief that acne is caused by masturbation is utterly untrue. Even mild cases of acne are often best seen by the family physician. He may refer severe cases to a skin specialist (dermatologist). Many physicians will forbid their acne patients to partake of chocolates, nuts (peanut butter), and soft drinks. The understandable emotional distress caused by severe acne makes professional counsel desirable.

13-5 The route
of a spermatozoon
from its origin to
its fertilization
of an ovum.

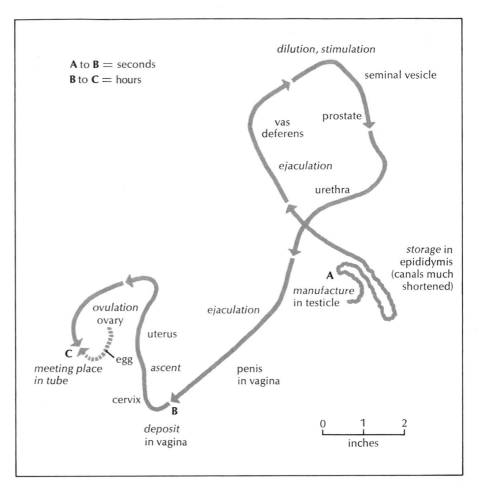

located between the bladder and rectum and produce a secretion that adds to the volume of the seminal fluid. The seminal vesicles empty their secretions into the *ejaculatory ducts* which, in turn, empty into the urethra. The urethra is the canal of the male organ for sexual intercourse, the *penis*. Through the penis, the semen is discharged and urine is passed from the bladder. Through a remarkable engineering mechanism, urine and semen never pass at the same time.

The first one and one-half inches of the urethra, as it leaves the bladder, is surrounded by the chestnut-sized *prostate gland,* which also contains many muscle fibers. The gland part secretes a thin fluid that helps carry the semen and provides it with a necessary alkaline medium. The muscle part of the prostate helps eject the semen out of the penis. On each side of the prostate glands is one of the two *Cowper's glands.* They look like peas and secrete the thick material characteristic of seminal fluid.

The penis hangs in front of the scrotum. At the tip of its head (*glans*) is the slitlike opening of the urethra. The thin skin of its body is loose.

At the neck of the penis, the skin folds upon itself to form the *prepuce* (foreskin). This is the portion of the skin removed at circumcision. Circumcision is associated with a decrease in the incidence of cancer of the penis. There is, moreover, some evidence that cancer of the cervix is more common among wives of uncircumcised men (see page 208). Nevertheless, not all physicians are agreed that routine circumcision is essential.

MECHANISM OF THE ERECTION OF THE PENIS AND EJACULATION   Penile erection results from a spinal reflex. First, there is a rapid inflow of blood into the cavernous space of the erectile tissue of the penis. This increased pressure compresses the veins, preventing return of most of the blood from the organ. Penile enlargement and stiffening result. (There is no relationship whatsoever between the size of the penis and either virility or fertility.) With erection, the Cowper's glands lubricate the urethra. Ejaculation occurs with peristaltic contractions of the muscles of the testes. These contractions spread to the epididymis and the vas deferens with resultant emptying of sperm and fluid.

SEMEN   The discharged material containing the sperm is about a teaspoonful in amount. In healthy men, the ejaculated amount is reestablished in about twenty-four hours or less. During ejaculation, the entire transit from testes to vagina occupies but a few seconds. Although sperm can remain motile in the vagina for as long as two hours, some can reach the cervix in seconds. Indeed, ejaculation may well take place directly on the cervix. However, hours may be required for ascent of the sperm through the uterus and part of the Fallopian tube in order to fertilize an ovum (a distance of about six inches). On an average, the journey probably requires about an hour (see Figure 13-5). Each spermatozoon has a bulbous head. Its long mobile tail propels it to its destination (see Figure 13-6).

The female reproductive system (Figure 13-7)

The essential glands of this system are the pair of female gonads (ovaries). The female reproductive *duct* system is composed of the Fallopian tubes,[13] uterus (womb), and vagina, and the associated structures— the external genitalia. The mammary glands (breasts) may also be considered as part of the female reproductive duct system (see Figure 13-11).

THE OVARIES AND OVA   The two ovaries (egg containers) are the fundamental organs of femininity. About the size and shape of a shelled almond, each ovary is situated on one side of the uterus and is attached to it by ligaments. Just as the organs of masculinity (the testes) produce male sperm, so do the ovaries produce mature *ova* in the female. When the female child is born, each of her ovaries contains about 200,000 tiny sacs or follicles.[14] In each follicle lies a microscopically small primordial

---

[13]Named after the Italian anatomist Gabriello Fallopio (1523–62). These structures are also called the *oviducts* or *uterine tubes.*

[14]Estimates of the number vary enormously. Some students believe that, at birth, there are as many as half a million follicles in each ovary.

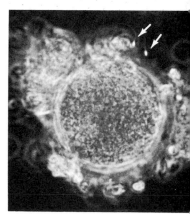

13-6 A spermatozoon (*top*) and spermatozoa (arrows) entering a human ovum. Only one will eventually complete fertilization.

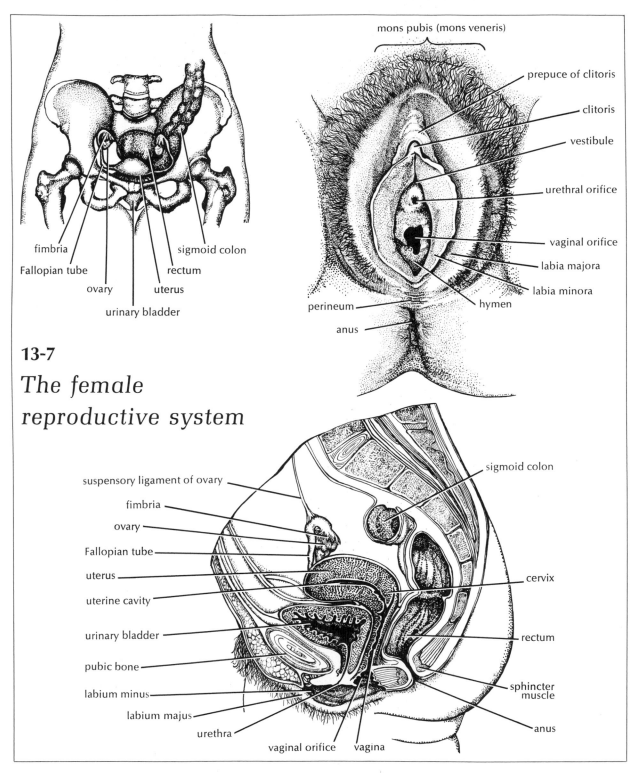

mons pubis (mons veneris)

prepuce of clitoris

clitoris

vestibule

urethral orifice

vaginal orifice

labia majora

labia minora

hymen

perineum

anus

fimbria

Fallopian tube

ovary

urinary bladder

rectum

uterus

sigmoid colon

13-7

The female reproductive system

suspensory ligament of ovary

fimbria

ovary

Fallopian tube

uterus

uterine cavity

urinary bladder

pubic bone

labium minus

labium majus

urethra

vaginal orifice

vagina

sigmoid colon

cervix

rectum

sphincter muscle

anus

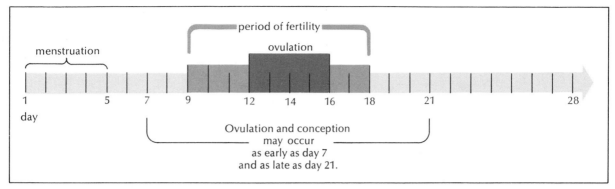

13-8 The menstrual cycle.

sex cell (or *oogonium*). Each woman is born with all the primordial sex cells she will ever have. At this primitive, unripened stage, no sex cell is capable of fertilization. The ripening process whereby a primordial sex cell becomes an ovum must await puberty. This usually occurs between the ninth and seventeenth year (twelve and one-half years is the average). During a woman's lifetime, only about 400 (perhaps 1 in 1,000) ova leave an ovary.

Every month the mature human female experiences a series of changes basically involving the pituitary gland, the ovaries, and the *endometrium* (the lining of the *uterus*). The purpose of these changes is to prepare for possible pregnancy. For pregnancy to occur, an egg must leave the ovary, be fertilized, and then be firmly implanted in the endometrium of the prepared uterus.[15]

What happens to the ovary (ovarian cycle) is related to what happens to the uterus (menstrual cycle). *Menstruation* and *ovulation* are different events, happening at different times, to different organs. But each is dependent on the other. Each intimately affects the other.

OVULATION   To follow the events leading to the release of a mature egg from the ovary (1–8 below), start with a landmark—day one, the beginning of the menstrual period. Why day one? Because a woman can observe the first day of her period more easily than her last. She can thus count from that day more reliably. Also assume that every twenty-eight days an average female menstruates five days. With different people these time periods vary normally. They are used here only as examples. Note, however, that the ovarian and menstrual cycles are correlated here.

1. Menstruation begins on day one and continues through day five (see Figures 13-8 and 13-9). The hypothalamus stimulates the pituitary gland to release a *follicle-stimulating hormone* (*FSH*) directly into the venous blood stream.

---

[15]The Roman Catholic church teaches that conception occurs with fertilization. Others, such as the American College of Obstetrics and Gynecology, consider biological life to begin with implantation.

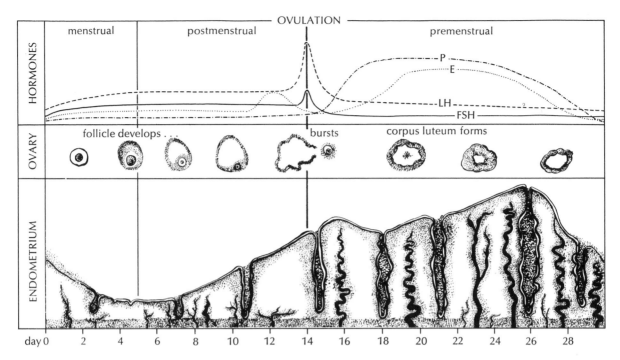

13-9 The menstrual and ovulatory cycles. (FSH = the follicle-stimulating hormone; E = estrogen; LH = the luteinizing hormone; P = progesterone.) Note that the progesterone level is detectably higher within twenty-four hours after ovulation occurs.

2. The FSH reaches and activates the ovaries. Not one but several (of the many thousands) of immature ovarian follicles in one or both ovaries respond to the FSH and begin to ripen. Which ovary is more affected is unpredictable. Estimates of the number of immature follicles that respond to the FSH usually vary from two to thirty-two.

3. The cells of those ovarian follicles that are ripening multiply greatly and the single maturing ovum within each follicle increases in size. The increased layers of follicular cells secrete a *follicular fluid*. This fluid forms tiny pools, which first separate groups of cells but which then run together to form a little lake within each follicle (see Figure 13-9). The follicles mature at different rates of speed, so some are at earlier stages of development than others. By about day ten, a few of the most mature follicles look like fluid-filled rounded sacks. The developing ovum is in the wall of the sack and is surrounded by follicular cells, which separate it from the lake. The follicle is now called a *Graafian follicle*, after a seventeenth-century Dutch anatomist, Regner de Graaf, who first described it.

4. As they ripen, the cells of maturing follicles also produce a hormone of their own called *estrogen*. Its function at this stage is to prepare the uterus for implantation of a fertilized ovum.

5. On about day ten, one (very rarely two) of the follicles undergoes a sudden spurt of growth. In three or four days it is completely mature. As a rule only one follicle and ovum will mature and only one ovum will leave the ovary. (If a woman has a tendency for multiple births there may be more than one.) No one knows what determines which follicle (and ovum) will be selected. The other follicles, and their contained ova that are not destined to leave the ovary, develop to varying extents, only to regress, die, and be replaced by small scars. No other trace of them remains.

6. A few hours before the ovum is ready to leave, the follicle that contains it migrates to the surface of the ovary. By day thirteen or fourteen the ovum is ready to go. It has been seen at surgery as a tiny blisterlike protrusion from the ovarian surface.

7. The pituitary gland then releases a second hormone, the *luteinizing hormone (LH)*, directly into the venous blood.

8. The LH causes the follicle to rupture, and the ovum is released. This is *ovulation*. On the average, ovulation occurs on day fourteen. Ovulation, then, occurs at about the middle of the menstrual cycle.

To this point, it has been seen that the pituitary gland has produced two hormones. One, FSH, stimulated the growth of follicles that, as they developed, produced estrogen. The second pituitary hormone, LH, caused rupture of the follicle, releasing the egg.

Three parenthetical observations will be made here. *First, conception,* the fertilization of an ovum by a sperm, cannot occur unless both mature sex cells are viable. Upon being released from the ovary, the ovum usually survives between twenty-four to thirty-six hours. For the ovum, assume a maximal survival time of two days. Upon being deposited in the vagina, sperm usually survive one to three days. For sperm, assume a maximum survival time of three days. Usually ovulation occurs, in the average woman, about fourteen days before the onset of the next menstrual period, give or take two days. Keeping in mind the average maximum survival times of the ovum and of sperm, as well as the average day of occurrence of ovulation (with its two-day leeway), refer to Figure 13-8 for an illustration of the average period of fertility of a woman who menstruates every twenty-eight days. Counting from day one of the menstrual period, she will ovulate between day twelve and day sixteen. However, her ovum will survive about two days. A viable ovum may thus be available for fertilization until approximately day eighteen of the menstrual period. The woman may have ovulated as early as day twelve. For about three days a sperm can survive to fertilize an ovum. It then follows that conception can occur if a sperm is deposited in the vagina as early as three days before ovulation. If a woman menstruates regularly every twenty-eight days (and many do not), she will, on the average, be most likely to become pregnant if sperm are deposited in the vagina between day nine and day eighteen of her menstrual period. Throughout this book human individuality has been stressed. Menstruation and ovulation are hardly exceptions. Some women flow every twenty-one days. Others menstruate every thirty-five days. They should calculate their periods of maximum fertility accordingly. For example, the woman who menstruates every twenty-one days can set an ovulation date on day seven of the menstrual period. If she menstruates every thirty-fifth day she will usually ovulate on day twenty-one. In either case her calculations of maximum fertility must make allowances for a two-day leeway for ovulation and the viability of both ovum and sperm. There are women whose menstrual cycles from month to month are irregular. Without obtaining a reliable average over a year, they cannot calculate a reasonably reliable period of maximum fertility.

Second, when ovulation occurs, the rupture is accompanied by a small amount of ovarian bleeding. This blood may be irritating and may cause brief abdominal discomfort. With right-side middle-of-the-month pain, a woman may worry that she has appendicitis. Only the physician is equipped to differentiate between the two.

Third, as the follicle develops, its estrogen (step 4 above) affects the uterus. In preparation for implantation of the developing product of the fertilized egg (the embryo), the lining (endometrium) of this organ thickens, as does the muscle layer. Estrogen also affects the cervical secretions, making them more receptive for the sperm if it is there. It also causes the Fallopian tubes to contract more rapidly. (Estrogen, the basic female sex hormone, is responsible for many of the female sex characteristics, such as the growth of breast tissue.)

THE DESTINY OF THE RELEASED OVUM Where does the ovum go? It enters the *Fallopian tube* (see Figure 13-10)[16] nearest the ovary from which the egg came. At its lower end, each of these three- to five-inch tubes opens into the upper uterine cavity. At its upper end, each Fallopian tube lies close but not directly attached to its corresponding ovary. This free end of the Fallopian tube ends in fingerlike projections called *fimbria.* And it is the fimbria that draw the escaped ovum into the Fallopian tube. Now the ovum is ready to be fertilized, to make the journey to the uterus. Unlike the male sperm, however, it cannot move alone. By the gentle sweeping motions of hairlike cilia lining the Fallopian tube, the ovum is helped along its way.

As the ovum begins its journey down the Fallopian tube, what goes on in the emptied follicle that remains behind in the ovary? Under the influence of LH it closes, grows to the size of a lima bean, and turns yellow. Now it is called the *corpus luteum* (Latin *corporis,* body + *luteum,* yellow). Its future function depends on whether or not the ovum is fertilized.

If the ovum is not fertilized within forty-eight hours, it continues down the Fallopian tube to the uterus. There it disintegrates. Any remnant of

---

[16]Obstruction of these tubes by inflammation is one of the most common causes of sterility, for the egg cannot reach the uterus. Sometimes, with a partially blocked tube, the sperm does reach the egg to fertilize it. But then the larger fertilized egg cannot get through the tubes to the uterus. A tubal pregnancy results, which can be terminated surgically.

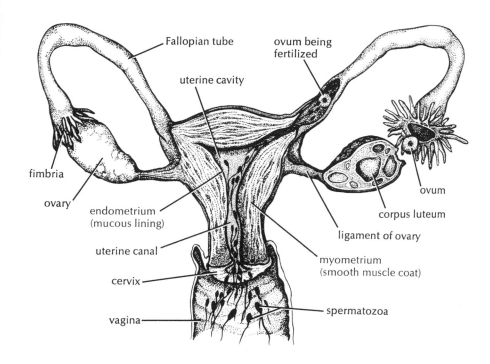

13-10 An ovum is shown leaving the ovary. The same ovum is shown later being fertilized in the upper Fallopian tube. The fertilized ovum (zygote) will cleave daily as it continues down the Fallopian tube to the uterus. After floating in the uterus for several days, it will be implanted in the uterine wall. It should be noted that this is a highly schematic representation.

it is eliminated through the vagina with the menstrual flow. The time period of ovum viability (its ability to be fertilized) has not been exactly determined. It is somewhere between twenty-four hours and about two days. In the ovary, triggered by LH, the corpus luteum produces the hormone *progesterone,* which means "to promote pregnancy." Indeed, this is its function. Acting upon the uterine endometrium, progesterone causes it to mature in preparation for a fertilized ovum. In the absence of fertilization, the corpus luteum continues to produce progesterone until late in the menstrual cycle. Not until about day twenty-five does the corpus luteum begin to degenerate to become a small depressed scar in the ovarian tissue. Progesterone is then diminished. Fragments of the uterine endometrium and mucus from the uterine glands slough off with an average of one to three ounces of menstrual blood. A new ovarian cycle is ready to begin.

If the ovum is fertilized (usually this happens in the upper portion of a Fallopian tube),[17] the sequence of events is somewhat different. Between two to four days are required for the trip of the fertilized ovum (the zygote) down the tube to the uterus. Once there, it is not immediately implanted. Several days may go by before the uterine endometrium is entirely ready. So it is about five to seven days following ovulation that implantation occurs. The elaborately prepared uterine endometrium receives the new life. The zygote is now an embryo. Implantation usually happens between day eighteen and day twenty-two. It may, however, occur as late as day twenty-three of the menstrual cycle.[18] After implantation, the embryo produces a *gonadotropic hormone.* This hormone, like LH, stimulates the corpus luteum to produce progesterone.

Indeed, with pregnancy the corpus luteum in the ovary continues its activity for twelve weeks before some of its functions are taken over by the *placenta* (afterbirth). By its timely continued production of estrogen and progesterone, it promotes persistent endometrial growth, so essential in sustaining the intrauterine being. It also prevents the maturation of new follicles. And this last fact makes possible the contraceptive "pill"—a synthetic chemical combination of progesterone and estrogen. Properly taken, the pill prevents ovulation.

The uterus and menstruation

The hollow uterus, about the size and shape of a pear, is a muscular pelvic organ. Nourished and sheltered in this abode, the developing child is an *embryo* for two months, then a *fetus,* and, upon birth, an *infant.* The upper part of the uterus, its *body,* is mostly muscle. During pregnancy, the uterus enlarges to about sixteen times its normal size. Its muscle must enlarge enough to produce contractions adequate to expel the baby. The smaller lower end of the uterus, the *cervix,* points downward into the vagina. It can be felt by the woman and has the consistency of the tip of the nose. Its identification is important to the woman who uses a diaphragm for birth control. The physician can both see and feel the cervix with ease. This is fortunate, for it affords early diagnosis of cancer of the womb, which most commonly begins at this site. There are small mucous glands in the cervix that may become infected. Sometimes they become clogged, causing a mucoid discharge.

The uterus is loosely moored to the bony pelvis by tough fibrous bands called *ligaments.* It is thus suspended in the pelvic cavity between the bladder, in front, and the rectum, behind. The stretching of these ligaments during pregnancy may cause a pulling sensation in the groin. An enlarging pregnant uterus diminishes space for the bladder and rectum (see Figure

---

[17] For the route of the sperm to the ovum see Figure 13-5.

[18] This assumes ovulation occurs on about day fourteen. Add approximately two to four days in the Fallopian tube, and about another two to four days in the uterus. The subsequent history of the embryo is described in Chapter 16.

13-7). This explains the frequent urinary dribbling that occurs during late pregnancy and the importance of emptying both bladder and rectum to facilitate delivery of the child.

As has been mentioned, the endometrium (the lining of the uterine cavity) is elaborately prepared in anticipation of a viable fertilized egg. Hospitality for the fertilized egg is the basic function of the uterus. Under the influence of estrogen from the maturing ovarian follicle, the endometrium thickens. Fluid accumulates. Blood engorges the tissue. When, however, these preparations are met with naught but an unfertilized and, therefore, degenerating egg, the uterus bleeds. With *menstruation,* the excess endometrium loosens and is discharged, with the mucus from the uterine glands, through the cervical opening and vagina as blood-filled tissue.

SOME UNTRUTHS ABOUT MENSTRUATION   The Greeks, wrongly considering menstruation to be a cleansing process, called it "katharsis." In the first century, Pliny the Elder wrote that menstrual blood dulled razors, and Aristotle thought menstruating women ruined mirrors. The early Hebrews punished those who had intercourse during menstruation (Leviticus 20:18). During medieval times, menstruating women were excluded from churches and wine cellars alike. In the latter case it was believed they would spoil the wine. Menstruating women are still segregated in "blood huts" by some African tribes. Child marriage developed among the Hindus because they incorrectly believed that the menstrual blood is essential for the embryo. To lose menstrual blood before pregnancy is still considered irreligious by many Hindus. Not long ago, in rural Russia, menstrual blood was collected in a flask by an unmarried girl from as many village women as possible. It was then used by the village witch to determine fertility. Elsewhere in Europe a drop of menstrual blood used to be placed in a swain's wine to help him win the love of its owner.

SOME TRUTHS ABOUT MENSTRUATION   During menstruation an absorbent pad is used to absorb the *menses,* or menstrual flow. It may be worn externally, although many women prefer an internal tampon. There is no reason whatsover to limit physical activity during menstruation. Some couples have sexual intercourse during menstruation and there is usually no contraindication to this. The mild abdominal cramping that sometimes occurs during menstruation may require an aspirin or two, but usually even this is not necessary. Douching at the end of menstruation is neither necessary nor recommended. The action of normal vaginal bacteria maintains vaginal cleanliness and health. Because of fluid retention some women may gain a pound or two during the week before the onset of menstruation. This does not call for a change in diet; with the onset the weight is lost, as is an occasional heavy feeling in the pelvis and legs. *Premenstrual tension,* manifested by increased moodiness and irritability, even mild depression, is not uncommonly experienced during the few days prior to the onset of menstruation. These are not usually significant symptoms. In the case of a very few women, the mild physical discomfort and increased emotional sensitivity combine to make her a trial both to herself and to others. An occasional woman will even use this situation to gain sympathy. But such instances are quite rare. The very rare personality change associated with menstruation usually indicates other deeply rooted problems. The vast majority of young women handle their monthly menstrual periods as what they are—an entirely normal indication of femininity during the reproductive years.

Dysmenorrhea, or painful menstruation, does not refer to the ordinary discomfort mentioned above; it is more severe. It may have a wide variety of causes, either physical, psychological, or both. *Menorrhagia* refers to excessive and usually prolonged uterine bleeding occurring at regular intervals. *Metrorrhagia* is uterine bleeding at completely irregular intervals. The amount may be normal; the flow may be prolonged. *Amenorrhea* refers to the cessation of menstruation before the menopause. Sudden changes in climate or emotional distress are among the variables that may cause a change in the amount of menstrual flow; a period may be delayed or may even be skipped because of such factors. Amenorrhea of longer duration is, of course, most commonly due to pregnancy. However, endocrine disorders or severe malnutrition and anemia may cause amenorrhea. Dysmenorrhea, menorrhagia, metrorrhagia, and prolonged amenorrhea all indicate prompt consultation with the family physician.

NORMAL DIFFERENCES AMONG WOMEN   Women who desire to be different from other women surely accomplish this with their menstrual histories. The onset of menstruation (*menarche*) varies. On the average, as noted above, it occurs at about twelve and one-half years. First menstruations are usually irregular. They may not be associated with ovulation. Some girls menstruate for months or even years without ovulating; so the onset of menstruation does not always mean fertility has begun. Abnormally early onsets of menstruation and ovulation do occur, but rarely. Lena Medina, a classic case in medical history, was delivered of a healthy child when she was only five years and nine months old. An ovarian tumor accelerated her sexual maturity. Lena's pregnancy had been caused by rape.

Women normally differ as to the duration (one to six days, with an average of four or five days) and the amount (one to eight ounces, with an average of about two or three ounces) of menstrual bleeding. Individual women also vary from month to month in their onsets of bleeding. For women who calculate "safe periods" based on the first day of menstruation, it is essential to keep an accurate record of monthly onsets for at least a year.

An important note: *it is vital for a particular individual to know what is ordinary for her. Any marked departure is the signal for an immediate visit to a physician.* A gross change in menstruation, such as excessive bleeding or spotting between periods, may be of minor significance. It may, however, signify disease such as cancer that, treated early, is easily curable.

The menopause

The age of the cessation of menstruation (*menopause*) varies widely. The average is about forty-seven years. Some women may normally cease menstruating even before forty, though this is not common. As many as twenty-five percent continue after fifty. With the menopause, the ovaries cease to function. Ovulation stops. Menstruation may stop abruptly. However, the amount of bleeding usually tapers off. Failure to realize this has resulted in pregnancy. Just as puberty is accompanied by body changes and the beginning of menstruation so is the menopause accompanied by body changes and the cessation of the function. The period in a woman's life that is begun by the menopause and during which she enters her postreproductive years is called the *climacteric*. (The normal diminution of male sexual activity is also called the climacteric.)

Two grossly cruel and senseless untruths about the menopause should be dismissed. First, the menopause does not herald old age. Second, it is not a common cause of insanity. Most menopausal women need no medical treatment. As a rule, sexual life continues. Frequently it improves. For many women, hot flashes and sweating are merely annoyances. With a considerable number, they do not occur. For a few, the symptoms, which occasionally include headaches and depression, do require some medical attention. Results of treatment are generally excellent. Her brood raised, her fear of pregnancy gone, relieved of some of her pressures, the postmenopausal woman can anticipate thirty or more happy, productive years.

A second important note: *the "flooding" of the menopause is not normal. To repeat: excessive bleeding and bleeding between periods (whether menopausal or not) always indicate immediate consultation with a physician. Delay has cost many a woman her life.*

The vagina

The vagina is a tube about three and one-half inches long. The vaginal walls are composed of muscle. The inner surface of the vagina is lined with transverse folds. During childbirth both muscle and folds expand tremendously. Cells from vaginal fluid are useful in determining not only the time of ovulation but also cancer of the uterus. In both instances the cells characteristically reflect these changes. In the virgin, the external opening of the vagina may be partially closed by a fold of mucous membrane called the *hymen* (see Figure 13-7). The hymen is frequently absent in females who have never had sexual intercourse. Rarely, the hymen interferes with the passage of menstrual blood. This is easily corrected by the physician. The normal reaction of the vagina is acid. A bacillus is involved in maintaining this normal reaction. If this acid reaction is not maintained, the vagina is prone to infection. Douching may be advised by a physician to encourage the acidity of the vagina. A woman should not douche unless so directed by her physician. Some popular douches not only harm delicate tissues but remove beneficial bacteria.

The external genitalia (see Figure 13-7)

The *mons pubis* is a rounded fatty pad above the labia majora and over the front pubic region. The *pubes* refer to the hair growing over the pubic region.[19] The *labia majora* are skin folds that pass backward from the mons pubis. Like the mons they are fatty pads covered, in the adult, with hair. The *clitoris,* at the upper end of the labia minora, is extremely sensitive. Its sole purpose is to stimulate sexual desire. The *labia minora* are about as thick as a large rubber band. They arise from the clitoris and then pass backward and enclose an area called the *vestibule.* The *urethra* (leading from the urinary bladder) and *vagina* open into the vestibule, as do the *Bartholin's glands* (vulvovaginal glands). During sexual excitement, the Bartholin's glands secrete a lubricating material. On either side of the opening of the female urethra are the several small *Skene's ducts.* These and the Bartholin's glands may easily become infected, particularly by the gonococcus.

The mammary glands

Before puberty there is little difference between the male and female breasts. In adult males they remain rudimentary. However, with the onset of puberty in the girl and the production of certain hormones by the ovaries, the breasts begin to develop. With each menstrual cycle the breasts enlarge slightly; they feel heavier, and the nipples are more sensitive. Just below the center of the adult female mammary gland is the raised *nipple,* surrounded by the circular pigmented *areola* (see Figure 13-11). Small openings on the surface of the nipple mark the openings of the ducts of the underlying glandular elements. With pregnancy, these are quite visible during the secretion of milk (*lactation*). The numerous small elevations on the areolar area are due to sebaceous glands. The breast structure is composed of about twenty distinct tubular glands or *lobes,* which, in turn, are composed of many *lobules.* The lobes are embedded in loose connective tissue and fat, which give the breast its shape. Each lobe eventually drains into the *lactiferous duct* of the nipple. Just before the duct terminates into the nipple it is dilated as a *lactiferous sinus.*

During pregnancy the nipples and areolae darken. Around the areola a secondary, lighter areola usually develops. The sebaceous glands of the areola enlarge. They are then called *Montgomery's glands.* They secrete an oily material that keeps the nipple supple and prevents the skin from cracking. Early in pregnancy a thin, scanty, yellow-white precursor of milk is secreted. This continues throughout the entire pregnant period. This secretion is called *colostrum.* During the first days of the baby's life, colostrum is a good food. Before the milk is produced, colostrum may be drawn off to stimulate milk flow. The sense of fullness and the tingling of the breasts, sometimes felt in the early months of pregnancy, soon abates.

---

[19] *Pubes* is also the plural of *pubis,* which refers to the pubic bone.

13-11   *The mature female breast*

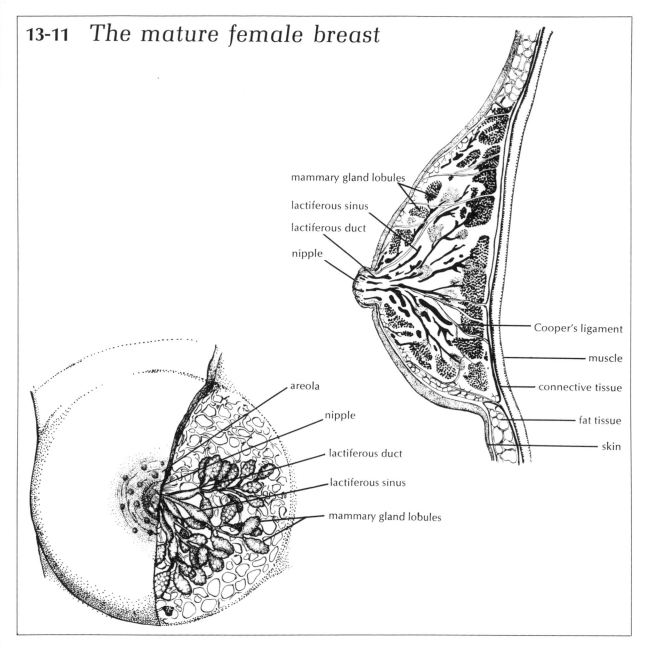

mammary gland lobules

lactiferous sinus

lactiferous duct

nipple

Cooper's ligament

muscle

connective tissue

fat tissue

skin

areola

nipple

lactiferous duct

lactiferous sinus

mammary gland lobules

Breast development of the pregnant woman does not usually cause her any discomfort whatsoever. As pregnancy continues into the later months, the growing baby presses upward and the woman's chest enlarges slightly. After delivery, the enlarged chest cavity returns to its normal size.

Having considered human overproduction and some aspects of reproduction, attention is now turned to certain social and biological aspects of human mating.

14

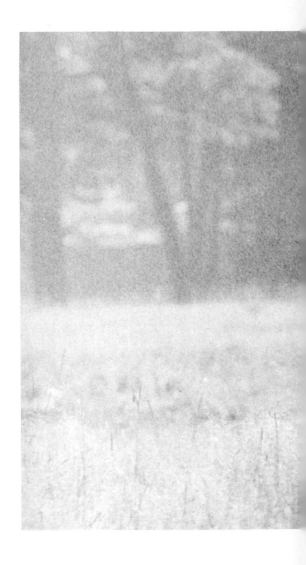

Some premarital considerations and advisements

Courtship and conquest: animal instinct, human learning

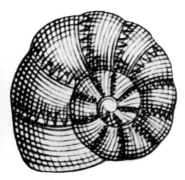

14-1 The hermaphroditic snail.

"The snail is a hermaphrodite: male and female are incorporated into one; there is no he and no she. Perhaps that is why snails are so sluggish; they have nothing to stir them, nothing to fight for, nothing to pursue, nothing to win."[1] Almost all other creatures, however, actively differentiate between the sexes and engage in elaborate mating rituals too. The index of neither Kinsey volume on human sexual behavior contains the

[1] James Kemble, *Hero Dust* (London, 1936), p. xiii. "Hermaphrodite" derives from the names Hermes (the Greek god who served as messenger to the gods) and Aphrodite (the Greek goddess of love and beauty).

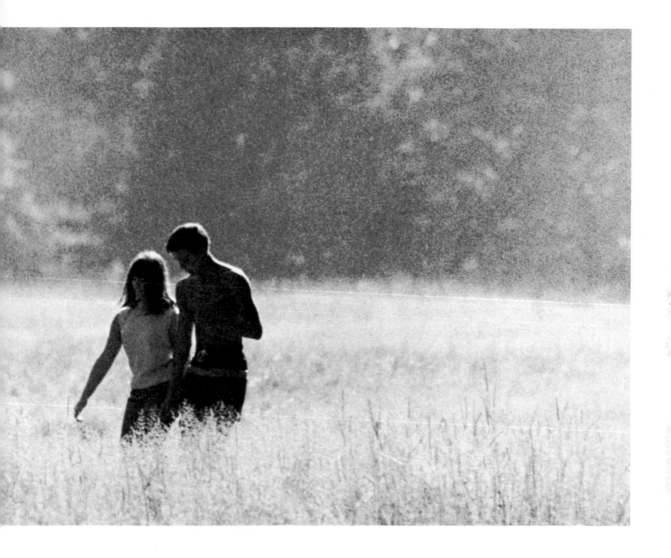

word "courtship." In a discussion of animal sexuality, such an omission would be impossible. For elegance and variety, nonhuman love-planning is both instructive and humbling. The fighting fish of Siam do an underwater courtship ballet, of which the color, grace, and timing would delight the most exacting choreographer. And the female cricket knows true devotion. Responding to a phonograph record playing the ardent chirp of a long-dead male cricket, she will desert locally available swains. Hurrying a considerable distance, she will lovingly seek an approach into the record player.[2] Gift-giving, too, is not unknown to creatures that go courting. Indeed, with some species of spider, an empty-handed male may become a snack. So, instinctively, he often arrives with a fly, carefully

[2] R. H. Smythe, *The Female of the Species* (London, 1960), p. 58.

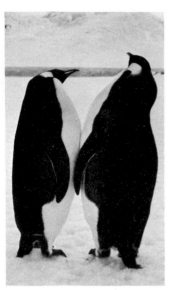

14-2 Penguins courting.

gift-wrapped in silk. Dancing a specific pattern and carefully displaying his markings, he can only trust to luck. As for higher animals, the complex courtship that goes on among penguins, for example (Figure 14-2), or among monkeys and apes, has long fascinated zoologists.

And so, all in season, the nonhuman world is a rhythmic maneuvering of love, a pervasive, instinctive planning for new life. Instinctive, not learned. But people need to be taught the art of love. One classic "textbook" is the third-century novel by Longus, *Daphnis & Chloe*. It tells the story of two innocent child lovers, a goatherd and a shepherdess, who needed instruction in the art of love. In his Introduction, Longus holds out this promise to his readers:

> *For this will cure him that is sick, and rouse him that is in dumps; one that has loved, it will remember of it; one that has not, it will instruct. For there was never any yet that wholly could escape love, and never shall there be any, never so long as beauty shall be, never so long as eyes can see.* [3]

Among earth's creatures, man is almost alone in becoming confused by such matters. His confusion is created by his culture, for in no other aspect of his life are his self-imposed regulations more rigid.

On the establishment of marital codes

Three hundred years ago, John Garland and his wife stood at the bar of justice in Suffolk County, Massachusetts. They had come all the way from Salisbury County to appeal their conviction by the local court, of a crime against man and God. Mrs. Garland had been delivered of a child eleven weeks too early. For this event, unblessed by their community, they had been fined five pounds.

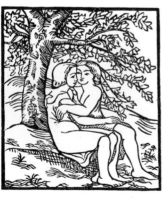

14-3 Daphnis and Chloe, a woodcut by Aristide Maillol (1861–1944).

"I and She had parents Concent to marry," John Garland protested, "had any Such Act been comited by us we could haue preuented it by marrying sooner." The untimely birth, he insisted, was due to a fall.

The prosecutor pointed a scornful finger. Garland, he rasped, hid his guilt behind a learning hardly suited to him. His contemptible quotes from "Aristottle" to prove that a child could come in the seventh month were mere deceptions. "Please to Cast an eye vpon John garland," the prosecutor exhorted the court, "they will judge Him to be no deepe man in philosophie."

The judge pondered. This was his decision:

> *It was well known to the Honored Court at Salisbury that the usuall time of woman was a set time As in genesis the 18 and the 10 compared with 2 of kings the 4th & the 16 verse, the Honored*

[3]Longus, "Proem," *Daphnis & Chloe*, tr. by George Thornley (New York, 1906), p. 9.

*Court likewise knew that that time was aboue seaven month as is
the first of luke the 36 vers compared with the 39 & 40 & 57 verse
of that chapter.* [4]

The decision of the lower court at Salisbury was reversed. John Garland
paid no fine. Today, despite having more accurate biological knowledge
than the judge in the Garland case had, most members of this culture
still live by Biblical codes. Why did they develop and persist? And
how are marital codes involved with health?

Family life of this culture is based on Judeo-Christian traditions. These **Stability and decay**
can be traced to the age of the biblical Hebrew patriarchs. The family **as sources**
was established as an institution to provide stability and protection for **of marital codes**
the group. In the home of the ancient Hebrews, the father was the head
and the mother the heart.

From the Hebrews, the early Christians got a model for building a stable
family structure. From the Romans, they learned the price of excessive
societal laxity and disruption of normal family life. Three Punic Wars
against Carthage (in the second and third centuries B.C.) occupied Rome
for over a century. These had made many Roman families enormously
rich. Roman sons were constantly off at war. Fathers consequently placed
their daughters in positions of wealth and indirect power. Roman women
of leading families began to vie among one another and with men for
power. The Elder Cato complained bitterly: "All men rule over women,
we Romans rule over all men, and our wives rule over us." Even the
Roman mother reflected the times. "Return with your shield, or on it,"
she sternly told her war-bound son. The new preoccupations of women
led them to neglect their families. Contemptuously, Roman men rejected
marriage. "Why do I not marry a rich wife?" asks a Roman writer. "Because I do not wish to be my wife's maid." [5] Laws penalizing celibacy
were to no avail. The upper classes, remaining childless, customarily
adopted children for purposes of inheritance. Divorce, previously rare,
became widespread. Marriage became a cynicism. Slaves cared for children. Children were spoiled. "Expressions which would not be tolerated
even from the effeminate youths of Alexandria," wrote Quintilian, "we
hear from them with a smile and a kiss." [6] With the family structure
crumbling, morals declined. Rome underwent a sexual revolution. Luxury
and sloth replaced the formerly strict family life. The public amorality
of the highborn also became a way of life for the middle classes. Other
factors, such as widespread malaria and an overextended economy, also
enfeebled the once mighty empire. But a basic flaw marred Rome. The
vitality of the family had been wasted. Rome collapsed. Upon its ruin,
Christianity began to build.

[4] From the manuscript *Early Court Files of Suffolk* (1675), No. 1412, quoted in George Elliott Howard,
   A History of Matrimonial Institutions, Vol. II (Chicago, 1904), p. 187.
[5] Quoted in Willystine Goodsell, *A History of Marriage and the Family* (New York, 1934), p. 136.
[6] *Ibid.*, p. 152.

Why the rigidity?
Why the guilt?

The year 312 saw Christianity legally recognized by the decaying Roman Empire. Observing the social disarray about them, the early Christians were determined not to repeat the errors of their predecessors. Polygamy, practiced by the Hebrews, was rejected. Roman sexual laxity was anathema. The abortion and infanticide, the divorce and adultery of the Greeks and Romans were condemned. In this atmosphere, sexual permissiveness was out of the question. Sex was sin. Centuries passed before even marital sex became more than a base need, to be tolerated only because it provided children.

Yet, as sex gradually did become a sanctified part of marriage, restrictive rules were retained. Those who took short cuts found society harsh indeed. Why? Because their actions threatened the family as the basic unit of society and, therefore, threatened society itself. If men were to survive, it was essential that sex and mating be controlled.

The Judeo-Christian culture, then established basic marriage codes that have endured for the Western world. Often, these codes have been supported by threat and guilt, two powerful tools of Western society. "In the last analysis, guilt feelings, for most people, are simply a realization that they have failed to follow societal convictions of right and wrong."[7]

But guilt promotes anxiety. Many people who ignore marital codes may reject their own sense of guilt, but it does not go away. Prolonged, unresolved guilt may become disease. That is why the origins of marital codes merit some exploration in a health book.

The lover, whom all the world does not love

Primitive
courtships

The tribulations of love and courtship vary from culture to culture. Among the Macusis of British Guiana, a young swain may not choose a wife until he has proved his courage. One way to demonstrate it is by allowing himself "to be sewn up in a hammock full of fire ants."[8] The hopeful Arab bridegroom of Upper Egypt displays his valor by undergoing a severe whipping by the bride's relatives.[9] The romantic maneuvering among the young of one Bolivian Indian tribe is no less hazardous:

> *Ordinarily young people of nubile age are supposed to be shy of one another, and while tending herds pass one another by many times without apparently seeing each other. Around Camata, if a boy in such a situation wishes to take notice of a girl, he picks up a handful of fine earth or dust and throws it at her. This is a first step of courtship in the Jesús de Machaca region. The next time they meet, the boy picks up some fine gravel, and the girl may do likewise. If they continue to be interested this goes on until finally they*

[7] William M. Kephart, *The Family, Society, and the Individual* (Boston, 1961), p. 117.
[8] Edward Westermarck, *The History of Human Marriage*, 5th ed., Vol. I (New York, 1921), p. 49.
[9] *Ibid.*, p. 51.

throw rocks at each other. Informants told me that there were two cases of deaths in Camata during the last four years from such a cause; one woman received a fractured skull and the other a broken back.[10]

In 1700, the British Parliament enacted the following:

That all women of whatever age, rank, profession or degree, whether virgin maid or widow, that shall from and after such Act impose upon, seduce and betray into matrimony any of His Majesty's subjects by means of scent, paints, cosmetic washes, artificial teeth, false hair, Spanish wool, iron stays, hoops, high-heeled shoes or bolstered hips, shall incur the penalty of the law now in force against witchcraft and like misdemeanors, and that the marriage upon conviction shall stand null and void.[11]

It was perhaps such legislation that prompted the degree of cautious honesty, if not outright optimism, so often proclaimed as proper in eighteenth-century English books on model letter-writing. One such volume, the *New London Letter Writer,* includes a model letter entitled, "From a Young Lady After Having Smallpox to her Lover." Apparently, the young man had led her to believe that "the beauties of my person were only exceeded by the perfection of my mind." She was, therefore, not regretting too much the loss of her good looks, for "it gives you a happy opportunity to prove yourself to be a man of truth and veracity."[12]

Many years later, in the nineteenth century, English lovers, for reasons of their own, were wont to go skating. Since chaperones rarely skated, they were benched on the sidelines. In 1876, *Punch* published a cartoon of these scandalous goings-on (Figure 14-4).[13] Not all was raucous humor, however. A Mrs. Burton Kingsland, composing for the *Ladies Home Journal* (*circa* 1900), prepared this brief, but presumably effective, speech to be made by a young lady whose debauched swain had slipped his arm about her waist: "Don't you think it rather cowardly for a man to act toward a girl as you are doing when she has trusted him and is in a measure powerless to resist such familiarity?"[14]

Things have changed.

In this culture, basic training for mating begins early, with group dating. This is followed by random dating. Perhaps it is during a shopping tour with their mothers that modern children gain the first unconscious tips for random dating. Random dating is just shopping around. One does not have to buy. There is time for window-shopping. If one chooses, one may

[10] Weston La Barre, "The Aymara Indians of the Lake Titicaca Plateau, Bolivia," *American Anthropologist,* Vol. 50, No. 1, Part 2 (January 1948), p. 129.
[11] Quoted in Henry A. Bowman, *Marriage for Moderns* (New York, 1960), p. 129.
[12] E. S. Turner, *A History of Courting* (London, 1954), p. 121.
[13] *Ibid.,* p. 178.
[14] *Ibid.,* p. 195.

14-4 "Rink to me only with thine eyes" (from *Punch,* 1876).

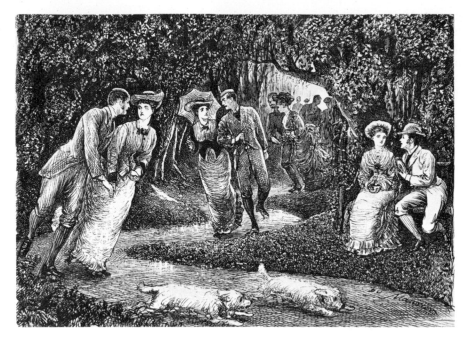

come in and browse. Sometimes, a small investment is made. By telephone, one learns a lot and overcomes much. Everybody gets stung a little, some more than others. But one gets to know the game. And, in the end (hopefully), one sees enough and adds up enough experience to get some idea of what one needs, what to look for, and what commitment may be safely made. People of other countries view random dating with astonishment. For them, the sheer number of dates per teen-ager is fickleness amounting to immorality. And the absence of a chaperone—an open invitation to family dishonor.

Admittedly superficial and often hurtfully competitive, random dating is instructive as a prelude to the next stage of mating, "going steady" (a status anxiously sought both by high school and by many college students). Since the random dater is but a recent graduate of the shy group-dating system, his sexual behavior is usually not a serious problem. It is not until the going-steady stage that the difficult problems associated with sexual relationships arise. Fearful that their children will drift or be forced into a poor marriage, many parents who regarded random dating with tolerance are suspicious of the going-steady stage of courtship. Nevertheless, going steady does relieve the competitive pressures of random dating. Moreover, it gives priceless training in such virtues as faithfulness, patience, and gentleness that will be useful in the married state.

Characteristic of some college attachments is a form of trial engagement called "pinning." Many, perhaps most, students do not consider pinning of significance. For some, however, it does provide an opportunity to become better acquainted before the more formal social step of an engagement is made. Since the commitment is not as binding, most girls will remove a pin without embarrassment. On the debit side, pinning provides an opportunity for sexual or other exploitation. A "big man on campus," for example, may trade his pin for sexual privileges with an otherwise unnoticed girl. He is like the lover described in Shakespeare's *Taming of the Shrew,* "who wooed in haste and means to wed at leisure."

It is in the turbulent, searching years of adolescence that a person must begin learning the mating game. In this anxious time of searching for a self-acceptable self, of trying to settle on a life's work, of attempting to cope with overwhelming bodily changes, and of beginning a separation from one's parents—it is in these years that the dating dilemma occurs. The dilemma is this: without being clearly told what is expected of him, the teen-ager is nevertheless given to understand that much is expected of him. "Grow up," he is told, yet he is forbidden to do what he sees grownups do. Driven by urges he has not yet learned to understand or control, he attempts to answer them as grownups do. With the paraphernalia of sexual activity, such as cars and condoms, readily available, what is missing? A chaperone? In this society, she is all but extinct.

Premarital sex

> Strephon kissed me in the spring,
>   Robin in the fall,
> But Colin only looked at me
>   And never kissed at all.
>
> Strephon's kiss was lost in jest,
>   Robin's lost in play,
> But the kiss in Colin's eyes
>   Haunts me night and day.[15]

This poem tells of emotions of a distant day. But it also tells something about people. In this age of laboratory-observed sex and a welter of sexual statistics, it has its place. People, not numbers, do the loving. No matter how informative the numbers seem to be about people, each person has a secret heart. Discussions of premarital sex are incomplete without an exploration of individual answers to a variety of questions. What does premarital sex do to the relationship of the participants? How much love is involved? The uses and abuses of sex are numerous. Valid uses of sex vary from reproduction and pleasure to deep desires to share and cooperate with and to give and belong to someone. Its abuses range from destructive domination to sheer revenge. How much premarital sex is based on emotional problems having little to do with love needs? How

[15]Sara Teasdale (1884–1938). "The Look," in Marjorie Barrows, ed., *The Quintessence of Beauty and Romance* (Chicago, 1955), p. 151.

much results from genuine mutual caring and how much from attempts to rebel or to escape anxiety or other problems, such as loneliness or a sense of personal worthlessness? How often does a young person engage in a premarital sexual experience because of the conviction that any pain or humiliation must be endured to get love? When is premarital sex an exploitation of one person by another? Does premarital sex relieve these nonsexual problems or merely accentuate them? Is the young person who has just terminated a first premarital sexual experience more vulnerable to becoming promiscuous? Is the decision to engage in a premarital sexual experience based on a realistic appraisal of the self, or is it part of a glamorized view of a constantly shifting "scene"? Statistics of coital rates among the unmarried hardly reveal adequate information about the causes of these rates. More research in this latter area is greatly needed.

The incidence of premarital sex

Do anxieties from societal and sexual pressures combine to force marriage? Or has the so-called sexual revolution relieved these pressures, reducing the need for marriage, or, at least, the need for early marriage?

One study[16] of college students and their parents indicates that the "sexual revolution" may, for many, be more verbal than active. This report indicates that a majority of girls (66 percent) and boys (52 percent) considered sexual intercourse between engaged couples acceptable. This compared with only 20 percent of their fathers and 17 percent of their mothers approving. That so many of the boys—48 percent of them—considered premarital intercourse unacceptable is not surprising. Some young men still expect to marry a virgin yet attempt to seduce every girl they date. In *Hamlet,* Ophelia notes this male paradox in a little song that relates a lovers' conversation:

> *Young men will do't, if they come to 't,*
>
> *. . .*
>
> *Quoth she, before you tumbled me,*
> *You promised me to wed."*
> He answers:
> *"So would I ha' done, by yonder sun,*
> *An thou hadst not come to my bed."*[17]

Another college study[18] emphasizes the difference in opinion between the generations. Only 55 percent of coeds questioned considered virginity at marriage very important. Eighty-eight percent of the coeds' mothers considered it very important.

This increased percentage of college students sanctioning sexual permissiveness is emphasized by their frank approach to the discussion of

---

[16]Seymour L. Halleck, "Sex and Mental Health on the Campus," *Journal of the American Medical Association,* Vol. 200, No. 8 (May 22, 1967), pp. 684–90.
[17]William Shakespeare, *Hamlet,* IV.v.61–66.
[18]Seymour L. Halleck, "Sex and Mental Health on the Campus," pp. 684–90.

sex. In this they do have a fortunate advantage over their elders. On many college campuses, subjects such as masturbation, oral-genital relations, and homosexuality are no longer taboo in group discussions. This is healthy. Nonetheless, most young people still get much of their sex information, and pressures, from contemporaries. Both can be damaging. Those who desire to help the sexually ignorant must add informed reason to rules. An increasing number of young people, on and off campuses, recognize this as a responsibility of future parenthood.

Do college students today carry out their permissive opinions about premarital sex? One investigator recently wrote:

> Since approximately the time of World War I, there is no strong evidence that the rates of premarital coitus have been increasing. Therefore, the belief that premarital sexual experience is much more common, especially for girls, since the end of World War II, is not supported by available research evidence . . . For the female, premarital coitus usually depends on strong emotional commitment and plans for marriage. The Terman, Burgess and Wallin, and Kinsey studies reported premarital coitus only with men they eventually married. [19]

But it should be emphasized that this and other studies were made some years ago. They relate not to today's college students but to their parents and grandparents. The sexual activities of young people today cannot be measured by data gathered decades ago by varying sampling techniques.

In a study reported in 1968 by Vance Packard, an attempt was made to ascertain premarital coitus rates among juniors and seniors from all regions of the United States. [20] A "College Checklist" was distributed to 2,100 junior and senior students at twenty-one U.S. colleges and universities. At each of the twenty-one institutions 100 students received the checklist. If the schools were coeducational, 50 of the checklists went to males and 50 to females. Of the schools, seven were in the East, five in the Midwest, three in the South, four in the Southwest, and two in the Northwest. Two all-male and two all-female colleges were included. Although these were located in the East, all four drew their students from the entire country. Two schools were church-related—one Protestant, the other Catholic. Both were in the Midwest. The mean age of the students was just under twenty-one. Great care was exercised to respect privacy and insure accuracy of reporting. Sixty-seven percent of the questionnaires were returned—1,393 of the 2,100—of which 665 were from males and 728 from females. The work lacks much in method and as interpretative social science. Some results, to be viewed within these limitations, are:

---

[19]Robert Bell, *Premarital Sex in a Changing Society,* quoted in Lillian Cohen Kovar, *Faces of the Adolescent Girl* (Englewood Cliffs, N.J., 1968), p. 30.
[20]Summarized from Vance Packard, *The Sexual Wilderness* (New York, 1967), Chapters 9–11 and Appendixes.

1. The coital experience of today's college male seems to have increased little since earlier studies. In the 1940s, for example, 51 percent of Alfred Kinsey's group of college-educated "younger generation" had reported that they were coitally experienced by age twenty-one. In the Packard report, the percentage was only slightly higher, 57.

2. Among the junior and senior female respondents, 43 percent reported coital experience. Bearing in mind the hazard of comparing results of present and earlier studies, one can nevertheless suggest that this represents a 60 percent increase over any data gathered before 1960. Only 27 percent of the college-educated females in the Kinsey group had reported coitus by the time they were twenty-one. Despite this, it should be noted that most junior and senior women today remain virgins, as do 43 percent of junior and senior men. This hardly supports the concept that promiscuity is a general practice among U.S. college students.

3. Coital rates by regions, as reported by this study, are as follows:

	MEN	WOMEN
South	69%	32%
East	64%	47%
West	62%	48%
Midwest	46%	25%
National totals	57%	43%

The variance by region is striking. The "double standard" in the South, for example, is apparent. In that region more than twice as many college men as women experience coitus. The relatively low rates in the Midwest support results from regional studies in that area. Several previous studies, wrongly applied by some to the enture U.S. college population, were merely based on regional results. The unreliability of such a procedure can be illustrated by comparing the regional percentages with the national percentages in the Packard report.

More limited data are available from a California study.[21] They indicate the lower incidence of sexual intercourse in early college years (these students were interviewed in the middle of their junior year); in the case of the women, the percentages—26 percent at Berkeley and 23 percent at Stanford—are only slightly more than half the percentage (43 percent nationally) shown in the Packard study of juniors and seniors. These are the coital rates in the California study, as reported to the interviewers:

	MEN			WOMEN		
	Yes	No	Information uncertain	Yes	No	Information uncertain
Berkeley (41 men, 39 women)	39%	61%		26%	72%	2%
Stanford (47 men, 39 women)	36%	60%	4%	23%	62%	15%

[21]Joseph Katz, "Four Years of Growth, Conflict, and Compliance," in *No Time for Youth* (San Francisco, 1968), p. 54.

In the Packard study, 53 percent of the nonvirginal girls had already had coitus with more than one man. More than a third of the nonvirgins had experienced coitus with "several" or many males. However, there are little data to support the picture of the wholly "immoral campus" presented in some newspapers and magazines. Of ninety girls recently queried at the University of Wisconsin, only four felt that casual coitus with many partners should be condoned.[22] And there is data, albeit scanty, to suggest that, for most college girls, sex and affection remain closely linked. (This feeling is, however, not shared by men to the same extent.) In this regard, the small California survey is of interest. According to the interviewers' ratings, sex and affection were strongly linked by the following percentages of those interviewed:[23]

	MEN	WOMEN
Berkeley	32%	62%
(40 men, 36 women)		
Stanford	48%	86%
(39 men, 36 women)		

It is apparent that the majority of today's college girls are more permissive in thought than in action. One may wonder what will happen to their permissive views twenty years hence. Did not their mothers (now so overwhelmingly opposed to premarital sexual intercourse) not have similar liberal opinions about sex? One might recall not only the "sexual revolution" of the middle thirties but also that of the twenties. To the forgetful adult, each new generation seems a heavy burden. And in every generation, elders find the sexual problems of youth easy to solve. Nevertheless, there is some limited evidence that sexual mores may be changing. "The current trend appears to be toward early engagment, followed by coitus, followed by marriage."[24] Many young people will want to carefully evaluate the extent and the meaning of their commitment to each other. The pressures are formidable.

As was the case with their parents and grandparents, this generation of college students has not escaped the accusatory press. Some newspapers, conveniently ignoring the behavior of most students, publish the flamboyant opinions or actions of the smaller percentage. But as one student counselor of long experience recently noted:

> The much-publicized growing sexual promiscuity is not general practice on the campus. Shyness, introversion, vestigial guilt, self-doubt, and the fear of rejection keep students from the practice of their preaching, even with pills and intrauterine devices to reduce their fear of pregnancy. Actually, premarital pregnancies are on the wane, "sleeping around" is not admired and premarital sex is practiced most often in a semiresponsible and monogamous relationship."[25]

[22] Seymour L. Halleck, "Sex and Mental Health on the Campus," pp. 684–90.
[23] Joseph Katz, "Four Years of Growth, Conflict, and Compliance," p. 55.
[24] George Schaefer, "Sex in the Family Milieu," GP, Vol. 36, No. 1 (July 1967), p. 114.
[25] Robert E. Kavanaugh, "The Grim Generation," Psychology Today, Vol. 2, No. 5 (October 1968), p. 55.

TABLE 14-1 *Impact of Premarital Sexual Experience on Two Hundred Young Men*

FEMALE PARTNER (by types)	REACTION OF MALES TO THE EXPERIENCE (by numbers)					RESULTS IN TERMS OF COMMUNICATION
	Satis-factory	Mixed feelings	Unsatis-factory	No feelings	No infor-mation	
TYPE I Prostitutes	8	9	19	2	2	No comment.
TYPE II Pick-ups	8	9	22	15	6	Negative hostility at part-ner.
TYPE III Casual ac-quaintances	28	14	19	4	33	Negative hostility at part-ner.
TYPE IV Dating partners (no affection)	No statistics—23 out of 87 subjects lost respect for partners.					Some hostility but em-phasis of subjects' com-ments stress total re-lationship more than previous types.
TYPE V Dating partners (much affection)	Over one-half expressed some kind of negative per-sonal feelings concerning effect of premarital inter-course.					More mutuality than in previous types. Some guilt reactions.
TYPE VI Fiancées	10	6	3	4	5	Varying effects: inter-course sometimes re-mains integrated into relationship, sometimes weakens it. One-third expressed guilt.

Source: Lester A. Kirkendall, *Premarital Intercourse and Interpersonal Relationships* (New York, 1961), summarized in James A. Peterson, *Education for Marriage*, 2nd ed. (New York, 1964), p. 166. This table is not found in Kirkendall's book but represents Peterson's effort at summarizing various aspects studied by Kirkendall.

How do young men feel about premarital sex?

In the 1968 Packard report,[26] more than half the respondents of both sexes reported that they would not be "seriously" troubled by their future partner having had intercourse with someone else. Nevertheless, a ma-jority of males reported that it would trouble them "some." This study did not reveal whether their feeling troubled would later create problems in their marriage. That a considerable number of college men defer sexual intercourse is significant.

Kirkendall's study of the reaction of two hundred young men to their

[26] Vance Packard, *The Sexual Wilderness*, p. 505.

own premarital sexual experience is summarized by Peterson in Table 14-1. Although this table must be viewed in the light of another time (the late 1950's), it does add to some of the Packard impressions. As affection for the girl develops, male guilt replaces indifference. (With affection, there was more male concern with his partner's possible pregnancy.) Moreover, the young people studied revealed immaturities such as a confusion of passion for love.

In over half the engaged couples, premarital sex was essentially disappointing. Although hardly true of all, those indulging in premarital sexual experience may face greater problems of marital adjustment. It is here pertinent to mention the distinct association between premarital pregnancy and high divorce rates.[27] (Note: data for this last statement were published in the early 1950's.)

A somewhat later study[28] by Reevy revealed that girls who had experienced premarital intercourse were twice as likely to score low on an inventory used to predict marital happiness as girls who had not. Moreover, "there seems to be a general acceptance among investigators that the girl who has premarital coitus before marriage is substantially more likely at some point to become unfaithful after marriage."[29] Some investigators, however, do not agree with this concept, finding it both extreme and unproven.

Young people today are constantly exposed to much argument favoring sexual experience solely on a physical basis. The mere fact that such experiences are pleasurable seems reason enough to casually engage in them. For many, the deferment of sexual pleasures for a more profound relationship, such as marriage, seems "out."

Some misinformed girls believe that almost all unmarried girls have coitus. In possibly being an exception, they feel odd. Frequently, they express surprise at studies showing otherwise. Others feel obliged to have sexual intercourse with young men about to leave for the war zone. Insecure, they are moved by fears of possible loneliness, or a need to make up for rejection, or guilt. This may be partly responsible for the increased coital rates shown in the Packard study (discussed on pages 475–76).

A considerable number of young women are concerned about the ill effects of chastity on their health. There is no doubt that, for some, prolonged sexual repression may give rise to emotional problems. For most women, this is simply not the case. An extremely high percentage of patients under psychiatric care have hardly experienced such repression. A recent survey conducted by two dozen psychiatrists caring for 107 unmarried female students at a Midwestern university revealed that "86

Premarital sex: some concluding reflections

[27] Harold T. Christenson and Hannah H. Meissner, "Premarital Pregnancy as a Factor in Divorce," in Robert F. Winch, Robert McGinnis, and Herbert R. Barringer, *Selected Studies in Marriage and the Family* (New York, 1968), p. 620.
[28] William Reevy, "Premarital Petting Behavior and Marital Happiness Prediction," cited in Vance Packard, *The Sexual Wilderness*, p. 434.
[29] *Ibid.*, p. 432.

percent had had sexual relations with at least one person, and almost three-fourths (72 percent) had relations with more than one person . . . Patients may be promiscuous but the population is not."[30] In this respect, however, further study of some of the nonvirginal college women of the Packard report[31] might have been helpful. As was stated above, a considerable percentage had reported coitus with "several" or "many" males. Whether any of these young women were receiving psychiatric therapy is not known.

It is not here inferred that either premarital sexual intercourse or promiscuity inevitably lead to severe emotional distress for everyone. Indeed, Kinsey found that most women did not regret their premarital sexual experience.[32] Yet, he went on to write: "The clinician might very well advise the individual who is strongly convinced that coitus before marriage is morally wrong to hesitate about having such experience, for she is more likely to be emotionally disturbed by it."[33] The idea that premarital sexual intercourse prevents emotional illness is not valid. The former president of the Academy of Psychoanalysis recently wrote: "There is no reason to believe that one will develop a mental or physical illness unless one's sex needs are satisfied, or that an individual patient's sex life must be paramount in his emotional adjustment."[34] Still another psychiatrist supports this statement in these words: "The proposition that gratification of sexual needs is highly correlated with mental health seems to be at least questionable."[35]

Although, in Kinsey's study, girls pregnant as a result of premarital sexual intercourse "registered little or no regret,"[36] there are those who would regret the potential problems the mothers and their children (and their society) face.

Promiscuity often compounds existing emotional problems. Defensive about flouting a basic societal rule, often ridden by guilt and anxiety, basically lonely, living through uninvolved, indifferent relationships without true intimacy, often committed to neither a past nor a future, the promiscuous person frequently feels a gnawing alienation. Some might say, "As long as nobody else gets hurt it's nobody else's business." But this may be an impractical point of view. One rueful young woman voiced it this way: "What has it all taught me?" she said. "This—when I hurt someone else, they could leave me. When I hurt myself, I couldn't leave me. So that's the real immorality. Hurting yourself. It's lots worse than hurting someone else."

[30] Seymour L. Halleck, 'Sex and Mental Health on the Campus" pp. 684–90.

[31] Vance Packard, The Sexual Wilderness, p. 163.

[32] Alfred C. Kinsey, Wardell B. Pomeroy, Clyde E. Martin, and Paul H. Gebhard, Sexual Behavior in the Human Female (Philadelphia, 1953), p. 316.

[33] Ibid., p. 319.

[34] Leon Salzman, "Recently Exploded Sexual Myths," Medical Aspects of Human Sexuality, Vol. 1, No. 1 (September 1967), p. 9.

[35] Seymour L. Halleck, "Sex and Mental Health on the Campus," pp. 684–90.

[36] Alfred C. Kinsey et al., Sexual Behavior in the Human Female, p. 318. The increased risk to both mother and child of extramarital pregnancy is further discussed in Chapter 11.

Sex without passion

In recently examining the causes of student despair, a Midwestern psychiatrist discussed the campus "elite" group. They are so named because of their considerable influence on other students. Devoted to the present, apprehensive of the future, the members of this group work actively, if intermittently, for political causes. Their attitude toward sex is certainly more casual than that of the average student. Halleck writes of them:

> *No one doubts . . . that the elite group (in contrast to the student population as a whole) are having intimate relations with a greater variety of partners than ever before. Elite students insist that they do so only if a relationship is meaningful. Sometimes this is true. More often, however, this is a pious rationalization . . . Rollo May, professor of graduate psychology at New York University, has described the new sexuality as sex without passion . . . There is reason to doubt the capacity of such students to make successful marriages . . . The student psychiatrist sees more and more recently married couples who find themselves unable to tolerate the possibility of loving one person intimately or remaining faithful to that person . . . The new era of promiscuity seems to have done little to enhance the female student's image of herself as a productive and responsible person. The elite female student shows little inclination to seek a career but seems to be trapped in a new feminine mystique which deprives her of meaningful goals and self-respect. Her status as a whole person is subtly degraded.*[37]

Almost five hundred years ago, the Dutch theologian Erasmus may have best described the true pain of the promiscuous: "I ask you: will he who hates himself love anyone? Will he who does not get along with himself agree with another? Or will he who is disagreeable and irksome to himself bring pleasure to any? No one would say so, unless he were himself more foolish than Folly."[38]

Searching for someone to marry

Why marry?

"We who dwell in the heart of solitude are always the victims of self-doubt. Forever and forever in our loneliness, shameful feelings of inferiority will rise up suddenly to overwhelm us in a poisonous flood of horror, disbelief, and desolation, to sicken and corrupt our health and confidence.[39]

[37] Seymour L. Halleck, "The Roots of Student Despair," *Think*, Vol. 33, No. 2 (March–April 1967), pp. 22–23.

[38] Erasmus, "The Praise of Folly," in Louis Kronenberger, ed., *The Pleasure of Their Company* (New York, 1946), p. 564.

[39] Thomas Wolfe, "God's Lonely Man," in *The Hills Beyond* (Garden City, N.Y., 1941), p. 187.

Thomas Wolfe could make the despair of solitude seem to be a stimulating episode. It may be. But as a way of life solitude is nothing to be desired. As the Creator observed, "It is not good that the man should be alone" (Genesis 2:18).

Basically, men who are alone seek wives, and single women husbands, so that they will not be alone. True, there are other reasons, such as societal pressure. But, by far the greatest majority of ordinary people seek a meaningful, sharing relationship with another person.

There are studies in which respondents rated "the relief of loneliness" last as a need they wanted satisfied. But to be loved, to have someone to confide in, to show affection—these were mentioned most often. Without these, one is indeed lonely. But marriage is not merely an escape from a self-centered downbeat emotion. It is a positive and creative way to work for self-realization. Successfully married people can take and give affection. They confide in one another without fear of harsh judgment. They can cry together and not be ashamed. They can disagree, even quarrel violently, and know it is not the end. They are busy, not only with one another, but with a variety of life's challenges. In no other human relationship can this kind of mutuality be developed. But the skills involved in building and sustaining such a relationship are not inherent, nor are they easily acquired. They require effort. So to conquer loneliness through marriage is to gain many things. One should seek not a person with whom to share loneliness but one to help dispel it.

Courtship: reflexive? reflective? or both?
The right person means contentment. The wrong one can indeed entwine two lives in grief. "Though thou canst not forbear to love," wrote Sir Walter Raleigh to his son, "yet forbear to link."[40] The brilliant Elizabethan knight did not advise against marriage. He advised caution. Of the three most elemental events in human life—birth, death, and marriage—marriage is most open to intelligent personal decision. Love has been too simply defined as a conflict between reflex and reflection.[41] Reflection can enrich the expression of love that molds a good marriage.

At twenty, one can hardly contemplate fifty years of living. A marriage choice is thus all the more difficult. It is not easy to make one decision do for half a century. The wonder is not that one of five marriages in this country ends in divorce. The wonder is that there are not more failures.

There are those, like H. G. Wells, who considered it foolhardly to leave so vital a decision "to flushed and blundering youth . . . with nothing to guide it but shocked looks and sentimental twaddle and base whisperings and cant-smeared examples."[42] Samuel Johnson grumbled that all marriages should be arranged by the Lord Chancellor "without the parties

[40] Quoted in Alan C. Valentine, ed., *Fathers to Sons: Advice Without Consent* (Oklahoma City, 1963), p. 16.
[41] *Szpilki* (Warsaw, Poland), cited in *Atlas*, Vol. 16, No. 3 (September 1968), p. 58.
[42] H. G. Wells, *Tono-Bungay*, quoted in E. S. Turner, *A History of Courting*, p. 15.

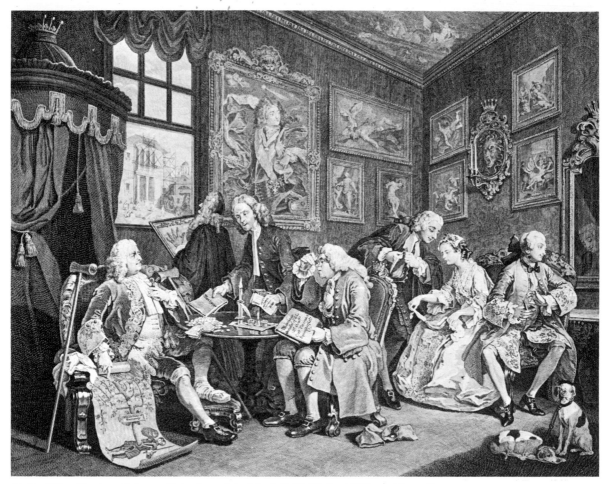

14-5 "The Contract" from "Marriage à la Mode" (1745) by William Hogarth (1697–1764). The wealthy, socially ambitious merchant and his lawyer offer gold, bonds, and mortgages, while the impoverished earl points to his impeccable family tree and favors his aristocratically gouty foot. As for the bartered couple, the merchant's daughter seems less than ecstatic at the match; the future groom admires himself in the mirror.

having any choice in the matter.[43] Some sixteen centuries ago, Father Tertullian (160?–230?) gloomily regarded the corrupt Roman society and its tottering empire. "Divorce," he said, "was now looked upon as one fruit of marriage."[44]

To avoid tasting of that bitter fruit, what thoughts, and questions should occur to the person who is considering someone as a potential mate?

---

[43] Boswell's *Life of Johnson*, quoted in Holbrook Jackson, *Bookman's Pleasure* (New York, 1947), p. 77.
[44] Willystine Goodsell, *A History of Marriage and the Family*, p. 145.

Some general pointers

1. Does the relationship survive loss of glamor? In the moonlight most girls look lovely. In a similar light most young men get by pretty well. However, how do matters seem when one of the parties is miserable with a bad cold?

2. How is conflict handled? Do the inevitable problems that erupt during a disagreement always get buried only by mutual physical attraction? Or do conflicts teach insight and better understanding of each other? It is as important to learn from a quarrel as it is to make up.

3. Is conversation easy? Perhaps the pair have never really talked to each other. Can one endure the occasional long silence of the other when necessary?

4. What happens to the pair in a group? Does either of them embarrass or persistently criticize the other? Is one ashamed of the other? Do they avoid groups altogether? Why? Courting is a private affair, but most married people have get-togethers with friends.

5. How are decisions made? Does one member of the pair expect the other to "like it or lump it"? Some couples say that "we have been married for forty years and have never had a word of disagreement." When two people agree on everything, only one is thinking.

6. Is that knitting or stamp collecting or pro football or interminable chatter on the telephone going to be bearable for fifty whole years?

7. What is the home life of the possible life partner like? Repeated studies have shown that people from relatively happy homes are the best marriage risks. (There is the exception, of course, of the child of divorced parents who works all the harder to make a marriage succeed. Too, there is the occasional case of the marital partner who sacrifices an entire life to the wounding memory of a parental divorce. Fearful of marriage failure, he or she may scrupulously avoid all disagreement and never express his or her individuality.) Moreover, although it need not be decisive, the attitude of the family toward the prospective mate is important.

8. What are his or her best friends like? "Kookie"? If so, it is well for the marriage partner to be a trifle "kookie" too. Or are they all conservative Republicans who treasure their used Goldwater buttons? In that case, matters will be more pleasant if the other partner is, at least, an admirer of President Nixon.

9. What is the physical health of the potential marital partner? A slight anemia may add a bewitching pallor to the complexion, but it may become wearing after a few years of marriage.

10. How self-sufficient is the proposed mate? How dependent? How much dependency does one need of the other? The following excerpt from a case history is pertinent:

She dreamed that she was holding her son in her arms and that suddenly he began to increase in size while she began to decrease in height. Within a few seconds her child was standing, holding her in his arms. This patient unconsciously wanted to continue to be the child, to prolong indefinitely the dependency relationship that she had with her father and the father image. [45]

Overdependency can become an illness. That it is an illness only when carried beyond a certain point is not well understood. It is degree that often determines mental aberration. To some extent all normal people are dependent. Marriage provides the individual with one way of satisfying this normal need. However, as is noted from the above case, dependency may be extreme and unresolved. Manifesting itself in marriage, overdependency may cause one partner to unconsciously expect the other to be a substitute parent. This role the second partner may summarily reject. Frustrated, the dependent partner may seek attention by becoming a hypochondriac or an alcoholic. When this happens, the marriage is endangered.

The knowledge that marriage must satisfy both unconscious and conscious needs should stimulate some analysis of the unconscious needs. "Lay yourself open to yourself." [46] So, in about 1654, wrote William Russell to his son Frank. It is good advice that is hard to follow. But, in the seeking of a marriage partner, it is essential. One man, for example, needs to be submissive. Unconsciously ashamed of this need, he hides it. Consequently, he behaves dominantly. And, worse, he does not realize it. It is in his unconscious self-deception that he is confounded, that he betrays himself. Another man is submissive. He is uncomfortable with domineering women so he marries a girl as submissive as he. When each looks to the other for the final word, who will make a decision?

11. What role does each potential marital partner expect the other to play? There is the man who wants to marry a pretty girl who is a good housekeeper. He understands and wants the responsibility of making money to support his family. Other men have a less traditional approach. They emphasize companionship and education. Those who contemplate marriage need, then, to examine the role they expect to play and the role they want their intended partner to perform in the marriage situation.

Mixed marriages

A paradox in this nation's culture is this: the attributes of which the nation is proudest endanger an institution on which it depends—marriage. Individualism is revered, yet marriage is hardly an individual enterprise. The people of this country draw strength from the cultural melting pot. Yet from this same pot come mixed marriages. And mixed marriages are risky.

There are, in this nation, at least a dozen Protestant denominations with memberships totalling over sixty-nine million people. The Roman Catholic church includes in its membership forty-six million people with

[45] James A. Peterson, *Education for Marriage*, 2nd ed. (New York, 1964), p. 187.
[46] Quoted in Alan C. Valentine, *Fathers to Sons: Advice Without Consent*, p. 33.

an almost bewildering variety of tongues and customs. Other Christians belong to such groups as the Eastern Orthodox church and the Polish National Catholic church. The Jews—Orthodox, Conservative, and Reform—number five and a half million. There are also quite a few Buddhists and Mohammedans in this country. Then, there are those who believe in not believing in God or in any divine personality or meaning. It may be the opinion of some that when they die and lie in state, they are indeed all dressed up with no place to go. But they rightfully expect their opinions to be respected.

In 1967, the great majority (87.9 percent) of the U.S. population was white. There were over twenty million blacks, hundreds of thousands of American Indians, Chinese, and Japanese. Filipinos, Hindus, Koreans, Hawaiians, and Malayans all add spice to the melting pot. And total racial amalgamation is unlikely to occur during the lifetime of anyone alive today.[47]

In the past century and a half, some 42 million immigrants came to this country. Over that long period of time, Ireland, Germany, and Great Britain contributed the greatest numbers. However, in 1960, Italy was the leading country of origin of foreign-born U.S. inhabitants. Most countries of the world have added some stock to the mixture.

This wonderful conglomeration of people marry and reproduce in a society dominated by one belief—the sanctity of the individual. A clash of interests is inevitable. The demand for the satisfaction of individual needs is opposed by the demands imposed on each individual by his cultural background. Too often the resulting conflicts lead to divorce.

Interfaith marriages   People of different religious faiths often fall in love. Rebellion or status-seeking by no means accounts for all interfaith marriages. But those who contemplate marrying someone outside their own faith should comprehend their chances of happiness. Unfortunately, there have been methodological problems in the study of this matter. Still, the following data do provide food for thought.

Interfaith couples are less likely to adjust well to marriage. One study showed the following percentages of low-adjustment scores for married couples:[48]

Protestant-Protestant	20%
Non-church marriages	29%
Catholic-Catholic	39%
Protestant-Catholic	50%

To look at it the other way, only 50 percent of Protestant-Catholic marriages scored *high* adjustments in this study, while 61 percent of

[47]David M. Heer, "Intermarriage and Racial Amalgamation in the United States," *Eugenics Quarterly,* Vol. 14, No. 2 (April 1967), p. 120.
[48]James A. Peterson, *Education for Marriage,* 2nd ed., p. 223.

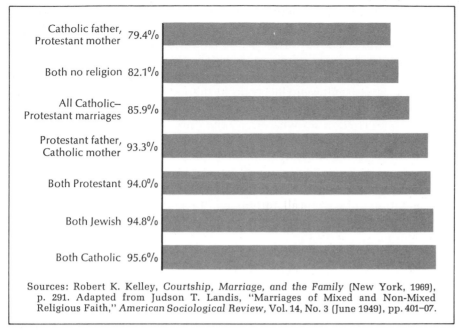

Catholic father, Protestant mother	79.4%
Both no religion	82.1%
All Catholic–Protestant marriages	85.9%
Protestant father, Catholic mother	93.3%
Both Protestant	94.0%
Both Jewish	94.8%
Both Catholic	95.6%

Sources: Robert K. Kelley, *Courtship, Marriage, and the Family* (New York, 1969), p. 291. Adapted from Judson T. Landis, "Marriages of Mixed and Non-Mixed Religious Faith," *American Sociological Review*, Vol. 14, No. 3 (June 1949), pp. 401–07.

14-6 Marriage stability: the religious factor.

Catholic-Catholic marriages, 71 percent of non-church marriages, and 80 percent of Protestant-Protestant marriages scored high.

Another study indicates that, by marrying a non-Catholic, a Catholic woman increases her chances of divorce or separation by about 50 percent. A Protestant woman, by marrying outside her religion, increases her risks of divorce or separation by more than 300 percent.[49]

Other research gives similar results (Figure 14-6). Some five percent of unmixed Jewish and Catholic marriages end in divorce or separation. This increases to about six percent in unmixed Protestant marriages. However, some fifteen percent of mixed Catholic-Protestant marriages end in divorce. The most hazardous of all is the marriage of a Catholic man to a Protestant woman. More than one in five, over twenty percent, end in divorce. The same study indicates too that the marriage of a Catholic woman to a man without a religion is only half as risky as a Protestant woman marrying a man who does not profess a religion.[50]

A 1960 study also revealed a markedly higher (three times the average) divorce rate in Catholic-Protestant marriages. It is true that tolerance is growing in this nation. How far this will go to reversing figures pointing to the increased risk of Protestant-Catholic marriages remains to be seen.

[49] *4,108 Marriages of Parents of Michigan State University Students,* cited in Robert O. Blood, *Marriage* (New York, 1964), p. 83.
[50] Judson T. Landis, "Marriages of Mixed and Non-Mixed Religious Faith," *American Sociological Review*, Vol. 14, No. 3 (June 1949), pp. 401–07.

There are isolated signs of permissiveness among individual members of the major religious bodies. However, the general reaction of the religious leadership in the United States to interfaith marriage is negative.

Although the Jewish intermarriage rate is the lowest of the three major faiths in this country, it is certainly increasing. In 1963, Rosenthal[51] reported the Jewish intermarriage rate in the nation's capital to have risen from 1 percent with first-generation Jewish marriages to 10.2 percent for those of the second to 17.9 percent by the third generation. It is of interest that the number of children of these marriages raised in the Jewish religion fell spectacularly when compared to earlier generations. In 1964, Sklare[52] accepted the 17.9 percent figure as "probably very close to the current rate." Reform Jewish congregations are more tolerant of Jewish intermarriage than those of the Orthodox or Conservative tradition. Although a large number of such marriages are known to be successful, more adequate studies are indicated.

What are some major sources of disharmony in interfaith marriages? Despite ardent premarital agreements, conflicts often occur over the religious training of children. (This may account for the very high divorce rates of Protestant mothers from Catholic fathers.) Artificial birth control, a practice opposed by the Catholic religion, is another source of deep disagreement. Then, there are the multitudinous cultural differences. Religion is a way of life. Even those whose relationship to their own faith has been casual may find the rituals of another church an imposition.

Many interfaith marriages succeed. Nevertheless, it is well to remember that love alone does not necessarily conquer all.

Interracial marriages   In 1967, the U.S. Supreme Court invalidated a Virginia law forbidding marriages between whites and blacks. That Virginia and sixteen other states had passed such laws testifies to the considerable hostility against such marriages. Nevertheless, they are increasing. In one recent study[53] of data from Hawaii, Michigan, Nebraska, and California, it was found that the rate of white-black marriages rose during the period studied. Hawaii had the highest reported incidence of black-white marriages, with California, Michigan, and Nebraska following. Interestingly enough, 1959 data, the latest available from California and Michigan, showed that the black-white marriage rate in Michigan was half that of California. Both are industrial states with similar proportions of black populations. An exploratory study in Indiana[54] indicated that such marriages generally occur among people who are, by and large, equals in education, economics,

---

[51]Erich Rosenthal, "Studies of Jewish Intermarriage in the United States," *American Jewish Year Book* (New York, 1963), pp. 3–53.

[52]Marshall Sklare, "Intermarriage & the Jewish Future," *Commentary*, Vol. 37, No. 4 (April 1964), pp. 46–52.

[53]David M. Heer, "Negro-White Marriage in the United States," *Journal of Marriage and the Family*, Vol. 28, No. 3 (August 1966), pp. 262–73.

[54]Todd H. Pavela, "An Exploratory Study of Negro-White Intermarriage in Indiana," *Journal of Marriage and the Family*, Vol. 26, No. 5 (May, 1964), pp. 209–11.

and culture. Kelley[55] suggests that those contemplating an interracial marriage would do well to carefully consider all the issues, varying from personal motivations to the possibilities of varying values, whether they be social, ethical, educational, or religious. Of course, these considerations, among others, are important in all marriages. As to the potential for marital success of these and other interracial marriages, adequate appraisal awaits more intensive study.

Interclass marriages

Numerous studies show that adjustment rates are poor in marriages in which the partners come from widely separated social classes. The wider the class difference between husband and wife, the lower is the percentage of good adjustment.[56]

Men are more likely than women to have a successful marriage with a partner slightly below their own class. The college English professor may marry the colorful truck driver and get away with it. She is more likely to end by criticizing his fingernails, and he will puzzle why she never noticed them before. Each will be right about the other and wrong for the other.

Money

> *"My other piece of advice, Copperfield," said Mr. Micawber, "you know. Annual income twenty pounds, annual expenditure nineteen nineteen six, result happiness. Annual income twenty pounds, annual expenditure twenty pounds ought and six, result misery. The blossom is blighted, the leaf is withered, the god of day goes down upon the dreary scene, and—and, in short, you are for ever floored. As I am!"[57]*

In this, the most affluent of nations, countless couples attribute their marriage failures to "money problems." One major study[58] points out that it is not the amount but the manner of expenditures that is the major cause of marital friction. Tearfully, one young wife told this story:

> *It's twenty years ago, but it's like yesterday. I was seven. I knew my father had just lost his job, but I pretended I didn't. He came out of the bedroom and told my mother, "I don't know. I just don't know where our next piece of bread is coming from." Sometimes, I can still hear him. His voice was quiet. In two years he was dead.*
>
> *What's this got to do with my husband? He doesn't understand. He'll go out and spend two hundred dollars on a suit. Or he'll buy white-wall tires. He just doesn't know that being poor can kill a person like it killed my father. He doesn't know what it's like not to know where your next piece of bread is coming from.*

[55] Robert K. Kelley, *Courtship, Marriage, and the Family* (New York, 1969), pp. 270–71.
[56] Ruth Shonle Cavan, *The American Family*, 2nd ed. (New York, 1953), p. 232.
[57] Charles Dickens, *David Copperfield* (London, 1849–50), Chapter 12.
[58] Lewis M. Terman, *Psychological Factors in Marital Happiness* (New York, 1938), pp. 167–71.

It is true; he does not know. And the danger to their marriage is that he does not want to know. He has never known a day of financial want. His side of the story is typical:

> We've been married eleven years. I've never made less than twenty thousand a year. We've got money in the bank. Even if we didn't, my folks could help. They have always had more than they need. What's she so scared about?

The problems of this couple spring from their widely disparate economic pasts. Spending patterns are learned in childhood from family experience. She will forever tighten the purse strings that he will forever loosen.

Similar tensions overtake the rich girl-poor boy marriage. The woman who once drove her own expensive car may well find a crowded bus irksome. The early fun of making a budget work often becomes a weary trial. Sadly, she may soon see the sum of her expenditures as the dreary sum of her marriage.

How can these pitfalls be avoided? One should know not only the financial behavior pattern of the proposed mate, but also his or her ability to plan expenditures. How one fits finances into married life is often critical.

Age   In no other Western country do people marry so young as in the United States. Prosperity, the income of the working girl, the changing role of the teen-ager from a family financial asset to a costly burden—all these promote marriage at an early age. In the United States, in 1965, more girls were married at eighteen than at any other age.

Teen-age marriages are particularly prone to failure. Numerous studies repeatedly emphasize the high divorce and poor adjustment rates of teen-age unions. One investigator found "that the proportion of remarried women among those who first married below the age of 18 years was about three times as high as that for women who first married between the ages of 22 to 24 years."[59] Particularly hazardous are marriages between the very young. The divorce rates of marriages between people sixteen or younger is 400 percent higher than for marriages in which husbands were from twenty to twenty-six years old and wives twenty-two to twenty-four.[60]

How old should one be before getting married? Some students of marriage recommend twenty-nine for the man and twenty-four for the woman. Others suggest twenty-five and twenty-two. Setting the same age for everyone is pointless. Emotional stability and maturity are better

---

[59] Paul C. Glick, "Stability of Marriage in Relation to Age at Marriage," in Robert F. Winch et al., eds., Selected Studies in Marriage and the Family, rev. ed. (New York, 1962), p. 624.
[60] Thomas P. Monahan, "Does Age of Marriage Matter in Divorce?" Social Forces, Vol. 32, No. 10 (October 1953), p. 86.

indices of marital success than chronological age. One good way of deferring a possibly premature marriage while at the same time learning more about a potential partner is a reasonably long engagement. How long should the engagement period be? A year should tell the couple enough. "The best insurance policy against divorce in our society is a thorough engagement."[61] As Chaucer wrote:

> It is no childes pley
> To take a wyf with-oute avysement.[62]

Seek, then, advisement for marriage.

[61] Ersel Earl LeMasters, *Modern Courtship and Marriage* (New York, 1957), p. 168.
[62] Geoffrey Chaucer, *The Merchant's Tale,* lines 1530–31.

15

Marriage: "the craft so long to lerne"

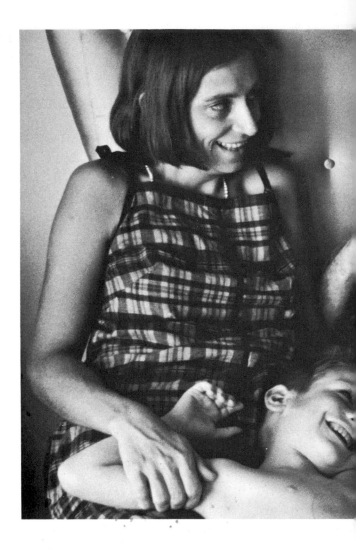

Prologue

Next, when they had got them huts and skins and fire and woman was appropriately mated to one man, and the laws of wedlock became known and they saw offspring born of them, then first mankind begun to soften. For the fire saw to it that their shivering bodies were less able to endure cold under the canopy of heaven and Venus sapped their strength and children easily broke their parents' proud spirit by coaxing. Then also neighbors began eagerly to join in a league of friendship amongst themselves to do no hurt and suffer no violence, and asked protection for their children and womankind, signifying by voice and gesture, with stammering tongue, that it was right for all to pity the weak. Nevertheless concord could not altogether be established, but a good part, nay the most part, kept the covenant in good faith or else the race of mankind would even

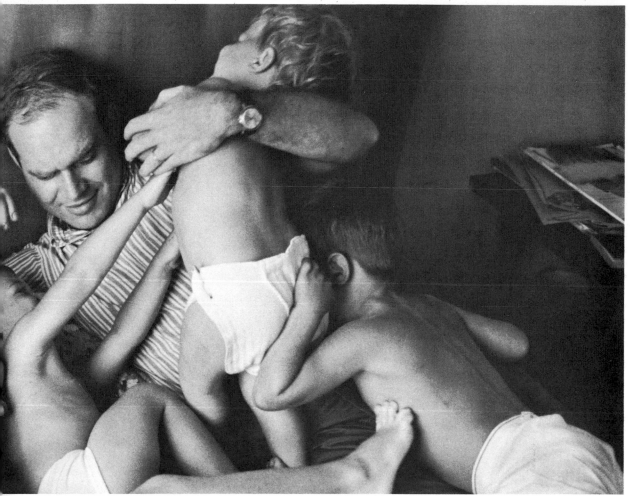

then have been completely destroyed, nor would birth and begetting have availed to prolong their posterity.[1]

So did the Roman poet Lucretius (96?–55 B.C.) tell about the beginnings of the family of man. As noted in the previous chapter, families banded together and established protective societal rules. Those breaking the rules imperiled the group and were punished. Sex and love, and marriage too, were essentially controlled by the group. In that sense, man's deepest intimacy was public business. So it is today. Although marriage has ancient origins, it remains as rich and complex an adventure as life itself. And just as six centuries ago the poet Chaucer described life as "the craft so long to lerne," so is marriage a craft no less quickly learned.

[1]Lucretius, *On the Nature of Things,* quoted in Felding H. Garrison, *Contributions to the History of Medicine* (New York, 1966), p. 25.

No known human society allows promiscuity—sexual life without rules—to be its governing way of life. In every society, marriage and the family exist. All societies, moreover, have chosen marriage as the arrangement for having children. And "in every known human society, there is a prohibition against incest."[2] These pervasive behavior patterns prevent social convulsions that would be inimical to child-rearing. Without such restrictions, the group would die, the victim of its own rulelessness. "It is marriage which is the basic social instrument of man's survival . . . for survival there must be an accommodation between the sexes . . . enduring enough to provide protection, care, and reasonable security for the offspring."[3]

Marriage serves man's needs to resolve loneliness and to perpetuate his kind. And society pressures him to resolve these needs through marriage. In relatively recent years, however, new dimensions of marriage have developed. Have they weakened the married state?

Today, the date of the marriage does not await the completion of either education or military service. Never before have so many students and soldiers married. And they share with all recently married people a new awareness of sexual relationships. No longer, for example, are woman's sexual needs incidental. Rapid social change, moreover, has added threats to the stability of marriage. The mobility of the family and the emancipation of the woman are but two of the factors contributing to fresh perspectives of marriage. What are some of the aspects of marriage so characteristic of these times?

War and marriage

War is the youth's premature introduction to age. On the battlefield he is old enough to die. Escaping death, it is there that he leaves his youth. Nobody ever returned young from a war. This the young today share with the young of yesterday. And both young men and women today ask an old question: how can we cope with a separating war?

During the First World War, British posters urged young women to jilt men who failed to volunteer for military service. How effective this method of obtaining soldiers was is unknown. Today, draft boards seem to do well enough. But even a little more than a generation ago there were no seemingly permanent draft boards. In the public mind, war and peace were curiously separated from each other. When war came, it was but a temporary tragedy to be gotten over with. It was peacetime that lasted long enough for planning. After a war was over, the arena of conflict was returned to politicians. Except for a few nostalgic songs such as "It's a Long Way to Tipperary" or "Lili Marlene," the war was fought to be forgotten.

[2] Bernard Berelson and Gary A. Steiner, *Human Behavior* (New York, 1964), pp. 313–16.
[3] William M. Kephart, *The Family, Society, and the Individual* (Boston, 1961), p. 64.

This is all over. Perhaps it is why there is no true promise of peace. To prevent one biggest war, modern man seems destined to agonize over smaller wars. The draft board is the culminating sickness of the times. It will not go away soon. How can young people deal with the anxiety it creates? How can they fit the draft board in their need to love and to marry?

The draft board may inadvertently help decide the date of a wedding. But it should never decide whether a marriage will take place. The decision to marry should not await the decision of a draft board. The suitability of the couple, the adequacy of the courtship—such factors, not "better times in which to get married," should determine the course of action. Some people spend their lives preparing for hurdles they never meet. When, at long last, they are forced to meet life's obstacles, they are alone. Impending military service is not a signal to ignore caution. There are many valid reasons to defer marriage. However, military service is not necessarily one of them.

In this, most parents will need help. Fathers and mothers remember the fragile marriages during the Second World War and the Korean "police action." Sometimes they will use the man's military service as an excuse because they oppose the marriage itself. However, parents can be remarkably sympathetic and helpful and should be consulted.

Whether the young wife should follow her enlisted husband to his post will depend on circumstances. If at all possible, the wife should live with or near her husband. On or around military bases, living costs are high. Housing may be inadequate. Transportation may be a trial. Overcrowding is usual. Competition for jobs is great. Recreational facilities are often poor. Social contacts may be limited. Yet the problems are not comparable to those that may occur with prolonged separation. If a baby is expected, the young wife may well choose to live with her parents temporarily. Those who go into marriage secure in their love and willing to work at making their marriage a success will find even the hardships on or near a military post an enrichment. On the other hand, the insecure will not usually find security in a marriage, no matter where they live.

Nonetheless, there are those for whom war means long separation. Are intimacy, love, closeness—the meanings of marriage—transmissible over great distances of time and space? In one study[4] of Iowa couples separated during the Second World War, these factors were found to ease the pain of separation:

1. Frequent, even daily, letters were exchanged detailing daily doings and hopes. These letters were more than mere reiterations of love. The sender communicated. The receiver shared.

2. Snapshots of each other, family, and friends were frequently exchanged.

3. Gifts were exchanged often between the couple and their families.

[4]Reuben Hill, *Families Under Stress,* cited in E. E. Le Masters, *Modern Courtship and Marriage* (New York, 1957), p. 218.

To the Young Women of London.

Is your "Best Boy" wearing Khaki? If not, don't you think he should be?

If he does not think that you and your country are worth fighting for—do you think he is worthy of you?

Don't pity the girl who is alone—her young man is probably a soldier—fighting for her and her country—and for you.

If your young man neglects his duty to his King and Country, the time may come when he will neglect you.

Think it over—then ask your young man to

JOIN THE ARMY TO-DAY.

15-1 A First World War British recruiting poster.

4. Special occasions, such as anniversaries and birthdays, were celebrated by cablegram and long-distance telephone.

Should a married woman date while her husband is away on military duty? No. Jealousy and gossip would result. Eventually, moreover, the jealousy could become justified; the gossip, true. If an engaged couple agreed upon it beforehand, the girl may date randomly while her fiancé is away on military duty. Such random dating may test an inadequate courtship. This is fair. Few engaged servicemen refrain from dating.

For some, war hastens marriage. A hasty marriage is a risky one. "Married in haste, we may repent at leisure," wrote William Congreve. Those considering hasty service marriages will do well to examine their motives. Some young women panic, fearful that all eligible men will be gone. Others desire "to have his baby so he will have something to remember while he's gone." Such immaturity resulted in numerous Second World War marriages. Many failed.

Service marriages are more successful if time has been taken for courtship and if the marriage takes place at least several months before or after the induction. A new marriage, combined with boot camp, demands too much adjustment in too little time.

Even the trial of unkind separation can be turned to some advantage. Seasoned by a major mark of maturity—the deferment of gratification— the bonds between the partners are deepened. So it is with many campus marriages. Again, gratification is deferred. But in the very planning together for a mutual future, there are opportunities for sharing. Of course, there are problems to be considered and solved. What are some of them?

The campus marriage

At the turn of this century the average boy left school at fourteen. Not until twelve years later, not until he had settled into his life work and had saved a tidy sum, did he chance marriage. The dictum of Benjamin Franklin, "First thrive, then wive," was the order of that day. Furthermore, in 1890 only 63.1 percent of the population of this country ever married. In this country today more than 80 percent of all people over eighteen are married. The average man now marries at about twenty-two rather than twenty-six. In 1967 half of the men in the United States who married did so between twenty and twenty-six (one-fourth by twenty, and three-fourths by twenty-six). About half of all women who married did so between nineteen and twenty-three (one-fourth are married by nineteen, and three-fourths by twenty-three).[5] So permanent a commitment by the college students in these groups poses singular problems.

It was not until the Second World War was over that married students were first seen in appreciable numbers on the nation's college campuses.

[5] Clark E. Vincent, "Sex and the Young Married," *Medical Aspects of Human Sexuality*, Vol. 3, No. 3 (March 1969), p. 13.

Thousands of veterans used their benefits to obtain an education. Today's graying professors remember them well. They were not college boys. They were older, tougher men. Some were filled with a speechless anger. Most were intensely purposeful. They had no time to fool around. They had been through a war and knew something about time. Many were married. Their wives worked. There was always pregnancy to think about. It was, for most vets, a difficult time. It was, for their wives, a time for marking time. Veterans were used to waiting. Their wives quickly learned.

One of the chief concerns of married students is money. A recent nation-wide survey showed that parents pay for 61 percent of students' expenses.[6] Marriage changes that picture. Some married students want to make it on their own. Often parents are reluctant to help because of a sincere belief that such a prolonged dependency might harm the marriage. Others are more abrupt: "If you're old enough to get married, you're old enough to support yourself." Many parents do help. Nevertheless, married students receive much less parental cash than do single students. Some married students are aided by the GI Bill. Most work. Not uncommonly the wife supports her student husband. Whatever the plan, it is beset with risks. That the vast majority of campus marriages succeed speaks well for the maturity of those who venture into them.

It is the campus wife's education that is at greatest risk. Marriage may dilute her motivation; the purchase of an economics text cannot compare with her first investment in a Picasso reproduction for the bedroom wall. No philosophy professor will gain her attention as a whimpering baby will. Yet, occasionally, an educationally mixed marriage may result, and her sacrifice multiplies. Her husband becomes involved in the world of the slide rule or the stethoscope or Byzantine art. Her world may become a matter of warming a typewriter or yesterday's stew. Or she may seek contentment in recipes and afternoon TV shows. (There is no evening TV. He has to study.) A conversation gap occurs and widens. In a class in Russian literature, the student husband hears a quote: "If you are afraid of loneliness, do not marry."[7] But he is already married. He studies guiltily. She is lonely too. "If it hadn't been for you . . ." they both think. The bubble of love bursts, and mutual blame takes over.

Moreover, the married student is pressed for time. He may need to devote every evening of the week to study. Restlessly, his wife remembers the ruthless exclusion of the married from campus activity. She seeks to be busy. She may read or do mechanical things or perhaps go to the movies alone. She worries about their inadequate sexual relationship, a surprisingly common problem among married college students.[8] To maintain her aspect of the mutual vision of an educational investment, she will need to draw from the deepest wellsprings of her maturity. For the wife, handling spare time may become an issue. Her youth does not

[6] Robert O. Blood, *Marriage* (New York, 1964), p. 163.
[7] *The Personal Papers of Anton Chekhov*, intro. by Matthew Josephson (New York, 1948), p. 75.
[8] James A. Peterson, *Education for Marriage*, 2nd ed. (New York, 1964), p. 216.

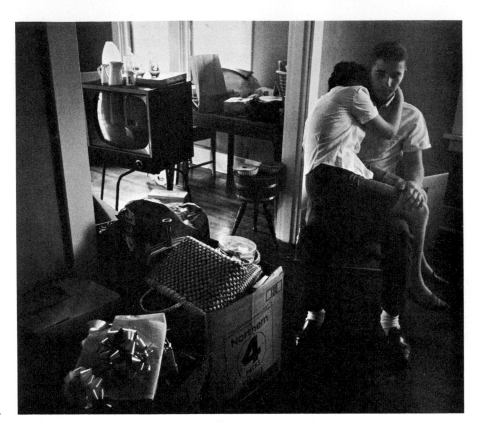

15-2 Move-in day.

help the situation. Conflicts over leisure time are a major cause of marriage failure among college students. Campus marriages now occur at an earlier age than they used to. The college student must bring security into a student marriage. To count on finding security within marriage is a mistake.

Pregnancy may also complicate the student marriage. It ends the wife's immediate plan for a college education. Often it concludes her husband's schooling. Some college fathers successfully lead a tripartite life. Their time is divided between job, school, and family. In one study it was found that "only 52 percent of the graduate-student fathers were going to school full-time compared to 79 percent of the childless graduate students."[9]

Grades may be a problem. Some studies do indicate that married-student grades are equal to, or even better than, those of single students. However, marriage can hardly be recommended as a means of improving grades. There is a significant lack of data regarding the number of married students who drop out of school because of poor grades. The relationship between the married student's age and grades needs further study. Sometimes grades, as such, create dissension. The wife who consistently does

[9]Robert O. Blood, *Marriage*, p. 166.

better than her husband may find herself in the same position as the unmarried coed who feels it necessary "to play dumb" with her dates. The young, nonbreadwinning husband, his masculine role further diminished, may add resentment to regret. It will require a tactful wife to weather the storm.

Premarital planning helps. Realism must temper romanticism. What must be accomplished? What resources will be needed? From whom will help come? What about pregnancy? For those who wish to marry while in college, at least these questions should first be objectively answered.

And so it is apparent that student marriages demand much from the young couple. By far the greatest majority do have what it takes.

So far in this chapter two circumstances of marriage that must be dealt with early have been considered. Indeed, they are best discussed and planned for before the marriage takes place. The next problem is rarely considered, even expected. So insidiously does it develop that neither partner clearly sees it as a threat to their future. Too, for some it hardly exists. Others accept it. Still others resent it. It is the problem of monotony in marriage.

Marriage, monotony, and the appreciation of both

> And may her bride-groom bring her to a house
> Where all's accustomed, ceremonious;
> For arrogance and hatred are the wares
> Peddled in the thoroughfares.
> How but in custom and in ceremony
> Are innocence and beauty born?[10]

In the pattern of everyday married life, there is much that is honored by time. Custom and ceremony, no matter how subtle, add to the richness of the marital fabric. But mere repetition makes for a drab cloth. Individuality and custom can, however, be compatible. Indeed, customs provide an opportunity for sharing individuality. Her custom may be as simple as a best tablecloth for dinner. But unless he occasionally brings a bunch of flowers to decorate the table too, the time will come when neither sees the tablecloth. What is left? Monotony.

Many people find some marriage monotony a comfort, not a problem. They see it as a mark of their certainty about each other. Whether one can count on the other is a valid test of courtship. In marriage it is part of the loving. Life cannot be perpetual excitement. There is surely some truth in this reasoning.

Others refuse to even recognize tedium as a possible part of marriage. They hark back to the "good old days," when people (meaning women) had no time for nonsense like boredom. "In the past," they say, "women

---

[10] William Butler Yeats, "A Prayer for My Daughter."

knew their place; they never thought about being bored, and they never got a divorce either." Just how far back the good old days go for such philosophers is never clear. That Grandpa was a kindly soul, in whose beneficent light Grandma was ever content, may be true. Maybe. For those, however, who forever seek improvement only from the distant past, a code of sixteenth-century Russian family practices, called *The Domostroy* (Domestic Ordinance), will be enlightening. It was prepared by Pope Sylvester in the reign of the first Tsar of Russia, that monstrous murderer Ivan IV (1530–80), called "The Terrible." This is an excerpt:

> *If she does not obey . . . then the husband should punish his wife and fill her with fear, and punish her with love.*

Gentleness, however, is urged.

> *The husband should not hit her eyes or ears nor beat her with his fists or feet under the heart . . . whoever beats her that way . . . causes much trouble; blindness, deafness, broken hands and feet . . . But to beat carefully, with a whip, is sensible . . . healthy . . . In case of grave offense, pull off her shirt and whip politely . . . saying "Don't be angry."*[11]

Before a young man married in those days, and in that part of Russia, the father-in-law presented the groom with a whip. It was a symbol of authority. Often it was hung over the bridal bed.

Such bizarre brutality diminished with time, but the wife's essential situation in society did not improve. In the early nineteenth century, *The Ladies' Book* quoted the following advice of a minister to a bride: "Your duty is submission . . . Your husband is, by the Laws of God and of man, your superior; do not ever give him cause to remind you of it."[12] So wifely self-expression continued to be discouraged and her total obedience to be expected. But the role of woman changed (not surprisingly, Russian women were among the leaders of this revolution). The shackling notion of feminine obedience was discarded. Millions of women in this country found work outside the home. (Some of their singular problems are discussed on pages 359–61.) But a great number of those who remain at home are bored. This is not to say that the working woman is never oppressed by monotony. Nor is homemaking a tedious occupation for most women. But many a stay-at-home woman certainly finds little opportunity to relieve the monotony of housekeeping. Sheer boredom then erodes her marriage. And her husband, tired and perhaps also bored with his work, joins her in an unrelieved tedium.

Many marriages, then, die on the vine. Husband and wife simply stop noticing each other. True, the arithmetic of living—the baby's allergy, the

---

[11] Elaine Elnett, *Historical Origin and Social Development of Family Life in Russia*, cited in Austin L. Porterfield, *Marriage and Family Living as Self–Other Fulfillment* (Philadelphia, 1962), p. 39.
[12] Cited in Vance Packard, *The Sexual Wilderness* (New York, 1967), p. 244.

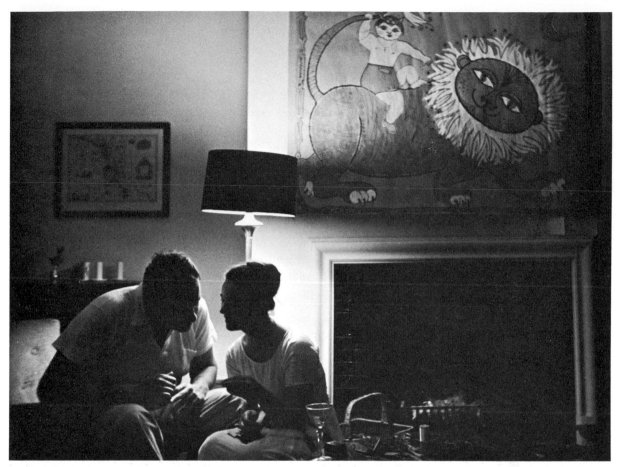

15-3 Being alone together takes planning.

leaking roof, the plugged sink—does not add up to romance. But to keep a marriage alive takes work and planning. The couple must make time to do things together both at home and away from the home and office. Daily opportunities to share thoughts and feelings must be created. Privacy is not always easy to achieve. But no home needs to be the private preserve of a small child. Often a good babysitter will help. Timing is also crucial. A woman, exhausted by a toddler, may find it hard to end the day by concentrating on her husband's office difficulties. In turn, he may be too weary, at the moment, to be concerned about the TV repairman. And so, at times, silence is the wisest and most appreciated course.

In a marriage marred by boredom, a word of appreciation is usually long overdue. Sincere praise for accomplishment is a need of both marital partners. There is the story of the unhappy man who ran around with other women, not because his wife did not understand him, but because she understood him only too well. To her, knowing him meant undermining

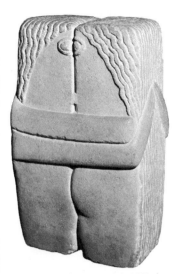

15-4 "The Kiss" (1908) by Constantin Brancusi (1876–1957).

him. The woman who cannot regard her husband without foil in hand, ready to pierce his ego, will destroy her marriage. Marriage is not a competition. One does not gain by the other's loss. Between the married, "one-upmanship" is a dangerous game. There is no victim in a good marriage. Moreover, the husband who does not accentuate his marriage with expressed appreciation may reap (and deserve) a bitter harvest.

"It was a lot of little things," then, explains many a happy marriage as well as many a divorce. The difference is that the happily married couple, having worked at it, will know what happened to them. They will know why it was that the customs and ceremonies of their marriage never lost freshness and meaning.

War marriage, campus marriage, monotonous marriage—all marriage is profoundly influenced by the next topic of this chapter, sexuality. As has been pointed out (see page 468), human beings are unique in needing instruction in the art of love. Complex products of this demanding culture, moderns usually bring into their marriage a long accumulation of information and misinformation about sexuality. Everywhere, the cultural influence on sexual behavior is profound. Some primitive cultures (the Muria of India, for example) expect women to be as sexually aggressive as men. In other cultures, the women are frigid and find coitus humiliating. In this country, only recently have a growing number of males felt the need to sexually gratify their partners. In Samoa this attitude has long existed.[13] Sexual mores are not often directly changed as a result of biological discovery, but such changes may yet come about in Western culture. Consider sexual mutuality in marriage.

Sexuality in marriage

The biological logic of mutuality

"In the beginning, we were all created females; and if this were not so, we would not be here at all."[14] This remarkable statement is the culmination of years of sophisticated biological research. It has been found that after the egg has been fertilized by the sperm, and during the first five or six weeks of development, all human beings are morphologically (structurally) female. At the fifth or sixth week, and not before, the sex genes exert their first influence. Then, if the genetic instruction is to produce a male, the primordial germ cells stimulate the production of a substance that, in turn, stimulates the growth of certain cells that elaborate the male hormone, *androgen*. Androgen suppresses the already present female germ cells (ovaries and Fallopian tubes). The male hormone overcomes the female pattern. Male patterns (male sex glands) develop. This is not evident until the seventh week of the embryo or a little later.

---

[13] Harvey D. Strassman, "Sex and the Work of Masters and Johnson," *GP*, Vol. 38, No. 4 (October 1968), p. 111.

[14] Mary Jane Sherfey, "The Evolution and Nature of Female Sexuality in Relation to Psychoanalytic Theory," *Journal of the American Psychoanalytic Association*, Vol. 14, No. 1 (January 1966), p. 43.

If the genetic instruction is to produce a female, the process by which androgen is produced does not take place, nor do the subsequent events. Instead, the female cellular potential remains unchanged. A female results.

"Only the male embryo is required to undergo a differentiating transformation of the sexual anatomy; and only one hormone, androgen, is necessary for the masculinization of the originally female genital tract."[15] The female genital tract develops independently, without cellular transformation by a hormone.

Thus, the female sex organs are not rudimentary, imperfect, inadequate versions of the male sex organs. On the contrary, it is she whose tissue is primordial; and the sex organs of the male are an outgrowth of her original tissue. The penis develops from the primordia of the clitoris; the scrotum, from the primordia of the labia; the male, from the female. Embryologically, man comes from woman.[16]

Modern biological knowledge mitigates against the sexual subordination of women. In her vital, active attitude to her existence, today's woman finds support in her present culture and its science. She has many problems to solve. But, like her primordial tissue, her die is cast.

William H. Masters and Virginia E. Johnson, of the Reproductive Biology Research Foundation at St. Louis, have written the most authoritative recent account of the physiology of the human sexual response.[17] Most of the discussion in this section is based on their work. (For illustrations of the reproductive systems, see Chapter 13, pages 450 and 454.)

On the physiology of the human sexual response

In their discussion Masters and Johnson divided the sexual responses of both sexes into four phases: the *excitement phase,* varying from a few minutes to hours; the intense, shorter (thirty seconds to three minutes) *plateau phase;* the three- to ten-second *orgasmic phase* (sometimes longer in women); and the *resolution phase,* lasting ten to fifteen minutes with an orgasm, and, without orgasm, lasting as long as twelve to twenty-four hours.

It should be emphasized that sex is more than a total body experience. It is an experience of the whole personality. What follows immediately below, for example, is a consideration of the female orgasm. But it is critical to understand that "it is the manifestation of that all-pervading instinct for survival of the child that is the primary organizer of the woman's sexual drive and by this also of her personality."[18] Moreover, since there is no human equation, some normal individual variations are common and should be expected.

---

[15] *Ibid.,* p. 45.

[16] These findings lend themselves to speculation. Is woman "superior," since she was embryologically first? Is man "superior," since he is "furthest along the evolutionary line"? Doubtless it is most sensible to put aside the notion of "superiority" and, instead, to use this new information for a more mature, realistic, and therefore enjoyable appreciation of the opposite sex.

[17] William H. Masters and Virginia E. Johnson, *Human Sexual Response* (Boston, 1966).

[18] From "Female Sexuality," a panel meeting of the American Psychoanalytic Association held in Detroit, Michigan, May 6, 1967, and reported by Warren J. Barker, *Journal of the American Psychoanalytic Association,* Vol. 16, No. 1 (January 1968), p. 126.

Even the early feminine responses to adequate sexual stimulation (during the *excitement phase*) are not limited to the pelvis. They are widely distributed. From contracting great muscles of the thighs, abdomen, and back, to the tiny muscle fibers often erecting the nipples, the woman's sexual attention is total. The distention of the breast veins as they become engorged with blood and the marked increase in breast size is called *tumescence*—swelling. (Tumescence occurs in all distensible parts of the body and is the major feature of the sexual response in both sexes. It results from the enormous increase of blood in the surface circulation. In these areas blood is forced in through the arteries faster than it can leave via the capillaries and veins. The presence of a special erectile tissue in some areas—the walls of the inner nose, the nipples, vaginal entrance, clitoris, and penis—makes them particularly susceptible to the swelling stiffness of tumescence.) During the late excitement phase, or early in the plateau phase, in perhaps three-fourths of women and one-fourth of men, there begins the *sex-flush*. Much more noticeable in fair-skinned people, this temporary, measleslike rash first appears on the skin of the abdomen. As sexual excitement intensifies, the rash spreads but it will disappear immediately after coitus. Often it does not occur. The clitoris also undergoes tumescence, and the vagina begins to lubricate itself, secreting a fluid by a process not unlike sweating. This fluid will aid penetration of the penis, thereby facilitating coitus. As sexual excitement continues, a sudden contraction of muscles encircling the vagina may cause some of this accumulated fluid to spurt out. This has led to the completely mistaken notion that women ejaculate as do men. In this first phase, the inner two-thirds of the vagina increases in size and the uterus contracts rapidly and irregularly. The reaction of labia depends on whether the woman has had children. If she has not, the labia majora will thin and flatten; if she has had children, they will enlarge. In both instances the labia minora will increase in size. Bartholin's glands may, in this stage or the next, produce a slight secretion to ease the entrance of the penis. The heart rate quickens, and, as is to be expected with sexual excitement, the blood pressure rises.

In the second phase, the *plateau phase,* tumescence and the sex-flush reach their peak. From head to toe, muscle tension reflects the physical and emotional absorption with the impending climax. Evidence of this is in the facial expression, flaring nostrils, rigid neck, arched back, and tensed thighs and buttocks. Now respiration increases and the heart rate and blood pressure remain high. It is in the plateau phase that the clitoris withdraws from its normally overhanging position, pulling back deeply beneath its hood. Contraction of the encircling muscles of the vagina causes it to tighten about the penile shaft. Within these vaginal muscles, the veins become engorged with blood. Added to this venous congestion is that occurring in the veins of the irregularly contracting uterus as well as the other pelvic organs. *Pelvic congestion* results, which is relieved by the third level of the woman's sexual cycle, the *orgasmic phase.*

The orgasm is the pleasurable peak of the sexual experience. This explosive release of body-wide, purposively developed, neuromuscular tension lasts from three to ten seconds. Hearing, vision, taste—all the senses are diminished or lost. It was during the excitement phase that this loss of sensory awareness had begun. It has been said that only a sneeze is as physiologically all-absorbing as an orgasm. But a sneeze is mostly a local experience and an orgasm is not. Although the sensation of orgasm is centered in the pelvis, the whole body responds to it. Of all the widespread muscle responses, the muscle contractions in the floor of the pelvis that surround the lower third of the vagina cause the most unique phenomenon. These muscles contract against the engorged veins that surround that part of the vagina and force the blood out of them. This creates the orgasm. These contractions will, in turn, cause the lower third of the vagina and the nearby upper labia minora to contract between three to fifteen times. The strength and number of these orgasmic contractions vary greatly and normally, as does the whole sexual experience.

The *resolution phase* of the woman's sexual response is marked by prompt disappearance of the sex-flush, decline of muscle tension and tumescence (detumescence), and her general return to the prestimulated condition.

In the male

Masters and Johnson have emphasized the physiological similarities of the sexes in their sexual responses. All the phases and the general changes, such as muscle contractions and tumescence, also occur in the male. In the excitement phase, blood that is delivered to the penis enters the spaces of its spongy erectile tissue. The increased pressure compresses veins, preventing return of most of the blood from that organ into the general venous circulation. Penile enlargement and stiffening result. (To repeat what was said earlier: there is no relationship whatsoever between the size of the penis and either virility or fertility.) During the male's plateau phase, the tumescent testes are elevated and become so congested with blood that they increase in size from 50 to 100 percent.

In the male, orgasm and *ejaculation* occur simultaneously. Contractions of the vas deferens, seminal vesicles, and prostate produce the sensation of imminent ejaculation. It is mostly the prostatic contraction that causes the seminal fluid to squirt out of the penis. This ejaculation accompanying the male orgasm is the most singular physiological difference in the sexual response between the sexes.[19]

General detumescence of the male is rapid (*resolution phase*). Penile detumescence usually occurs in two stages. After ejaculation the penis quickly returns to be about 50 percent larger than its prestimulated flaccid

[19]See Chapter 13, pages 451–53, for further discussion of ejaculation and seminal fluid.

state. Since complete erection usually increases the actual size of the penis considerably less than an inch (see page 514) the initial stage of penile detumescence may not seem to have resulted in much diminution of the erection. Depending largely on the kind and duration of the stimuli of the excitement and plateau stages, final detumescence requires a longer time. After orgasm, the male experiences a *refractory period*—a temporary resistance to sexual stimulation. During this period, the sexual stimulation that excited him earlier is no longer effective. It may be distasteful. But restimulation of the woman after her orgasm may result in one or more orgasms. Nothing will help more in understanding this complex human difference than honest communication. The male, for example, may learn to delay his orgasm until his wife has been satisfied. Consistent premature ejaculation with loss of erection is a frequent problem that can be effectively helped.

Sex differences in sexuality

Most males respond almost immediately to sexual stimulation; most females, gradually. For the male, sex is a gratification that can be achieved independent of love. For many females, sex and love cannot be separated. For the male to bring casualness to the marital bed is to invite rejection, or worse, resentful submission. The wise male will "seduce his wife romantically rather than erotically, to put her in the right frame of mind by romantic words and settings that appeal to her and by veiling from her whatever erotic stimuli affect him."[20] He will do well to heed Balzac:

> *The order of the pleasures is from the couplet to the quatrain, from the quatrain to the sonnet, from the sonnet to the ballad, from the ballad to the ode, from the ode to the canto, from the canto to the dithyramb: the husband who begins with the dithyramb is a blunderer.*[21]

After sexual intercourse, a woman's pelvic congestion abates slowly. Her tender feelings linger. Her husband will not show his consideration of her by going to sleep, even if his feelings do end much more precipitously.

The sexes are not equally aroused by the same stimuli. Although the role of cultural conditioning has yet to be determined, it is believed that few women are as sexually stimulated by burlesque or night club floor shows as are most men. Kinsey, moreover, noted that by the age of twenty only 33 percent of the females in his sample had masturbated to the point of orgasm, as compared to 92 percent of the males.[22] His data also indicate that only about 10 percent of the total female population experiences orgastic sex dreams in any single year. About 40 percent of males have

[20]Robert O. Blood, *Marriage*, p. 360.
[21]Honoré de Balzac, *The Physiology of Marriage* (London, 1925), p. 57.
[22]Alfred C. Kinsey, Wardell B. Pomeroy, Clyde E. Martin, and Paul H. Gebhard, *Sexual Behavior in the Human Female* (Philadelphia, 1953), p. 173.

such dreams.[23] Men, then, are usually reminded of sex, think about it, and wish for it much more than do women. Usually, the sex drive of most males is considerably greater than that of most females. Certainly, the great majority of women enjoy sexual intercourse. However, feminine sexual interest between episodes of coitus is, compared to the male, relatively minimal. Why?

A basic reason for the difference in response to sexual stimulation between the male and female lies in the differences in sexual cell development. With the onset of the menstrual cycle, ova regularly mature singly and are discharged without accumulating. Unlike the female, the male adolescent is vexed by accumulated and trapped sexual fluids, which must escape by ejaculation. In the young girl, sexual stimulation results in a rather diffuse reaction that is dominated by the cerebral cortex. Her increased adolescent sexuality is socially oriented toward marriage. In the adolescent male, a similar amount of sexual stimulation results in the increased production of spermatozoa and the flow of secretions from the accessory sex glands. With this pressure the ejaculatory reflex is excited. His tensions can be relieved only by ejaculation. In the male this is not a diffuse but a local reaction. It is not as cerebral as it is genital. His increased adolescent sexuality is genitally orientated. Although he is capable of great tenderness at this age, only later does his sexuality become social. "This contrast points to a basic distinction between the developmental processes for males and females: males move from privatized personal sexuality to sociosexuality; females do the reverse and at a later stage in the life cycle." Combine this with the ordinarily greater sexual imagery of the young male and the reasons for his earlier interest in sexual relief become clear. And this also explains why the woman's interest in intercourse in marriage peaks so much later than the man's.[24]

Frequency of sexual intercourse

How often do most married couples have sexual intercourse? This depends on a wide variety of factors, such as how old they were when they got married and their individual needs. There are no rules. To establish one would be to ignore normal variations. The frequency of intercourse is not so significant as the frequency of rejection—and how rejection is handled.

> *A woman has a profound responsibility in maintaining an active marital relationship . . . A wife sometimes finds that her husband's spontaneous desire for intercourse occurs more often than she is able actively to respond, no matter how much she would like to . . . If she enjoys it most of the time, she should certainly participate whenever he needs her.*[25]

[23] William M. Kephart, *The Family, Society, and the Individual,* p. 455.
[24] William Simon and John Gagnon, "Psychosexual Development," *Trans-action,* Vol. 6, No. 5 (March 5, 1969), p. 13.
[25] Maxine Davis, *The Sexual Responsibility of Women,* quoted in Robert O. Blood, *Marriage,* p. 374.

What is normal?   Many married couples, completely normal, are nevertheless plagued by a too often unspoken worry. Is what we are doing normal?

> *A woman should be willing to learn. She should not cooperate in anything that proves to be actually distasteful or unpleasant for her after she has attempted it for a time, for it would tarnish their love. But she should have an open mind and adventurous spirit and be willing to try anything that might make the relationship more flexible and gratifying to them both.*[26]

By no means are these statements to be considered applicable to women only. Everything in the above lines is equally pertinent to the male. His responsibilities to learn about his wife's needs, and to respond to them, are no less vital to the success of the marriage.

The experimental range in sex has widened considerably in recent years. Today there is a widespread practice of various forms of sexual intercourse. Manual genital stimulation is now ordinary. Oral-genital sex, although by no means universal, is certainly common. The mutuality of making love requires that its variety be acceptable to both partners. The great seventeenth-century philosopher Spinoza wrote, "Pleasure in itself is not bad but good; contrariwise, pain in itself is bad . . . Mirth cannot be excessive, but it is always good; contrariwise, melancholy is always bad."[27] Sexual intercourse should be a pleasurable, not a painful, experience for both.

Some anxieties in   The modern interest in the orgasm should surprise nobody. In this
marital sexuality   technological age, it is the technique rather than the art of love that sells marriage manuals. Yet, apparently technique alone does not suffice. The promiscuous college girl, frequently considering herself sophisticated about sex, is often reduced to frustrated failure in achieving an orgasm. One psychiatrist writes:

> *An emphasis on orgasm pervades all age groups of our society . . . Among university students the search for the ultimate orgasm has become almost a competitive matter . . . the ultimate confession . . . I have seen girls who admitted cheating, stealing . . . and promiscuity with little shame but who wept violently when they confessed that they could not have orgasms.*[28]

It has been repeatedly observed that in this culture until recently the female half of the human species had much less experience with orgasm than the male. Not more than a hundred years ago, the opinion was held in Western cultures that only evil women ever admitted, even to them-

[26]*Ibid.*
[27]Benedict de Spinoza, *Ethics,* tr. from the Latin by R. H. M. Elwes (Washington, D.C., 1901), p. 211.
[28]Seymour L. Halleck, "Sex and Mental Health on the Campus," *Journal of the American Medical Association,* Vol. 200, No. 8 (May 22, 1967), p. 687.

selves, that they enjoyed the sexual act. Sexual anesthesia was the price most women paid for the protection and support of their home and children. Society supported the male as ruler of the roost, and the double standard extended to the double bed. The male's sexual needs were gratified according to his, not his wife's, wishes. He chose the time. He felt no need to give. Once satiated, he rarely gave his docile mate a second sexual thought. Moreover, he had deeply founded memories of another woman who, presumably, had also been a wife. She had provided for other hungers. With affection he remembered his mother. For such various reasons, then, did the male accept his monogamous arrangement.

The long overdue liberation of women changed all that. Enfranchised, and finding new employment and enjoyment opportunities open to them, women also, at last, expected equality in the marital bed. Many of their husbands then imposed upon themselves an unaccustomed husbandly duty—the sexual satisfaction of their wives. Many, but not all. College-matriculated men are apparently more concerned with wifely sexual gratification than are those with less education. In one study only 7 out of 51 men without college matriculation "expressed the slightest concern with responsibility for coital-partner satisfaction . . . Out of a total of 261 . . . subjects with college matriculation, 214 men expressed concern with coital-partner satisfaction."[29]

This concern of some men with the sexual satisfaction of their wives is to their credit; perhaps college is a civilizing influence, after all.[30] But, as occurs with all social progress, new problems arise. They come from a series of misconceptions.

Misconception No. 1: To have a satisfactory marital experience, the wife and husband must have an orgasm with each intercourse.

This generally unrealized ideal has been a hazard to many a marriage. The difference in the degree of sexual interest between the sexes has already been mentioned. As a marriage matures and intimacy deepens, the frequency of the wife's orgasms may increase. However, the wife will accomplish orgasm, and more often sooner, when she realizes that "the husband's enjoyment of the act has to take precedence over his efforts to please his wife. Otherwise, sooner or later, neither of them will have any pleasure at all."[31]

The fate of the frail male will be more thoroughly examined later (see pages 540–41). Compared to women, men are sick more often and die sooner. But there is yet another area in which the male is relatively feeble. Man is not as sexually potent as woman.

Aside from ejaculation, there are two major areas of physiological difference between male and female orgasmic expression. First, the

[29] William H. Masters and Virginia E. Johnson, *Human Sexual Response*, p. 202.
[30] Increased knowledge about female sexuality doubtless plays some part in the college male's interest in his sexual partner's satisfaction.
[31] Milton R. Sapirstein, *Paradoxes of Everyday Life* (New York, 1955), p. 28.

female is capable of rapid return to orgasm immediately following an orgasmic experience if restimulated before tensions have dropped below plateau-phase response levels. Second, the female is capable of maintaining an orgasmic experience for a relatively long period of time.[32]

Not only, then, are women able to be multiorgasmic, but they are also able to experience longer orgasms than men.[33] Moreover, they do not need to undergo profound nervous system coordinations to prepare themselves anatomically for sex. Men do. For a man, an erection is necessary.

With this seemingly obvious conclusion, consider the problem of some young couples on their first married night. Whether they admit it to themselves or not, they have placed themselves, and each other, on trial. Each feels an obligation to perform sexually. Why? And why might they expect trouble?

Both the young husband and the young wife approach their new roles with some guilt and anxiety. They do not suddenly awaken to maturity after a long period of sexual somnolence. Nevertheless, instead of preparing adolescents for their future sexual function, society merely controls them. Many of these controls are necessary. (Today, almost the only adult pleasure actively forbidden the unmarried teen-ager is sex.) But this sexual control is matched by a conspiracy of parental silence about the subject. The growing boy is not helped by the slick magazine, nor by the refusal of his parents to talk about sex, nor by the embarrassment of his teachers. Too often, his education is a compound of the sniggering anxieties of his comtemporaries and furtive, short-lived, basically uncomfortable liaisons. He drifts alone on the murky waters of opinionated misinformation. Sex is associated with something evil.[34] It may then be loaded with guilt and anxiety.

His young wife may be similarly ill-equipped. Her secret anxiety may be matched by her dreamy determination to equal the seemingly satisfactory creatures her husband sees in some magazine gatefolds. She owes it to him, the man she loves, to be the responsive and adequate wife.

No matter what their previous experience has been, marriage has ceremoniously thrust them into a new, often threatening role. They must prove themselves. Right now. Every time.

Thus does marriage pose anxieties that require patience, enormous understanding, and a sense of humor about oneself and one's mate. It

---

[32] William H. Masters and Virginia E. Johnson, *Human Sexual Response,* p. 131.

[33] The ability to have multiple and longer orgasms should not be confused with actual sexual activity. During the teens and early twenties, the sexual activity of the male is usually much greater (see page 506). Nor should the female ability to be multiorgasmic lead one to assume that more than one orgasm is desired by all women. There is as much variability in orgasmic wants as in any other complex human function. Moreover, many young men are able to have several ejaculations (and orgasms) closely following the first; however, this male capacity for multiple orgasms is generally lost by the age of thirty.

[34] This association may have begun long before adolescence—on the day the small child is punished for examining his genitalia.

will relax the couple to know that orgasm with each intercourse is not necessary to a happy marriage. Terman's research indicates that a wife's capacity for orgasm is not highly related to the couple's happiness.[35] And more recent research by Masters and Johnson suggests that the intensity and duration of a woman's orgasm is not necessarily related to her sense of sexual gratification. An orgasm of relatively low intensity and short duration, during a sexual experience with a husband she loves, may indeed be evaluated by the wife as a complete and fulfilling sexual experience.[36] The consistent sexual competency of the wife is not as important to marital happiness as understanding and patient communication. Feeling safe and feeling a sense of trust are more profoundly involved with marital happiness than the orgasm.

Misconception No. 2: Simultaneous orgasm is absolutely essential for ultimate and satisfactory sexual expression.

This nonsense, a favorite of some marriage manuals, is another anxiety producer. The woman must, after all, either begin to have, or have, an orgasm before the man. If the former is true, simultaneous orgasms are possible. These are delightful experiences. However, many couples never have them, nor do they miss them. To insist on a simultaneous orgasm is, again, a way of putting oneself on trial. A man who is on constant trial does not relax. He may become unable to have an erection. This failure may, in turn, make him fear that he has lost his sexual prowess. Shame torments him. Sometimes a man may become impotent (lose the ability to have sexual intercourse) with a wife with whom he feels on trial. Instead he finds himself potent with an "other woman." Or, with his wife, he may have premature ejaculations, with attendant guilt feelings. As has been pointed out: "Problems of premature ejaculation . . . disturbed the younger members of the study-subject population." This was particularly true of college matriculated men: "with these men ejaculatory control sufficient to accomplish partner satisfaction was considered a coital technique that must be acquired before the personal security of coital effectiveness could be established."[37]

With premature ejaculation, there is anxiety. Again the male doubts his potency. It is well to be reminded that male sexual activity is circumscribed by a basic requirement. He must feel certain of his active role. He cannot, like his mate, submit to sex.

Some marriage manuals make effective chaperones.

Misconception No. 3: Direct clitoral stimulation during intercourse is essential.

There are some misguided writers who detail the crucial importance of direct clitoral stimulation to arouse sexual desire. Research disputes this

[35] L. M. Terman, "Correlates of Orgasm Adequacy in a Group of 556 Wives," in M. F. De Martino, ed., *Sexual Behavior and Personality Characteristics* (New York, 1966).
[36] Warren R. Johnson, *Human Sexual Behavior and Sex Education* (Philadelphia, 1968), pp. 50–51.
[37] William H. Masters and Virginia E. Johnson, *Human Sexual Response*, p. 202.

advice. The difference between clitoral excitement and irritation is slight. To their surprise (and in contradiction to many marriage manuals) many husbands will discover that their wives find manual clitoral stimulation distinctly disagreeable, if not painful. Many, instead, prefer manual stimulation of the general mons area. There is only one best way to find out. Ask.

Effective manual general-mons stimulation results in a clitoral *retraction reaction* (see page 504). The clitoris normally retracts upward.

> *This physiological reaction to high levels of female sexual tension creates a problem for the sexually inexperienced male. The clitoral-body retraction reactions frequently cause even an experienced male to lose manual contact with the organ. Having lost contact, the male partner usually ceases active stimulation of the general mons area and attempts manually to locate the clitoral body. During this "textbook" approach, marked frustration may develop in a highly excited sexual partner . . . Once . . . clitoral retraction has been established, manipulation of the general mons area is all that is necessary for effective clitoral-body stimulation.*[38]

Misconception No. 4: This is a double mistake: (1) that there is a vaginal orgasm distinct from the clitoral orgasm, and (2) that clitoral orgasm is immature; only vaginal orgasm is mature.

These false concepts go back to the outmoded idea that female sexual organs are but incomplete male organs, nothing more than a perpetual case of arrested genital development. Thus hopelessly sexually retarded, it was even thought impossible, if not indecent, for woman to enjoy, much less desire, sex. Freud did not fall into this trap, but he did fall for the idea of the female as an incomplete, hence inferior, male. He considered woman biologically dependent on the male. Lacking a penis, she was thought to be passively envious. "Freud's theories buttressed all the prevailing prejudices and promoted the notion that the female was a deficient male and a second-class citizen."[39] Reflecting the patriarchal culture of his time, he attributed to biology what was, in reality, culturally prescribed. To this was added another error. Girls who masturbated usually did so by manual clitoral stimulation. This, it was decreed by many early writers, was immature. Hence, manual clitoral stimulation to orgasm by adults was immature. Although clitoral stimulation during intercourse was acceptable, only vaginal orgasm was the mark of the normal and sexually mature woman.

The trouble with all this is that it is wrong. What are the facts?

1. The sexually sensitive areas of the female genitalia are the clitoris, labia minora, and the lower third of the vagina (see Figure 13-7).

[38] *Ibid.,* pp. 65–66.
[39] Leon Salzman, "Psychology of the Female," *Archives of General Psychiatry,* Vol. 17, No. 2 (August 1967), p. 195.

2. The upper two-thirds of the vagina has a different embryological origin than the lower third; that is, it arises from a different group of cells. The lower third of the vagina and the labia minora have the same embryological origin; they arise from the same group of cells. Nor are the clitoris and the lower third of the vagina separable structures.

3. The upper two-thirds of the vagina plays no part in the orgasm. Nor does it play a part in the development of erotic feelings.

4. During sexual arousal, the lower third of the vagina and labia minora function as a unit. They are thought to be about equally sensitive to sexual stimulation. The clitoris is more sensitive than either.

5. With one exception, there are no nerve or muscle or blood vessel connections between the clitoris and the vagina. The exception is a network of veins from the clitoris that merges into a network of veins lying along the walls of the vagina. During sexual excitement, these veins are engorged with blood, causing tumescence. Within ten to thirty seconds after sexual excitement, a lubricating fluid appears on the vaginal walls. This fluid seeps onto the vaginal walls directly from the plexus of veins surrounding the vaginal barrel.

6. Like the penis, the clitoris is generously endowed with nerves and is capable of tumescence, spasmodic contraction, and detumescence.

7. During sexual intercourse, the penis rarely comes in direct contact with the clitoris. This is because of the above-mentioned retraction reaction. The traction of the penis on the sensitive labia minora stimulates the enlarged, erect clitoris. (By varying positions during sexual intercourse, more direct contact may be achieved.) The thrusting movements of the penis

> create simultaneous stimulation of the lower third of the vagina, labia minora, and clitoral shaft and glans [the glans of the clitoris is the erectile tissue at the end of the clitoris] as an integrated, inseparable functioning unit with the glans being the most important and, in by far the majority of instances, the indispensable initiator of the orgasmic reaction ... it is a physical impossibility to separate the clitoral from the vaginal orgasm.[40]

8. During the female orgasm, the male often feels contractions on the shaft of his penis. What are they? Does the vagina produce these contractions of orgasm? No. Then what does contract? It was pointed out above that the orgastic contractions are of the muscles located in the floor of the pelvis which surround the lower third of the vagina. With female orgasm, these muscles contract, not directly against the vaginal wall, but against the network of engorged chambers of veins and blood channels

---

[40] A. M. Guhl, "Gonadal Hormones and Social Behavior in Infrahuman Vertebrates," cited in Mary Jane Sherfey, "The Evolution and Nature of Female Sexuality in Relation to Psychoanalytic Theory," *Journal of the American Psychoanalytic Association*, Vol. 14, No. 1 (January 1966), pp. 28–128.

about that part of the vagina.[41] In this way the venous passages are emptied of blood (detumescence). These muscle contractions about the vaginal veins cause the lower vaginal walls to be passively pushed in and out. Moreover, these muscle contractions cause the upper labia minora to contract. That is what the male feels. "Therefore there is no such thing as an orgasm of the vagina. What exists is an orgasm of the circumvaginal venous chambers."[42]

9. Thus, one cannot distinguish between vaginal orgasm and clitoral orgasm. Regardless of how it was stimulated, the nature of the orgasm is the same.

Present knowledge of the origin, anatomy, and function of the female genitalia should help to dispel many a female fear. Long depressed by the idea of the inferiority of the clitoral orgasm, many women blamed either themselves or their husbands for their failure to achieve "vaginal orgasm." The whole notion, however, of a vaginal orgasm separate from clitoral orgasm is biologically impossible and, therefore, utterly invalid. And to consider clitoral orgasm immature and vaginal orgasm mature is senseless. "The tendency to reduce clitoral eroticism to a level of psychopathology or immaturity because of its supposed masculine origin is a travesty of the facts and a misleading psychologic deduction."[43]

Misconception No. 5: The size of the genital organ (penis or vagina) is related to sexual prowess.

This is a common misconception. First, the size of the penis is not related to the development of the muscles or skeleton. Second, the relative increase in size of the erect penis over its size in the relaxed or flaccid state is only about 0.4 to 0.8 inches. Third, so distensible is the vagina that if penile insertion occurs at the right time of sexual excitement, any vagina can accommodate any penis. Fears about too large or too small a penis or too small or too large a vagina are a psychological, not anatomical, problem.

Misconception No. 6: Aged people are always (1) uninterested in sex and (2) impotent.

Kinsey's data revealed that, by seventy years of age, about 73 percent of white males remained sexually potent.[44] Masters and Johnson studied 61 menopausal and post-menopausal women. The oldest was seventy-eight years of age. All were able to reach orgasm. Of the 39 elderly males in the study, the oldest was eighty-nine. All achieved erection. All actively participated in coitus. However, with aging, the time necessary for erection increases. (It also takes older men longer to run a hundred yards.) In the young male, it usually takes about three to five seconds. The six

[41] Male orgasm is similar. Muscles, contracting against the network of engorged venous chambers, force them to empty.
[42] Mary Jane Sherfey, "The Evolution and Nature of Female Sexuality in Relation to Psychoanalytic Theory," p. 84.
[43] Leon Salzman, "Psychology of the Female," p. 196.
[44] Alfred C. Kinsey, Wardell B. Pomeroy, and Clyde E. Martin, *Sexual Behavior in the Human Male* (Philadelphia, 1948), p. 237.

to fifteen seconds required for erection by the older male may lead him to fear failure and to experience impotence.[45] Masters and Johnson have emphasized the limits of their sample and the need for more research.

Frigidity

This general term refers to an inadequate sexual response. Usually it is on the part of the female. Its causes are various. They may include vaginal damage due to childbirth, inadequate development of genitalia, and lack of adequate hormones. However, an exceedingly common cause of female frigidity is inadequate physical stimulation. But the importance of female receptivity must also be emphasized.

During premarital dating, many young couples try to neck their way out of their conflicts. For a while it may work. But marriage is another matter. No woman will enjoy her sexual life if the rest of her life is a nightmare. She cannot be deeply hurt at 9 P.M. and deeply loving at 10 P.M. Angry reminders of wifely duties accomplish nothing except, at times, indifferent submission, which is worse than nothing. Only a secure wife, sure of being loved, will find joy in sex.

The husband must understand, in addition, the wife's need, not only for prolonged and tender foreplay but, once intercourse has begun, of continuous stimulation. If stimulation is stopped, the level of the woman's sexual tension immediately falls. Even if stimulation is stopped at an extremely high plateau of sexual excitement, the orgasm may be delayed. The male must control his ejaculation, and thereby maintain his erection, long enough (four to five minutes) for the female pelvic congestion to reach a level sufficient for orgasm.[46]

Partial or total impotency

Occurring in the male, impotency refers to his inability to have or maintain an erection. Fatigue or stress contributes to it. Further, the tension of the man who feels he is sexually on trial may cause him to be either impotent or to ejaculate prematurely. Sometimes the problem is glandular. Such conditions are usually easily treated.

At times, however, impotency has deeper roots. Not uncommon is the prostitute-Madonna image. Consciously or subconsciously, the male believes that only "bad girls" have intercourse. Carrying this feeling to his marital bed, he both loves and rejects his wife. Such men can usually be aided by being helped to understand their attitudes toward women.

---

[45] William H. Masters and Virginia E. Johnson, *Human Sexual Response*, p. 251.

[46] For women who have borne children, the importance of orgasmic relief, once the considerable pelvic congestion of sexual stimulation is present, should not be underestimated. Competent medical authority considers that "chronic pelvic congestion furthered by inadequate or absent orgasmic release fosters a pelvic condition conducive to many disorders interfering with impregnation, pregnancies and general health." (E. S. Taylor, *Essentials of Gynecology*, cited in Mary Jane Sherfey, "The Evolution and Nature of Female Sexuality in Relation to Psychoanalytic Theory," p. 73.) This is especially true with formerly pregnant women who have intercourse often. Pregnancy may result in some varicosities and chronic congestion of the pelvic veins. For such women added chronic venous congestion is thus considered harmful.

By being impotent, some men subconsciously punish their wives or themselves. Occasionally the male thinks of his wife as a mother or sister. The age-old taboo against incest inhibits him. Psychotherapy often helps.

Premature ejaculation

Not uncommonly this occurs during the early anxious months of marriage. However, as experience is gained and the male relaxes his way out of the trial situation, matters improve. The wearing of two condoms frequently solves the problem. Sometimes the causes of premature ejaculation are due to profound emotional problems, for which psychiatric help is indicated.

Saving the marriage

Where can those with these and other marital problems seek help?

Family, friends, and relatives often must act as willing (or unwilling) family counselors. Doubtless, they are the ones most frequently asked for advice. Not enough are reluctant to give it. Some, however, are mindful that "marriage resembles a pair of shears, so joined that they cannot be separated; often moving in opposite directions, yet always punishing anyone who comes between them."[47] They are faced with the twin handicaps of involvement and lack of training—two serious shortcomings in an often explosive situation. In considering the intimate, interrelated complexity of the three elements of the ailing situation—the husband, the wife, and their marriage—one appreciates more clearly the need for professional objectivity and experience.

The family physician or gynecologist often acts as a marriage counselor. Particularly if the problem is physical, he is in an invaluable position to promptly discover its source and to give practical advice. The average physician is profoundly aware of the emotional needs of patients. He may feel that the services of a professional counselor are indicated.

The specialist marriage counselors have organized the highly professional American Association of Marriage Counselors, composed of sociologists, psychologists, lawyers, physicians, and clergymen. These counselors have both training and experience in a field requiring sensitivity and wisdom. Unfortunately, there are not enough of them. The more accessible Family Service Association of America is comprised of local Family Service agencies, which are found in most cities. Staffed by social caseworkers, these agencies charge fees based on ability to pay. Many such marriage counselors hope to explore the marital dilemma with both parties. Frequently, however, the tension between the two precludes this.

A basic first step is the acceptance by both partners that they need help. Sometimes "talking out" a problem, in the presence of an attentive

[47] Sydney Smith, "Lady Holland's Memoir," Vol. I, Chap. 10.

third party, opens a road to its solution. Often, the marriage counselor can guide a degree of interaction between marital partners that is a revelation to both of them. Many married people simply do not talk enough to each other. As the years go by, they tend to confide less and less in each other. Some couples do not talk—they quarrel. Fear and pride and the sheer habit of quarreling have shipwrecked many a marriage.

Should the marriage counselor discover a deep emotional base to the marital problem, he may urge the couple to seek the help of a psychiatrist. One person may have been taught that sex is dirty. Another may have had an acrimonious mother who taught her daughter only of the baseness of men. Still another may be frightened of giving or taking love. "She can't give. I can't take." This tragic dialogue has been expressed in many ways to more than one therapist.

A marriage cannot be put on and taken off like a coat. It must be mended and refitted. But it can wear well.

It can last a lifetime.

Epilogue

Then Almitra spoke again and said, And what of Marriage, master?

And he answered saying:

You were born together, and together you shall be forevermore.

You shall be together when the white wings of death scatter your days.

Ay, you shall be together even in the silent memory of God.

But let there be spaces in your togetherness,

And let the winds of the heavens dance between you.

Love one another, but make not a bond of love:

Let it rather be a moving sea between the shores of your souls.

Fill each other's cup but drink not from one cup.

Give one another of your bread but eat not from the same loaf.

Sing and dance together and be joyous, but let each one of you be alone,

Even as the strings of a lute are alone though they quiver with the same music.

Give your hearts but not into each other's keeping.

For only the hand of Life can contain your hearts.

And stand together yet not too near together:

For the pillars of the temple stand apart,

And the oak tree and the cypress grow not in each other's shadow.[48]

[48] Kahlil Gibran, *The Prophet* (New York, 1923), pp. 16–17.

16

On continuing the human beginning

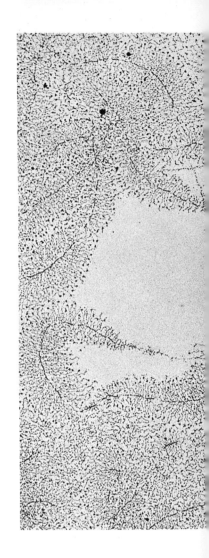

"In the beginning . . ."

Many millennia ago there was no life in the world. In a certain right time and environment, however, chemicals combined and were sparked into living fragments. That is, they reproduced themselves exactly. Sometimes they failed to do this and reproduced themselves inexactly. This accident was then duplicated exactly.

In time the living fragments became cells. Cells became tissue. Tissues

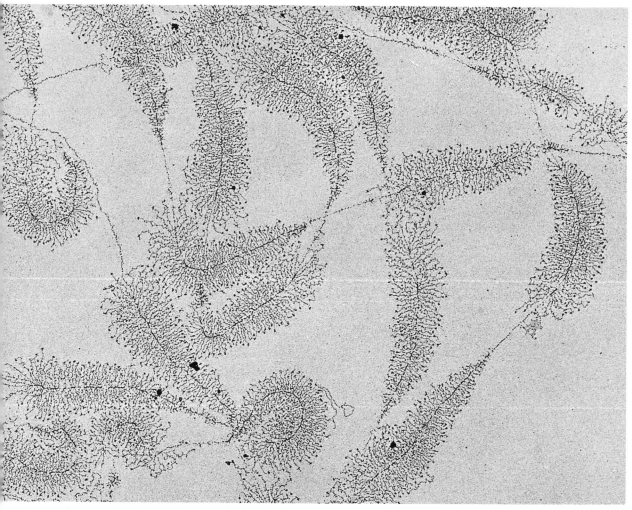

Genes from a salamander oocyte (×22,000). This photograph is one of the first to show genes (the spines of the carrot-shaped structures) in the process of producing molecules of ribosomal ribonucleic acid (rRNA), seen as the hairlike fibers extending from the genes. Each gene is simultaneously producing about one hundred molecules of rRNA. (See pages 527–29.)

were formed into creatures. Countless trillions of different individuals were born into a million species, and died. Some, like the dinosaur, perished forever. Others, like man, endured and became more complex. But, although man has found a way to get out of this world and back again, he still has, as an embryo, "gills" like a fish. His genes send ancestral messages, but his needs have modified the message. His "gills" become glands and major blood vessels. Genetic instruction and evolution dictate this.

Genetics: molding a new person

The reasons for interest in heredity are several. The chromosomes within the nucleus of the human cell give directions that help decide the characteristics of men. Change those directions and man can be changed. Many scientists are apprehensive that man will "tamper with heredity." To better understand its destiny, this generation must understand some genetics.

Atomic energy provides a second reason for concern with genetics. The fallout from atomic testing may produce an effect, most likely deleterious, on human genes. But more than bombs are involved. Future generations will see a greatly expanded industrial use of atomic energy. The effect of possible atomic radiation on the progeny of posterity is urgent health business, and only an informed public can influence government policy-makers to safeguard health.

The involvement of genetics with illness is yet a third reason the subject requires study. Over a thousand varieties of birth defects perplex man. Some, like flat feet, are minor. Others, like Mongolism, are more serious. In all such disorders, genes play a varying role. Sometimes it is the gene that is basically at fault. In other cases it is the environment that disturbs genetic processes. And there are conditions for which the primary cause is unclear. But one concept is clear: all genetic processes must be considered within their ecosystems. Every gene interacts with its environment and is inexorably influenced by it.

The cell, unit of life
The *cell* (Figure 16-1) is the basic unit of life. The cellular *protoplasm* is the chemical life of the cell. Protoplasm is composed mainly of cellular proteins, fats, carbohydrates, and inorganic salts in a watery medium. It contains thousands of *enzymes* (see footnote 5 and page 298). Many enzymes contain *vitamins.* Enzymes are eventually used up and must continuously be created anew by the cell from available nutrients. Their vitamin component must be made by the cell or taken in with food. Cells also contain special materials involved with their particular activity, such as the *glycogen* seen as granules in the liver cell.

The mini-structures in the cell's protoplasm, the *organelles,* function in concert with their intracellular environment. The membrane-encircled nucleus, the largest of the cell's organelles, contains and is surrounded by protoplasm. Protoplasm outside the nucleus is called *cytoplasm.* Thus, the two major parts of most cells are the nucleus and the cytoplasm. The events that occur in the cytoplasm, such as digestion, respiration, secretion, and excretion, depend on the activity within the nucleus. The nucleus is also essential for the reproduction of the cell.

The nucleus

Within the nucleus are the *chromosomes.* The chromosomes contain the *genes.* A gene is the unit of heredity. But it is even more. Because

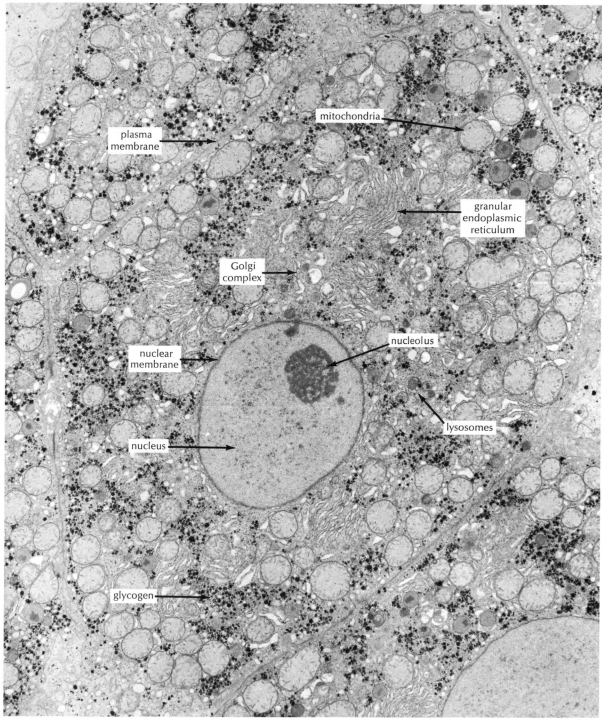

16-1 A mammalian cell. Visible in this liver cell are granules of glycogen.

16-2 Chromosomes of a normal human male (*left*) and of a whitefish (*right*). The chromosomes of this whitefish cell have duplicated themselves, and the cell itself is dividing into two cells (see mitosis, pages 525–26).

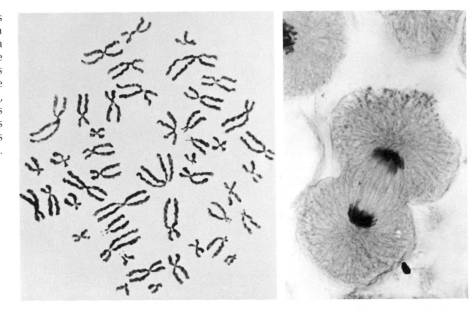

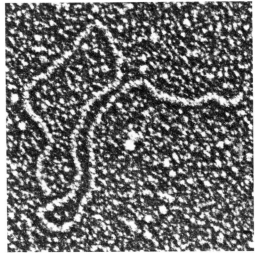

16-3 A single gene, isolated from a common intestinal bacterium. This technical triumph has troubled the youthful Harvard scientists who achieved it. They question whether man is mature enough to deal wisely with discoveries that may eventually enable him to tamper with human genetic processes.

each gene is composed of *DNA,* it governs the life of the cell. Because DNA can reproduce itself during cell division, its code is transmitted to subsequent cells. The *nucleolus,* or "little nucleus," is an organelle that is not visible in some stages of cell division. It has no membrane. It may be a storehouse of chemicals for the reproduction of DNA.

In the cell community, red blood cells are unique. During their maturation in the bone marrow they lose their nuclei. Bereft of DNA, these cells cannot synthesize protein. Red blood cells live only so long as their enzymes last—about 120 days. Every second some 2.5 million red blood cells must be released into the circulation.

The cytoplasm, its membranous wall, and the endoplasmic reticulum

Policing the kind and amount of material entering the cell is its enveloping, porous *plasma membrane*. The plasma membrane admits some molecules that seek to enter the cell; it rebuffs others. It also permits the escape of waste materials from the cell but fastidiously retains essential substances. At various places the plasma cell membrane folds inward to extend into the cytoplasm of the cell as the *endoplasmic reticulum*. Thus is created a membranous transportation system of canals along which needed materials move deep into the cell's cytoplasm. The endoplasmic reticulum communicates with the nuclear membrane. By this route nutrients for the nucleus are delivered. Wastes can be carried out via these canals too.

The organelles within the cytoplasm

On part of the endoplasmic reticulum granules are clustered; these are *ribosomes*—the sites of protein synthesis. Seemingly continuous with the nongranular endoplasmic reticulum is the *Golgi complex*. This may be a sort of enzyme storage bin; protein enzymes, completed at the ribosomes, penetrate the membrane of the endoplasmic reticulum and possibly migrate, via its channels, to the Golgi complexes, to be kept and released when needed by the cell. Also in the cytoplasm of most cells are the *mitochondria* and *lysosomes*. Mitochondria are the cell's energy sources. Like tiny fuel furnaces distributed throughout the cellular cytoplasm, they convert the chemical energy of cellular nutrients into a high-energy compound called *adenosine triphosphate* (*ATP*). ATP is released as needed for the cell's work. Mitochondria are enclosed by a membrane. So are the lysosomes, the cell's digestive organelles. Each lysosome contains enzymes that break down complex nutrients into simpler substances. Another duty of the lysosome is to act as a minute garbage disposal, ridding the cell of bacteria or worn-out materials.

Consider the treasure of past and future generations contained within the cell: the nucleus, the power-packed mitochondria, the digesting lysosomes, the Golgi complex of storage facilities for completed protein enzymes, the membranous network of endoplasmic reticulum that provides a transportation system for cellular nutrients and wastes and a ribosomal site for protein synthesis—all these active islands surrounded by a small sea of protoplasm, which, in turn, is enveloped by the meticulously selective plasma membrane. They speak of the balanced organization within the cellular ecosystem. Two tools have made the cell more accessible to scientific scrutiny—the *electron microscope* and the *ultracentrifuge*. The first has afforded magnifications of over 100,000. The ultracentrifuge can whirl treated cell suspensions at speeds of 60,000 revolutions per minute. Trapped in such an intense separating force, the microlayers of the cells separate to provide materials for the study of

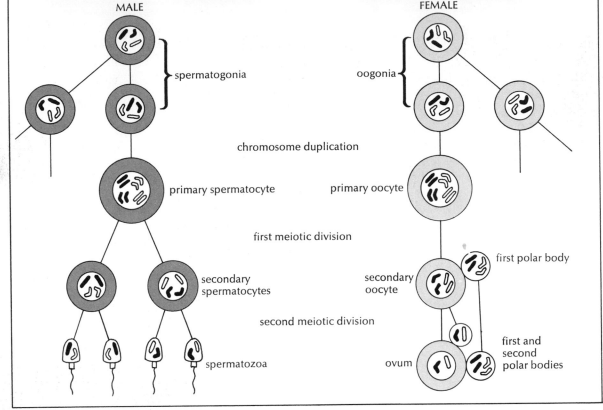

16-4 Meiosis. The mature gametes (spermatozoa or ova) have half the number of chromosomes that the primordial sex cells (spermatogonia or oogonia) had. During the maturation process, polar bodies simply degenerate. For simplicity, cells shown here have only four chromosomes.

organelles. A new science, *molecular biology*, reveals both the normal and the abnormal at this level. Scientists in this field may soon discover what, for example, causes cancer, a disease of the cell.

Meiosis and mitosis   There are two basic kinds of cells in the human body: germ cells (or *gametes*) and somatic cells (Greek *soma*, body). A germ cell is a cell of an organism the function of which is to reproduce the kind; these are the ova (eggs) and the sperm.[1] All other body cells are somatic.

When a mature sperm fertilizes a mature ovum, the resultant fusion is a cell called the *zygote*. To achieve the maturity necessary to participate in zygote formation, the germ cells, starting from *primordial sex cells*, must go through a special process of cell division called *meiosis*. Primordial sex cells have forty-six chromosomes, but when meiosis of a primordial sex cell is complete, the mature gamete has only twenty-three chromosomes (see Figure 16-4). Twenty-two of these are single, nonsex chromosomes and are called *autosomes*. The remaining chromosome is either an X or a Y sex *chromosome*. At the end of meiosis, the ma-

[1]Women are born with their total supply of primitive eggs, which nestle immature in the ovary until puberty. Beginning at puberty, men continually replenish their supply of sperm cells.

ture ovum carries a single X-chromosome; the mature sperm either an X-chromosome or a Y-chromosome (see Figure 16-5). It is a basic (although not the only) function of the Y-chromosome to direct the production of the male sex glands (testes).

When fertilization of the mature ovum by the mature sperm occurs, each parent contributes twenty-three chromosomes to the resultant zygote—twenty-two autosomes and one sex chromosome. A normal ovum always contains an X-chromosome. If an ovum is fertilized by a normal sperm containing an X-chromosome, the result is XX (female):

$$X \text{ (ovum)} + X \text{ (sperm)} = XX \text{ (female)}$$

If an ovum is fertilized by a sperm containing a Y-chromosome, the result is XY (male):

$$X \text{ (ovum)} + Y \text{ (sperm)} = XY \text{ (male)}$$

So the zygote and all subsequent body (somatic) cells will normally always contain twenty-three pairs of chromosomes (a total of forty-six chromosomes), of which twenty-two pairs are autosomes and one pair are sex chromosomes. Each autosomal pair is different in genetic content and usually in appearance from all other pairs. Figure 16-6 shows the chromosomes arranged in pairs to form a chromosomal chart called a *karyotype*. Note that each autosomal pair is numbered from 1 to 22 and the sex chromosomes are appropriately labeled X or Y.

As noted above, only the primordial sex cells multiply by meiosis. The zygote and all subsequent body (somatic) cells multiply by *mitosis*. In the process of mitosis, the threadlike chromosomes in the nucleus of a

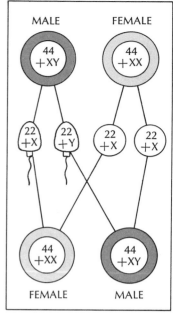

16-5 If a sperm carrying an X-chromosome fertilizes an ovum, a female (XX) results; if a sperm carrying a Y-chromosome fertilizes an ovum, a male (XY) results.

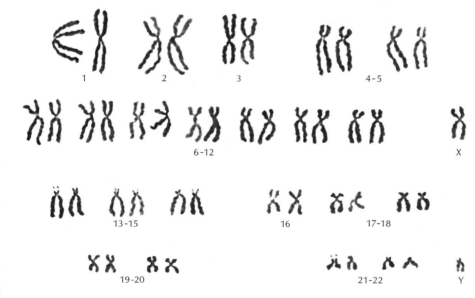

16-6 Karyotype (chromosomal chart) of a normal human male. The karyotype of a female has two X-chromosomes where the X- and Y-chromosomes appear here.

GENETICS: MOLDING A NEW PERSON **525**

cell duplicate themselves; the duplicate sets are separated, with one set going to each of the two "daughter" cells produced by the division of the original cell. Thus in *mitosis* each of the two cells produced by the division of a single cell has a full set of chromosomes, whereas in *meiosis* each of the cells has *half* the number of chromosomes the original cell had. By mitosis the body replaces discarded cells, and by mitosis the body grows. In both meiosis and mitosis there are plenty of chances for errors. Should a cell, be it germ or somatic, fail to receive its proper share or composition of chromosomes, abnormality results.

Cellular engineering: genetic order

By their union in the Fallopian tube (see pages 458–60) the mature sperm and egg contribute their twenty-three single chromosomes to the fertilized egg to form a zygote with its full normal complement of forty-six. Mitosis begins. The zygote prepares to divide. Each of the forty-six chromosomes splits into two parts, which are exact replicas of one another. The cell divides. Now there are two body cells. Normally, each has its full share of forty-six chromosomes. Several hours later the two somatic or body cells cleave again. There are then four body cells. Normally, each still contains forty-six chromosomes. And so cell multiplication continues. Every day the somatic cell cluster continues to divide as it travels down the Fallopian tube toward the uterus. With each division these cells double in number. Normally, they never have fewer or more than forty-six chromosomes. At last, the tiny multiplying cellular mass[2] is implanted in the uterine endometrium. Membranes begin to form. Within two or three weeks after fertilization, the embryo is being fed via these membranes. In another week there is a heart. A week later the heart begins to beat. Now cell differentiation continues rapidly, and so does organ development. Differentiation began with the earliest division. For each cell must multiply in the limited space allotted to it and it is influenced by pressures from every other cell. And, as will be seen, each cell is instructed as to its future function. This is the nature of the cellular ecosystem.[3]

The cells of various organs are specific for those organs. In other words, the cells of the heart are different from those of the gut which, in turn, are different from those of the nerves, and so on. By birth, there have been about forty-four successive cell divisions resulting in trillions of marvelously organized cells. With normal cell division, every one of those trillions of cells contains the identical number of chromosomes as the original individual single zygote contained. How did this happen? How does one kind of cell end up as a part of a bladder muscle, another kind in the eye, still another in a toenail, and yet a fourth in a mole on the left cheek? How does each cell get the message telling it what to become?

The answer lies within the nucleus of the cell, in the chromosomes.

---

[2] In the human, one week after ferilization, the developing organism is called an *embryo*; this term is applicable until the end of the second month; then the term *fetus* is used.

[3] *Embryology*, the science dealing with the development of the embryo, is discussed in this chapter, pages 556–63.

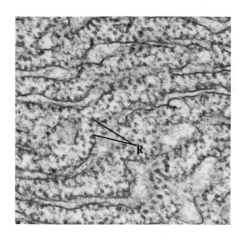

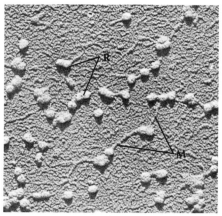

16-7 Ribosomes: the sites of protein synthesis. The photo on the left shows granular endoplasmic reticulum (×60,000), on which ribosomes (R) are located (see also Figure 16-1 and page 523). The photo on the right shows ribosomes (R) at a higher magnification (×88,000). Numbers of ribosomes are connected by filaments (M), which are believed to be messenger RNA (see page 529).

DNA, the master plan; RNA, the obedient worker

Chemically, a chromosome consists mostly of proteins combined with a substance called *deoxyribonucleic acid* (abbreviated as DNA). The chromosomal DNA is the material of the gene. Within it is stored the genetic information. Chromosomal DNA cannot itself leave the nucleus. It remains imprisoned within it, capable of duplicating itself with each cell division, and serving as a blueprint for the formation of *ribonucleic acid* (RNA) molecules. Thus, chromosomes also contain RNA. As will be seen, several kinds of RNA are made, and each plays a specific role in the building of cell proteins.

Outside the nucleus, as part of the cell's cytoplasm, there are still other proteins. Like all body proteins they are originally derived from food. Like all other proteins they are composed of amino acids. It is from this nutrient pool of cytoplasmic proteins that amino acids are taken and brought to the *ribosomes* (see Figure 16-7).

How the ribosomal factory is made

Peering through the electron microscope at an amphibian oocyte,[4] biologists believe they have discovered how ribosomes originate. Study the photograph of amphibian genes on pages 518–19. Each gene is shaped like a carrot or spindle. Each gene is linked with every other gene like the beads of a necklace. The spindle-shaped gene is actually three-dimensional; technical limitations make possible only a two-dimensional view. Running from the broad base of the spindle to its tip is a thread. This thread is DNA—a tiny segment of a chromosome. In this picture, genes are producing molecules of ribonucleic acid (RNA). The RNA molecule is seen as an individual hairlike fiber extending from the gene. One gene is producing about one hundred molecules of RNA. These molecules spiral

[4]An *amphibian* is a vertebrate animal (a frog or a toad, for example) able to live both on land and in water; an *oocyte* is a female gamete that has not reached full development; mature, it is an ovum.

GENETICS: MOLDING A NEW PERSON **527**

about the DNA thread decreasing in size from the base to the tip of the spool. (The RNA is not an inherent part of DNA; the DNA merely governs the synthesis of RNA according to its preset code.) Every single RNA fiber or molecule has reached a particular stage of maturity as evidenced by its length. Its length, indeed, its very structure, has been dictated by the DNA, which directed its synthesis from cytoplasmic amino acids. During its synthesis, the RNA molecule apposed itself to the DNA pattern in such a way as to reflect specific chemical configurations. It is thus instructed by the DNA. According to DNA instructions, each RNA fiber will break off and, when free in the nucleus, will be broken up into segments, probably by an enzyme.[5] First one, and then a second part of the original RNA fiber will leave the nucleus, deserting the nuclear DNA, which cannot leave. Bearing the specific instructions of the DNA, these segments of the RNA fiber will meet in the cellular cytoplasm to together form a single ribosome. Lear has described this remarkable process:

> *According to the biochemical evidence, the opening event in the sequence of the spindle's operation is the extrusion of the RNA fiber from the main thread of DNA. As the extrusion proceeds, the fiber is strung with a protein coat according to coded instructions from the DNA. This process goes on until each fiber reaches a predetermined length (note in the photograph [on pages 518–19] that the maximum length is remarkably uniform), after which that particular RNA fiber separates from the DNA thread like a quill from a porcupine's back. The fibers depart individually after attaining individual maturity. En route they pass under an unidentified biological knife (presumably an enzyme) that chops each fiber into segments. The first segment to be severed is about one-sixth the length of the whole fiber. This segment moves into the cytoplasm very quickly and at once coils into a tiny sphere. The coiling apparently occurs in response to instructions the DNA thread imprinted on the RNA fiber before setting the fiber loose. That part of the fiber that remains in the nucleus is subsequently chopped several times, until the surviving segment is about one-third as long as the original fiber had been. The final segment then moves out through the nuclear membrane into the cytoplasm, finds a tiny sphere formed by an earlier segment of fiber, and coils into a larger sphere alongside the tiny sphere. The two spheres together make a ribosome.[6]*

How body protein is made

Consider what happens at a single ribosome.

An amino acid is brought and attached to it. Then a second amino acid is brought to it. With the assistance of an enzyme, the second amino acid

[5] As noted in Chapter 9, an enzyme is frequently a protein and has the power to initiate or accelerate certain chemical reactions in plant or animal metabolism.
[6] John Lear, "Spinning the Thread of Life," *Saturday Review* (April 5, 1969), pp. 63–64.

is linked to the first. But only in a predetermined way. A third amino acid is brought to the ribosome. It is linked to the second—again in a manner previously decided, and helped by an enzyme. A fourth amino acid then reaches the assembly line at the ribosomal factory. It is linked to its predecessor. Still another follows it. Then another and another. To all the ribosomal depots, in all the body cells, whether in a developing embryo or in an aging man, amino acids, derived from the nutrient pool of cytoplasmic proteins, are brought and linked one to the other. At each ribosome, then, a series of linked amino acids, a chain, is formed. Bonds between these amino acid chains form complex proteins. The manner of arrangement of the amino acids determines protein structure. And protein structure decides body structure and, therefore, function. So the chemical arrangement of the amino acids at the ribosomes results in proteins that will become blue eyes or black eyes, liver or heart, a short or tall person. The variations in the arrangement of amino acids at the ribosomal workbench are no less endless than the variations of hereditary characteristics.

How do the amino acids get selected out of the cytoplasmic protein? How is their sequence determined? How are they brought to the ribosome? And, once at the ribosome, how does it happen that amino acids are so properly arranged? It is the nuclear DNA that governs all this. Only the DNA contains the genetic formula, so only the DNA can impart the genetic code, the hereditary instructions. But how can these DNA instructions reach the ribosome? It has been seen that the DNA cannot itself leave the nucleus to direct protein construction at the ribosome. It is imprisoned within the nucleus, irrevocably locked within the chromosomal pattern. It is fixed, a die, a stamp, a mold, a template of chemicals. Since the DNA is unable to carry its own message outside the nucleus, an intermediary is needed—a messenger.

That messenger must somehow obtain the exact complex message, the specific instructions, of the DNA. Like the ribosomal RNA before it, that messenger must, therefore, in turn become a template, a mold of the DNA code. And unlike DNA, that messenger must then be able to leave the nucleus. Obediently that messenger must wend its way to the waiting ribosome, bringing to it the DNA message of instructions. A special kind of RNA is that messenger. Somehow, *messenger RNA* (as it is called) must obtain the patterned message, established by the coded position of certain chemical elements in the DNA. (As will be seen, the message obtained by the messenger RNA is for a different purpose than that obtained by ribosomal RNA.)

Within the cell's nucleus, messenger RNA places itself in apposition to the DNA template. It arranges its own chemical structure to exactly match that of the DNA. The RNA transcription of the DNA template is thus formed.[7] In this way the messenger RNA has itself become a template,

---

[7]The *rate* at which messenger RNA is transcribed from the DNA is determined by the arrangement or sequence of the chemicals of the DNA. In some manner light affects this rate. It sets the biological clock.

a mold, a momentous master copy of the DNA basic chemical structure. Having incorporated within itself the instruction of the DNA, having acquired within its very structure the position of the coded chemical elements of the DNA, the messenger RNA deserts the DNA. It traverses the nuclear membrane. It enters into the midst of the cellular cytoplasm. There the DNA-code-carrying messenger RNA heads for a waiting ribosome. For, as has been stated, it is at the ribosomal workbench that protein will be manufactured. And these synthesized proteins will contribute to the specific characteristics of the creature-to-be.

Upon finding a ribosome, the messenger RNA is associated with it. Thus is established, at the ribosome, the DNA-patterned code of instructions. Now amino acids, taken from the surrounding cytoplasmic protein, may be brought to the ribosome. And now, with DNA instructions awaiting their arrival, the amino acids will be properly arranged at the ribosome. They can only be arranged as determined by the DNA. For although the DNA remains in the nucleus, it remains the master. The traveling messenger RNA, associated with a ribosome, remains but a copy, a slave. And now the readied ribosomal workbench (the synthesis of which was also specifically directed by the DNA) awaits amino acid delivery. To construct specific proteins, to create specific tissue as instructed, amino acid building blocks must be brought to the ribosomal factory from the nutrient cytoplasmic protein pool.

How is this accomplished?

While the ribosome was receiving its instructing messenger RNA, the DNA in the nucleus was not idle. It kept busy directing the production of still another, smaller type of RNA. This third RNA is called *transfer RNA*. Also instructed by the DNA, in a predetermined sequence, transfer RNA leaves the nucleus and enters the cytoplasmic protein pool of amino acids. For each separate amino acid there is a separate transfer RNA. On its way to the ribosome the transfer RNA picks up its selected amino acid from the protein pool. On reaching the ribosome, the amino acid leaves the transfer RNA and, helped by enzymes, attaches itself to the ribosome. One after another, in assembly line fashion, and as instructed by the messenger RNA, the amino acids are linked one to the other.

So transfer RNA keeps leaving the nucleus, picking up selected amino acids from the cytoplasmic protein pool, and delivering them to be linked to the growing amino acid chain at the ribosomal protein factory. But recent work suggests that this factory is not merely an inert organelle—that it is more than a passive building site. It is postulated that the ribosome moves. The message that is brought to the ribosome from the DNA by the messenger RNA is in the form of a string of chemicals arranged in a specific sequence. Along this messenger RNA these chemicals are arranged in groups of three and each group is called a *codon*. Each codon specifies a particular amino acid. So the messenger RNA associated with a ribosome is like a string of beads; each bead is a codon, which is composed of an exact sequence of three chemicals. And

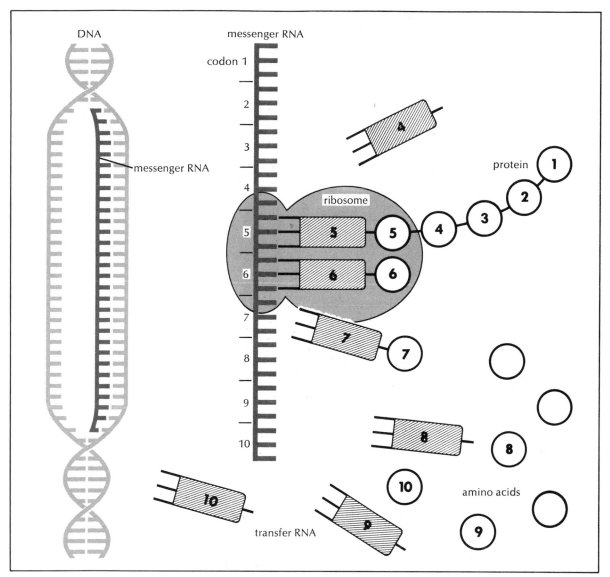

16-8 The synthesis of proteins. The diagram at the left represents the transcription of genetic information from DNA to messenger RNA. The rest of the illustration schematizes the process by which transfer RNA brings its specified amino acid to the ribosome, which is situated at the codon specifying that particular amino acid. Here amino acid number 6, specified by codon number 6, has just been bound to its site on the ribosome by the corresponding transfer RNA. Amino acid number 6 will bond to amino acid number 5, adding to the growing chain. Then the ribosome will move along the messenger RNA to codon number 7. In this example, the chain will be complete when amino acid number 10 has been bonded to it. (Most proteins, however, consist of two or more chains of amino acids.)

each codon waits for transfer RNA to bring to it an allocated amino acid. It is the codon, then, that the transfer RNA must recognize to know at what point at the ribosome to bring its amino acid. Imagine such a string of messenger RNA beads or codons (Figure 16-8) and, for the present purpose, give each codon a number from 1 through 10. (There are many more, and this is done for the sake of explanation.) Also for convenience, number each molecule of transfer RNA carrying its particular amino acid. Transfer RNA number 1 brings its specific amino acid, number 1, from the cytoplasmic pool to the ribosome, which is now located at codon number 1 of the messenger RNA. There, amino acid number 1 is attached to the ribosome. Transfer RNA number 1 is then released to seek another of its specific amino acids. Carrying its first amino acid, the ribosome moves on to codon number 2. There another transfer RNA (number 2) waits with its amino acid number 2. Amino acid number 2 is then bound to amino acid number 1. The ribosome moves on to the third bead (or codon) of the string of messenger RNA. The process is repeated and amino acid number 3 is bound to amino acid number 2. In this way one after another specific amino acids are bound to one another, as shown in Figure 16-8. In this sense the ribosome makes its own string of beads, and each bead is an amino acid. The completed amino acid chains are the components of complex proteins. Thus, the ribosome conducts the synthesis of proteins. Finally, and, as always, according to DNA instructions,[8] the ribosome has had enough. There are no more codons for it to move along. The ribosome then rids itself of its linked chain of amino acids—of its protein component. What becomes of the complete protein? It contributes to the body structure and function. It will contribute to the eye, or to the heart, or to an enzyme. Multiplied billions of times, this process accounts for the creation of a unique person.[9] The wonder is not that an occasional error or defect occurs. The wonder is that it occurs so rarely.

How extensive is all this activity?

> If it were possible to assemble the DNA in a single human cell into one continuous thread, it would be about a yard long. This three-foot set of instructions for each individual cell is produced by the fusion of egg and sperm at conception and must be precisely replicated billions of times as the embryo develops.[10]

After birth too, and so long as the individual grows, develops, and ages,

---

[8] Recent research indicates "that genetic messages are produced not only in the cell nucleus but also in the cytoplasm outside the nucleus." (*Science News*, Vol. 92, No. 17 [October 21, 1967], p. 394.) The significance of this discovery awaits further work.

[9] Here can one best comprehend the individuality of the single being. Within each new zygote formed by the union of sperm and ovum is a completely new organization of DNA, a new master plan, a new set of instructions. Never before, never again, will there be another zygote with exactly the same DNA code.

[10] Marshall W. Nirenberg, "The Genetic Code; II," *Scientific American*, Vol. 208, No. 3 (March 1963), p. 82.

the genetic process by which cellular proteins are manufactured is repeated still more billions of times. So long as the person lives, it goes on.

The new person: product of genetics? environment? or both?

DNA instructions are many and they are related one to the other. And the whole genetic process takes place in, and is affected by, an all-encompassing environment. Each cell, each nucleus within the cell, each strand of DNA within the nucleus, each chemical component within the DNA, functions within the context of its environment. So there are genetic ecosystems.

If the whole genetic process operates in an environment, it is inexorably influenced by it. An individual is not merely the result of the *genotype*. "The genotype is the sum total of the heredity the individual has received, mainly . . . in the form of DNA in the chromosomes of the sex cells. The cytoplasm may also contain some heredity determinants; if so, they are likewise constituents of the genotype."[11] But with cell division and the resultant increase in the number of cells, with the growth of the organism, the constituents of the genotype must continuously reproduce themselves (replication). The material for this replication is taken from the environment. Consider just the change in size that occurs from man's beginning as a fertilized ovum to full adulthood.

> *A human egg cell weighs roughly one twenty-millionth of an ounce; a spermatozoon weighs much less; an adult person weighs, let us say, 160 pounds, or some fifty billion times more than an egg cell . . . The phenotype is, then a result of interactions between the genotype and the sequence of the environments in which the individual lives . . . The 'environments' include, of course, everything that can influence man in any way. They include the physical environment—climate, soil, nutrition—and, most important in human development, the cultural environment—all that a person learns, gains, or suffers in his relations with other people in the family, community, and society to which he belongs.*[12]

Thus, to say that an individual is genetically predetermined is more than an unjustified limitation on human potential. It is also scientifically invalid. And there is an element of absurdity to the "heredity versus environment" argument. For whatever happens in the genetic system is a happening in an environment. Genes are not fateful. By themselves, they decide little.

---

[11] Theodosius Grigorievich Dobzhansky, *Heredity and the Nature of Man* (New York, 1964), pp. 49–50.
[12] *Ibid.*, pp. 50–51. The *phenotype* is the appearance of the trait; the *genotype* is the genetic basis of the trait.

Nevertheless, practicality does require an answer to the question, "To what extent can genes predispose an individual to develop certain illnesses?" Some disorders are dependent on the presence of a particular genetic error (though not all individuals who carry such errors will necessarily manifest the disorders). Then what is the role of the surrounding environment? This varies. In some instances, such as hemophilia (see page 250), the environmental influence, compared to the genetic, is rather small. With other conditions, the environment plays a more distinct role. Coronary artery disease, as an example, is greatly influenced by both genetic instruction and environment. Short stocky men with a history of heart attacks in the family are more prone to coronary heart disease than tall thin men without such a history (see page 264). But diet (environment) plays an important role too. How long the condition remains latent and, when revealed, how severely it is manifested—these may be profoundly influenced by the environment. Another example: much has been written of the relationship between an XYY chromosomal pattern and aggressive behavior (see page 538). And the association appears to be valid. Yet, most aggressive behavior is unrelated to the XYY chromosome. Moreover, a gentle, well-adjusted person may carry an XYY chromosomal aberration and harm nobody. Another, with the same genetic disorder will be a violent, homicidal menace. The difference may be in the environment.

A few years ago, Charles J. Whitman, a twenty-five-year-old architectural engineering major, climbed to the observation deck of the University of Texas tower in Austin. He shot and killed fourteen persons who were on the campus below. Thirty-one others were injured. A few hours before, he had killed his wife and mother. Whitman's chromosomal pattern is unknown. This, however, is known: at autopsy, he revealed a highly malignant brain tumor. Could his brain tumor have contributed to his aggression? Perhaps. (He had presented no known neurological abnormality.) The chromosomal patterns of Lee Harvey Oswald and Jack Ruby are also unknown. But the terrible childhood of the former certainly helped lay the groundwork for the terrible act of his adulthood.[13] On the other hand, Ruby suffered from psychomotor epilepsy—a seizure disorder singularly resistant to treatment. During a seizure from this type of epilepsy, violence is not uncommon. Twice in his lifetime Ruby had been struck on the head by a pistol butt. Where did genetic influence begin? Where did the environment enter the behavioral picture? It is now impossible to tell. But neither factor can be ignored. What is needed is more alert study.

Genetic disorder   Human genetic problems are related either to (1) an error in the physical or chemical *structure* of a chromosome or (2) an error in the *amount* of chromosomal material in the cell. This is generally expressed in terms of the *number* of chromosomes in the cell.

[13]David Abrahamsen, "A Study of Lee Harvey Oswald: Psychological Capability of Murder," *Bulletin of the New York Academy of Medicine*, Second Series, Vol. 43, No. 10 (October 1967), pp. 861–88.

Disorders of chromosomal structure

SPONTANEOUS MUTATIONS Man was once a fish and within the uterus he still lives submerged in water like a fish. Slowly, over millions of years, he left the sea, and over still more millions of years he adapted to a new environment. All his adaptive changes were made possible by infinitely gradual gene changes or mutations (Latin *mutare,* to change). There are much more rapid changes due to environmental influence, as occurs when the German measles virus attacks the embryo. However, some genetic changes, although occurring in the environment, do not seem to be primarily caused by it. These are called *spontaneous.* A spontaneous change of some part of the chemical structure of the DNA takes place. If the change is not basically molded by the surrounding environment, how, then, may one account for the existence of a mutation in chromosomal structure? What causes a spontaneous change in DNA? The answer to this question remains unknown. Yet even one spontaneously mutant gene can result in profound developmental changes and hereditary health problems. Anatomical and, therefore, functional deviations from the normal ensue. There may be inborn errors of metabolism. Disorders of carbohydrate metabolism such as diabetes mellitus (see page 239) and of amino acid metabolism (phenylketonuria—PKU, see page 552) are examples. Or disease of the blood or blood-forming organs may result. Hemophilia is one of these. By no means are all mutations spontaneous, however. Some are plainly *induced* by an external environmental stimulus. An example is Mongolism (see below) caused by radiation.

CHROMOSOMAL TRANSLOCATION AND DELETION This, too, may occur spontaneously, or there may be a direct external cause, such as radiation. Sometimes a chromosome breaks. DNA structure is disrupted. The chromosome may heal into a new and different structure. Or it may remain in fragments. Or it may be just partly repaired, leaving a piece out of its structure. Or two chromosomes may exchange pieces. *Translocation* occurs when a segment or a fragment of one chromosome shifts into another part of a noncorresponding chromosome. Sometimes, one of the products of such an exchange is so small it gets lost. This is called *deletion.* Whatever occurs the chromosome is adversely altered. Genetic instruction by the DNA of the affected chromosomes is awry. Usually a fertilized egg, containing a broken or wrongly formed chromosome, will die. Occasionally, the zygote lives. The individual develops to suffer various deficiencies.

Disorders of chromosome number during meiosis or early mitosis

Sometimes it is not a changed chromosomal structure that results in disease. Rather it is an error in the total number of chromosomes that find their way into the cells. Normally, there are forty-six. With genetically related sickness, there may be too many or too few. How can this happen?

16-9 Nondisjunction in the mother, resulting in ova with either two X-chromosomes or none. When fertilized, these ova can give rise to the four chromosome combinations shown here. Three of them are abnormal; the fourth is nonviable—the complete absence of an X-chromosome is lethal to a zygote. (This diagram presents an abbreviated view of the development of spermatozoa and ova from the primordial sex cells. The process of meiosis is shown in greater detail in Figure 16-4.)

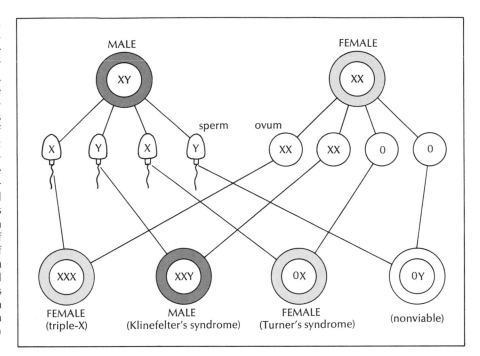

ERRORS DURING MEIOSIS   Study again Figure 16-4 illustrating meiosis. This shows how the chromosomes, having duplicated themselves, separate. Consequently, after the first cell division, when two cells are formed, each cell normally has duplicates of only a single member of each original pair of chromosomes. Sometimes, though, something goes wrong. Nobody really knows why. During meiosis, the chromosomes of a pair do not separate. This is the basic error. One cell receives both chromosomes of the pair, while the other gamete receives none. This is called *meiotic nondisjunction.*

It will be further noted in Figure 16-4 that there are two meiotic divisions. Meiotic nondisjunction can also occur during the second meiotic division after a normal first division. Upon fertilization, should a gamete with a missing chromosome unite with a normal gamete, the zygote and all the cells consequent to its multiplication will have forty-five chromosomes instead of the normal forty-six. This condition is called *monosomy.* Should a gamete with an extra chromosome unite with a normal gamete, the zygote will have forty-seven chromosomes. This is *trisomy.* The trisomy and monosomy of meiotic nondisjunction can affect both the autosomal chromosomes and the sex chromosomes.

Trisomy 21. The most common trisomy affects the twenty-first autosome of the karyotype. *Trisomy 21* is one of the causes of *Mongolism* or *Down's syndrome.* In this illness nondisjunction occurs with chromosomes other than the X and Y. As a result of this autosomal aberration, the individual has forty-seven instead of forty-six chromosomes. Children with Down's

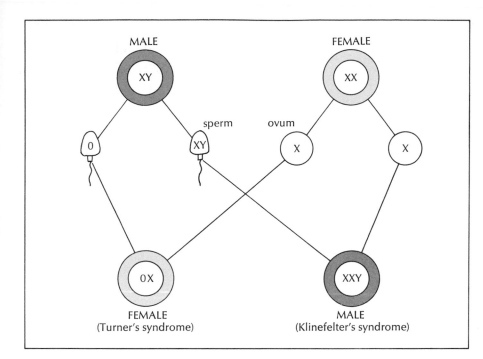

16-10 Nondisjunction in the father, resulting in spermatozoa with either no sex chromosomes or both an X- and a Y-chromosome. Ova fertilized by such spermatozoa can give rise to the two chromosome combinations shown here. Both of them are abnormal. (As in Figure 16-9, this diagram omits the step-by-step process of meiosis, which is shown in Figure 16-4.)

syndrome[14] (named after a nineteenth-century English physician, John Down) are physically and mentally retarded. Muscle tone is poor. The tongue is large. The eyes are slanted, which accounts for the other name of the condition—*Mongolism*. Palm and footprints are abnormal. As the age of the mother increases, so do her chances of giving birth to a child with Mongolism.

Meiotic nondisjunction involving the X and Y sex chromosomes can result in gametes that may unite to produce zygotes that manifest some aberrant sex chromosome arrangements. How do these disorders occur?

Turner's syndrome (Figures 16-9 and 16-10). Illness may result from nondisjunction of sex chromosomes during meiosis. Assume that during an error in meiotic division an ovum receives no X-chromosome. It is fertilized by a normal sperm containing an X-chromosome. The resultant individual acquires a chromosomal pattern as follows:

$$\text{No X (ovum)} + \text{X (sperm)} = \text{0X}$$

(0 refers to the missing X chromosome.)

An 0X zygote develops into an individual with a combination of characteristics called *Turner's syndrome (monosomy X)*. At birth the baby appears to be a female. But the child has tiny ovaries. Nor does the child develop secondary sexual characteristics. She is abnormally short and never menstruates. Turner's syndrome also results if a sperm with no X-chromosome fertilizes a normal ovum.

[14]A syndrome refers to a set of signs and symptoms occurring together, as a group, in a disease state.

Klinefelter's syndrome (Figures 16-9 and 16-10). Sometimes, during meiosis, a single ovum receives both (XX) chromosomes. With fertilization by a sperm carrying the Y chromosome, what happens? This:

$$XX \text{ (ovum)} + Y \text{ (sperm)} = XXY$$

Here there is an excess X (female) chromosome (*intersex*[15]). The result: a *Klinefelter male,* as this individual is called. These people may appear normal, or be quite tall. They may have underdeveloped sexual structures. Ordinarily, they are sterile and are often mentally retarded.

Illness from nondisjunction of sex chromosomes during male meiosis can also result in the Klinefelter male.

Chromosomes and crime. Another abnormal arrangement of chromosomes that can result from nondisjunction of sex chromosomes in male meiosis involves an extra Y-chromosome. Figure 16-11 shows how a sperm carrying two Y-chromosomes is produced. When such a sperm fertilizes a normal ovum the *XYY syndrome* occurs. Recent research has brought considerable attention to individuals manifesting this syndrome. Tentative results indicate a startling association between the XYY disorder and criminal insanity.[16] Richard Speck, the 1966 murderer of eight Chicago nurses, was found to have the XYY disorder. The XYY chromosomal error is by no means an absolute indicator of criminal behavior. Only a portion of XYY males develop criminal behavior. But it does appear much more commonly in prison populations. Its victims are unusually tall males,[17] often mentally retarded, with histories of aggressive violence. Should they be punished for their crimes? A French court has ruled affirmatively. An Australian court has said "no" and acquitted an XYY murderer. In this country, a final decision has yet to be made. Although society must be protected, many suggest that XYY aggressiveness should no more be punished than the genetic gentleness of the Mongoloid is rewarded. Everything possible should be done for the known XYY carrier. With such an individual, environmental conditions encouraging crime take on a special meaning.

Configurations with three, four, or no X-chromosomes. Rarely a person is born with an XXX configuration—the so-called "super-" or "hyper-" female. However, they are often nonfunctional mental defectives. Males with two extra X-chromosomes (XXXY) have also been found. Even more rarely, males and females with four X-chromosomes have been noted by investigators (XXXXY and XXXX). The complete absence of an X-chromosome in a zygote is lethal.

Chromosomes and competition in athletics. Abnormal chromosome arrangements can become a matter for concern in international female athletic events. Disputes arise when a performance is thought to be due

---

[15]Intersexuality should not be confused with homosexuality. The former is a genetic disorder. It refers to the abnormal intermingling, in varying degrees, of the characters of each sex. The incidence of homosexuality among intersexually abnormal patients is not higher than in the general population.

[16]Fathers and children of XYY are no more likely to have abnormal chromosomes than the average person in the population. The condition is innate, but not hereditary.

[17]Extraordinary height is not necessarily due to chromosomal abnormality.

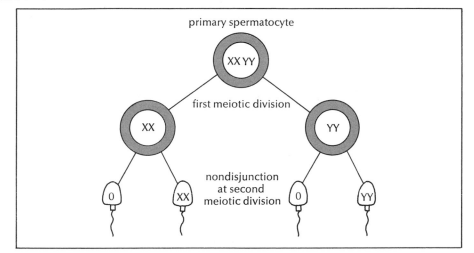

primary spermatocyte

XX YY

first meiotic division

XX

YY

nondisjunction
at second
meiotic division

0

XX

0

YY

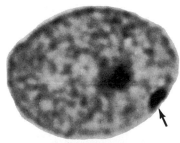

16-11 The XYY syn-drome. Nondisjunction in the father may pro-duce spermatozoa with two Y-chromosomes, as shown here. When such a sperm fertilizes a normal ovum (which has an X-chromosome), the result is the XYY male.

to chromosomal maleness. Microscopic examination of cells usually settles the argument. Most experts disagree with this superficial approach.[18]

Chromosomal analysis alone does not determine sex. Also to be considered is *nuclear sex*. In the cell nuclei of female mammals (including the human) is a structure not present in males (see Figure 16-12). Yet, even these two—chromosomal sex and nuclear sex—are not adequate to definitely determine the appropriate sex of some people. Other important criteria include genital appearance, internal reproductive organs, structure of the gonads, influence of other endocrine glands, psychological sex, and social sex.[19] Thus, it is the opinion of some that it was unfair to disqualify the Polish track star Ewa Klobukowska from the 1967 Women's European Athletic Cup competition.[20] In her case, apparently only nuclear and chromosomal sex indicators were used. (Incidentally, there have been instances of males who, disguised as females, won Olympic medals. "Claire," the bronze-medal winner in the 100-meter dash in the 1946 competition at Oslo, today answers to the name of Pierre, is a father, and lives on a farm near Metz, France.)

ERRORS DURING MITOSIS   Although most abnormalities from non-disjunction occur during meiosis, nondisjunction can also occur during mitosis. A normal sperm fertilizes a normal ovum. But during the early mitotic cellular multiplication following fertilization two chromosomes may fail to separate. In this way half the body cells of the affected individual have three rather than two of a particular chromosome (forty-seven total) and the other half of his body cells have one instead of the normal

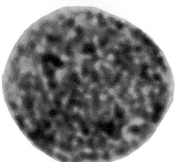

16-12 Nucleus of a human female cell (*top*), showing characteristic Barr body (arrow); nucleus of a human male cell (*bottom*).

[18] Some tests used in detecting abnormalities in chromosomes are mentioned in the section on genetic counseling on page 555.

[19] Sometimes sex is determined by surgical exploration, but only after all these and other factors have been carefully weighed.

[20] "Olympics: Sex Test Inconclusive," *Science News*, Vol. 94, No. 13 (September 28, 1968), p. 312.

two (forty-five total). This is called *mosaicism*. Sometimes three types of cells may occur in one person's body, normal (forty-six chromosomes), trisomic (forty-seven), and monosomic (forty-five). Mosaicism can also result, not from failure of separation of chromosomes, but from the loss of a chromosome during the cell division of mitosis. In all these mitotic variables there is the potential of grave illness.

Illness and the genes of sex and race

Illness patterns are profoundly influenced by such genetic factors as sex and race.

SEX   Fortunately, the union of the human sperm and egg results in about 140 males for every 100 females. Fortunately indeed. The male hold on life is relatively feeble. Even within the safety of the uterus, fifty percent more males than females perish. In all age groups up to the age of eighty, there is a consistent excess of male over female deaths (see Table 16-1). In 1968 over two and a half times as many males between fifteen and twenty-four died as did females in the same age group. Neither U.S. civilians nor members of the armed forces who died outside this country were included in these data. Moreover, the ratios were similar in 1960, a year in which the United States was not engaged in hostilities. For the

TABLE 16-1   *Male Deaths Per 100 Female Deaths by Age Groups, United States, 1968**

AGE	MALE DEATHS PER 100 FEMALE DEATHS
Under 1	138.7
1–4	120.5
5–14	166.9
15–24	257.2
25–34	189.2
35–44	161.4
45–54	174.3
55–59	188.1
60–64	187.2
65–69	159.4
70–74	139.4
75–79	111.0
80–84	88.5
85 and over	65.3
Total all ages	128.6

*These data do not cover deaths of U.S. civilians or members of the armed forces that occurred outside the United States.

Source: National Center for Health Statistics, *Monthly Vital Statistics Report*, Provisional Statistics, Annual Summary for the United States, 1968.

fragile male, almost all disease categories are more lethal. Aside from the complications of childbirth, it is only in a relatively few disease categories that females die more frequently (see Table 16-2). Syphilis has been called "the chivalric disease." It surely shows special consideration for the female. For her, the disease is milder and is less likely to involve the heart and central nervous system. Syphilis kills less than half as many females as males. When suitable antibiotics are given to a male child with bacterial meningitis, his chances for survival are less than those of a female child of about the same age and in the same circumstances. Adverse effects of atomic radiation are more frequent in boys than girls.

Why the disparity? There is a good theory. It has been stated that, of the forty-six chromosomes in the primordial sex cell of the ovum or sperm, two are sex chromosomes. The female has two X-chromosomes. These are equal. The male, however, has one X-chromosome and one puny Y-chromosome. Thus, the arrangement of the X- and Y-chromosomes is probably to the advantage of the female. If something goes wrong with one of her chromosomes, perhaps she can rely upon the other. The male is denied such possible insurance. There is evidence, at present inconclusive, that this biological inequality may be gradually equalizing because of the inactivation of one of the female X-chromosomes. Nonetheless, the male is indeed the weaker sex.

RACE   As noted on page 29, sickle-cell anemia is much more frequent among Negroes than Caucasians. In the United States, tooth decay is more common among Caucasians than Negroes. Among women in Japan, cancer of the breast is rare. One should, however, view with caution the varying frequency of diseases in races. True, heredity helps decide body reactions to disease. But socioeconomics rather than genes accounts for the comparatively greater frequency of such illnesses as tuberculosis and syphilis among blacks in this country. Moreover, recent studies emphasize the association between the malnutrition of poverty and mental retardation.

Within the nucleus of the cell, the basic genetic chemicals are arranged in relation to one another. And they are dependent on one another. So, inside the very nucleus there is environment with ecological balance or imbalance.

The genetic ecosystem: the fertilized ovum in the environment

Within the no longer secret nucleus, the genes contain a pattern set to direct development. But no amount of healthy genetic instruction can bid cytoplasm, sickened by an abnormal environment, to be normal. Nor can a healthy cytoplasm expect beneficial patterns of instruction from a gene made deviant by environment. Normal genetic action depends on a normal environment inside and outside the cell. The internal drama of the cell will be disarranged not only when the chromosomal players unaccountably neglect their proper parts but also when they are surrounded by destructive microorganisms, or hostile drugs, or searing radiation. That is why German measles (rubella) and thalidomide and atomic radiation kill and cripple the unborn. Consider now these and other influences.

TABLE 16-2 *Deaths in the United States Due to Selected Causes, 1967*

(according to sex)

CAUSE OF DEATH	TOTAL		MALE		FEMALE	
	NUMBER	RATE (per 100,000 population)	NUMBER	RATE (per 100,000 population)	NUMBER	RATE (per 100,000 population)
Tuberculosis, all forms	6,901	3.5	5,002	5.2	1,899	1.9
Syphilis and its sequelae	2,381	1.2	1,684	1.7	697	0.7
Meningococcal infections	635	0.3	355	0.4	280	0.3
Malignant neoplasms (cancers)	310,983	157.2	169,164	174.9	141,819	140.2
Benign neoplasms and neoplasms of unspecified nature	5,013	2.5	2,450	2.5	2,563	2.5
Asthma	4,137	2.1	2,286	2.4	1,851	1.8
Diabetes mellitus	35,049	17.7	14,421	14.9	20,628	20.4
Anemias	3,460	1.7	1,738	1.8	1,722	1.7
Major cardiovascular-renal diseases	1,012,047	511.5	554,242	573.2	457,805	452.5
Influenza and pneumonia (except pneumonia of the newborn)	56,892	28.8	31,904	33.0	24,988	24.7
Bronchitis	6,264	3.2	4,598	4.8	1,666	1.6
Other bronchopulmonic diseases	29,360	14.8	23,556	24.4	5,804	5.7
Ulcer of the stomach and duodenum	9,825	5.0	6,783	7.0	3,042	3.0
Appendicitis	1,526	0.8	928	1.0	598	0.6
Hernia and intestinal obstruction	9,814	5.0	4,462	4.6	5,352	5.3
Gastritis, duodenitis, enteritis, and colitis (inflammation of the stomach, intestine, or colon), excluding diarrhea of the newborn	7,504	3.8	3,489	3.6	4,015	4.0
Cirrhosis of the liver	27,816	14.1	17,930	18.5	9,886	9.8
Gallstones and inflammation of the gallbladder or bile duct	4,383	2.2	1,967	2.0	2,416	2.4
Infections of the kidney	9,006	4.6	4,179	4.3	4,827	4.8
Congenital malformations	17,328	8.8	9,346	9.7	7,982	7.9
Certain diseases of early infancy (birth injuries, postnatal suffocation, infections, etc.)	48,314	24.4	28,261	29.2	20,053	19.8
Symptoms, senility, and ill-defined conditions	24,098	12.2	14,394	14.9	9,704	9.6
Accidents	113,169	57.2	77,879	80.5	35,290	34.9
Suicide	21,325	10.8	15,187	15.7	6,138	6.1
Homicide	13,425	6.8	10,236	10.6	3,189	3.2
Total deaths due to all causes	1,851,323	935.7	1,045,945	1,081.7	805,378	796.1

Source: National Center for Health Statistics, *Monthly Vital Statistics Report*, Advance Report, Final Mortality Statistics, 1967.

TABLE 16-3   Mean Birth Weights According to Socioeconomic Status

PLACE	POPULATION	SUBJECTS	MEAN BIRTH WEIGHTS (in grams)
Madras	Indian	Well-to-do	2985
		"Mostly poor"	2736
South India	Indian	Wealthy	3182
		Poor	2810
Bombay	Indian	Upper class	3247
		Upper-middle class	2945
		Lower-middle class	2796
		Lower class	2578
Calcutta	Indian	Paying patients	2851
		Poor class	2656
Congo	Bantu	"Very well nourished"	3026
		"Well nourished"	2965
		"Badly nourished"	2850
Ghana (Accra)	African	Prosperous	3188
		General population	2879
Indonesia	Javanese	Well-to-do	3022
		Poor	2816

Source: *World Health Organization, Nutrition in Pregnancy and Lactation,* cited in Miriam E. Lowenberg *et al., Food and Man* (New York, 1968).

Nutrition

Pregnant women may need extra calories, proteins, minerals, and vitamins. However, dietary decisions, including vitamins and iron therapy, should be made only by the physician. Deficient maternal diets mean more stillborn babies and more deaths among babies less than one month old. The child is affected by the mother's diet not only during his residence in the uterus but also long after birth. Babies born to poorly nourished mothers are more susceptible to infections in early life and have more birth defects. A child surviving a mother's poor nutrition may be smaller at birth and often will grow into a small adolescent and adult. There is a direct relationship between the economic status of the mother and the birth weight of her baby (see Table 16-3). Children born of poor mothers weigh less. And children with lower-than-normal birth weights have a greater tendency to physical defects in later life.

Should the mother fail to provide enough food for the child within her, will he suffer shortages? Or will he be able to avoid malnourishment by

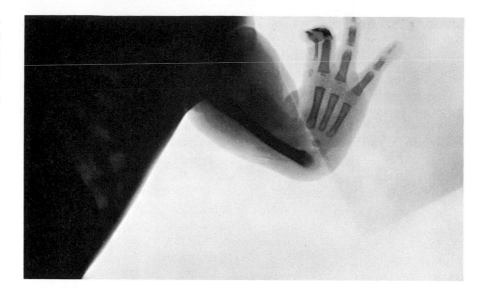

16-13 X-ray photograph showing the deformed arm of a one-year-old child whose mother had taken the drug thalidomide during early pregnancy.

helping himself to whatever is available from his mother's reserve? The availability of the mother's reserve has been overestimated. Daily nourishment for the developing child comes from the daily nourishment of the mother. Even a temporarily inadequate diet, unnoticed by the mother, may wreak irreparable damage to an unborn child. With maternal malnutrition, the unborn infant suffers before, and more, than the mother.

A maternal diet that is poor in calcium may result in a child born with poor bone development and teeth. Inadequate iron results in anemia for both mother and child. Severe protein deficiency retards growth and development. Vitamin diseases, such as beriberi, rickets, and scurvy, are seen in the babies of mothers deprived of vitamins B, D, and C respectively. An iodine-deficient maternal diet may result in the birth of a child that will show the distressing signs of cretinism by the sixth to the eighth month of life. Marked by severe physical and mental retardation, cretinism is always a threat when the mother uses plain salt without added iodine. Animal experiments indicate that maternal diets deficient in zinc and manganese result in deformed babies. The effects of such shortages on human beings is unknown. A malnourished mother may not carry her child full term, and she is more inclined to develop complications of pregnancy.

Drugs

Knowledge about the effect of drugs on the unborn child is incomplete. Animal experiments may be inconclusive, and their results do not always apply to humans. The calamitous crippling of unborn children, in 1961 and 1962, by a German-made sleeping pill containing thalidomide,[21] will

[21]Nevertheless, although initially associated with tragedy, thalidomide shows great promise in helping people with an ancient disease; it apparently prevents acute reactions in leprosy patients.

long be a mournful reminder of the dangers in the use of inadequately tested drugs. LSD and tobacco effects are discussed on pages 410 and 553.

Infection

Women who develop *German measles* (rubella) during the first three months of pregnancy are over five times (15 percent) more likely to give birth to a defective child than woman who do not have the disease (2.8 percent). The heart, hearing, and vision (cataracts) are most commonly affected. *Regular measles* (rubeola) should not be confused with German measles (rubella). There is some medical opinion that a woman who contracts regular measles also has a greater chance of having a defective child. But many physicians think that this contention is unproved. There are now available effective vaccines to prevent both regular measles and German measles. There is limited evidence that *infectious hepatitis,* a third viral illness, can adversely affect chromosomes. Because *smallpox vaccine* is composed of a living virus, it may affect the unborn child. Consequently, pregnant women are not usually vaccinated against smallpox. *Syphilis* can also be transmitted from mother to unborn child. Adequate treatment of the mother can prevent tragedy for both.[22]

Direct radiation

Excessive exposure of a pregnant woman to X-rays can result in either fetal death or a malformed child. Women should, therefore, always advise a doctor who plans to X-ray them of a possible, still unapparent, pregnancy.

There have been large-scale experiences with radiation. Seven out of eleven Hiroshima children were born retarded if, within the first twenty weeks of conception, their mothers stood within 1,200 meters of absolute center of the atomic bomb blast. Others, whose mothers were at a greater distance, had malformed hips, eyes, and hearts. Some, symptomless at birth, developed poorly.

In Chapter 4, mention was made of the U.S. experimental explosion of a nuclear device at Bikini. An unpredictable wind deposited significant amounts of radioactive material on the residents of four nearby islands as well as on twenty-three Japanese fishermen. Years later, children of the islands who were less than five years old at the time of exposure were found to be retarded in physical growth.

Why does radiation cause abnormal babies? The baby is a triumph of recent cellular multiplication. And radiation has a predilection for multiplying cells. It requires more radiation to kill a fly than a mouse. Why? As a maggot, the fly passes through all its phases of growth and development. As an adult, it has few dividing cells. Adult mice and men have many dividing cells. It is these that are sensitive to radiation.[23]

[22] See also Chapter 6, pp. 175–76.
[23] Charlotte Auerbach, *Genetics in the Atomic Age,* 2nd ed. (New York, 1965), pp. 4–5.

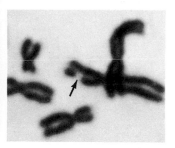

16-14 A chromosomal break (arrow) due to radiation.

Radiation reaching the testes or ovaries, and thereby the reproductive cells, can cause changes in the structure of the DNA (genes). Mutation rates are increased by radiation. Since over ninety-nine percent of mutations are harmful and since they do accumulate in man, the threat to future generations is apparent. Depending on the amount, moreover, radiation may cause chromosomal breaks and translocations. So another danger of radiation, more recently recognized, is related to chromosomal aberrations. Thus, radiation may be one of the causes of a wide variety of genetic disorders, ranging from the mental retardation of phenylketonuria to the mental retardation of Mongolism.

Endocrine influences

The *pancreas,* lying in the abdomen behind the stomach, is a gland producing a juice that passes into the upper intestine through a duct (see body chart 14 in the color section). However, another of its products, *insulin,* is produced by specialized islands of cells (*islets of Langerhans*) and is released directly into the blood. Insulin regulates carbohydrate metabolism. Without enough insulin, diabetes develops.

Diabetes is a genetically transmitted disorder of metabolism. (See pages 239–41.) Diabetic mothers have malformed children ten times more frequently than the average. The reasons are undetermined. They may be genetic or endocrine or nutritional or, perhaps, all three.

The Rh factor

In 1967, in this country, about ten thousand babies died of *Rh blood disease.* The condition is also known as *erythroblastosis fetalis* (Greek *erythros,* red + *blastos,* germ + *osis,* increase). The increase in red germ cells refers to the numerous immature primitive red blood cells seen in the circulation of the affected child. Their development in the fetus accounts for the term "fetalis." Why do they occur? To make up for the normal red cells that are destroyed. Why are the normal red blood cells destroyed? In this the Rh factor is involved. What is Rh?

Rh is a chemical substance. Its exact structure is unknown. It sits on the surface of the red blood cells of 85 percent of all people. They are then Rh positive. The 15 percent who do not carry it are Rh negative. Why is it called Rh? The *Rh*esus monkey also has the factor. Has Rh a known purpose? No. It just causes trouble. How?

One in eight marriages is between an Rh-negative woman and an Rh-positive man. If the child is Rh negative, like the mother, there is no problem. But the child may inherit the Rh-positive factor from the father. The Rh-negative mother thus carries an Rh-positive child. Erythroblastosis fetalis occurs when the Rh-positive blood of the child enters the mother's blood. The baby's Rh-positive factor is a foreigner to the mother. It is an antigen (see Chapter 6, page 158), an antibody generator. To neutralize her baby's Rh-positive antigens, the mother produces antibodies in her blood. When these antibodies enter the child, they destroy red blood cells. There are two ways in which a child's antibody-stimulating Rh-positive factor reaches the mother's circulation. One way is through the placenta during pregnancy. Usually only small amounts of baby-antigen reach the mother in this fashion. During the time that she is carrying her first child, these minimal amounts are not thought to be enough to cause the mother to manufacture antibody. The second way that the child's Rh antigen enters the mother occurs during delivery. Indeed, most of the child's Rh-positive blood reaches the mother during delivery, since, at that time, the afterbirth loosens and bleeds. Therefore, it is after delivery that she manufactures antibodies. Once she has manufactured such antibodies, she will be restimulated, in future pregnancies involving an Rh-positive fetus, to produce antibody with only the small amount of antigen that enters through the placenta. That is why erythroblastosis fetalis will usually affect the child of a later pregnancy more severely than an earlier one; a third child, for example, will be more adversely affected than a second; a fourth child, more than a third; and so on.

To repeat, then, in most cases the mother usually does not produce enough antibodies to harm the child during a first pregnancy. During the actual delivery of her first child, however, she receives enough Rh-positive blood to manufacture a high level of antibodies. These antibodies remain in the mother's blood. With the second child, harm is likely. As with the first child, the second may inherit the father's RH-positive blood factor. The mother's antibodies, formed in response to the Rh-positive antigen of the first baby, now pass through the placenta of the second baby. The antibodies destroy the unborn second child's red blood cells. To recoup, the child hastily makes new cells. These are the primitive red blood cells of erythroblastosis fetalis. But, as immature cells, they do not make up for the destroyed mature red blood cells. Anemia results. Products from the child's red cell destruction seep into the skin. Jaundice occurs.

Well over 90 percent of babies with erythroblastosis are saved. Complete replacement of their blood is necessary. Of the most severely affected, only about 25 percent are salvaged. A relatively new technique has sometimes been helpful. Rh-negative blood is introduced directly into the unborn child. This may maintain life within the uterus long enough to result in a baby who, at delivery, is adequately mature for transfusion. To the baby with erythroblastosis fetalis, the new era of the surgery of unborn babies has brought renewed hope. It is now even possible to temporarily remove a child from the uterus, replace the child's blood, and then return that child to the womb to complete the intrauterine life. Although such spectacular fetal surgery is not generally needed in the treatment of erythroblastosis fetalis, the very fact that it has been accomplished successfully opens further the whole new field of the surgery of the unborn.

But in some cases erythroblastosis fetalis can now be prevented. Recently, a product containing antibodies against Rh-positive blood has

TABLE 16-4 *Childbearing Children in the United States, 1965*			
Number of Babies Born to Mothers Ten to Fourteen Years of Age			
NUMBER OF CHILDREN BORN	WHITE	NONWHITE	TOTAL
One child	2,450	4,984	7,434
Two children	72	248	320
Three children	2	10	12
Four children	2	0	2
Total	2,526	5,242	7,768

Source: Lucille B. Hurley, "The Consequences of Fetal Impoverishment," *Nutrition Today*, Vol. 3, No. 4 (December 1968), p. 9.

proved successful. Within 72 hours of delivery of her first Rh-positive baby, the mother's blood is tested for antibodies. If she already has them in considerable amount, the product is useless. But if she does not have a significant level of antibodies, because not enough of the baby's Rh-positive antigen had passed through the placenta into her circulation, the mother is injected with the medicine containing antibodies against Rh-positive blood. These medicine-antibodies quickly combine with the baby's Rh-positive antigen that had reached the mother's blood during delivery. This happens before the mother has a chance to make her own Rh-positive antibodies. The Rh-positive antigen-antibody mixture is then washed out through the kidney. The mother does not have any antibody against Rh-positive blood to threaten her next baby.

The mother's age

As a rule, young mothers (under thirty) provide a relatively safer intra-uterine environment for their children. Perhaps older women do not produce adequate endocrine secretions to guarantee proper development of ova. (In animals, both aged ova and sperm appear less likely to combine to produce healthy offspring than do fresh ones.) With increase in the mother's age, for example, the frequency of Mongolism, as well as some other rare abnormalities, increases (see page 554).

It should not be concluded that the younger mother needs less medical attention than the older. Table 16-4 shows that child marriages and pregnancies in this country are but a small percentage of the total but they are by no means rare. The young-teen-aged mother presents a special problem. She is less likely to obtain early professional care and is more prone to be improperly nourished. Consequently, both her life and that of her baby are at greater risk.

The mother's emotions

Emotional stress, particularly early in pregnancy, may be related to cleft palates. Some emotions cause a hyperactivity of the outer part (cortex) of the adrenal glands. This hyperactivity causes the adrenals to produce the hormone hydrocortisone, which can pass through the placenta. If hydrocortisone is injected into mice while their upper palates are being formed, over 90 percent are born with cleft palates.

Many other factors such as abnormal fetal position or a faulty placenta may adversely affect the environment of the child developing in the uterus. A mother's high blood pressure and hyperactivity of the thyroid gland also detract from the safety of the embryonic and fetal ecosystem.

So, even within the environment of the uterus, there are numerous ways in which that delicate individual, the developing human, may be threatened. Heredity and environment interact. Both may be improved.

About birth defects

More babies die of defective development before they are born than after. Such defective embryos account for most of the million miscarriages in this country every year. Most occur early in pregnancy—the period of greatest vulnerability of the developing child. Some miscarriages occur so early that the woman may never have known she was pregnant. Others occur after a few months. "Many [of such deaths] are nature's way of getting rid of an abnormally developing fetus in order that a new and better one can be started."[24] Of every sixteen babies born alive in this country, one is found to be defective within the first year. (Some birth defects, such as gout and diabetes, may not be apparent for years.) This amounts to about a quarter of a million babies a year. Eighteen thousand of these die in the first year of life.

It may be estimated conservatively that 15 million persons in the United States have one or more congenital defects which affect their daily lives. Included are an estimated 4 million with clinical diabetes, 2,900,000 with mental retardation of prenatal origin, 1 million with congenital orthopedic impairments, 500,000 who were born blind or with serious loss of vision, 750,000 with congenital hearing impairment, at least 350,000 with congenital heart disease, and more than 100,000 with speech defects of prenatal origin.[25]

As the population grows, the number of babies born with birth defects increases. Moreover, modern surgery, newer drugs, and more research combine to keep many defective children alive to adolescence and maturity. Though this kind of effort will always be a basic purpose of medicine, such survival, nevertheless, means problems.

[24] Edith L. Potter, "Defective Babies Who Die Before Birth," in Morris Fishbein, ed., *Birth Defects* (Philadelphia, 1963), p. 46.
[25] V. Apgar and G. Stickle, "Birth Defects: Their Significance as a Public Health Problem," *Journal of the American Medical Association*, Vol. 204, No. 5 (April 29, 1968), pp. 79–82.

TABLE 16-5 The More Common Birth Defects

TYPE OF DEFECT	APPROXIMATE FREQUENCY	DESCRIPTION	CAUSES AND TREATMENT
Birthmarks	Very common.	The disfiguring ones are red or wine-colored patches of small dilated blood vessels.	Cause unknown. Treatments include plastic surgery, skin grafts, or tattooing of normal skin colors over the purple area.
Cleft lip (harelip)	About 1 in 1,000 babies born in the U.S. has a cleft lip; two-thirds of these also have cleft palate. Frequency seems lower in blacks than in whites.	If embryonic swellings that will become the upper lip do not fuse at the right time, the gap remains and the baby will have a cleft lip.	Sometimes related to genetic defects. Influence of intrauterine environment and of some drugs given during pregnancy are being studied. Harelip can be repaired in the first few weeks after birth, and cleft palate before age fourteen months in most cases.
Cleft palate	About 1 in every 2,500 babies has a cleft palate without cleft lip. The two conditions are not genetically related.	A cleft palate is a hole in the roof of the mouth.	
Clubfoot	1 in 250.	The foot turns inward (usually) or outward and is fixed in a tip-toe position.	Possibly due to position of child in uterus or to maldevelopment of the limb bud. Treatments include shoe splints, braces, corrective shoes, plaster casts, or surgery. Tends to recur, so treatment must begin early and is often prolonged.
Congenital heart disease (see also page 261)	1 in 200.	Some are so slight as to cause little strain on the heart; others are fatal. In some abnormalities, the baby appears blue.	German measles during pregnancy is one cause. Many heart conditions can now be repaired by surgery, saving lives and preventing invalidism.
Congenital urinary tract defects	1 in 250.	May involve kidneys, ureters, bladder, and genitalia. Organs may be absent, fused, or obstructed.	Causes include certain hormones given during pregnancy. Some hereditary tendency. Most conditions are correctable by surgery.
Diabetes (see also page 239)	About 1 in 4 carries the trait. Clinical diabetes (actual cases) seen in about 1 in 2,500 persons between ages one and twenty; in 1 in 50 persons over sixty years old.	A metabolic disorder. The body cannot handle sugar normally, and high glucose levels in the blood and urine result. This familial condition is related in some unknown way to abnormal utilization of insulin. Long-standing diabetics may develop complications involving blood vessels, kidneys, heart, eyes and peripheral nerves. Obesity predisposes individuals to the disease.	Marked hereditary tendency. Persons with family history of diabetes should seek periodic check-up. Doctors can recognize symptoms, make positive diagnosis, and prescribe specific treatment. Special diets, oral medication, and injections of insulin are measures that will usually keep condition under control and permit normal activity. Good prenatal care is especially important for known or suspected diabetics.

Table 16-5   Continued

TYPE OF DEFECT	APPROXIMATE FREQUENCY	DESCRIPTION	CAUSES AND TREATMENT
Erythroblastosis fetalis (see also pages 546–548)	About 10 percent of babies of Rh-negative mothers married to Rh-positive fathers were, until preventive medication became available, threatened by this condition. In U.S. population, 1 in 7 whites and 1 in 16 blacks has Rh-negative blood.	Without preventive medication—and among infants of mothers sensitized during previous deliveries—baby is often yellow soon after birth. Anemia is a common symptom. Mental retardation may be severe. Erythroblastosis is a common cause of stillbirth.	Baby inherits Rh-positive gene from his father, and the mother is Rh negative. Red blood cells of fetus reach mother's blood, causing her blood to form antibodies which pass back through the placenta to the baby and destroy his red cells in varying degrees. First pregnancy is usually uneventful. Preventive medication prevents sensitization of mother, if given soon after birth of each baby. Intrauterine or exchange transfusion, replacing baby's blood with compatible blood right after birth, prevents severe damage to babies of sensitized mothers.
Extra fingers and toes (polydactyly)	Extra digits are twice as frequent as fused digits. Incidence is 1 in 100 among blacks; 1 in 600 among whites.	Extra fingers or toes.	Cause unknown; frequently hereditary. Cure is amputation of the extra digits. This can often be done at birth or at about age three.
Fused fingers and toes (syndactyly)	Fused digits do not have such racial variation.	Too few digits.	Surgery can improve the function and appearance of the hand or foot.
Fibrocystic disease (cystic fibrosis; see also pages 238–239)	About 1 in 1,000 births. Rare among blacks; infrequent in Orientals.	A sickly, malnourished child with persistent intestinal difficulties and chronic respiratory problems. Death usually due to pneumonia or other lung complications.	Hereditary. New tests detect carriers. Mucus blocks the exit of digestive juices from the pancreas into the intestinal tract. Excess mucus is also secreted by lungs. Treatments have extended life.
Galactosemia	Somewhat more rare than PKU (see below).	Causes eye cataracts and severe damage to liver and brain, resulting in mental retardation.	Hereditary. Caused by absence of an enzyme required to convert galactose to glucose. Experiments show that early recognition and dietary treatment can arrest the disease. Diagnosis can be made at birth.
Hydrocephaly (water on the brain)	1 in 500.	Enlargement of the head due to excessive fluid within the brain. Fluid's pressure often causes compression of the brain with resulting mental retardation.	Cause unknown. May result from prenatal infection or abnormality in development. Treatment is an operation to lead fluid from brain into blood stream or some other body cavity. Frequently fatal if not treated.
Missing limbs	Very rare.	One to four limbs missing or seriously deformed.	Cause unknown. A recent international outbreak was due to thalidomide used by pregnant mothers. Great strides have been made in prosthetic (artificial) devices.

Table 16-5 Continued

TYPE OF DEFECT	APPROXIMATE FREQUENCY	DESCRIPTION	CAUSES AND TREATMENT
Mongolism (Down's syndrome; see also pages 536–537)	1 in 600. Women twenty-five years old have about 1 chance in 2,000 of producing a mongoloid child. Women of forty-five have about 1 chance in 50.	Short stature, slightly slanted eyes, and varying degrees of mental retardation.	All patients have an extra chromosome or its equivalent. Causes can be hereditary or environmental. No known cure, but IQ can be improved by special training.
Open spine (spina bifida)	Approximately 1 in every 500 births. More common among whites than blacks. About half of the patients are also victims of hydrocephaly (see above).	Failure of the spine to close permits the protrusion of spinal cord or nerves; often leads to total dysfunction of legs, bladder, and rectum. Often the child has other serious defects.	Cause unknown. Sometimes surgery in the early months of life can correct or arrest the condition, preventing other complications. Several new surgical techniques are being used on the bladder, rectum, and spinal cord.
Phenylketonuria (PKU)	Approximately 1 in 10,000.	Child appears normal at birth, but his mind stops developing during the first year. Retardation is severe. One-third never learn to walk; two-thirds never learn to talk. Pigment of skin and hair is decreased.	Hereditary metabolic defect. The liver enzyme that changes the protein phenylalanine to tyrosine is inactive or absent; phenylalanine accumulates. PKU can be detected within the first few days of life. Treatment is special low-phenylalanine diet for the infant, which can prevent further retardation. Early treatment important. Some experiments show that after a few years PKU children can be fed normal diets.
Sickle-cell trait (see also page 29)	Low among whites; very high (about 40 percent) in some black African populations and high (10 percent) among American blacks.	When red blood cells of people with this trait are exposed to low-oxygen atmosphere their red blood cells become crescent or sickle-shaped. Usually fatal when accompanied by severe anemia. Carries some resistance to malaria.	Hereditary. Severe anemia results if the child receives the abnormal trait from both parents.

Source: Adapted from a booklet published by The National Foundation–March of Dimes, New York.

For too long birth defects have been associated with stigma and superstition. "If a woman gives birth, and the abdomen of the child is open, there will be a dwindling of the suburbs." So predicts an ancient Babylonian tablet. Greek mythology makes frequent reference to half-human, half-animal centaurs and minotaurs. Believing fertility between species to be possible, and birth defect the result, many Greeks were contemptuous of malformed children. In early Judeo-Christian cultures, the parents of defective children were ostracized. Even today, the expression "harelip" is used. Mothers of such children were once thought to have been frightened by a rabbit. But modern science has brought mankind a long way from such ignorance.

How to avoid some birth defects

1. A physician should be seen as soon as pregnancy is suspected because (a) the baby is most vulnerable during early pregnancy (the first 20 weeks), and (b) delay increases the chances of premature birth and a defective child.

2. No medication, not even vitamins, may be taken unless prescribed by the family doctor. Drugs may pass through the placenta and the child may be injured.

3. Except in emergencies, abdominal X-rays early in pregnancy should be avoided. Any physician about to X-ray a female patient, therefore, will want to know if she is pregnant.

4. Cigarette smoking should be discontinued. At the very least, excessive cigarette smoking must be avoided. The mother who smokes may have an underweight baby. Such a baby may thus pay dearly for the cigarette habit. Recent studies showed that nicotine injected into a pregnant monkey swiftly crossed the placental barrier. In the monkey fetus the nicotine level declined slowly. Both the heart rate and blood pressure of the monkey fetus were depressed. Potentially harmful disturbances in the unborn monkey's acid-base state and oxygen supply were noted.[26]

5. If possible, elective surgery should be delayed until after pregnancy. Abrupt changes to high altitudes should be avoided. In both instances, even temporary oxygen depletion might injure the embryo. In commercial airliners this is not ordinarily a problem.

6. An adequate diet must be followed.

7. Relatives should never marry. Even rare hereditary disorders occur much more commonly among the children of such unions. Except in Georgia, state laws forbid a person from marrying a parent, grandparent, child, or grandchild. In Georgia a man may marry his daughter or grandmother. Generally, marriages between persons with a relatedness equivalent to first cousins or closer are not legally sanctioned.[27]

[26] Karlis Adamsons et al., "Effects of Nicotine on the Unborn," cited in Briefs: Footnotes on Maternity Care, Vol. 33, No. 7 (September 1969), pp. 99–100.
[27] Michael G. Farrow and Richard C. Juberg, "Genetics and Laws Prohibiting Marriage in the United States," Journal of the American Medical Association, Vol. 209, No. 4 (July 28, 1969), p. 534.

8. Many physicians feel that the relationship between the older mother and the occurrence of Mongolism (and a few other rare abnormalities) should never alone deter childbearing.

9. Under some circumstances, the advice of a genetic counselor is indicated. The family physician will know if such help is necessary.

Some interesting relationships

Is there any relationship between survival of a fetus and a child and the spacing of pregnancies? What, if any, are the relationships between fetal and child survivals and the age of parents? In attempting to find answers to these questions, Day[28] surveyed the statistical literature. Although his findings by no means necessarily apply to individual cases, they are nonetheless of significance.

1. The ideal age for maternity seemed to be between the ages of twenty and thirty.

2. An interval of about two years between the end of one pregnancy and the beginning of another was associated with the lowest incidence of late fetal and newborn (up to one month of age) mortality as well as prematurity. Since prematurely born babies have a higher mortality than those born with a normal weight, this finding takes on added significance.

3. If pregnancy intervals are three years or more, survival through childhood is statistically more likely.

4. If the mother is over thirty-five, the first-born is more likely to be a stillbirth than if she is younger. On the other hand, the very young mother also shows a higher rate of stillborn babies. Very young mothers present special problems, as was noted earlier.

5. Children of small families grow taller and weigh more than children of large families.

6. It is the young mother, who has already had at least one child and whose baby is at greatest risk from preventable conditions, who is apparently most likely to profit from medical care (including contraceptive advice). Special efforts to improve her health, particularly if she is poor, would result in a great improvement in statistics that are used to describe the outcome of pregnancy.

7. An older father, regardless of the age of his wife, is statistically more likely to beget a stillborn child than a younger father.

8. Certain birth defects seem to occur more frequently in children with older parents than in those whose parents are young.

Genetic counseling

Second cousins want to marry. They share three diabetic parents. What are the genetic dangers? A couple have a second child that is Mongoloid. Can they hope for a normal child? A young man's sister has been incapacitated for ten years with severe muscular dystrophy. He is engaged and deeply troubled. An agency brings a pretty child, the product of an incestuous union. What are the risks to adopting parents? Parents bring

[28]Richard L. Day, "Factors Influencing Offspring," *American Journal of Diseases of Children,* Vol. 113, No. 2 (February 1967), pp. 179–85.

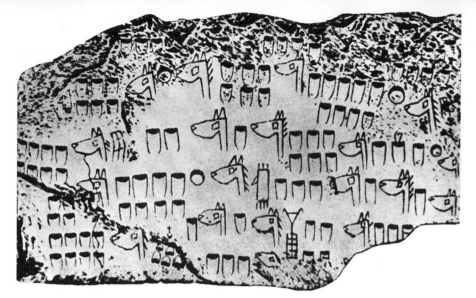

16-15 Heredity: an ancient concern. This 6,000-year-old horse pedigree was unearthed in the Middle East.

their baby. They have been putting it off, but something is wrong. Their family doctor has suggested that they come here.

Such are some of the intensely human problems brought to the genetic counselor. He can help as no one else can. He may discuss risks with those who inquire. In the event a diagnosis of a possible genetic illness is required, more detailed work is necessary. *The International Directory of Genetic Services,* 2nd ed. (September 1969), compiled by Henry T. Lynch, has been published by the National Foundation. It is of great professional value.

From the patient's medical and genetic history, the genetic counselor (usually a physician with special training in genetics) will construct a *pedigree* of the patient going back at least three generations. Detailed information on such matters as spontaneous abortion or previously discovered defects are thus charted. Blood samples provide cells for study. These will be taken from the patient, both parents, and other relatives likely to be carrying an abnormality. To diagnose most defects this is all that is necessary. Usually two to six weeks are required. Other procedures besides blood studies are also helpful. A few cells scraped from the inside of a patient's mouth can help determine the number of X-chromosomes a patient has. Normal females have a dark area called the *Barr body* in these cells. It is absent in the male. The greatest number of Barr bodies in a buccal cell equals the number of patient's X chromosomes minus one. Thus abnormal females with no Barr body have only one X-chromosome and abnormal XXY males have one Barr body. Since bone marrow provides most of the circulating blood cells, it also may provide much valuable information.

At most large medical centers, the diagnosis of Mongolism can be confirmed by a chromosome count (see page 525). Moreover, through the use of special techniques it is possible to discover Mongolism (and other genetic defects) while the child is still in the womb. The developing fetus floats in amniotic fluid. As he grows, he sheds cells into the fluid. Some of these are withdrawn through a needle and examined for chromosomal aberrations. Moreover, physicians at the University of California Medical Center have reported successful prediction that nineteen unborn infants were male through a blood test taken early in pregnancy. Such information may be of value in families with a history of sex-linked diseases.[29]

Pregnancy

The ovum is one of the body's largest cells; the sperm, the smallest. Alone, they are just potential. Together, they can fuse, and the product of their fusion can multiply to form a creature that can wonder. But even in the earliest phases this product is already remarkable. "Every child starts as an invisible unit with a weight of only 5/1000 of a milligram and gains during the first weeks of life more than a million percent in weight. Which industry, whatever direction or planning boards there may be, can claim such an increase in output?"[30]

The duration of a pregnancy

Counting from the time of fertilization of the egg by the sperm (*conception*), the duration of the pregnancy is $9\frac{1}{2}$ lunar months (38 weeks or 266 days). A "lunar" month is 28 days because there is a full moon every 28 days. Counting from the first day of the last menstrual period, the average pregnancy lasts 10 lunar months (40 weeks or 280 days).

In calculating the expected date of confinement (birth), three months are subtracted from the date of the beginning of the last normal menstrual period. Then seven days are added. For example, if the first day of the last normal period was June 17, the expected date of confinement would be March 24.

But these calculations are only based on averages. Perhaps ten percent of all pregnancies end 280 days after the beginning of the last menstrual period; less than half end within one week of the 280th day. The time required for the individual in the uterus is individual. Extreme but normal variances of 240 days to 300 days in the uterus occur. The calculated expected date of confinement is not often exact. There is less than a fifty percent chance that the child will be born within a week of that date and a ten percent chance that labor will occur about two weeks later.

The child within the uterus

Before pregnancy the uterus weighs one ounce. At the end of pregnancy, the empty uterus weighs 2.2 pounds and its capacity has increased more than five hundred times. (A short time after delivery, it returns to almost its original size.) The remarkable events occurring during the development of the child in the uterus are described in the science of embryology—the story of a new individual.

The new individual is the zygote—the fertilized egg. It is unique and no larger than the tiniest sand speck. It does not wait long in the uterine

---

[29]"Big Step in Sex Prediction," *Science News,* Vol. 96, No. 4 (July 26, 1969), p. 76.
[30]G. M. H. Veeneklass, cited in *Physicians Bulletin,* Vol. 24, No. 8 (November 15, 1959), p. B/8.

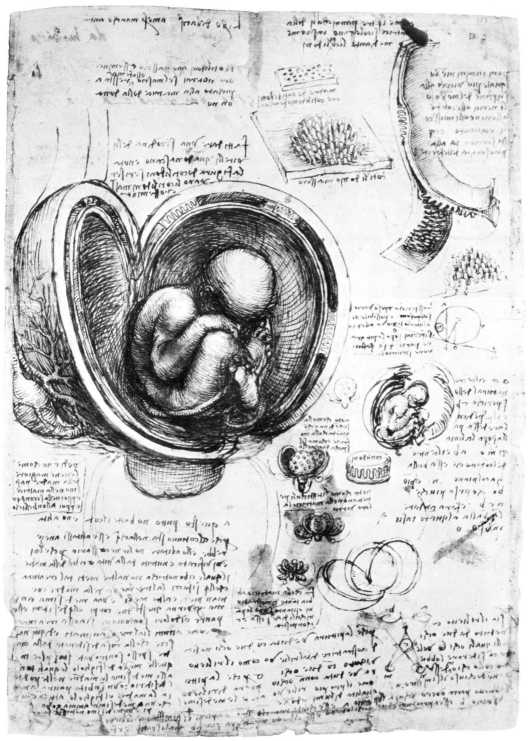

16-16 "Embryo in the Womb" (c. 1510) by Leonardo da Vinci (1452–1519).

tube. While on its two- to four-day, four- to five-inch journey to the uterus, the zygote cleaves daily. When it arrives the uterus is not yet ready for it. About two to four more days pass as the small, continuously multiplying cell mass floats in the uterus. Meanwhile, as described in Chapter 13, the uterine lining continues to prepare for it. At last, as early as day 18 and as late as day 23 of the menstrual cycle and as much as eight days following fertilization, implantation occurs.[31]

When implantation occurs, the cellular mass (called a *blastocyst*) is a fluid-filled sphere of cells. Cell multiplication continues until, on the internal surface of the blastocyst, a layer of cells separates; this is the *entoderm*. It will contribute heavily to such inner body parts as the digestive and respiratory systems. Cells of the outer layer also multiply. These comprise the *ectoderm* destined for outer structures such as the skin, hair, and nervous tissue. A middle layer of cells multiplies to push in between ectoderm and entoderm. This intermediate *mesoderm* will be muscle and bone, marrow and blood, kidney and gonad. These three layers will further differentiate to become the organized human creature. After the first week of development following fertilization, the cell mass is called an *embryo;* the youngest human embryo is about seven and a half days old. Not until the beginning of the third month will the embryo be a *fetus.*

The firm establishment of the new life

But not all of the fertilized egg becomes an embryo. Some is destined to be auxiliary embryonic equipment which will not only protect the embryo but will also provide a means of nourishment, excretion, and respiration. Even in the blastocyst two cell masses differentiate: the *inner cell mass,* which is to become the embryo, and an outer cellular wall, the *trophoblast,* which is the beginning of the auxiliary tissue. (Later in pregnancy the trophoblast is called the *chorion.*) The cells of the trophoblast have the ability to digest or dissolve both the wall of the uterine endometrial lining and the walls of small blood vessels in that area. The multiplying and digesting cells of the trophoblast extend into the endometrium and around them occur slight uterine bleedings. From the little lakes of mother's blood seepages of nutriments feed the growing cellular mass. Via these early maternal blood lakes, then, the mother offers the first food to the parasitic cell mass imbedded in the lining of the uterus. Then the inner layer of the trophoblast grows out to push fingerlike projections into the endometrium. These are the *villi;* their encroaching cells continue to digest the cells of uterine endometrium and small adjacent blood vessels.

Some villi extend not only into the endometrium but also into the maternal lakes in which they float free. Soon the maternal lakes are so crowded by villi that there are now only *intervillous spaces.* It is primarily

---

[31] The American College of Obstetricians and Gynecology considers implantation and conception to be synonymous. The reason for this is that implantation cannot be diagnosed unless conception has occurred.

in these intervillous spaces that the physiological exchanges occur between mother and child during pregnancy. Each mature villus eventually contains fetal blood vessels connected with the circulation of the child.

By a month after fertilization, the inner cell mass that is the embryo is encircled by a *chorionic membrane* and this membrane is surrounded by *chorionic villi.* A fluid-filled sac, or vesicle, has been created. The embryo is attached to the wall of this *chorionic vesicle* by a *body stalk,* which will elongate to become a cable containing blood vessels, the *umbilical cord.* As the last part of the second month of pregnancy approaches, many of the villi on the surface of the chorionic membrane begin to degenerate. Only about twenty percent of the villi remain as the *fetal placenta.* It is apparent that the mother contributes to the placenta and, via her placental arteries, the mother brings oxygen and nourishment to the blood lakes. The placenta is attached to the fetus by the umbilical cord. Within the umbilical cord are two arteries and one vein. Through the arteries waste-laden blood is carried from the fetus to the villi of the placenta. From the villi, these fetal waste products are then lost to the blood lakes. (The mother will take them up into her placental veins and excrete them with her own venous wastes.) At the same time, oxygen and nourishment are taken up into the villi from the blood lakes. The single umbilical vein carries these from the villi of the placenta to the fetus. At no time will there normally be a direct connection between maternal and fetal blood. The fetal circulation of blood in the placenta is a system that is closed to the mother.

Other extraembryonic equipment is also formed. At the age of two weeks the embryo is tucked beneath the surface of the uterine lining. A hollow beneath it will enlarge to a fluid-filled cavity surrounded by a sac called the *amnion.* This sac will be filled with *amniotic fluid;* by the fifth month the fetus is swallowing some amniotic fluid. As long as the fetus remains within this sac in the uterus, it will live the aquatic life of a fish. Also during early development, the extraembryonic membranous *yolk sac* and *allantois* appear. After the second month the yolk sac begins to wither and becomes quite useless, but not until it has contributed to the gut as well as early blood cells and vessels. The allantois becomes the blood vessels in the umbilical cord. It is well to now summarize the functions of the placenta and the amnion.

A versatile temporary organ, the placenta (Figure 16-17) is derived, then, from a fertilized ovum, but the mother contributes too. It serves as a gland, intestine, kidney, lung, sieve, and barrier. Also, the placenta separates two genetically different individuals. When the placenta is by-passed in laboratory animals, the fetus is rejected.[32] This is not unlike the process that occurs when a recipient rejects a transplanted heart. From the maternal side of the placenta, projections branch into the endometrium and into the mother's blood. By osmosis, nutrients from the mother's blood

[32] Joseph Dancis, Symposium on "Homeostasis of the Intrauterine Patient," cited in "The Purpose of the Placenta," *Briefs: Footnotes on Maternity Care,* Vol. 33, No. 4 (April 1969), pp. 54–55.

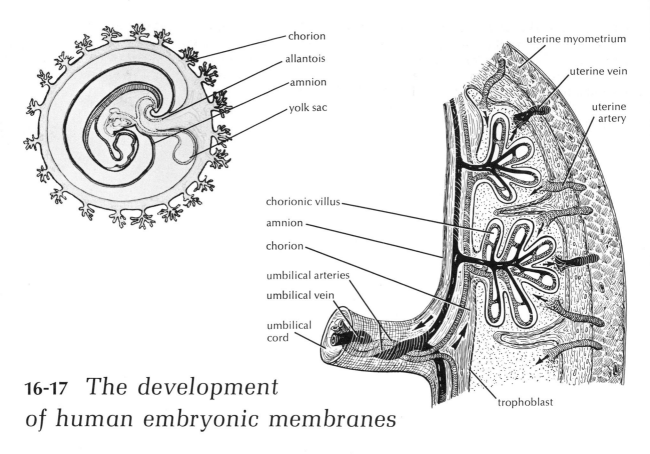

chorion
allantois
amnion
yolk sac

uterine myometrium
uterine vein
uterine artery

chorionic villus
amnion
chorion
umbilical arteries
umbilical vein
umbilical cord

trophoblast

16-17 The development
of human embryonic membranes

Two stages of embryonic development, showing the interrelationship of embryo
and membranes (*top left* and *bottom*) and a cross section of the placenta
(*right*).

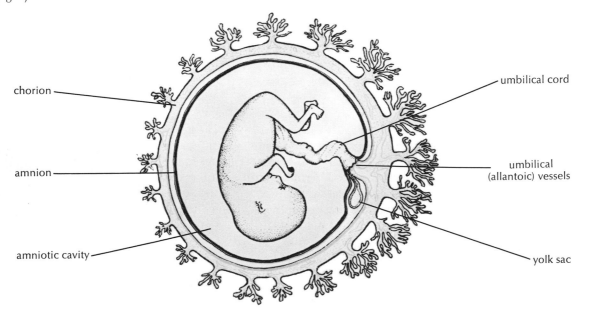

chorion

amnion

amniotic cavity

umbilical cord

umbilical
(allantoic) vessels

yolk sac

ooze through the placenta. In a reverse manner, the child eliminates wastes. Attached to the fetal surface of the placenta is an umbilical cord and fused membranes. Through the cord circulation, exchanges are made to and from the placenta. Together, the membranes form a bag or sac, completely encompassing the child. In the bag are the "waters" or amniotic fluid. Throughout intrauterine life the child is submerged in these waters. Like an astronaut in a space capsule, the fetus within the amniotic sac is in a state of weightlessness. Therefore, the child is able to move about without expenditure of energy that is needed for growth and development. In addition, the fluid protects delicate tissues, provides a stable temperature, and is of some help in the dilatation of the cervix in early labor.[33] It is not true that a baby born in the membranes of the amniotic sac is lucky. Unless unassisted by a doctor, this does not happen. To enable the baby to breathe immediately at birth, the doctor will, if necessary, rupture the membranes.

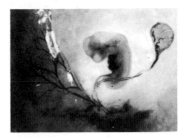

16-18 Human embryo 6 weeks after conception. Note the clear amniotic sac with the yolk sac lying outside it.

The month-by-month changes in the human being during intrauterine residence are now related.

END OF THE FIRST LUNAR MONTH By the end of the first lunar month, the embryo is about one-quarter of an inch long (smaller than a BB shot) and resembles a sea urchin. About one-third of the embryo is the head, which almost touches the tail. The bulging, beating heart propels blood through primitive vessels. From a developing mouth leads a tube that will become the digestive tract. Rudiments of eyes, ears, and nose appear, and buds that will become extremities are all visible. Soon the umbilical cord will develop, not as an outgrowth from the baby's body but from accessory tissue.

END OF THE SECOND LUNAR MONTH Every week the embryo has grown one-fourth of an inch and is now a fetus weighing one-thirtieth of an ounce. Sex organs are apparent, but the sex of the fetus is difficult to determine. The developing brain causes the head to be disproportionately large. Pawlike hands have appeared. The half-closed eyes will soon close completely; they will remain closed until the end of the seventh month. A few muscles are developing and the feet may kick a few times (but much too feebly to be felt by the mother). The tail begins to regress. At the end of two months, almost all the internal organs have begun to develop. The changes now will mostly be related to growth and tissue differentiation.

END OF THE THIRD LUNAR MONTH The three-inch fetus weighs about an ounce but the placenta weighs more. The ears rise to the level of the eyes and the eyelids are fused. Soft nails appear on the stubby fingers and toes. Sex can be distinguished. From rudimentary kidneys, small amounts of urine are excreted into the amniotic fluid. Tooth sockets and buds are apparent. Now the mother's enlarging uterus can be felt below the umbilicus.

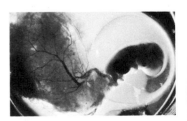

16-19 Human fetus at 10 weeks. Note the persistence of the yolk sac.

[33] Peter J. Huntingford, "The Fetus in Its Aquatic Environment," cited in "Amnion: Protector of the Unborn Baby," *Briefs: Footnotes on Maternity Care*, Vol. 32, No. 9 (November 1968), pp. 131–32.

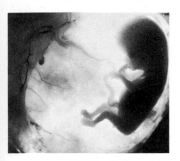

16-20 Fetus at 14 weeks. Note the enlarging amniotic sac.

END OF THE FOURTH LUNAR MONTH   The four-ounce fetus is not quite seven inches long. On the scalp a few hairs may sprout. Soon there will be a fine downy whorl-like growth of hair called *lanugo* covering the whole body. The mother may feel the first subtle movements of the fetus at the end of this period (quickening) but usually these do not occur until the following month.

END OF THE FIFTH LUNAR MONTH   The ten-inch fetus weighs about eight ounces. The heart can be heard through the stethoscope. The baby moves actively. Later in pregnancy movements may become quite vigorous but they do not hurt. Since the lungs are not sufficiently developed, babies born prematurely at this time do not survive; they may live but a few minutes. Many states require legal notification of the delivery of a fetus at this age.

END OF THE SIXTH LUNAR MONTH   Now the fetus weighs a pound and a half and is about a foot long. The fetus is not idle. Sucking an available thumb, swallowing amniotic fluid, exercising developing muscles, even an occasional spasmodic chest movement—these are some activities. Noise will startle the child in the uterus. When the mother rocks, the child may go to sleep. The child's activity may waken the mother. Intrauterine quarters are crowded and some children are more restless than others. The sebaceous glands and cells that are shed from the wrinkled skin combine to provide a protective *vernix caseosa* or "cheesy varnish." At birth this may be an eighth of an inch thick. At the end of this month, the eyelids separate and eyelashes form. If born at this stage, the child is still too undeveloped to survive. The medical literature has recorded the rare case of a thirteen-ounce child born at this age who lived three months.

END OF THE SEVENTH LUNAR MONTH   The two-and-a-half-pound fetus is about fifteen inches long. The eyes are open and the child can appreciate light. The testicles are usually in the scrotum. Fat begins to flatten out a few wrinkles. Every day in the uterus at this stage is vital. A baby born at this time has only a fair chance of survival because the lungs and intestinal canal are incompletely developed.

END OF THE EIGHTH LUNAR MONTH   The fetus now weighs about four pounds and measures some sixteen and a half inches. The bones of the head are soft. The fetus looks like a little old man. If provided with good nursing and medical care, a baby born now has a much better chance of surviving than one born in the previous month.

END OF THE NINTH LUNAR MONTH   The fetus, weighing about six pounds and measuring about nineteen inches, begins to make ready to leave the weightless watery ecosystem within the uterus. As if to prepare for the new environment, the fetus gains half a pound a week and wrinkles now disappear. The fingernails need cutting and the fetus may be born with harmless scratch marks. If born prematurely during this month, the chances for survival are good.

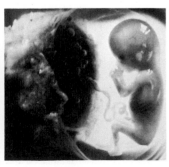

16-21 Fetus at mid-pregnancy.

THE TENTH LUNAR MONTH By about the middle of the tenth lunar month, the full-term twenty-inch fetus is born, weighing about seven pounds (girls) or about seven and one-half pounds (boys). The umbilical cord is about as long as the baby. The placenta weighs about one and one-quarter pounds; it is a disc that is about six to eight inches in diameter. There is from one-half to two quarts of amniotic fluid. Most of the lanugo is gone, although some may remain about the shoulders. The vernix caseosa remains and will need to be wiped away. The hormones that cause the mother's breasts to enlarge cause the unborn child's breasts to protrude a little. The newborn may secrete milk ("witch's milk"). Within a few days after birth, the breast enlargement subsides and there is no further secretion of milk. The final hue of the slate-colored eyes cannot be predicted.

The mother

Some married women, perhaps too long denied, eagerly await a first child. Many others want a baby, but not at the moment. Some will feel a trifle taken in by their pregnancy. Frequently, a first-time mother may need time to accept the idea. She has about three months to do so. During that time, she weighs herself often. But the scales say little. Her pregnancy is not very real. Nothing much changes.

In the second three months, she grows, and not just physically. The emotional preparations may be more profound than the physical ones.

For many a woman, the last three months of pregnancy drag. A dozen discomforts plague her. This ordeal, she thinks, will be capped by still another. She may wish to be rid of her pregnancy. Yet, she may fear its end. She is weary of glossy magazine pictures of overjoyed women hurrying to the hospital without a care in the world. She wishes she could control her urinary bladder better. And she may worry that her husband, too, is tiring of her pregnant condition.

During pregnancy, some women (not all) are somewhat less responsive to sex. Knowing this, the husband will not feel rejected. The sensitive husband will, moreover, understand that his wife's emotional state profoundly affects the pregnancy. It is here that his responsibility is so considerable. As never before, she needs his love, patience, and confidence.

Some changes and rules

A regularly menstruating woman's first, most common sign of pregnancy is a missed menstrual period. The breasts are sensitive. The nipples enlarge and become pigmented. More than half of all pregnant women experience nausea. Vomiting is infrequent. This is not necessarily "morning sickness." It may occur at any time of the day. It may never occur at all. It is much less frequent than formerly. Serious vomiting of pregnancy hardly ever occurs anymore.

Within days after the first missed menstrual period, laboratory tests

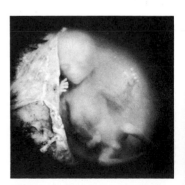

16-22 Fetus approaching viability.

indicating pregnancy are over 95 percent accurate.[34] Following implantation, a hormone is found in the woman's urine. Injection of that urine into immature female mice or rabbits causes ovarian changes. With a male frog, the hormone causes sperm to be released in the urine. Other such biological pregnancy tests are constantly under study. Several nonanimal chemical tests are also being used to diagnose pregnancy. Opinions as to their accuracy vary somewhat. However, they do have the advantage of providing a reading within a matter of hours.

Pregnancy has some cosmetic effects. Skin blemishes abate. The complexion glows. But pink stretch marks (striae) may appear, mostly on the abdomen. Neither massage nor costly oils will prevent them. Most (but not all) will disappear. There is also, temporarily, increased pigment on the abdominal midline, around the nipples, and on the face. The breasts fill. By three months, colostrum, the precursor to milk, is secreted. During pregnancy, an average of twenty pounds is gained. Much of this occurs in the last two months. The pregnant woman who, as a girl, ate intelligently and exercised, and continues these habits under a physician's direction during and after pregnancy, has the best chance of keeping her figure. Walking is good for her. During the first four months, she may, if she likes, play golf. In the first few months, she may be permitted to swim. Some physicians permit swimming in later months. Surf bathing, horseback riding, and tennis are not advisable. Activities that involve bumping and compression are ill-advised. Only absolutely necessary long trips should be made. Nonfatiguing employment is acceptable. In considering the amount and kind of activity that is best for the patient, the physician always considers the individual. Some pregnant women seem able to do more than others. One recent Olympic swimmer was not much handicapped by her three-and-a-half-month pregnancy; she placed third in her class. It has been reported that of the twenty-six female Soviet Olympic champions of the Sixteenth Olympiad, in Melbourne, Australia, ten were pregnant.[35]

Extra rest is essential. Although showers are preferable in the last month, a daily tepid bath adds to comfort. The teeth, although more vulnerable, are not demineralized. "For every pregnancy a tooth" is an untrue old wives' tale. The kidneys need special attention. The doctor will examine the urine often. Constipation may be relieved by fruits and vegetables; prunes, dates, and figs help.

---

[34] Before the days of pregnancy tests "imaginary" or "unconscious" pregnancy was not uncommon. Young brides hoping for a baby or older ladies who worried about having one often developed many of the symptoms of pregnancy without actually being pregnant. At thirty-nine, "Bloody" Queen Mary Stuart was so anxious for a child by her husband Phillip II of Spain that she developed many signs and symptoms including milk-filled breasts. Counting the months, she sewed baby clothes, fitted out a royal cradle, and had announcements made of the birth of her child. Her expected due date was calculated to be between May 23 and June 5, 1555. Surrounding her at Hampton Court were physicians, midwives, and wet nurses who were dismissed when, two months after her expected due date, she failed to deliver. (M.D., Medical Newsmagazine, Vol. 13, No. 3 [March 1969], p. 282.)

[35] Michael Bruser, "Sporting Activities During Pregnancy," cited in "Sports and Pregnancy," Briefs: Footnotes on Maternity Care, Vol. 33, No. 4 (April 1969), pp. 51–53.

In moderation, sexual intercourse is usually (not always) permitted until the last six weeks, to be resumed at about six weeks after delivery. The physician's advice will vary with the individual patient.

Two or three weeks after the first missed period, a doctor should be consulted. This marks the beginning of a relationship that, as much as any other single factor, has made pregnancy so safe. Compared to just a generation ago, decreased maternal (and infant) mortality rates have been spectacular.

Prenatal care

The pregnant woman must visit her doctor regularly. This *prenatal* (before-birth) *care* is essential to her wellbeing. The whole complex of physical examinations, laboratory examinations of the blood (for syphilis, blood types, Rh factor, and anemia), urine tests—all these, and more, create a constancy of communication between patient and doctor that has brought security to mother and child. Problems can be prevented. If trouble threatens, the doctor can then avert it.

Unless special problems arise, visits to the doctor are scheduled every three or four weeks during the first six months. In the next two months, these are usually increased to every two or three weeks. Visits thereafter are usually weekly.

A few days before the onset of true labor, "false labor" may occur. However, it is the onset of regular, rhythmic contractions that heralds true labor. Discomfort, beginning in the lower abdomen, spreads to the back and thighs. The bag of water may break. (A "dry birth" does not prolong labor. Indeed, it may shorten it.) The "show" is another common sign of early labor. This pink vaginal discharge occurs with the onset of cervical dilation. Most first-time mothers may start for the hospital when contractions occur every ten minutes. Others should pay no attention to timing. When contractions are regular, they should go to the hospital. Long before, several reliable ways of transportation should have been arranged.

Labor

The stages of labor

There are three stages of labor (see Table 16-6). The first stage is the longest. The upper part of the uterus contracts. The lower cervix dilates. To allow passage of the infant into the vagina, dilation of the cervix must be complete (four inches). In this stage the baby, assisted by uterine contractions, does the work. Both mother and doctor must await dilation of the cervix and the descent of the baby into the proper position. To minimize possible infection, the pubic hair will have been shaved. To increase the space in the pelvic cavity, an enema may have been given. As the first stage progresses, the uterine contractions become more frequent and of longer duration. When the cervix is fully dilated, the mother is taken from the labor room to the delivery room. If for any reason the child cannot do his job, if he cannot adequately act as a wedge, the doctor will perform a *cesarean section*. By this safe surgical procedure, the infant is removed through an incision in the abdomen and uterus.

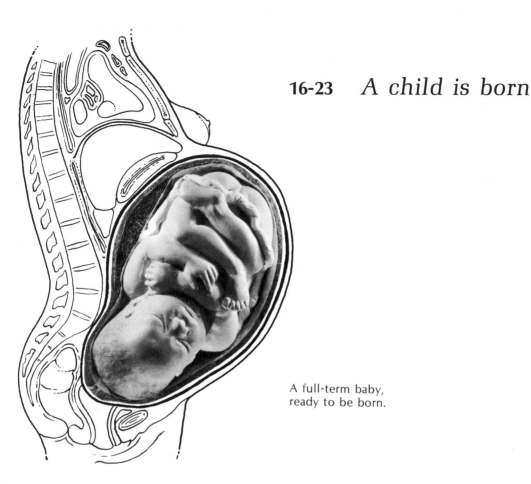

16-23 *A child is born*

A full-term baby,
ready to be born.

		DURATION		WHO DOES THE WORK*
STAGE	TASK	FIRST BABY	SECOND OR LATER BABY	
First stage	Dilation of cervix	8 to 20 hours	3 to 8 hours	Baby
Second stage	Delivery of infant	20 minutes to 2 hours	20 minutes to 2 hours	Mother
Third stage	Delivery of placenta	5 to 20 minutes	5 to 20 minutes	Obstetrician

TABLE 16-6 *Stages of Labor*

*In some cases the physician may decide to do a cesarean section during the first stage or to apply forceps during the second.

Source: Adapted from M. Edward Davis and Reva Rubin, *De Lee's Obstetrics for Nurses,* 18th ed. (Philadelphia, 1966), p. 273.

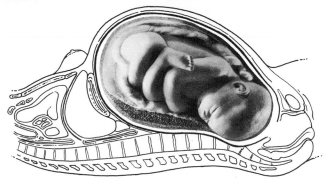

Early first stage. Strong uterine contractions cause the cervix to dilate.

Early second stage. Pains every two minutes; membranes ruptured; cervix completely dilated; head has begun to extend.

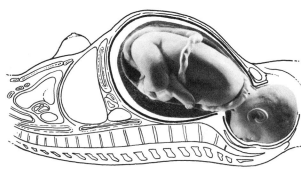

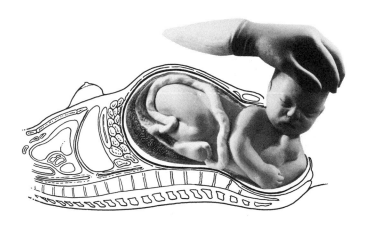

End of second stage. Head is born; shoulders have rotated in birth canal.

Third stage. Uterus expels placenta and cord.

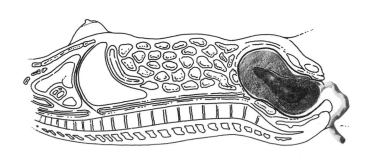

It is in the second stage of labor that the mother works. By bearing down only with each contraction, the mother adds her fifteen pounds of pressure to the twenty-five pounds of the uterine contraction. Very occasionally, for special medical reasons, such as a premature baby, the physician will shorten this stage. For the mother who desires to see her baby born, a mirror can be arranged.

After the birth of the baby, the afterbirth (placenta) is delivered. This is the third stage. A drug is given to further contract the uterus.

About the pain of childbirth

Normal labor pain is as old as humanity. The Bible (Genesis 3:16) reads, "in sorrow thou shalt bring forth children." Surely it is life's briefest and most rewarding sorrow.

The human is the only mammal that has pain with the expulsion of the fetus.[36] Uterine contractions do not hurt. What does hurt is the pressure of the descending baby on lower pelvic structures and the stretching of the cervix. In 1857, Queen Victoria was given the anesthetic chloroform for childbirth. A resultant controversy about the morality of this was largely limited to men. Today, most women expect, and receive, relief from the pain of childbirth. No woman need endure more than she can bear. Today, there are adequate safe pharmaceuticals to control pain.

Dr. Grantly Dick Read correctly taught that ignorance breeds fear and fear impedes labor. Although fear is not responsible for all the pain of childbirth, it can cause much of it. The pregnant woman is not helped by those who exaggerate those pains, which, in any case, vary greatly with the individual. Read's concepts of natural childbirth include education, plus exercise in relaxation and breathing. All this is commendable. Pain may occur. Drugs may be used. For some couples, there is much in favor of natural childbirth. Not only the mother but also the expectant father may derive considerable psychological benefit from the experience.[37] There is a long overdue, growing awareness of the father's opportunities to participate in the birth experience.

Postnatal care Before leaving the hospital the mother is examined. In six to eight weeks she should be examined again. Of particular interest to the physician will be such matters as her weight, blood pressure, the condition of her breasts, uterus, cervix, vagina, and genitalia. He will advise her that the first menstruation may normally be somewhat profuse. Some women are troubled by a vaginal discharge. This is easily treated. The busy mother may forget or defer the examination. This is unwise. She cannot adequately take care of anyone else unless she also takes care of herself.

[36] Dorothy V. Whipple, *Dynamics of Development: Euthenic Pediatrics* (New York, 1966), p. 74.
[37] Deborah Tanzer, "Natural Childbirth: Pain or Peak Experience?" *Psychology Today*, Vol. 2, No. 5 (October 1968), p. 63.

Abortion

A viable fetus is one that has reached such a stage of development that it can live outside the uterus. The premature expulsion from the uterus of a nonviable fetus or an embryo is considered an *abortion*. Abortions are not just *criminal* or *therapeutic* (medically indicated). For a variety of reasons, many occur *spontaneously*. Lay people refer to a spontaneous abortion as a "miscarriage." Ten to fifteen percent of pregnancies end in abortion or miscarriage.

The causes of spontaneous abortions are numerous and sometimes unclear. Maternal illnesses, such as malnourishment, German measles, and possibly influenza, are often causative. Of the traumas that cause abortion, only one in a thousand is nondeliberate.

Indications for therapeutic abortions are diminishing. Heart disease was once a common reason for medical interruption of pregnancy. Heart surgery has changed this; that reason for the interruption of a pregnancy has become less frequent. Nevertheless, chronic hypertension and kidney disease, breast and uterine cancers are considered valid indications by many physicians. Most hospitals have a *therapeutic abortion committee* composed of distinguished medical staff specialists. They review each case. Their decision is final. Therapeutic abortions are not done in Catholic hospitals.

Only a generation ago, abortion, like contraception, was rarely discussed in public. There are ample reasons for this change. (1) *The sheer number of abortions* makes the procedure a major concern. Throughout the world, every year, some twenty-five million legal and illegal abortions are performed. Illegal abortions are the major cause of maternal deaths. In Latin America half of all pregnancies end in illegal abortions. The resultant cost of mothers' lives is a shocking tragedy. It is fully four times greater than in countries in which abortions are legal. In the United States, the estimated one million abortions a year result in over ten thousand maternal deaths. For countless women, infection, the most common complication of illegal abortions, results in sterility. The criminal abortionist is often an incompetent, operating in atrociously unsanitary conditions. (2) *Medical knowledge now warns of possible abnormal babies.* Maternal infection with German measles (rubella) virus in the first trimester, for example, results in a high percentage (20 percent) of abnormal babies. Such information has stimulated interest in legal abortion. (3) *The failure of contraception in overpopulated countries* has brought about a reevaluation of abortion. (4) Some think present *abortion laws* penalize the poor, are unenforceable, and are less applicable to married than to unmarried women[38]—these impressions have added to the widespread discussion. Moreover, limited objective studies so far indicate that "there was little new psychiatric illness that appeared after therapeutic abortion that could

[38] *M.D., Medical Newsmagazine*, Vol. 12, No. 2 (February 1968), p. 105.

be related to the abortion."[39] As a result of such considerations, new state legislation has been passed.

In 1962, a model law, proposed by the American Law Institute, allowed therapeutic abortion to (1) save the life or health of the mother, (2) prevent the birth of a deformed or mentally deficient child, or (3) prevent the birth of a child conceived as a result of rape or incest. In June 1967, the American Medical Association Committee on Human Reproduction approved of these. However, they added two more prerequisites: two consulting doctors were to approve the abortion and, if agreed upon, the abortion was to be performed in an approved hospital.[40] A majority, though not all, of U.S. physicians agree. Based on the model law of the Law Institute, some liberalizing state legislation has been passed. Colorado was one of the states that passed such a law. During the first year of operation of the law there was an eightfold increase in the legal abortions in the state. Only 32 percent were from out-of-state. Of the 407 women who were aborted in the first year, only 138 were married; 12.7 percent were under sixteen; one-third were between sixteen and twenty-one. Seventy-two percent of the abortions were done for psychiatric reasons. Forty-six percent of the legal terminations of pregnancy were performed on patients with a family income of less than $6,000 yearly.[41]

Numerous ethical and theological problems arise when fallible men attempt to define indications for abortion. One of these is the scientific limitation in predicting abnormal births. Another lies in the variable interpretation of "health" of the mother. The family of a poor woman would suffer more, perhaps, with the addition of another child. Her health might thus be adversely affected. Should she be more eligible for abortion than the wealthy woman? Complicating the issue even more is the present gulf between some scientists and some theologians.

"Life is a continuum," the scientists say;

it has evolved and survived over billions of years by the provision of fantastic margins of safety in terms of excess sperms and ova; the particular conjunction of sperm and ovum that leads to conception is not a unique event but is rather a matter of chance, the development of the individual from conception to full humanity is an unbroken process—who is to say when "life" began?[42]

Opponents of abortion place a sacred and infinite value on each separate beginning, on each potential life. Many consider that this value must be protected even beyond the mother's life. Threats to this concept, such

---

[39] R. Bruce Sloane, "The Unwanted Pregnancy," *New England Journal of Medicine*, Vol. 280, No. 22 (May 29, 1969), p. 1209.

[40] "AMA Policy on Therapeutic Abortion," *Journal of the American Medical Association*, Vol. 201, No. 7 (August 14, 1967), p. 544.

[41] William Droegemueller, Stewart E. Taylor, and Vera E. Drose, "The First Year of Experience in Colorado with the New Abortion Law," cited in "The First Year of the 'Modernized' Colorado Abortion Law," *Briefs: Footnotes on Maternity Care*, Vol. 33, No. 5 (May 1969), pp. 67–69.

[42] "Abortion and the Doctor," *Annals of Internal Medicine*, Vol. 67, No. 5 (November 1967), pp. 1111–13.

as selfishness, irresponsibility, and sexual promiscuity, are especially condemned.

Both theologians and scientists revere life. To the responsible, both concepts surely have much to offer. Abortion laws, meticulously respectful of every human being's conscience, are now being considered.

Subfertility

Among the married, the threat of childlessness often begins with suspicion, which may grow to anxious doubt, and end in sad resignation. Fully 20 to 25 percent of couples in this country fail to have as many children as they wish. Only 10 percent seek adequate help.

In this culture, many people incorrectly consider subfertility[43] to be primarily a fault within the woman. In the Bible, it is the sterile woman who is regarded with pity, if not scorn. The "adversary" of Hannah "provoked her sore, for to make her fret, because the Lord had shut up her womb" (I Samuel 1:6). Of course, the problem occurs just as often within men.

The cause of subfertility may be easily discovered or it may require a long investigation. Sometimes it will be necessary to consult various medical specialists.

Severe nutritional deficiencies have been known to cause reduced fertility. Both ovulation and menstruation may be impaired in this way. Alcoholism, drug dependence, chronic infections—all may contribute to a subfertile marriage. Physical problems may range all the way from excess obesity of both marital partners (interfering with actual consummation of the marriage) to an occluded uterine tube. Malfunction of the uterine tube accounts for no less than 25 percent of all cases of subfertility. A kinked tube, or one blocked as a result of an infection, may be unable to receive the ovum and permit its passage to the uterus. Or it may stop the sperm's ascent to the ovum.

Emotional problems may impede conception. A young wife, forced to live with an interfering mother-in-law, may learn to bide her time. But, while she is biding her time, her vagina, uterus and tubes tense. She may be unable to conceive. Moving to her own apartment might cure her. Spasm of the vagina and tubes may disappear. The quality of her cervical mucus improves and becomes more receptive of her husband's sperm. She will then more likely conceive.

How long should it take before a normal couple may expect conception? Usually six months of ordinary cohabitation results in pregnancy. If conception does not occur within a year of marriage, the couple would do well to seek the advice of the family doctor.

Psychological factors account for perhaps a quarter of subfertility cases.

---

[43] *Subfertility* refers to a state of being less than normally fertile. It is relative sterility. *Sterility* refers to the inability to conceive or to induce conception.

A prolonged sense of guilt over a previous sexual misfortune, such as a venereal infection, combined with lack of knowledge, has resulted not only in subfertility but in serious marital problems. The erroneous idea "V.D. germs kill sperms" has, at times, been eradicated by showing a young husband his own sperm darting about under the microscope. Too many girls, subjected to exaggerated and lurid stories by "well-meaning" mothers and acquaintances fear both intercourse and childbearing. Resultant tensions may well interfere with fertility. Knowledge of the reassuring facts about both will help her. The husband who is sensitive to his wife's sexual needs will enrich his marriage. He is also more likely to enhance her fertility.

The physician will usually first investigate the man, since the cause can often be more easily established in the male. After a thorough physical examination, there are several tests to be done. Spermatozoa will be examined for numbers, motility, appearance, and other features.

The search for the cause of female subfertility is usually more complex. It may be a persistent, simply treated, vaginal inflammation. Or the physician may find that his patient encourages intercourse but once every month or two and then without attending to her ovulation cycle. Some physicians feel that *coitus interruptus* (see Table 16-7) establishes a reflex that results in withdrawal just before male ejaculation. The causes of a woman's inability to conceive may be multiple and complex, and patience is needed in investigating them. Only with the discovery of the cause of the problem may rational approach to its solution be made.

Adoption

The ancient Greeks and Romans adopted children to assure continuance of the family line, thereby protecting property. The child was secondary. Today, he is primary. He needs a secure home and love. The adopting parents must be able to give both.

The depth of relationship between adopted child and parents is no less profound than that with the biological parents. The risk is mutual.

Every year over a hundred thousand legal adoptions occur in this country. One half are by persons unrelated to the child. Most children placed in nonrelated homes are illegitimate. Unfortunately, many an unmarried mother is unaware of the strict privacy available at social welfare agencies. Her child is then placed through a "black market" agency. In this way, she disadvantages both herself and her child. There is yet another problem. Twice as many nonwhite children are illegitimate than white. Yet, most adopted children are white.

A couple considering adoption should seek help from the social welfare agency in their community. They will further profit from conferences with the family attorney and physician.

Contraception

Birth control is not a modern development of a civilized society. Primitive societies limit population in various ways. Although less common than formerly, *infanticide* still occurs. Some African tribes practice *coitus interruptus* (coitus in which the penis is withdrawn from the vagina before ejaculation). The primitive Achinese of Sumatra use a vaginal suppository containing tannic acid. This primitive group has hit upon a valid scientific principle; tannic acid is an effective spermicide.[44]

Ancient writings are replete with instructions on birth control. In the Petri papyrus (1850 B.C.), crocodile dung is recommended. Twenty-seven hundred years later, the Arabian physician Qusta ibn Tuqa substituted elephant dung for that of the crocodile. Few if any prescriptions, contraceptive or otherwise, persisted for as many years as did dung.[45]

Coitus interruptus is described in the Bible (Genesis 38:9). It was practiced by the ancient Hebrews. Infanticide is also mentioned in the Bible.[46] It was condemned by Jew and Christian alike.[47]

The views of St. Thomas Aquinas have been vastly influential. In the *Summa Theologica,* he wrote: "In so far as the generation of offspring is impeded, it is a vice against nature which happens in every carnal act from which generation cannot follow."

An Englishman, Francis Place (1771–1854), was the first to attempt mass education concerning contraception. Place was followed by many disciples, but none is better known than Margaret Sanger. As a nurse among the poor of the lower East Side of New York, she had been moved by the poverty of large families. She became an ardent worker for contraception. Her first contraceptive advice station in Brooklyn, in 1916, and her constant brushes with the law[48] testify to her militance. When she died, some years ago, she was widely mourned.

Table 16-7 presents the most common contraceptive devices available today. Oral contraceptives merit special discussion. Recent research indicates that oral contraceptives increase the risk of disturbances of the blood coagulation mechanism. Clots, apparently due to oral contraceptives, can obstruct vital body blood vessels. Rarely, this results in death. For example, the pulmonary (lung) artery, or one of its branches, may be plugged. In one major study,[49] death from pulmonary embolism occurred in fifteen

---

[44] Norman E. Himes, *Medical History of Contraception* (Baltimore, 1936), p. 63.

[45] *Ibid.*

[46] See, for example, Ezekiel 16:21; Leviticus 18:21; Deuteronomy 12:31; II Kings 3:27, 16:3; II Chronicles 28:3, 33:6; Psalms 106:38; Isaiah 57:5; Jeremiah 19:5.

[47] In China's first official document against infanticide, in 1659, Choen Tche (1633–62) wrote: "I have heard that the sad cry uttered by these girl babies as they plunged into a vase of water and drowned is inexpressible. Alas! that the heart of a father or mother should be so cruel." (Fielding H. Garrison, "History of Pediatrics," in Arthur Frederick Abt and Fielding H. Garrison, *History of Pediatrics* (Philadelphia, 1965), p. 3.

[48] In 1915, she was jailed in New York for trying to distribute her pamphlet *Family Limitation.*

[49] W. H. M. Inman and M. P. Vessey, "Investigation of Deaths from Pulmonary, Coronary, and Cerebral Thrombosis and Embolism in Women of Child-bearing Age," *British Medical Journal,* Vol. 2 (April 27, 1968), p. 193.

TABLE 16-7 A Summary of Contraceptive Methods

METHOD	WHAT IT IS AND HOW IT WORKS	EFFECTIVENESS AND ACCEPTABILITY
Cervical cap	Small deep cup placed directly over cervix to block sperm from entering uterus. Used with contraceptive cream or jelly. Must be fitted by physician.	Used very little in this country. Among women who can use them, effectiveness is about the same as for diaphragm.
Chemical methods	Products inserted into vagina. Purpose is to coat vaginal surfaces and cervical opening, and to destroy sperm cells; may act as mechanical barrier as well. Provide protection for about an hour.	The effectiveness of chemical contraceptives used alone is believed to be lower than the effectiveness of the chemical preparations used in combination with a diaphragm or a condom. Nevertheless, significant reductions in pregnancy rates may be obtained by the use of these simple methods.
Vaginal foams	Cream packed under pressure (like foam shaving cream); inserted with applicator.	
Vaginal jellies and creams	Inserted into vagina with applicator.	
Vaginal suppositories	Small cone-shaped objects that melt in vagina. Must be inserted in sufficient time to melt before the sex act.	
Vaginal tablets	Moistened slightly and inserted into vagina; foam is produced. Must be inserted in sufficient time for tablet to disintegrate before the sex act.	
Coitus interruptus (withdrawal)	Man withdraws sex organ from woman's vagina before emission of semen. Requires that husband practice great self-control. Even then, some sperm may escape before the climax.	Coitus interruptus has been responsible for many failures in family planning probably because semen may be deposited without the man being aware of it. However, statistical studies have also shown coitus interruptus to be relatively effective. This is the principal method by which the decline of the birth rate in western Europe was achieved from the late 18th century onward. This method is unacceptable to a large number of couples because it may limit sexual gratification of the husband or wife or both.
Condom	Thin, strong sheath or cover, made of rubber or similar material, worn by husband to prevent sperm from entering vagina. (Wife may also use a vaginal foam, cream, or jelly to provide added protection.)	Offers a high degree of protection if husband will use it correctly and consistently. Some couples find the use of condoms objectionable. Failures are due to tearing of the sheath or its slipping off after climax. The condom rates in effectiveness with the diaphragm.

Table 16-7 Continued

METHOD	WHAT IT IS AND HOW IT WORKS	EFFECTIVENESS AND ACCEPTABILITY
Diaphragm	Flexible hemispherical rubber dome used in combination with cream or jelly; woman inserts into vagina to cover cervix, providing barrier to sperm. Must be left in place at least six hours after intercourse and may be left in place as long as twenty-four hours. Must be fitted by physician; refitted every 2 years and after each pregnancy.	Offers a high level of protection although occasional method failures may be expected because of improper insertion or displacement of the diaphragm during sex relations. A rate of 2 to 3 pregnancies per 100 women per year would seem to be a generous estimate for consistent users. If motivation is weak, much higher pregnancy rates must be expected. Many women use the diaphragm successfully. Others have difficulty inserting it correctly, or dislike the procedure required.
Douche	Flushing of vagina immediately after intercourse to remove or destroy sperm.	A poor method of contraception because sperm enter the cervical canal within 90 seconds after ejaculation. Statistical studies have confirmed this low level of effectiveness.
Intrauterine devices	Small objects (loops, spirals, rings) made of plastic or stainless steel; inserted into uterus by physician. May be left in place indefinitely. How the devices prevent pregnancy is not completely understood. They do not prevent the ovary from releasing eggs. The evidence suggests they probably speed descent of the egg so that the sperm cannot fertilize it, or the egg may reach the uterus at a time when it cannot nest there.	These devices do not require continued attention on the part of the user. Some women who try the devices cannot use them satisfactorily because of expulsion, bleeding, or discomfort. The level of protection offered is probably not greater than with such "traditional" methods as the diaphragm or condom if these methods are used with perfect regularity. Intrauterine devices are less effective than the pill when the latter is used according to direction.
Oral contraceptive (the pill)	The synthetic hormones contained in oral contraceptives (estrogens and progestins) inhibit ovulation, mimicking the actions of the body's own estrogen and progesterone. When no egg is released from an ovary, a woman cannot become pregnant. The pills are usually taken for 20 or 21 consecutive days in each menstrual cycle.	Except for total abstinence or surgical sterilization, the combination pill is the most effective contraceptive known. Approximately one-third of women experience one or more commonly observed side effects during the first cycle or two of use. These side effects (nausea or other gastrointestinal distress; spotting or "unexpected" breakthrough bleeding; breast tenderness, enlargement or secretion; weight gain) are usually quite mild and transient, and tend to diminish sharply in incidence and severity or disappear completely after the first cycles.

Table 16-7 Continued

METHOD	WHAT IT IS AND HOW IT WORKS	EFFECTIVENESS AND ACCEPTABILITY
Rhythm	Depends on abstinence from intercourse during time of month when woman is fertile. Due to menstrual irregularity in many women and inability to accurately determine time of egg release, success with the method may require abstinence for as long as half the month.	Correctly taught, correctly understood, and correctly practiced, the effectiveness of the rhythm method in women with regular menstrual cycles may approach that of mechanical and chemical contraceptives. However, such successful use implies periods of abstinence longer than many couples find acceptable. Self-taught "rhythm," haphazardly practiced, is one of the most ineffective methods of family planning. While some couples have successfully worked out this system for themselves, most will require assistance from a doctor or rhythm clinic.
Sponge and foam	Spermicidal powder or fluid is placed on small moistened sponge, which is squeezed to develop a foam; sponge is placed in vagina. Must remain in place 6 hours after intercourse.	Used successfully by some women. Bulkiness of sponge and drainage from vagina sometimes objectionable to husband or wife.

Source: Adapted from "A Summary of Contraceptive Methods," G. D. Searle & Co.

women who took oral contraceptives. For that age, this was four times the expected number.[50] Although the death risk from oral contraceptives is even less than the extremely low death rate from pregnancy, further investigation of their safety is indicated. Extensive studies are today being conducted on any possible relationship between oral contraceptives and stroke, cancer, high blood pressure, and atherosclerosis. So far results are certainly inconclusive. Oral contraceptives should never be taken without medical supervision.

Long-acting contraceptives are being researched. A single monthly injection of a contraceptive agent is promising.[51] By midsummer of 1968, "a long-acting contraceptive administered to women by injection once every three months . . . proved effective during three years of clinical

[50] Other investigators reported that "in the absence of other predisposing causes the risk of developing deep vein thrombosis, pulmonary embolism, or cerebral thrombosis is increased about eight times by the use of oral contraceptives, while the risk of developing coronary thrombosis is apparently unchanged." (R. Doll, cited in *Second Report of the Advisory Committee on Obstetrics and Gynecology*, Food and Drug Administration [August 1, 1969], Chairman's Summary, Louis M. Hellman, M.D.) Despite the absence of comparable U.S. data, the Food and Drug Administration has ordered labeling changes that warn of these possibilities. By early 1969, twenty different preparations of oral contraceptive were being used by millions of women in this country.

[51] "The Long-Acting Contraceptives: Quarterly Injections Pass Three-Year Trials," *Journal of the American Medical Association*, Vol. 204, No. 11 (June 10, 1968), p. 35.

trial."[52] Under investigation is a capsule that, once inserted under the skin, slowly releases birth-controlling medication. Other studies are concerned with "morning-after" drugs. These may be effective in ending pregnancy when taken as late as five days after intercourse, perhaps even a month afterwards. A new device being tested is a vaginal ring made of rubber or Silastic. Inserted by the woman at the end of the menstrual period, the ring releases the hormone progestin (also used in oral contraceptives). A much smaller amount is absorbed from the ring by the body than is taken orally. A steady concentration of hormone is maintained in the blood. The ring is left in the vagina for three weeks and then is thrown away. Male contraceptive drugs are also being studied. Although their development is, at present, slow, they will doubtless become available.

[52] Arturo Esquivel and Leonard E. Laufe, "Contraception Control by a Single Monthly Injection," *Obstetrics and Gynecology*, Vol. 31, No. 5 (May 1968), pp. 634–36.

17

The last chapter: health for the freeman

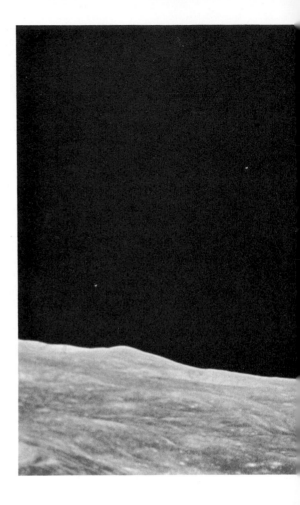

In health there is freedom. Health is the first of all liberties.[1]

Modern miracles

Engineers join the health team

In a San Francisco hospital, a young patient intently watches a television screen. Beside him sits his psychiatrist. There is a close-up of hands gesticulating jerkily, then of eyes, troubled and suspicious. The camera

[1]Henri Frédéric Amiel, quoted in *M.D., Medical Newsmagazine,* Vol. 7, No. 4 (April 1963), p. 109. In his *Journal,* the Swiss philosopher wrote on Easter Monday, April 14, 1879: "Sickness makes one dependent . . . sickness is a blow to our freedom and our dignity." (*The Private Journal of Henri Frédéric Amiel,* tr. by Van Wyck Brooks and Charles Wyck Brooks [New York, 1935], p. 569.)

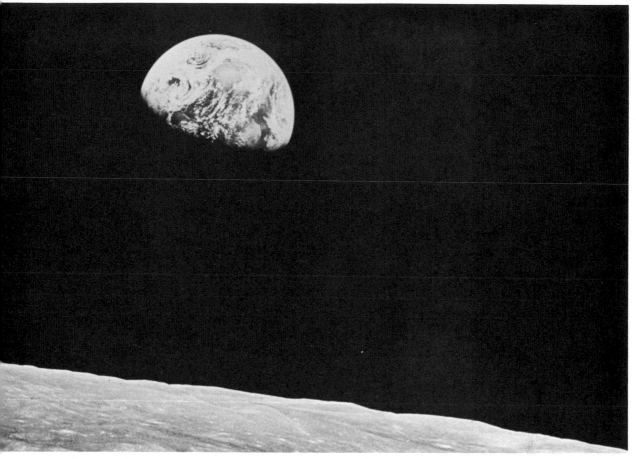

A view from another ecosystem: earth seen from the moon (an Apollo 8 photograph).

lengthens the shot and includes the entire figure of the main character. Almost oblivious to other people seated in the room about him, he talks incessantly. Slowly, the camera picks up the expressions of the silent onlookers. The patient watches, absorbed. For it is he who is the main character. Only a few moments before he was in the waiting room. Instant replay television is showing him himself.

After two centuries the wish of an eighteenth-century poet becomes reality:

> Oh wad some power the giftie gie us
> To see oursels as others see us!
> It wad frae monie a blunder free us.[2]

[2] Robert Burns, "To a Louse."

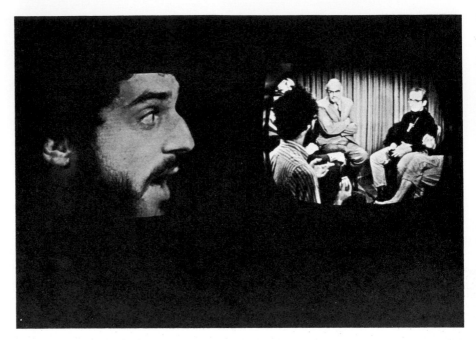

17-1 Videotape in psychotherapy. Two TV monitors placed side by side simultaneously record a close-up of a patient talking and a group shot showing the reactions of those around him.

Uninvolved, the electronic device has involved the patient. And yet the patient sees himself apart from himself and as others see him. He confronts himself. Perhaps now, with his view uncluttered, he will improve.[3]

Four hundred miles to the south, in Los Angeles, a medical specialist ponders a patient's heart problem. To improve the heart muscle tone, to strengthen the heart's action, the drug digitalis has been prescribed. But digitalis tends to accumulate in body tissues. Now the patient complains of a loss of appetite—one sign of early digitalis intoxication. Of critical importance is how well the kidneys function. Impaired kidney function means diminished digitalis excretion. Consequently, within the body, the drug rises to poisonous levels.

Carefully, the internist reviews the patient's chart. Finally, he telephones the University of California at Los Angeles Medical Center. He tells a fellow physician there about the type of digitalis used and results of the patient's kidney function tests. The information is fed into a computer. Previously, the machine had been programmed to receive and correlate such information. Within moments it has computed the ability of this particular patient's pair of kidneys to eliminate this particular kind of digitalis. Then it tells how much digitalis accumulates in his body. From this information the doctor decides the best level of digitalis for the patient. "The computer then prints a suggested dose program, tailored to the patient's kidney function, to achieve and maintain that level."[4]

---

[3]Harry A. Wilmer, "Innovative Uses of Videotape on a Psychiatric Ward," cited in "Videotaping in Psychiatric Evaluation," *Modern Medicine*, Vol. 36, No. 23 (November 4, 1968), p. 88.
[4]"Clicking Clinicians," *M.D., Medical Newsmagazine*, Vol. 12, No. 11 (November 1968), p. 91.

The marriage of medicine and engineering has produced a variety of useful offspring. Surgery, television, computer—all combine to bring lifesaving emergency care. In a Swedish hospital a man's cancerous lung is removed. In his recovery room is an input terminal. Via the input terminal, the nurse promptly feeds vital information—temperature, blood pressure, laboratory test results—into a computer. In the doctor's office, or his home, there is an output terminal, which is connected to a television screen. The doctor receives information immediately. Perhaps a laboratory test indicates that a certain medication might help the patient. Into his computer connection the doctor feeds certain specific information. From it he expects an organized answer. "What," for example, he may ask, "is the hospital experience with this new drug?" Within moments the answer is formulated on his screen. From his office he relays instructions to the hospital room. In an emergency, time is the enemy. Computers speed accurate help to the sick.[5]

From all these innovations a new and urgent discipline has developed —*biomedical engineering*. Just as there are engineering systems, there are also biological systems. The diffusion of a fluid, for example, through a semipermeable membrane resulting in pressure equalization on both sides is *osmosis*. That basic bioengineering fact is being put to good experimental use. By osmosis some anesthetics may seep through tubes into the blood. Many patients will eventually receive anesthetics in this way. Pain relief without sleep is a possibility.[6] Body repair will be easier. And miraculous, too. Consider this case.

The date: April 10, 1965. Near Denver, a twenty-one-month-old girl is picked from a car-train wreck. She is still conscious. Her entire left arm is severed. A state patrolman looks for the arm and finds it alongside a railway track. In twenty minutes both the child and her amputated arm are at the University of Colorado Medical Center. With deliberate speed surgeons work to replant the arm. Much later they will report, "Recirculation of the extremity was instituted 4 hours and fifty minutes after the accident and resulted in return of color to the arm," and, in eighteen months, the little patient "would use her left hand to . . . comb a doll's hair."[7]

Replanting, replacing, repairing

It was not the first successful replantation of a human arm. That had been accomplished in 1962. But five years later an even more startling surgical first was performed.

A team of Cape Town surgeons had completed a singularly taxing operation. While relaxing with a postoperative cup of tea one of them said,

"Perhaps we should tell someone what we've done."

[5]A. Marcus, "The Computer Comes to the Patient's Bedside," *World Health* (August 1968), pp. 8–15.
[6]"Engineering the Body," *Science News*, Vol. 94, No. 20 (November 16, 1968), p. 493.
[7]Jens G. Rosenkrantz, Robert G. Sullivan, Keasley Welch, James S. Miles, Keith M. Sadler, and Bruce C. Paton, "Replantation of an Infant's Arm," *New England Journal of Medicine*, Vol. 277, No. 11 (March 16, 1967), pp. 609–11. Before the accident the little girl's mother considered her to be left-handed.

It was agreed to tell the hospital superintendent.

"Was it on a dog?" the superintendent asked.

"No, on a human," was the reply.[8]

Thus did Christiaan Barnard announce the first heart transplant. Throughout the world physicians soon read about it in this brief scientific reference:

Barnard, C. N.: A Human Cardiac Transplant: An Interim Report of a Successful Operation Performed at Grotte Schuur Hospital, Cape Town, S. Afr. Med. J., 41:1271–74 (Dec. 30) 1967.

Today's success is tomorrow's commonplace. Artificial heart valves and portions of blood vessels have brought a healthier life to scores of the otherwise disabled. Figure 17-2 shows an aneurysm of the abdominal aorta and a Dacron graft that has replaced and taken over the work of the damaged segment. Those photographs were taken at Baylor Univer-

17-2 An aneurysm of the abdominal aorta (*left*) and a Dacron graft (*right*), which has replaced portions of the abdominal aorta (the large tube), the iliac arteries (the bottom branches), and the renal arteries (the top branches). An aneurysm is the sac formed by abnormal dilation of the weakened wall of a blood-filled blood vessel. The wall is impaired by disease, such as advanced atherosclerosis or syphilis.

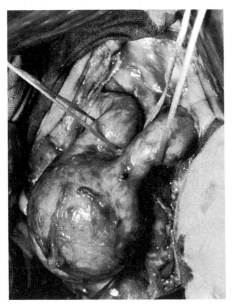
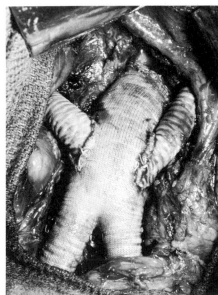

sity, where, too, an artificial heart pump temporarily assumes the vital function of an ailing, failing heart. The exhausted organ rests and heals. Then the artificial pump is removed. In a few weeks the rescued patient goes home, his lease on life renewed. At times another technique may be indicated. To control an erratic heart, a pacemaker may need to be inserted beneath the skin. Its impulses bring regularity to the heart beat, life to its beneficiary. Every four or five years, batteries for the electric pacemaker have to be replaced. Recently a new radioisotope battery was

[8]*Medical Tribune,* Vol. 10, No. 68 (August 25, 1969), p. 2.

developed. For a decade or more this battery—a small nuclear power plant—may safely generate electrical impulses. Still another electrical unit, worn by the selected heart patient, brings relief from the suffocating pain of angina pectoris.[9] When he feels the impending attack, the patient presses a button. Electrical stimulation of certain nerves brings almost instant relief. Nor have the possibilities of electrical stimulation been neglected elsewhere. Several physicans recently reported the successful use of electrical brain stimulation to relieve the pain of an inoperable cancer. In one such patient, electrodes were inserted in precisely selected brain areas.

> *We . . . constructed for him a small battery powered stimulator which could be carried in his shirt pocket and connected to his electrodes at will . . . He became quite dependent on this stimulation, felt it an important aspect of this alleviation of both his pain and to some extent his subjective suffering and used it as the primary control rather than drugs for about the last six weeks before his death from carcinoma.*[10]

The patient "described the subjective effects of stimulation as being like 'two martinis.' "

Does this remarkable surgical event threaten to produce an electrically controlled society? How is the electrical threat related to the drug threat? Creating, if not answering, such basic societal enigmas, the scientific quest for new knowledge continues. Kidney transplants? They are almost common. So are artificial kidneys. In this country some eighteen hundred people depend on them to survive.

Triumphs vie with one another. Perhaps the greatest are occurring in the laboratories of the molecular biologist.

In the laboratories of the world, men have been learning about DNA and RNA. In 1961, at the National Institutes of Health, Marshall Nirenberg learned to read the code, the message that DNA sends to RNA. It is the RNA, carrying the DNA instruction, that prescribes new protein manufacture at the ribosomes in cellular cytoplasm (see Chapter 16, p. 527). Limitless possibilities tantalize the inquisitive scientists. Will they not someday make genetic materials, which are, after all, only complex chemical compounds? Will it not then be possible to manipulate DNA and to modify living cells? Perhaps chromosomal error can then be corrected before it warps cellular harmony. Or the malignant messages of cancer DNA may be thwarted and replaced by man-made DNA. However, scientists issue a warning: "When man becomes capable of instructing

**"For nothing is secret, that shall not be made manifest"
(Luke 8:17)**

---

[9] Angina pectoris is the pain in the chest, accompanied by a feeling of suffocation, due to a lack of blood supply (and therfore oxygen) to the heart muscle (see Chapter 8).

[10] "Striatal Influence on Facial Pain," cited in Donald B. Louria, "Some Aspects of the Current Drug Scene," *Pediatrics,* Vol. 42, No. 6 (December 1968), pp. 904–11.

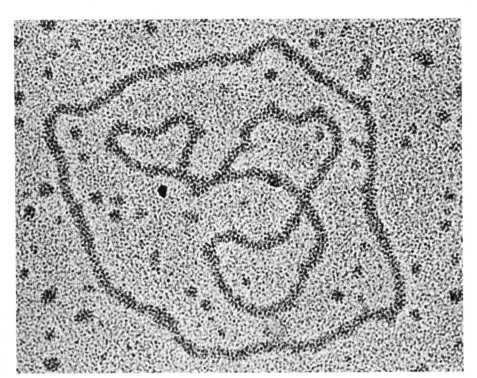

17-3 This biologically active DNA virus was synthesized from inert test-tube chemicals.

his own cells, he must refrain from doing so until he has sufficient wisdom to use his knowledge for the benefit of mankind." [11]

At Stanford University researchers labored to create an artificial DNA —the code-containing genetic instructor of the cell. It might be done by making a DNA virus. In the laboratories at the University of Illinois, biologically active RNA virus had already been synthesized. Magnificent as this accomplishment was, the synthesis of DNA virus would overshadow it because RNA genes occur in a limited group of specialized cells, while DNA genes are found in many known viruses and living cells.

On December 15, 1967, the Stanford scientists made a startling announcement: after eleven years of work, they had succeeded in producing biologically active DNA from inert chemicals (see Figure 17-3). This DNA was, indeed, the genetic material, the inner core, of a virus. And, like the genetic material of ordinary natural virus, the synthetic DNA infected cells and caused them to participate in making more DNA virus. Some scientists do not consider viruses living particles. Viruses cannot reproduce themselves. To reproduce they depend on living cells. But one of the manifestations of virus existence is the ability to infect. Another is the capacity to seduce cells into helping make more virus. These criteria the Stanford University laboratory-created virus met. A long step had been taken toward creating life in the test tube.

[11]"Nobel Prizes in Medicine. Geneticists Rewarded," *Science News,* Vol. 94, No. 17 (October 26, 1968), p. 411.

Scientists are edging toward realities undreamed of a generation ago. The following experiment has been performed:[12] Using a powerful microscope and minute surgical tools, the nucleus is extracted from a skin cell of a frog. With ultraviolet radiation the nucleus in an unfertilized egg of a second frog is destroyed. The naked nucleus from the first frog's skin cell is transplanted into the denucleated frog egg. Originally the unfertilized frog egg had had only half the number of chromosomes as the skin cell nucleus now residing in it. Now containing a full set of chromosomes, the egg is tricked. The transplanted skin cell nucleus causes the frog egg to behave as if it had been fertilized. The result: from the egg develops a new frog that is exactly like the frog whose skin nucleus was transplanted. No sperm was necessary.

Such work with higher animals is in progress. A transplant scientist has said, "An Einstein could literally be made immortal. One may envision a transplant generation," which would be composed of "individuals born from eggs fertilized by nuclei transplanted from body cells rather than by sperm."[13]

When one considers the implications of these experiments, scientifically altered genes seem but a part of the whole biological revolution. To alter the chemical structure of DNA, to create artificial genes so as to correct genetic defects, to eventually modify tumor DNA with alternate DNA—these are not fanciful visions of science. They are likelihoods.

Problems: a price of progress

The exploration of outer space and the exploration of the oceans are complex undertakings. But scientists can be concerned about simple problems even under the most esoteric circumstances. Before actual space flights were made, they were worried about details that might affect the astronauts' health. Every ninety minutes astronauts would be subjected to a day and night. Ordinary intercontinental travellers are often sickened by interference with their normal circadian rhythms (see Chapter 1, pp. 9–10). What grave consequences might ensue when astronauts endured forty-five minutes of day followed by forty-five minutes of night? How, for example, could they sleep? How could this threat to their health be diminished?

The solution? Like a cloth over a bird-cage, "the spacecraft was artificially darkened by covering the windows, and, as far as the crew was concerned, it was night."[14] Few health problems are so easily solved. The efforts to avoid contamination of the moon by germ-laden earthly spacecraft are more complicated. Spacecraft sterilization is now under study. The problem goes both ways. Upon returning from its moon-landing, the

Searching space above and space below

---

[12] Anthony Blackler, quoted in "Protecting Man from Man," *Science News*, Vol. 95, No. 2 (January 11, 1969), p. 32.

[13] *Ibid.*, pp. 31–33.

[14] Charles A. Berry, "Space Medicine in Perspective," *Journal of the American Medical Association*, Vol. 201, No. 4 (July 24, 1967), p. 234.

Apollo 11 spacecraft, its astronauts, and moon samples needed to undergo a period of quarantine and testing to safeguard against the possibility of introducing stowaway, immigrant, moon organisms to earth.

There remains another vast ecosystem to explore. It lies beneath the ocean. "Do you know," says one fish to another "that over a quarter of the earth is covered by land?" Beneath the seas, the mountains are greater and the canyons are deeper than those above. But inner space is even less hospitable than outer space. Astronauts feel freer, see vast distances, are moved by overwhelming beauties, and can easily communicate with earthlings. But under just two hundred feet of water, life is miserable. Visibility is almost zero. At great depths, radio waves do not travel far. Communication with the world above remains impossible. Astronauts and aquanauts share some problems. Pressure, weightlessness, cold—these hazards vary with the ecology. In space, the astronaut is weightless. In deep water, the aquanaut is nearly so. The astronaut works in a vacuum. Every square inch of the aquanaut's body is under enormous pressure. Yet one can feel secure that science will solve these problems. (It is the ruination of man's natural environment that causes concern.)

For various reasons the space above and the space below are being explored. Man's need to penetrate the unknown, to solve the mystery of his life on earth, to understand his relationship with all else—these drive him to search. He seeks unity, to be part of a greater whole, to fit into an encompassing order and purpose. Jedáleddin wrote: "All that is not One must ever suffer with the wound of Absence."[15] It is this wound that man needs to heal. He seeks one unified idea of himself. Thus, reflected Einstein, "the story goes on until we have arrived at a system of the greatest conceivable unity."[16] Man wants order. Without its sense, he is not quite well.

And in his search there is serendipity. In "serendipity," there is meaning that merits digression. In 1754, the English writer and wit Horace Walpole told a tale of three travellers, *The Three Princes of Serendip*. Being blessed by a mixture of luck and keen observation, the three made all sorts of valuable discoveries they were not looking for. So the word *serendipity* refers to the faculty of happening on valuable findings when not searching for them. But as Louis Pasteur succinctly said, "Chance favors the prepared mind."

Formidable indeed are the serendipitous results of oceanography. Submarine rescue (pitifully inadequate in 1963, when the nuclear submarine *Thresher* disappeared) is now a realistic hope. From the surfaces and crevices of the ocean floor come valuable minerals. But perhaps the greatest dividend of sea science is the promise of food. Today, whole populations hunger. Between water depths ranging from thirty to nine hundred feet there live succulent sea plants. These are consumed by minute animal organisms, which are in turn consumed by flesh-eating fish.

[15]Quoted in John M. Dorsey, *Illness or Allness* (Detroit, 1965), p. 540.
[16]Albert Einstein, "Physics and Reality," *Out of My Later Years* (New York, 1950), p. 63.

By using new understandings of sea science, oceanographers can now help the world's fishermen find their catch. This is but the beginning of the scientific exploration of a vast food source. To a world expecting a population of six billion in a generation, this is hopeful news. But without research that hope will remain unreality.

Examine the charts on page 588. Regular measles (and poliomyelitis too) has become a relatively rare disease. The vaccine for German measles (rubella) will soon relegate that crippler of the unborn to a melancholy memory. In the period from 1963 through 1968, drugs (streptomycin and isoniazid) helped cut the tuberculosis death rate by twenty-nine percent. And antibiotics also reduced the death rates from pneumonia and rheumatic fever. Nor were the victories of those several years limited to infectious diseases. The control of infectious diseases has provided longer life in which to develop chronic ailments. Nevertheless, drugs lowered death rates from hypertensive heart disease by thirty-two percent. Strokes killed two percent fewer people. Deaths from stomach and duodenal ulcers lessened twenty percent. Although in the period from 1963 through the first nine months of 1967 mortality from all causes declined only three percent, infant death rates[17] fell thirteen percent. Maternal mortality dropped by one-fourth from 1963 to 1968. These declines are continuing.

In the United States, more health for more people; more problems with progress

Even in so affluent a country as the United States, these are major accomplishments. But they do not tell the whole story. Closer examination reveals a less heartening picture. In terms of longevity, how do the people of this nation compare to those of other industrial societies?[18]

In 1949, an average male child born in the United States could be expected to live 65.2 years, a female, 70.7. In this statistical measure of longevity, the *average remaining lifetime at birth,*[19] the U.S. male ranked fourteenth among males of other nations; the female, ninth.

Could the U.S. health dollar buy more?

In 1964, an average male child born in the United States could be expected to live 66.9 years; a female, 73.7. The 1949–64 improvement: an increase of 1.7 and 3 years respectively. But, compared to other nations, in those fifteen years the U.S. male longevity slipped to thirty-first place and the female to eleventh. And, by 1966, preliminary figures indicated that, in terms of average remaining lifetime at birth, the U.S. male's rank had further fallen to thirty-fifth. Females were thirteenth. So, compared to longevity in other affluent countries, U.S. longevity ranks low. And it is losing ground.

A few more figures: in 1955, the average remaining lifetime at birth for

[17]The infant mortality rate is the number of deaths occurring among children less than one year of age, divided by the number of births.

[18]Much of the following section (pages 587–91) is based on an article by William H. Forbes, "Longevity and Medical Costs," *New England Journal of Medicine*, Vol. 277, No. 2 (July 13, 1967), pp. 71–78.

[19]*Longevity* refers to the average remaining lifetime at various ages. For example, in 1962, the average remaining lifetime for the new-born male in Sweden was 71.32 years. For ten-year-old Swedish males it was 63.05 years. In the United States in 1964, it was 66.9 and 59.2 for the two ages respectively.

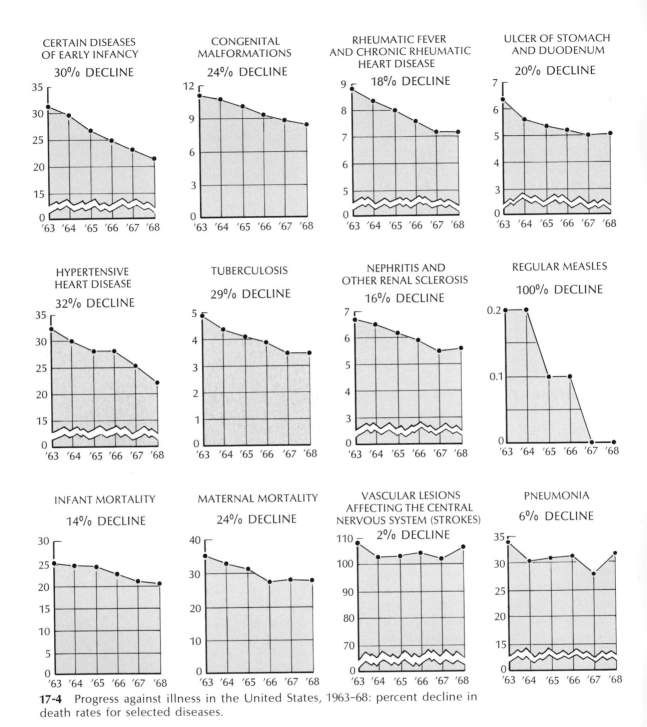

17-4 Progress against illness in the United States, 1963–68: percent decline in death rates for selected diseases.

All rates are per 100,000 population except for infant mortality (infant deaths per 1,000 live births) and maternal deaths (deaths from maternal causes per 100,000 live births). Figures for 1968 are provisional.

Sources: *What Are the Pay-Offs from Our Federal Health Programs?* National Health Education Committee (New York, 1968), and *Monthly Vital Statistics Report,* Provisional Statistics, Annual Summary for the United States, 1968, Table 8. Data from Division of Vital Statistics, National Center for Health Statistics, Public Health Service, Department of Health, Education, and Welfare.

U.S. males was 66.6 years; for females, 72.7. Thus, in the period 1955–64, a statistically insignificant 0.3 years had been added to male life expectancy at birth. A barely significant one year had been added to the U.S. female expectancy. Compared to previous ten-year periods a virtual plateau has been reached.

The difference between the average remaining lifetime of the male and that of the female is greater in the United States than in thirty-one other industrial countries studied. (In France, however, the difference is even greater than in the United States.) "The six countries at the top of the list have an average difference of 3.45 years—half of ours."[20]

What do these data mean? U.S. health expenditures rose from $12 billion a year in 1949 to $44 billion in 1964. So, despite an enormous annual increase of health expenditures extending over fifteen years, male longevity failed to significantly increase, and female longevity increased but slightly. Is longevity at least a partial measure of health? Yes. There are exceptions—a healthy child, killed in an auto accident, for example. But, generally, healthy people live longer.

In this affluent nation can one correlate sheer expenditure with better health? More than one expert thinks not. Forbes wrote:

> In the United States there is no longer any significant relation between the money spent on health and the results achieved . . . the main determinants of longevity are cultural rather than medical . . . That is why the undoubted progress of medicine in the last fifteen years has had such a very small effect on longevity in this country and why many countries with less highly developed medicine have greater life expectancy than the United States.[21]

That this statement could come from so reliable a source is, in itself, remarkable. Correlation between expenditure and health was not always so questionable. At the turn of this century human life was abbreviated, mostly by communicable disease. Leading the list of lethal ailments were influenza, pneumonia, tuberculosis, and gastroenteritis. Arrayed against these costly killers were vast monies and efforts. Sewage systems routed danger away from human beings. Water, food, and milk were purified. Too, effective and better medical drugs and surgical procedures were developed. Prevention of communicable illness became a way of life. An outbreak of typhoid, for example, was preventable. Its occurrence was a correctable failure. A death from tuberculosis was needless. Not even the existence of one case of tuberculosis was excusable. And pneumonia? To cure many cases of pneumonia what was necessary? A few cents' worth of penicillin? Or aureomycin? Or terramycin? The money was spent. Whether by prevention or cure, communicable disease was curtailed. If a disease could not be prevented or cured death from it was

[20] William H. Forbes, "Longevity and Medical Costs," p. 76.
[21] Ibid., p. 78.

delayed. Longevity increased. And, while all these benefits were happening, health, in terms of longevity, could be equated with expenditures. In developing countries, this is still possible. In the United States, according to some experts, this statistical correlation no longer seems possible. Why? The answer lies in the changed nature of the U.S. health problem.

Communicable diseases still sap the nation's strength (see Chapter 6). "In fact, flu is such a thief of life among the elderly that the National Center for Health Statistics attributed a .3 of a year increase in life expectancy between 1963 and 1964 largely to the fact that there was no influenza epidemic in the latter year."[22] As the major executioners, however, the communicable diseases have been replaced by heart disease, malignancies, and stroke. All need research. But even now it is apparent to some experts that this deadly trio will not be conquered by the same kind of expenditures as in the past. By the separation of man from his microbes, typhoid fever has been almost eliminated in this country. But lung cancer is another matter. Methods of diagnosing lung cancer have improved. Its surgery is superb. Yet, it kills more than ever before. In fifteen years it has increased almost 90 percent. Today, it accounts for over 2.5 percent of all deaths. There is no gainsaying that routine physical examinations, early diagnosis, and more efficient organization and delivery of medical care will help reduce its death rate. But more effort must surely be expended in behavioral science. Why do people smoke? What can be done to induce them to stop this fatal dependency? Another example of the need to study behavioral science is accidents. As a cause of death in this nation, they rank fourth. For people under the age of 25, they are the leading cause of death. Like lung cancer, they, too, are responsible for over 2.5 percent of all fatalities. How may they be reduced? By education? Yes. But behavioral science can teach many a secret about causes of accidents and their prevention.

Increased knowledge in the behavioral sciences will hardly provide all the answers needed to increase U.S. longevity. Money for research is essential. The unequal distribution of health services must be corrected. Constant improvement of health service organization and of delivery of health services to those in greatest need—these are prime priorities.[23] (One would wish that organization and delivery of health were as easy as that of automobiles!) But if the average longevity of the people of this nation is to be increased, more study of their behavior in their complex ecosystem is essential.

It is not only in the longevity of its citizens that the United States

[22]Hollis S. Ingraham, "Long Life and Good Health," a paper presented at the symposium on "Advances in Medical Care of the Aging," State Medical Society, February 17, 1966, New York. Indeed the fluctuations in U.S. death rates between 1954 (9.2) and 1963 (9.6) are attributed to the presence or absence of epidemic influenza. Influenza epidemics invariably increase death rates.

[23]The importance of these should be stressed. "Now we are waking up to the fact that emphasis on financing research, although desirable in itself, has been at the expense of equal attention to the training and other health manpower to deliver, to a growing and more demanding population, the medical knowledge and skills already existing." (Greer Williams, "Needed: A New Strategy for Health Promotion," *New England Journal of Medicine*, Vol. 279, No. 19 [November 7, 1968], p. 1033.)

compares poorly with other industrial countries. In more than a dozen industrial nations infant mortality rates are also lower than those in the United States. U.S. infant mortality rates are almost double those of Sweden (see Table 13-4).[24] Thus do data from life's opposites—infant mortality and longevity—indicate to this nation's health workers that there is much work to do. Yet work creates work. As health success brings more infants to adulthood, the more adults to old age, the problems of older people come to the forefront. Legislation such as Medicare testifies to societal concern for the economic and health needs of the elderly. Nevertheless, how well do the aged fit into modern cultural patterns? This question suggests a tale.

Once upon a time in Asia Minor, it was the custom for people who had reached the age of sixty to be taken away to a cave. There they might live in peace the rest of their lives, and, of course, would be out of people's way.

Aging: man's common denominator

It was considered most proper that when the time came for a man to leave for the cave, his son should contribute the necessary food and "chull," a goat-haired woven blanket.

One day a middle-aged man asked his own little boy to take the chull and come with him and grandpa, for they were taking the latter to the cave from which none returned. Though the grandson was brokenhearted at his grandfather's departure, he was about to shoulder the chull obediently when suddenly he was struck by an idea. Cutting the chull in half, he took one part with him and left the other part at home. When the grandfather had been deposited with due filial piety in the cave, son and grandson returned home.

Then it was that the son discovered what had happened to the chull. He scolded the boy severely. "Look what you've done. Everyone would say we were too stingy to give grandpa the whole blanket!" "No, father," the boy replied, "I wasn't being stingy, but I thought it was better to give grandpa only half . . . Then I could keep the other half for you." [25]

If mankind has failed to escape eventual aging, it has not been for want of trying. By drinking the warm blood of dying gladiators, elderly Romans sought to partake of youth. Others bathed in young people's blood. Those violent Roman emperors, Nero and Caligula, hopefully ingested male gland preparations.[26] In the twentieth century, Serge Voronoff made a fortune by surgically implanting monkey glands. John Brinkman got rich by transplanting goat glands. His profits helped pay for an almost suc-

---

[24] In the United States, infant mortality is slowly decreasing. The 1960 rate was 26.0 per 1,000 live births. In 1966, it was 23.7, in 1967, 22.1—less than half the 1940 rate. Although the nonwhite infant mortality rate has declined substantially, it remains 80 percent higher than the white rate. (Myron E. Wegman, "Annual Summary of Vital Statistics," *Pediatrics*, Vol. 42, No. 6 [December 1968], pp. 1005–09.)

[25] George Lawton, ed., *New Goals for Old Age* (New York, 1943), p. v.

[26] "Quest for Youth," *M.D., Medical Newsmagazine*, Vol. 2, No. 8 (August 1958), p. 86.

cessful campaign to a governor's chair. There have been phony pills, creams, and "sera." But man continues to age.

Science has now entered the quest for prolonged youth. The process of growing old (*senescence*) is being avidly studied. *Gerontology* is the science of the physical and psychological changes incident to old age. *Geriatrics* is concerned with the treatment of the problems of the aged. Perhaps the determinants of aging lie in the chromosomal pattern. This pattern possibly dictates the time schedule of cellular aging. Maybe this is why the heart and blood vessels wear out more often and earlier than other body parts. If (as has been theorized) aging speed is predetermined in the configuration of genetic structure, perhaps the chemical program can be changed. Already scientists have transplanted DNA (genes) from one bacterial cell to another. Those bacteria that received transplanted DNA transmitted the new genetic characteristics to their progeny.[27] Can DNA transplants be accomplished in man? Can young genes be transplanted into old cells? Those who peremptorily dismiss this possibility are out of step with the scientific strides of the past twenty years.

To increase the life span, to bring more people to older age—these are agelong efforts by civilized communities. As has been seen, in the latter decades of this century longevity has leveled off. Nevertheless, the number of people attaining old age continues to multiply. In 1900, only 4 percent of the U.S. population was sixty-five years of age or older. In 1968, about 9.5 percent were. In 1970, that proportion was over 10 percent.

In various cultures age has had various meanings. Among the Ainos of Japan, it was recorded that the "old women show themselves the most vigorous and wildest dancers."[28] Montaigne wrote that "there is nothing more notable in Socrates than that he found time, when he was an old man, to learn music and dancing, and thought it time well spent."[29]

Some members of the youth-oriented society of today have a harsh view of age. It is the image described by the Chief Justice in Shakespeare's *The Second Part of King Henry the Fourth*:

> *Do you set down your name in the scroll of youth, that are written down old with all the characters of age? Have you not a moist eye? A dry hand? A yellow cheek? A white beard? A decreasing leg? An increasing belly? Is not your voice broken? Your wind short? Your chin double? Your wit single? And every part about you blasted with antiquity? And will you yet call yourself young? Fie, fie, fie, Sir John!*[30]

Perhaps the greatest pain of the aged is thinking that this is youth's view of them.

---

[27] "Scientist Says Senility May Be Controlled," *Geriatric Focus*, Vol. 4, No. 10 (June 15, 1965), pp. 1–6.

[28] R. Hitchcock, "The Ainos of Yezo, Japan," quoted in Leo W. Simmons, *The Role of the Aged in Primitive Society* (New Haven, Conn., 1945), p. 97.

[29] Michel de Montaigne, "Living to the Point," quoted in J. Donald Adams, ed., *The New Treasure Chest* (New York, 1953), p. 2.

[30] William Shakespeare, *The Second Part of King Henry the Fourth* (I.ii.204–12).

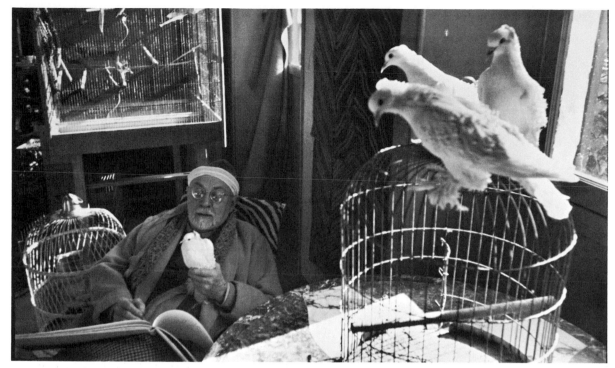

17-5 Henri Matisse in 1944.

The extra gift

In 1940, the great painter Henri Matisse lay dying. He was then seventy-one. But he did not die. Confined to his bed or to a chair, he could sit up for only brief periods. Yet, he lived to create some of his greatest work. About his illness he said this:

> I was extremely ill and had to have an operation. I had hardly regained consciousness, and still seemed to be sleeping, when I heard the doctors gathered at the foot of my bed, speaking among themselves: "We cannot do any more for him; if he gets over this, he has himself to thank for it; all depends on the way his body reacts." I did get over it. Since that day I have had the impression of having started a new life. My previous life was terminated at the moment when theoretically I was going to die. The life I am now enjoying is an extra gift; I have the right to do as I please, to try any experience, no longer seeking a link with a completed past. Moreover, I have a sense of total liberty in my experiments. [31]

[31]Quoted in Raymond Cogniat, "Art and Longevity," *Abbottempo*, Vol. 1, No. 1 (March 22, 1963), pp. 9–13.

The extra gift also came to Oliver Wendell Holmes, Jr. He had fought in the Civil War. He had fought for civil rights. In 1882, at forty-one, he had been made a Justice of the Supreme Court. There, for over half a century, he fought for the law as a living instrument. In 1931, he was ninety years old. This was his birthday message to the nation:

> In this symposium my part is only to sit in silence. To express one's feelings as the end draws near is too intimate a task.
> But I may mention one thought that comes to me as a listener-in. The riders in a race do not stop short when they reach the goal. There is a little finishing canter before coming to a standstill. There is time to hear the kind voice of friends and to say to one's self: "The work is done."
> But just as one says that, the answer comes: "The race is over, but the work never is done while the power to work remains."
> The canter that brings you to a standstill need not be only coming to rest. It cannot be while you still live. For to live is to function. That is all there is to living.
> And so I end with a line from a Latin poet who uttered the message more than fifteen hundred years ago:
>
> "Death plucks my ears and says, Live—I am coming."[32]

But what about the average man? As he survives, he has a predictable chance of a longer life. In this country, retiring at sixty-five, a man has a 50-50 chance of living twelve more years. Today, Western man experiences both a prolonged period of learning and a prolonged retirement. It is during the first that preparation should begin for the second. This is not to say that youth should be haunted by the spectre of old age. But it is during youth that the foundation for age is built. In the *Republic*, Plato puts these thoughts into the conversation of Cephalus with Socrates:

> How well do I remember the aged poet Sophocles, when in answer to the question, How does love suit with age, Sophocles,—are you still the man you were? Peace, he replied; most gladly have I escaped that, and I feel as if I had escaped from a mad and furious master . . . And of these regrets, as well as of the complaint about relations, Socrates, the cause is to be sought, not in men's ages, but in their characters and tempers; for he who is of a calm and happy nature will hardly feel the pressure of age, but he who is of an opposite disposition will find youth and age equally a burden.[33]

---

[32] Oliver Wendell Holmes, Jr., a radio talk on the occasion of a national celebration of his ninetieth birthday, quoted in Max Lerner, ed., *The Mind and Faith of Justice Holmes* (Boston, 1943), p. 451.
[33] *Dialogues of Plato*, tr. by Benjamin Jowett (Oxford, Eng., 1897), p. 14.

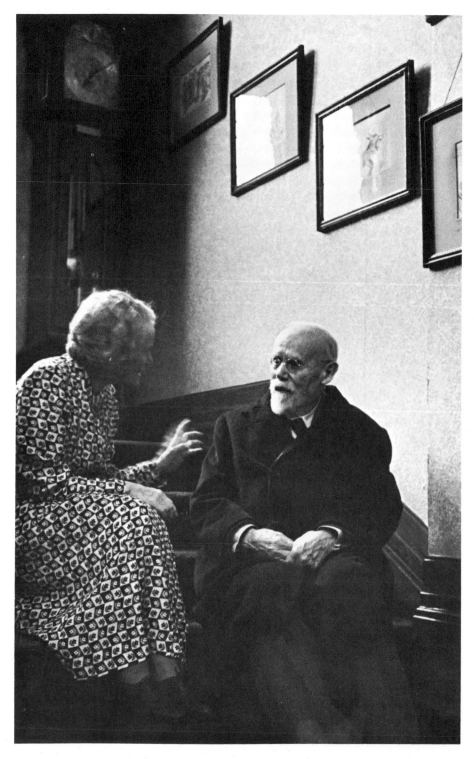

17-6 "There is time to hear the kind voice of friends."

The plight of the poor everywhere

To the poor of this nation sickness and death come sooner and oftener. Lack of prenatal care, for example, kills the poor infant a third more often than the baby born to parents in nonpoverty areas. Premature births, malnutrition, handicapping conditions—these are but a few of the prices of poverty paid by the helpless infant.

Other statistics add to this totally unacceptable picture. The white infant mortality rate is dropping more sharply than the nonwhite. Moreover, the poverty of racial inequality kills almost four times as many pregnant black women as white. And there is the inequality not only of race, but also of place. It is in the South that mothers and their babies are at greatest risk. For years Mississippi has had the nation's highest infant mortality rate, and Alabama is not far behind.[34] This is further evidence of the need for more equal distribution of medical care.

For many a nation, aging people are no issue. Not enough people live to be old. True, U.S. data give little reason for complacency. But the information on sickness from developing countries provides even less. Compared to the rates in industrial nations, infant mortality rates in developing countries are two to eight times greater. Yet, even in these struggling areas, infant mortality rates portray but a part of the childhood calamity. "Mortality for children 1 to 4 years of age is from 20 to 30 times higher, sometimes much more in underdeveloped nations."[35] Affliction is compounded by more affliction. In the developing countries:

Every year the twenty million people with active cases of *tuberculosis* infect two and one-half million people. Two million die of the disease.

Twelve million people suffer *leprosy,* and the number is increasing.

Plague, an ancient enemy, is on the rise (see Chapter 5).[36]

Diarrheal diseases, perpetuated by three tragic factors—poor sanitation, low economic development, and inadequate nutrition—afflict so many of the globe's inhabitants as to defy estimation. In many areas, for example, *typhoid fever* (rare in this country) is common. Other parasitic diseases, such as anemia-causing *hookworm* and the colic-producing *ascariasis* (a roundworm infestation) torment more than a billion and a half sufferers.[37]

---

[34] In 1967, the infant mortality rate in Mississippi was 34.7; in Alabama, 27.4. Nebraska (16.9) and Hawaii (16.8) had this nation's lowest infant mortality rates that year.

[35] Nevin S. Scrimshaw, "The Death Rate of One-Year-Old Children in Underdeveloped Countries," *Archives of Environmental Health,* Vol. 17, No. 5 (November 1968), p. 692.

[36] In Vietnam, for example, defoliation has deprived many a wild rodent of its natural habitat. Scurrying from the devastated woodlands, it makes its way to the devastated cities. There, war has unbalanced the human ecosystem, but not that of the domestic rat. In the disorder of war, the latter thrives. It, however, becomes plague-infested by its immigrant country cousins. The incidence of human plague in Vietnam has recently risen. (Alexander Alland, Jr., "War and Disease: An Anthropological Perspective," *Bulletin of the Atomic Scientists,* Vol. 24, No. 6 [June 1968], p. 29.) Due to U.S. interest in the reporting of plague, some of the dramatic rise is more apparent than real. (J. D. Marshall, Jr. *et al.,* "Plague in Vietnam 1965–1966," *American Journal of Epidemiology,* Vol. 86, No. 3 [November 1967], p. 616.)

[37] "The Second Ten Years of the World Health Organization," *WHO Chronicle,* Vol. 22, No. 7 (July 1968), pp. 267–312.

And, throughout the world, those who survive these endure cardio-vascular illness, cancer, emotional disabilities, malnutrition, and dental problems.

There is work to do. Who does it?

Organized participants in health work

Organized health work is done by *official* and *voluntary agencies.* Official agencies are governmental, have legal health responsibilities, and are tax-supported. Voluntary health agencies are not part of governmental structure, are not responsible for carrying out health laws, and are supported by voluntary contributions. Both types of agencies have paid staffs. Millions of unpaid workers help voluntary agencies. Without volunteers, official health agencies could function, albeit not so comprehensively. Without volunteers, voluntary agencies would not exist.

Who's WHO in health?   **Official agencies**

The World Health Organization is an agency of the United Nations. Today, over twenty years after it was founded in 1948, it includes 126 member states and 3 associate members. In WHO's governing body, the *World Health Assembly,* each member state has one vote. Not often in history have so many nations labored together so long and so harmoniously. Each WHO worker is witness to a world of woe. Yet hope, not despair, is his image. Clearly he sees his purpose and his vision in these lines:

And hold Humanity one man, whose universal agony
Still strains and strives to gain the goal, where agonies shall cease
    to be.[38]

Meeting annually, the World Health Assembly establishes its policy, program, and budget. It also selects the rotating membership of its executive arm—the *Executive Board.* This twenty-four member group, the representatives of twenty-four nations, effectuates assembly decisions. In case of an emergency plea—prompted perhaps by national trials such as earthquake, flood, or epidemic—the board is empowered to give immediate help. But it is through six regional field offices of WHO (in Brazzaville, Alexandria, Copenhagen, New Delhi, Manila, and Washington, D.C.) that most of the work of WHO reaches the people. Member nations apply to these offices for help, and from these offices field workers are assigned. The nerve center of WHO—its central headquarters—is located in Geneva.

WHO's basic purpose is to help applicant nations help themselves. Thus

[38] Richard Francis Burton, *The Kasîdah of Hâjî Abdû El-Yezdi,* Part 9, verse 31 (Portland, Me., 1896), p. 56.

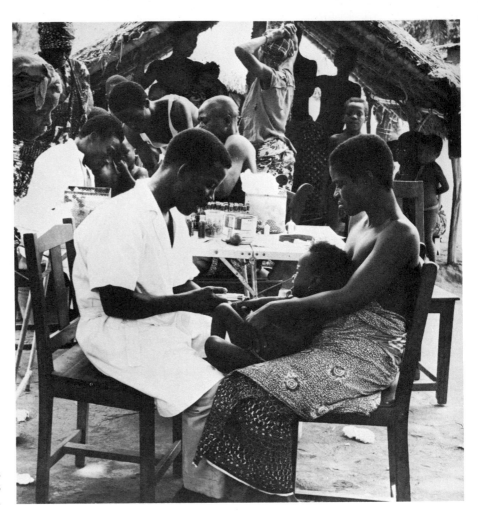

17-7 WHO workers taking blood samples in a Togolese village.

WHO assists nations in planning basic health services as an integral part of local development. Expert consultants on forty-four panels include 12,000 scientists, educators, and administrators. A permanent staff of 3,500 includes physicians, nurses, engineers, and other personnel. With WHO's world-wide intelligence system, world communicable disease control is a practical reality. It helps set international standards on foods, vaccines, drugs, diagnoses, and disease classifications. It is part of the counterspy system against the international drug racketeer. Its participation in training health personnel and in research is vast. It directs enormous campaigns against smallpox, malaria, tuberculosis, syphilis, and other plagues of mankind. It combats maternal and infant death. To old countries it has brought new concepts for dealing with water, soil, and air pollution; mental disease; accidents; heart disease; and cancer.

Its annual budget is less than the cost of a battleship.

Federal health work

It is from a broad interpretation of the Constitution that the federal government derives public health powers. The Constitutional phrase "promote the general welfare" establishes the basic philosophy. More specific is the federal *power to tax.* Consequently, the physician's annual $1 tax for his narcotic license provides the government with still another way of checking on drug use. Or federal tax monies may be eventually used for local health programs. By its *controls over foreign commerce,* other problems are contained, such as the exclusion of dangerous drugs (thalidomide, for example) or people (such as unvaccinated aliens from smallpox areas). *Interstate commerce regulations* empower the federal government to exert controls over food and drugs transported from one state to another. *The federal right to raise armies* makes possible soldier and veteran medical care. *Control over federal territories* (Indian reservations, the District of Columbia) and the *post office* system include extensive federal health powers. In making treaties (as with Canada and Mexico) the United States exerts wide public health influence. Recent years have seen much international health activity abroad without treaty involvement. Much U.S. health work abroad is done via the World Health Organization, Public Health Service, State Department Agency for International Development, Peace Corps, and the military. All have done distinguished work.

In various agencies throughout the federal establishment, a wide variety of health activities are dispersed. Examples: the provision of medical services to federal prisoners by the Department of Justice and the interest in industrial safety by the Department of Labor. There are many more. These have their counterparts in state and local government. But it is in the *Department of Health, Education, and Welfare* that the nation's greatest concentration of health program activity occurs. Table 17-1, depicting the organizational structure of the Department, reveals the extraordinary extent of its effort. Its budget: over $10 billion. Its major interest: health.

Table 17-1, also presenting the basic structure of the *Public Health Service,* provides a general concept of its activities. Its functions include education and research, assistance to state health departments, and provision of medical and hospital services to eligible persons. It is, moreover, responsible for protecting U.S. borders against the entry of communicable diseases. The *Bureau of Health Manpower* is particularly interested in training health personnel. Education and research are, however, common denominators of the service. Especially concerned with research are the *National Institutes of Health,* the *National Communicable Disease Center,* and the *National Institute of Mental Health.* And they are assisted in this work by the largest and most comprehensive collection of medical literature in the world—the collection located in the *National Library of Medicine.*

TABLE 17-1 *Organization of the U.S. Department of Health, Education, and Welfare**

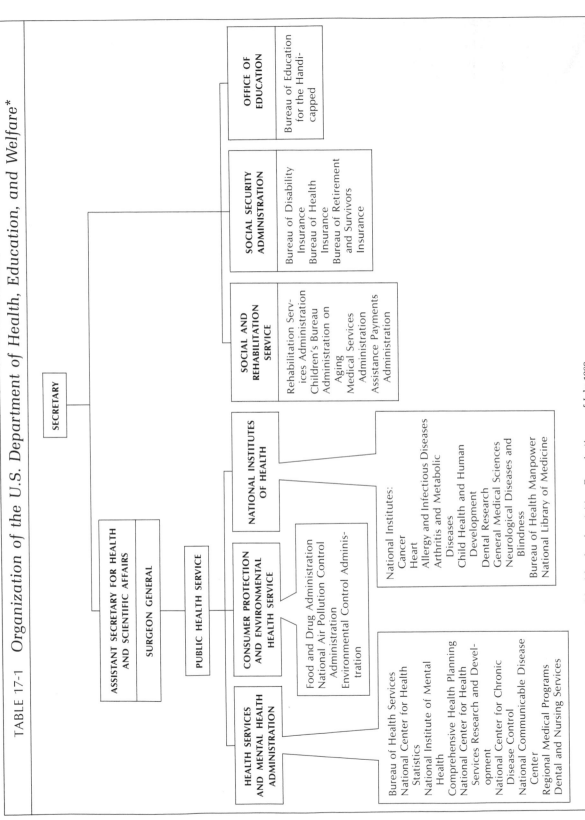

SECRETARY

ASSISTANT SECRETARY FOR HEALTH AND SCIENTIFIC AFFAIRS

SURGEON GENERAL

PUBLIC HEALTH SERVICE

HEALTH SERVICES AND MENTAL HEALTH ADMINISTRATION

Bureau of Health Services
National Center for Health Statistics
National Institute of Mental Health
Comprehensive Health Planning
National Center for Health Services Research and Development
National Center for Chronic Disease Control
National Communicable Disease Center
Regional Medical Programs
Dental and Nursing Services

CONSUMER PROTECTION AND ENVIRONMENTAL HEALTH SERVICE

Food and Drug Administration
National Air Pollution Control Administration
Environmental Control Administration

NATIONAL INSTITUTES OF HEALTH

National Institutes:
Cancer
Heart
Allergy and Infectious Diseases
Arthritis and Metabolic Diseases
Child Health and Human Development
Dental Research
General Medical Sciences
Neurological Diseases and Blindness
Bureau of Health Manpower
National Library of Medicine

SOCIAL AND REHABILITATION SERVICE

Rehabilitation Services Administration
Children's Bureau
Administration on Aging
Medical Services Administration
Assistance Payments Administration

SOCIAL SECURITY ADMINISTRATION

Bureau of Disability Insurance
Bureau of Health Insurance
Bureau of Retirement and Survivors Insurance

OFFICE OF EDUCATION

Bureau of Education for the Handicapped

* Partial listing, highlighting certain health and health-related activities. Organization as of July 1968.

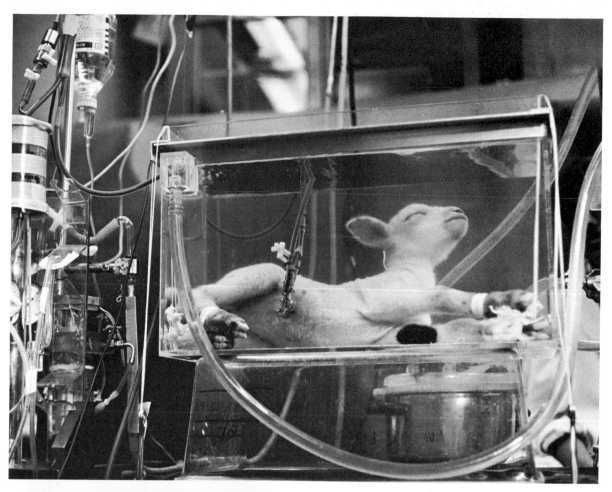

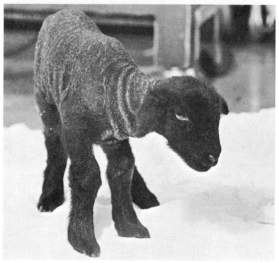

17-8 At the National Heart Institute, fetal lambs have been sustained for up to fifty-five hours in a womblike tank of synthetic amniotic fluid. The artificial "placenta" is the apparatus shown above. The healthy lamb (*left*) was weaned from such an apparatus.

Human premature babies, who need respiratory support while their lungs finish developing, and patients with serious lung problems may be among those who eventually profit from these experiments. However, this startling accomplishment suggests more than man's growing control over his ecosystems. Other basic experiments, such as the recent (1968) successful test-tube fertilization of mouse ova, will ultimately demand a higher order of human responsibility.

TABLE 17-2 *Organization of the County of Los Angeles Health Department*

BOARD OF SUPERVISORS

PUBLIC HEALTH ADVISORY COMMISSION

HEALTH OFFICER

PUBLIC INFORMATION OFFICER

ADMINISTRATIVE PUBLIC HEALTH ENGINEER

MEDICAL DEPUTY BUREAUS

ADMINISTRATIVE DEPUTY

MEDICAL DEPUTY DISTRICTS

PROGRAMS

SERVICES

DISTRICTS

BUREAU OF MATERNAL AND CHILD HEALTH

BUREAU OF MEDICAL SERVICES

ADMINISTRATIVE SERVICES

PERSONNEL AND TRAINING DIVISION

DISTRICT HEALTH OFFICES

Twenty-three major offices, each directed by a district health officer and manned by physicians, public health nurses, social workers, environmental sanitation specialists, and others. Emphasis is on disease prevention, with concentration on the individual district's primary health problems. Future plans are to broaden the scope of services. Together with other community resources, comprehensive health care—including prevention, diagnoses, treatment, and rehabilitation—will be offered.

Includes the divisions of venereal disease control, alcohol rehabilitation, chronic disease control, public health nutrition, occupational health, radiological health, tuberculosis control, acute communicable disease control, and drug abuse control. Plans and coordinates services offered through the district offices.

BUREAU OF ENVIRONMENTAL SANITATION

BUREAU OF PUBLIC HEALTH NURSING

RECORDS AND STATISTICS DIVISION

HEALTH EDUCATION DIVISION

BUREAU OF PUBLIC HEALTH LABORATORIES

BUREAU OF PUBLIC HEALTH SOCIAL WORK

PUBLIC HEALTH INVESTIGATION DIVISION

Source: Gerald A. Heidbreder, Health Officer, County of Los Angeles Health Department. Organization as of March 1, 1970.

State and local health departments

Protection of the public's health is part of the legal obligation of each state. The federal government may interfere only when it is invited or when problems between states occur. Examples: a state has an outbreak of viral encephalitis. The governor requests federal Public Health Service help. Or a contaminated vaccine manufactured in one state is sold in another. This offense is federal and action is taken by federal agents. Similarly, it is only by state authority that a local city or county health department exists. Should a local department fail in its duty, the state can assume control. This almost never happens.

The basic job of the state health department is to help the local health departments do a better job. State departments, consequently, are more concerned with health legislation, planning, and policy. They are consultants, helping to set the standards of the service-giving local city and county health departments. And, since local health departments provide the services detailed in their organization charts (Table 17-2), state health departments, to advise them best, are organized to help them.

Examine the present organization chart of the County of Los Angeles Health Department (Table 17-2). It seems complex and the different bureaus may seem to have little connection with each other. Yet, during a few duty hours, a public health nurse may perform functions directly related to every bureau, indeed every division. Before leaving her assigned district office for a home visit, she notes her mileage. Eventually relayed to the Bureau of Administrative Services, this information makes possible her reimbursement. During her home call she sees a child with whooping cough. The Division of Acute Communicable Disease Control (within the Bureau of Medical Services) is interested. And so is the Bureau of Maternal and Child Health. The child's mother is pregnant. "I can't afford the doctor," she tells the nurse. Mindful that delay in prenatal care means increased risks to both mother and child, the nurse arranges a health department prenatal clinic appointment. "I've got a rat problem," the mother may tell the nurse. This information will go to the Bureau of Environmental Sanitation. From their office a trained sanitarian will come to help. Within a few days, the mother-to-be will be seen by a department medical social worker. They will discuss such matters as her hospitalization and her husband's employment. Part of the examination period in the prenatal clinic will be given to obtaining a blood specimen. It will be tested for syphilis by the Bureau of Public Health Laboratories. Thus is the local health department organized to give service. But its basic purpose is health education. Modern health departments employ health education specialists. But that does not relieve the obligation of every health department professional to teach health.

It is clear that official agencies perform a variety of vital services. But they are not alone in attempting to meet the health needs of the public; major contributions are made by the voluntary health agencies.

**People care—
and organize**
During the long trial of his convalescence from tuberculosis, Lawrence Flick conceived an idea that led to the establishment of the first voluntary health agency in this country. Recovered at last from his illness, he set to work. Gathering together a small group of medical and lay people, he fired them with his own zeal. He told them this: a volunteer army, an organized community, could conquer consumption. Thus the Pennsylvania Society for the Prevention of Tuberculosis was founded in 1892 and later developed into the National Tuberculosis Association. And from its small beginnings came the whole voluntary health agency movement.

Other personal pain quickened similar activity against other problems. From the psychic sufferings of Clifford Beers, as told in his book *A Mind That Found Itself,* came a Connecticut mental health association and then one for the country. The loss of a son lent purpose to Edgar F. Allen's efforts to create a lasting memorial—the National Society for Crippled Children and Adults. The plight of Franklin Delano Roosevelt brought millions of dollars to a poliomyelitis foundation. That money helped Salk and Sabin to develop their vaccines. And Mrs. Rose Kennedy's quiet public reminder that she bore not only brilliant children but also a retarded child has brought wide citizen support for a society founded to attack that problem. Not the least important feature of the voluntary health agency movement is the willingness of these agencies to tackle seemingly insoluble problems. This gives hope to those afflicted with muscular dystrophy, multiple sclerosis, and a host of other robbers of human health and life.

In the United States today there are some seventy-five national voluntary health agencies. To their more than twenty-five thousand local chapters millions of citizens donate both time and money. So numerous are they that they have been classified according to their interest in:

1. *specific diseases* (American Cancer Society, American Diabetes Association);

2. *special organs or structures* (American Heart Association, National Society for the Prevention of Blindness);

3. *special groups or society as a whole* (Planned Parenthood Federation of America, Ford Foundation, Alcoholics Anonymous, National Safety Council).

Like official agencies, volunteer health agencies are organized on four levels. They are international, national, state, and local.

Of both national and international import are such volunteer philanthropies as the Rockefeller, Ford, W. K. Kellogg, and Markle Foundations, as well as the Commonwealth and Milbank Memorial Funds. And justly famed are the dedicated contributions of such church groups as the Seventh-Day Adventist and Roman Catholic. These usually offer direct service.

Some voluntary health agencies have been bitterly assailed for money competitiveness, others for high administrative costs, still others for overlapping functions. Their enduring contributions, however, are not to be denied. As health educators, as stimulators of official agencies and supplementors of their programs, as demonstrators of newer, better ways to health, as campaigners for improved health legislation, and as contributors to productive research, volunteer health agencies make a bright light. And they prove something important.

People care.

Epilogue, health: whose responsibility?

But people must care as individuals, as active participants. Without enough individual participation, the best health organization is enfeebled. In the individual lies the basic responsibility for health. That is what this book has to say. A parable, very old and completely modern, sums it up.

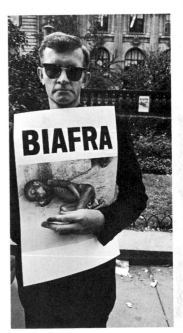

> *There was once a rabbi who had the reputation for knowing what was in a man's mind by reading his thoughts. A wicked boy came to see him and said: "Rabbi, I have in my hand a small bird. Is it alive, or is it dead?" And the boy thought to himself: If he says it is dead, I will open my hand and let it fly away; if he says it is alive, I will quickly squeeze it and show him it is dead. And the boy repeated the question: "Rabbi, I have in my hand a small bird. Is it alive, or is it dead?" And the rabbi gazed steadily at him, and said, quietly: "Whatever you will; whatever you will."*[39]

Man is neither a victim nor an innocent bystander. He is more than a casual collection of chromosomes. Sartre has written that man is "condemned to be free."[40] "Everything," Sartre continued, "takes place as if I were compelled to be responsible . . . engaged in a world for which I bear the whole responsibility without being able, whatever I do, to tear myself away from this responsibility for an instant. For I am responsible for my very desire of fleeing responsibilities."[41] So freedom means responsibility. This is the freeman's paradox, his reality, and his health.

17-9 Health: whose responsibility?

[39] From *The Talmud,* quoted in Daniel Bell, "The Year 2000—The Trajectory of an Idea," *Daedalus,* Vol. 96, No. 3 (Summer 1967), p. 697.
[40] Jean-Paul Sartre, *Of Human Freedom,* Wade Baskin, ed. (New York, 1966), p. 94.
[41] *Ibid.,* p. 97.

Bibliography

This selective bibliography is a guide for students who want to pursue the study of health on their own. It suggests some useful articles and books on general subjects and several on rather specialized topics. The many sources that are mentioned in the footnotes in the text, some of which are also included in this bibliography, provide further leads. It is well to remember that most footnotes refer to sources with their own bibliographies. Some of the bibliographic material in this book tends to be quite technical. To profit most from such sources the student will do well to explore them with the help of the faculty.

The card catalog in the library is another bibliography of sorts. Using its subject index, the student may copy down selected titles that appear relevant, or he may note some typical call numbers, which will indicate the location in the library of books on the subject. Going directly to the bookshelf, he may then examine the books themselves. In addition, there are a number of general guides to publications. The annual *Subject Guide to Books in Print* lists the most current books as they come into print. However, this book has three major drawbacks for the student: many of the books listed are likely to be unavailable in a given library; no information as to the quality of the book is given; and the choice is vast. The *Readers' Guide to Periodical Literature* indexes, by author and subject, the articles that have appeared in about 150 major popular magazines, from *Reader's Digest* to *Scientific American* and *Science News*. The *Cumulated Index Medicus* (published by the National Library of Medicine) amasses a much more technical group of articles from 2,300 medical journals published throughout the world. Articles are cross-indexed under subject headings and are also listed by author. A computerized service, MEDLARS, composed of the items from the *Cumulated Index Medicus*, conducts bibliographic searches of more refined and specific topics than are available in the published index. MEDLARS can be reached by writing to the National Library of Medicine, Guide to MEDLARS Services, 8600 Rockville Pike, Bethesda, Maryland 20014.

In seeking material on any subject, one should always keep in mind the inexpensive publications on a vast variety of subjects issued by the U.S. Government Printing Office in Washington, D.C. And the student will find it useful to keep abreast of the short reviews of books that are routinely published in the numerous journals. *Journal of the American Medical Association, Science News, Natural History,* and *Psychology Today* regularly list and briefly review the most recent books relating to human health.

1. Health: a fabric richly woven

Many books elaborate the basic concepts in this chapter. Roger J. Williams in his book *Free and Unequal* (Austin: University of Texas Press, 1953) presents a highly readable point of view of human individuality. His *Biochemical Individuality* (New York: John Wiley & Sons, 1956, also in paperback) is more technical. Curt Paul Richter has published extensively on human rhythms; his scholarly *Biological Clocks in Medicine and Psychiatry* (Springfield, Ill.: Charles C Thomas, 1965) presents some interesting examples. A rather advanced but relatively recent article by Michael Menaker, "Biological Clocks," was published in *Bioscience,* Vol. 19, No. 8 (August 1969), pp. 681–89.

The dangerous pollution of the human ecosystem has stimulated wide interest in the environment. Among the most prolific and prophetic writers in this area have been René Dubos and Marston Bates. Dubos' famous little book *Mirage of Health* (New York: Harper & Row, 1959, also in paperback, Doubleday) is must reading. Although his *Man Adapting* (New Haven, Conn.: Yale University Press, 1965, also in paperback) and *So Human an Animal* (New York: Charles Scribner's Sons, 1968) require more biological knowledge, they are recommended for a basic understanding of man in his ecosystems. Among Marston Bates's erudite contributions in this field are *Animal Worlds* (New York: Random House, 1960, also in paperback) and *Man in Nature,* 2nd ed. (Englewood Cliffs, N.J.: Prentice-Hall, 1964, also in paperback). Also highly recommended is Richard P. Dober, *Environmental Design* (Princeton, N.J.: Van Nostrand Reinhold, 1969). This book examines what man needs to live in harmony with his external ecosystems.

George L. Clarke's *Elements of Ecology,* rev. ed. (New York: John Wiley & Sons, 1965) is a carefully organized and lucid text. Redcliffe N. Salaman's *The History and Social Influence of the Potato* (Cambridge, Eng.: Cambridge University Press, 1949) remains a classic study of the effect of ecological change on the history of a whole people. Recommended also is Allen H. Barton's timely work *Communities in Disaster* (Garden City, N.Y.: Doubleday, 1969). The effects of a tornado, a famine (the Irish potato famines are described), and an atomic bomb in man's ecosystem are all explored. The following two articles are examples that show how the health of groups of people is influenced by a changing environment: Dugald Baird, "Perinatal Mortality," *Lancet,* Vol. 1, No. 7593 (March 8, 1969), pp. 511–15, and Paul T. Baker, "Human Adaptation to High Altitudes," *Science,* Vol. 163, No. 3872 (March 14, 1969), pp. 1149–56.

2. Health and the community

Published fifteen years ago, *Health, Culture, and Community* (New York: Russell Sage Foundation, 1955, also in paperback), ed. by Benjamin D. Paul, remains a significant collection of experiences by different health workers in various cultures. Leo J. Simmons and Harold G. Wolff also provide a study of culture and health in their *Social Science in Medicine* (New York: Russell Sage Foundation, 1954). There are many famous writings in cultural anthropology but one may begin with Ruth Benedict, *Patterns of Culture,* 2nd ed. (Boston: Houghton Mifflin, 1961, also in paperback); Bronislaw Malinowski, *Magic, Science and Religion* (Gar-

607

den City, N.Y.: Doubleday, 1954, paperback); and Margaret Mead, ed., *Cultural Patterns and Technical Change* (New York: New American Library, 1955, paperback).

For some recent articles describing various human responses to cultural elements, see Nathan S. Caplan and Jeffrey M. Paige, "A Study of Ghetto Rioters," *Scientific American,* Vol. 219, No. 2 (August 1968), pp. 15–21; Roy Menninger, "What Troubles Our Troubled Youth?" *Mental Hygiene,* Vol. 52, No. 3 (July 1968), pp. 324–27; and Irving Kenneth Zola, "Culture and Symptoms—An Analysis of Patients Presenting Complaints," *American Sociological Review,* Vol. 31, No. 5 (October 1966), pp. 615–30. T. A. Lambo has written a provocative article, "Adolescents Transplanted from Their Traditional Environment: Problems and Lessons out of Africa," *Clinical Pediatrics,* Vol. 6, No. 7 (July 1967), pp. 438–45, showing how adolescents change markedly when moved from an environment they understand to one that confuses them. And René and Jean Dubos have written a fascinating chapter in Berton Roueche, ed., *Curiosities of Medicine* (Boston: Little, Brown, 1963) that tells about tuberculosis and romanticism.

How cultural stress causes disease is explored in a rather technical fashion in *Harold G. Wolff's Stress and Disease,* rev. and ed. by Stewart Wolf and Helen Goodell, 2nd ed. (Springfield, Ill.: Charles C Thomas, 1968).

Too often, ill health is a problem of poverty. For an examination of poverty in this country, the following are suggested:

Arthur I. Blaustein and Roger R. Woock, eds., *Man Against Poverty: World War III* (New York: Random House, 1968, also in paperback).

Louis A. Ferman, Joyce L. Kornbluh, and Alan Haber, eds., *Poverty in America* (Ann Arbor: University of Michigan Press, 1966, also in paperback).

Martin Luther King, Jr., *Where Do We Go from Here: Chaos or Community* (New York: Harper & Row, 1967, also in paperback, Bantam).

Oscar Lewis, *The Children of Sánchez* (New York: Random House, 1961).

———, "The Culture of Poverty," *Scientific American,* Vol. 215, No. 4 (October 1966), pp. 20–25.

———, *Pedro Martinez: A Mexican Peasant and His Family* (New York: Random House, 1964).

———, *Study in Slum Control* (New York: Random House, 1968).

———, *La Vida* (New York: Random House, 1966, also in paperback).

A bibliography on poverty and health is available in Patricia A. Leo and George Rosen's "A Bookshelf on Poverty and Health," *American Journal of Public Health,* Vol. 59, No. 4 (April 1969), pp. 591–607. In addition, an interesting group of nine articles on poverty as it relates to emotional problems is to be found in a section appropriately titled "The Dark Side of the Moon: Poverty, Children, and Psychosis" in *Mental Hygiene,* Vol. 53, No. 4 (October 1969), pp. 497–549. Also suggested is an article by Lawrence Bergner and Alonzo S. Yerby, "Low Income and Barriers to Use of Health Services," *New England Journal of Medicine,* Vol. 278, No. 10 (March 7, 1968), pp. 541–46. Kenneth B. Clark and Jeannette Hopkins' *A Relevant War Against Poverty* (New York: Harper & Row, 1969) is a good descriptive discussion of a community action program to combat this "mother of all diseases." Nor may one disregard Gunnar Myrdal's monumental study of poverty, *Asian Drama,* 3 vols. (New York: Twentieth Century Fund, 1968).

3. Man versus man: waters of affliction and ill winds

A study of man's efforts to control the environment is provided by W. M. S. Russell in *Man, Nature and History* (Garden City, N.Y.: Doubleday, 1969). A general source for further study of environmental pollution is a compilation of articles ed. by William L. Thomas, Jr., *Man's Role in Changing the Face of the Earth* (Chicago: University of Chicago Press, 1956). Although dated, it is full of valuable information still applicable to today's problems. Other references of a general nature include two provocative articles: René Dubos, "Adapting to Pollution," *Scientist and Citizen,* Vol. 10, No. 1 (January–February 1968), pp. 1–8, and Philip H. Abelson, "Man-Made Environmental Hazards: How Man Shapes His Environment," *American Journal of Public Health,* Vol. 58, No. 11 (November 1968), pp. 2043–49. In the same issue of the latter journal, Ron M. Linton and Frank M. Stead have addressed themselves specifically to the problems of restoration of the ecological balance. Both Linton in "What We Must Do—Politically and Socially—to Restore the Environment," pp. 2055–59, and Stead in "What Man Can Do Technologically to Restore His Environment," pp. 2050–54, expose the complex nature of the problem of environmental control. Three recent volumes discussing environment and planning were published as a result of meetings of the American Institute of Planners' Fiftieth Year Consultation: *Environment for Man: The Next Fifty Years* (Bloomington: Indiana University Press, 1967, also in paperback), *Environment and Change: The Next Fifty Years* (Bloomington: Indiana University Press, 1968, also in paperback), and *Environment and Policy: The Next Fifty Years* (Bloomington: Indiana University Press, 1967, also in paperback), all ed. by William R. Ewald, Jr.

More specific treatment of air pollution can be obtained in Robert and Leona Train Rienow, *Moment in the Sun* (New York: Dial Press, 1967); a succinct presentation of the problem is found in Abel Wolman's article, "Air Pollution: Time for Appraisal," *Science,* Vol. 159, No. 3822 (March 29, 1968), pp. 1437–40. A fundamental article for research into solid wastes is Melvin W. First, "Urban Solid-Waste Management," *New England Journal of Medicine,* Vol. 275, No. 26 (December 29, 1966), pp. 1478–85. Athelstan Spilhaus' "Environmental Hazards, Urban Solid-Waste Management," *Scientist and Citizen,* Vol. 9, Nos. 9 and 10 (November and December 1967), pp. 219–23, is also available.

Students of water pollution would want to investigate the contents of three separate articles: Earl G. Howard's "That Dirty Mess: Water Pollution," *Today's Health,* Vol. 44, No. 3 (March 1966), pp. 53–60, is nontechnical; of a slightly more technical nature is Howard B. Gotas, "Outwitting the Patient Assassin: The Human Use of Lake Pollution," *Bulletin of the Atomic Scientists,* Vol. 25, No. 5 (May 1969), pp. 8–10, and Richard L. Woodward, "Environmental Hazards, Water Pollution," *New England Journal of Medicine,* Vol. 275, No. 15 (October 13, 1966), pp. 819–24.

Raymond L. Nace discusses the need for new directions in planning with regard to a precious resource in his article "Arrogance Toward the Landscape: A Problem in Water Planning," *Bulletin of the Atomic Scientists,* Vol. 25, No. 10 (December 1969), pp. 11–14. Robert H. Boyle has made a specific study of one river and its pollutions in *The Hudson River: A Natural and Unnatural History* (New York: W. W. Norton, 1969). A consideration of a recent water pollution problem is presented in a book ed. by David P. Hoult, *Oil on the Sea* (New York: Plenum, 1969). In this volume the Santa Barbara disaster is described and the latest developments in oil cleanup are discussed.

4. Man versus man: pesticides, radiation, noise, and accidents

For those interested in further study of pesticide effects and control, two supplements to the *American Journal of Public Health* may be helpful: *Man—His Environment and Health,* Vol. 54, No. 1 (January 1964), and *A Survey of Pesticide Problems and Control Activities,* Vol. 55, No. 7 (July 1965). Although both are dated, they still contain basic concepts of significance today. The recent publication of the 1968 Rochester Conference on Toxicity is especially valuable: *Chemical Fallout: Current Research on Persistent Pesticides,* by Morton W. Miller and George C. Berg (Springfield, Ill.: Charles C Thomas, 1969). The reasons for restricting the use of DDT are summarized in a brief article prepared by George Conway, "DDT on Balance," *Environment,* Vol. 11, No. 7 (September 1969), pp. 2–5. For some additional reading on the topic, the student may peruse Robert L. Rudd, *Pesticide and the Living Landscape* (Madison: University of Wisconsin Press, 1964, paperback); George M. Woodwell, "Toxic Substances and Ecological Cycles," *Scientific American,* Vol. 216, No. 3 (March 1967), pp. 24–31; and K. S. Khera and D. J. Clegg, "Perinatal Toxicity of Pesticides," *Canadian Medical Association Journal,* Vol. 100, No. 4 (January 25, 1969), pp. 167–72. The latter is particularly recommended.

Excellent discussions of radiation problems can be found in two articles: Ann B. Strong *et al.,* "Localization of Fallout in United States from the May 1966 Chinese Nuclear Test," *Public Health Reports,* Vol. 82, No. 6 (June 1967), pp. 487–95, and James G. Terrill, "Microwaves, Lasers, and X-rays," *Archives of Environmental Health,* Vol. 19, No. 2 (August 1969), pp. 265–71.

There is growing emphasis on the deleterious nature of some sound. Several concerned authors have imaginatively exposed some adverse consequences of conditions of unusual sound magnitudes. Suggested writings are:

Donald F. Anthrop, "Environmental Noise Pollution: A New Threat to Sanity," *Bulletin of the Atomic Scientists,* Vol. 25, No. 5 (May 1969), pp. 11–16.

Robert Alex Baron, "Noise and Urban Man," *American Journal of Public Health,* Vol. 58, No. 11 (November 1968), pp. 2060–66.

Clifford R. Bragdon, "Noise, a Syndrome of Modern Society," *Scientist and Citizen,* Vol. 10, No. 2 (March 1968), pp. 29–37.

Alan R. Freedman, "Rock 'n' Roll Music: Harmful?" *Clinical Pediatrics,* Vol. 8, No. 2 (February 1969), p. 58.

David P. Lipscomb, "High Intensity Sounds in the Recreational Environment: Hazard to Young Ears," *Clinical Pediatrics,* Vol. 8, No. 2 (February 1969), pp. 63–68.

John Gabriel Navarra, *Our Noisy World* (Garden City, N.Y.: Doubleday, 1969).

Colin A. Ronan, *The Meaning of Sound* (London: Weidenfeld & Nicolson, 1967).

Samuel Rosen *et al.,* "Presbycusis Study of a Relatively Noise-Free Population in the Sudan," *Annals of Otology, Rhinology and Laryngology,* Vol. 71, No. 3 (September 1962), pp. 727–43.

Ralph R. Rupp and Larry J. Koch, "Effects of Too-Loud Music on Human Ears. But, Mother, Rock 'n' Roll HAS to Be Loud!" *Clinical Pediatrics,* Vol. 8, No. 2 (February 1969), pp. 60–62.

Frank L. Seleney and Michael Streczyn, "Noise Characteristics in the Baby Compartment of Incubators," *American Journal of Diseases of Children,* Vol. 117, No. 10 (April 1969), pp. 445–50.

L. K. Smith, "Noise in the News," *Canadian Journal of Public Health,* Vol. 60, No. 8 (August 1969), pp. 299–306.

Further information on accidental injury and death can be found in such readings as Don Macdonald's article "All About Tires," *Westways,* Vol. 61, No. 3 (March 1969), pp. 28–31, 47, and a report on why the young male driver seems to be the perennial cause of high insurance rates: Stanley H. Schuman *et al.,* "Young Male Drivers: Impulse Expression, Accidents, and Violations," *Journal of the American Medical Association,* Vol. 200, No. 12 (June 19, 1967), pp. 1026–30. Also recommended are G. Anthony Ryan, "Injuries in Traffic Accidents," *New England Journal of Medicine,* Vol. 276, No. 19 (May 11, 1967), pp. 1066–76, and Melvin L. Selzer, Joseph E. Rogers, and Sue Kern, "Fatal Accidents: The Role of Psychopathology, Social Stress, and Acute Disturbance," *American Journal of Psychiatry,* Vol. 124, No. 8 (February 1968), pp. 1028–36.

Of interest to skiers is an article by Daniel E. Curtin, "Injuries Peculiar to Skiing," *Journal of School Health,* Vol. 37, No. 10 (December 1967), pp. 518–21. Another type of accident about which there ought to be required reading is poisoning among children. Henry L. Venhulst and John J. Crotty offer a valuable discussion in "Childhood Poisoning Accidents," *Journal of the American Medical Association,* Vol. 203, No. 12 (March 18, 1968), pp. 1049–50.

5. Disease and destiny

An excellent source of historical material about the effect of disease on history is the *Bulletin of the History of Medicine.* This journal began publication in 1939, having superseded the *Bulletin of the Institute of the History of Medicine* published by Johns Hopkins University from 1933 through 1938. Recommended useful books date back to S. H. Garrison, *Introduction to the History of Medicine,* 4th ed. (Philadelphia: W. B. Saunders, 1929). Other dated but informative volumes include Arturo Castiglioni, *A History of Medicine,* tr. and ed. by E. B. Krumbhaar, 2nd ed. rev. and enl. (New York: Alfred A. Knopf, 1947), and three books by Henry E. Sigerist: *Civilization and Disease* (Ithaca, N.Y.: Cornell University Press, 1944); *History of American Medicine* (New York: W. W. Norton, 1934); and *A History of*

Medicine (New York: Oxford University Press, 1951). Victor Robinson's *The Story of Medicine* (Philadelphia: Blakiston, 1943) is also valuable; it is a fascinating presentation that can be read with pleasure.

For more specific information about widespread disease movements, read Charles Creighton's classic *A History of Epidemics in Britain*, 2 vols., 2nd ed. (New York: Barnes & Noble, 1965); Paul H. De Kruif, *Man Against Death* (New York: Harcourt, Brace & World, 1932); and Berton Roueche, *Annals of Epidemiology* (Boston: Little, Brown, 1967, also in paperback). Evidence of residual existence of a once-devastating disease such as the plague crops up in occasional articles, for example, Joseph L. Caton and Leo Kartman, "Human Plague in the U.S.," *Journal of the American Medical Association*, Vol. 205, No. 6 (August 5, 1968), pp. 81–84, and J. D. Marshall *et al.*, "Plague in Vietnam 1965–66," *American Journal of Epidemiology*, Vol. 86, No. 3 (November 1967), pp. 603–16. For an earlier account of the plague, see W. G. Bell, *The Great Plague in London in 1665* (London: The Bodley Head, 1924).

Some instances of the impact of disease on the history of mankind, the central topic of this chapter, are intriguingly recounted in Philip Marshall Dale, ed., *Medical Biographies: The Ailments of Thirty-three Famous Persons* (Norman: University of Oklahoma Press, 1952); Ralph H. Major, *Fatal Partners, War and Disease* (New York: Doubleday, 1941); and Hans Zinsser, *Rats, Lice and History* (Boston: Little, Brown, 1935). James Westfall Thompson in an article entitled "The Aftermath of the Black Death and the Aftermath of the Great War," *American Journal of Sociology*, Vol. 26, No. 7 (January 1921), pp. 565–72 provides an excellent example of the effect of disasters upon society.

6. Man's smallest enemies: the agents of communicable sickness

A number of basic texts, though detailed, serve as fundamental references for the study of microorganism life and man's efforts at controlling it. Three are recommended: Lenor S. Goerke *et al.*, eds., *Mustard's Introduction to Public Health*, 5th ed. (New York: Macmillan, 1968), Chapters 8 and 9; Philip E. Sartwell, ed., *Preventive Medicine and Public Health*, 9th ed. (New York: Appleton-Century-Crofts, 1965), Section II; and Franklin H. Top, *Communicable and Infectious Diseases*, 6th ed. (St. Louis: C. V. Mosby, 1968).

A way of keeping up to date on late statistical compilations and recent discoveries in communicable diseases is through publications of the Public Health Service (U.S. Department of Health, Education, and Welfare) such as monographs, bulletins, and the *Morbidity and Mortality Weekly Reports*. Nation-wide and world-wide views in this field can be obtained through such associations as the National Tuberculosis and Respiratory Disease Association and through special editions of *World Health*, the magazine of the World Health Organization. WHO also publishes several technical health materials of value.

Some very readable presentations for the layman on microbiology are found in John M. Adams, *Viruses and Colds: The Modern Plague* (New York: American Elsevier, 1967); Hubert A. Lechevalier and Morris Solotorovsky, *Three Centuries of Microbiology* (New York: McGraw-Hill,

1965, also in paperback); and Paul D. Thompson, *The Virus Realm* (Philadelphia: J. B. Lippincott, 1968). All are pleasureable reading. For historical accounts of the discovery of specific microbes, the reader may wish to refer to Paul De Kruif, *Microbe Hunters* (New York: Harcourt, Brace & World, 1932, also in paperback); Richard Dunlop, *Doctors of the American Frontier* (Garden City, N.Y.: Doubleday, 1965); Berton Roueche, *Eleven Blue Men* (New York: Berkley, 1947, paperback) and his *The Incurable Wound* (New York: Berkley, 1954, paperback); and Greer Williams' now dated, but still informative, *Virus Hunters* (New York: Alfred A. Knopf, 1959).

Harry R. Hill *et al.* traced a specific epidemic, offering an excellent example of epidemiological methods of detection of communicable disease, in a recent article entitled "Food-borne Epidemic of Streptococcal Pharyngitis at the United States Air Force Academy," *New England Journal of Medicine*, Vol. 280, No. 17 (April 24, 1969), pp. 917–21.

A letter to the editor in the *American Review of Respiratory Diseases*, Vol. 96, No. 4 (October 1967), pp. 830–31, presents a specific statement of the position of twenty-one physicians who endorse BCG vaccination. A concise review of the clinical effects of viruses upon the unborn baby is offered in an article by Janet B. Hardy, "Viruses and the Fetus," *Postgraduate Medicine*, Vol. 43, No. 1 (January 1968), pp. 156–65. A much larger enemy of mankind is discussed in a rather technical book by P. F. Mattingly, *The Biology of Mosquito-Borne Disease* (New York: American Elsevier, 1970). And a nontechnical volume concerned with the infectious diseases of childhood by Samuel Karelitz, *When Your Child Is Ill* (New York: Random House, 1969), answers over 1,000 questions pertaining to childhood communicable diseases. Finally, for those who seek a sophisticated review of a single disease as it is being conquered in this country, a two-part book by Anthony M. Lowell, Lydia B. Edwards, and Carroll E. Palmer is recommended: *I. Tuberculosis Morbidity and Mortality and Its Control* and *II. Tuberculosis Infection* (Cambridge, Mass.: Harvard University Press, 1969).

7. Of structure, function, and chronic impairments thereto: part I

A scholarly, well-illustrated text on structural and functional physiology is Fritz Kahn, *Man in Structure and Function*, tr. and ed. by George Rosen, 2 vols. (New York: Alfred A. Knopf, 1960). A relatively small book (432 pages) ed. by Barry G. King and Mary Jane Showers, *Human Anatomy and Physiology* (Philadelphia: W. B. Saunders, 1969), concisely presents material that is excellently illustrated and is valuable to the beginning student. One might add to this list Helen Dawson's clear text *Basic Human Anatomy* (New York: Appleton-Century-Crofts, 1966); Ernest Gardner, Donald J. Gray, and Rohan O'Rahilly, *Anatomy* (Philadelphia: W. B. Saunders, 1961); and J. C. Boileau Grant and J. V. Basmajian, *Grant's Method of Anatomy*, 7th ed. (Baltimore: Williams & Wilkins, 1965).

Some famous anatomy texts for the advanced student include the following:

Charles H. Best and N. B. Taylor, *The Human Body: Its Anatomy and Physiology*, 4th ed. (New York: Holt, Rinehart and Winston, 1963).

Charles H. Best and N. B. Taylor, *The Living Body: A Text in Human Physiology,* 4th ed. (New York: Holt, Rinehart and Winston, 1958).

Daniel J. Cunningham, *Manual of Practical Anatomy,* 3 vols., rev. and ed. by G. J. Romanes, 13th ed. (New York: Oxford University Press, 1966–68).

Daniel J. Cunningham, *Textbook of Anatomy,* ed. by G. J. Romanes, 10th ed. (New York: Oxford University Press, 1964).

Henry Gray, *Anatomy of the Human Body,* 25th ed. (Philadelphia: Lea & Febiger, 1948).

Sir Henry Morris, *Human Anatomy: A Complete Systemic Treatise,* ed. by Barry J. Anson and Robert Laughlin Rea, 12th ed. (New York: McGraw-Hill, 1966).

For up-to-date references about chronic impairments, turn to the publications of such specialized organizations as the American Cancer Society, which publishes the monthly *CA—A Cancer Journal for Clinicians* and a yearly report, *Cancer Facts and Figures.* The National Advisory Cancer Council (U.S. Department of Health, Education, and Welfare) prepares a yearly report on the latest findings about cancer, easily understood by the intelligent layman and entitled *Progress Against Cancer.*

Up-to-date facts about incidence and control of cancer are to be found in specific articles. On cancer of the cervix, for example, the following writings are recommended: W. A. D. Anderson and Samuel A. Gunn, "Cancer of the Cervix. Further Studies of Patient-Obtained Vaginal Irrigation Smear," *CA—A Cancer Journal for Clinicians,* Vol. 17, No. 3 (May–June 1967), pp. 102–04; William M. Christopherson, "Sex Activity and Cancer of the Cervix," *CA—A Cancer Journal for Clinicians,* Vol. 15, No. 6 (November–December 1965), pp. 278–82; and Clyde E. Martin, "Marital and Coital Factors in Cervical Cancer," *American Journal of Public Health,* Vol. 57, No. 5 (May 1967), pp. 803–14. C. K. Wanebo *et al.* report on the relation of cancer and radiation in "Breast Cancer After Exposure to the Atomic Bombings of Hiroshima and Nagasaki," *New England Journal of Medicine,* Vol. 279, No. 13 (September 26, 1968), pp. 667–71. Robert G. Freeman and John M. Knox provide additional data on sun radiation in "Skin Cancer and the Sun," *CA—A Cancer Journal for Clinicians,* Vol. 17, No. 5 (September–October 1967), pp. 231–38.

Richard Doll's *Prevention of Cancer: Pointers from Epidemiology* (London: Whitefriars Press, 1967), a brief discourse for the serious student of patterns of occurrence of cancer, is recommended, although it is already out of date. Another already dated but excellent review is *A Synopsis of Cancer* (Baltimore: Williams & Wilkins, 1966). A succinct report of the new directions in cancer research is that of Fred Rapp and Joseph L. Melnick, "The Footprints of Tumor Viruses," *Scientific American,* Vol. 214, No. 3 (March 1966), pp. 34–41.

8. Of structure, function, and chronic impairments thereto: part II

A student who wishes to supplement fundamental information on structure and function of the circulatory and urinary systems should refer to two excellent basic texts: John Field, ed.-in-chief, *Handbook of Physiology,* 2 vols. (Baltimore: Williams & Wilkins, 1963) and R. F. Pitts, *Physiology of the Kidney and Body Fluids* (Chicago: Year Book Medical, 1968). Less technical general information on the heart can be obtained by perusing Alton L. Blakeslee and Jeremiah Stamler, *Your Heart Has Nine Lives* (Englewood Cliffs, N.J.: Prentice-Hall, 1963); this is a sound discussion aimed at the intelligent lay reader. Also informative is Menard Gertler, *You Can Predict Your Heart Attack and Prevent It* (New York: Random House, 1963). Lawrence E. Lamb's *Your Heart and How To Live with It* (New York: Viking Press, 1969) and Yehuda Kesten's *Diary of a Heart Patient* (New York: McGraw-Hill, 1968) are also interesting reading.

Some more limited topics are treated in specific articles. An editorial in the *Journal of the American Medical Association,* Vol. 200, No. 2 (April 10, 1967), pp. 173–74, discusses "Exercise and Heart Disease." A fine article by Bernard Lown, "Intensive Heart Care," *Scientific American,* Vol. 219, No. 1 (July 1968), pp. 19–27, details the considerations in intensive heart care. Atherosclerosis is discussed with clarity in Alfred Kershbaum and Samuel Bellet, "Smoking as a Factor in Atherosclerosis," *Geriatrics,* Vol. 21, No. 12 (December 1966), pp. 155–70, and in David M. Spain, "Atherosclerosis," *Scientific American,* Vol. 215, No. 2 (August 1966), pp. 49–56.

Some related features of coronary heart disease are those of emotional stress, smoking, and socioeconomic status. These relationships are considered in Lawrence E. Hinkle, Jr., "Occupation, Education, and Coronary Heart Disease," *Science,* Vol. 161 (July 19, 1968), pp. 238–46; in Henry I. Russek, "Role of Emotional Stress in the Etiology of Clinical Coronary Heart Disease," *Diseases of the Chest,* Vol. 52, No. 1 (July 1967), pp. 1–9; and in Carl C. Seltzer, "An Evaluation of the Effect of Smoking on Coronary Heart Disease," *Journal of the American Medical Association,* Vol. 203, No. 3 (January 15, 1968), pp. 127–34.

Three articles describe anatomical details in a highly readable fashion. The electrical system of the heart is graphically presented in E. F. Adolph, "The Heart's Pacemaker," *Scientific American,* Vol. 216, No. 3 (March 1967), pp. 32–37; the lung, in Julius H. Comroe, Jr., "The Lung," *Scientific American,* Vol. 214, No. 2 (February 1966), pp. 56–68; and the venous system, in J. Edwin Wood, "The Venous System," *Scientific American,* Vol. 218, No. 1 (January 1968), pp. 86–96.

Valuable, well researched (albeit technical) studies on heart disease include Len Hughes Andrus *et al.,* "Epidemiological Study of Coronary Disease Risk Factors," *American Journal of Epidemiology,* Vol. 87, No. 1 (January 1968), pp. 73–86; Frederick H. Epstein, "Predicting Coronary Heart Disease," *Journal of the American Medical Association,* Vol. 201, No. 11 (September 11, 1967), pp. 117–21; and Menard Gertler, H. H. Whiter, and J. J. Welsh, "Assessing the Coronary Profile," *Geriatrics,* Vol. 22, No. 2 (February 1967), pp. 121–32. All are methodologically interesting investigations.

Of unique interest are Edward F. Bland and Gilbert W. Beebe's article of traumatic injuries to the heart, "Missiles in the Heart, A Twenty-year Followup Report of World War II Cases," *New England Journal of Medicine,* Vol. 274, No. 19 (May 12, 1966), pp. 1039–46, and J. P. Merrill's article "The Artificial Kidney," *Scientific American,* Vol. 205, No. 1 (July 1961), pp. 56–65.

9. Nourishment

Hunger and malnutrition are world-wide problems. Two articles bring this international scope to the fore: Jacques M. May and Hoyt Lemons, "The Ecology of Malnutrition," *Journal of the American Medical Association,* Vol. 207, No. 13 (March 31, 1969), pp. 2401–05, and N. W. Pirie, "Orthodox and Unorthodox Methods of Meeting World Food Needs," *Scientific American,* Vol. 216, No. 2 (February 1967), pp. 27–35. Also highly recommended is T George Harris, "Affluence: The Fifth Horseman of the Apocalypse," *Psychology Today,* Vol. 3, No. 8 (January 1970); in this highly provocative interview one of this nation's leading nutritionists, Jean Mayer, states, "It's the spread of wealth that threatens the environment just as it's the spread of fat that threatens the lives of so many Americans . . . It's the rich who wreck the environment." This article is stimulating and worth much reflection.

General information is available in four books. Graham Lusk presents a brief history of nutrition in *Nutrition* (New York: Hafner, 1964, also in paperback). Ethel Austin Martin's *Nutrition in Action,* 2nd ed. (New York: Holt, Rinehart and Winston, 1965) is written in a relaxed, easily understandable style. Helen S. Mitchell *et al., Cooper's Nutrition in Health and Disease,* 15th ed. (Philadelphia: J. B. Lippincott, 1968) remains a basic text, as does the very important compilation of articles ed. by Nevin S. Scrimshaw and John E. Gordon, *Malnutrition, Learning, and Behavior* (Cambridge, Mass.: M.I.T. Press, 1968). Those who wish to explore one major aspect of nutrition thoroughly will find John Mark's small volume *The Vitamins in Health and Disease* (Boston: Little, Brown, 1969) worthwhile. Much less technical is David N. Locke, *Enzymes: The Agents of Life* (New York: Crown, 1969).

Overweight is provocatively discussed by Jean Mayer in *Overweight* (Englewood Cliffs, N.J.: Prentice-Hall, 1968, paperback). This book is highly recommended. Nevin S. Scrimshaw's "Infant Malnutrition and Adult Learning," *Saturday Review* (March 16, 1968), pp. 64–66 and 83–84, presents a discourse on the most recent studies in malnutrition. A discussion of body image disturbances can be found in Albert J. Stunkard, "Body Image Disturbance in Obesity," *Feelings and Their Medical Significance,* Vol. 10, No. 1 (January–February 1968), pp. 1–4.

Finally, those who wish entertaining reading on nutrition may peruse Hector Bolitho's compilation *The Glorious Oyster* (London: Sidgwick & Jackson, 1960) for an erudite, fascinating history of man's appetite for the oyster. A splendid, illustrated history of cooking is William Harlan Hale and the editors of *Horizon* Magazine, *The Horizon Cookbook and Illustrated History of Eating and Drinking Through the Ages* (Garden City, N.Y.: Doubleday, 1968). It is both entertaining and informative. Ronald M. Deutsch's *The Nuts Among the Berries: An Exposé of America's Food Fads* (New York: Ballantine, 1961, paperback) is an entertaining and accurate book on faddisms in foods.

A second topic of this chapter, dentistry, may be further investigated in Abraham E. Nizel, ed., *The Science of Nutrition and Its Application in Clinical Dentistry,* 2nd ed. (Philadelphia: W. B. Saunders, 1966). For historical background, John Menzies Campbell's *From a Trade to a Profession: Byways in Dental History* (Alva, Scot.: Robert Cunningham and Sons, 1958) can be recommended.

Further information about quackery can be found in Gerald Carson, *One for a Man, Two for a Horse* (Garden City, N.Y.: Doubleday, 1961). It is a superbly illustrated book on quacks of the past. Discussion of quackery in the present age is set forth in Viola W. Bernard, "Why People Become the Victims of Medical Quackery," *American Journal of Public Health,* Vol. 55, No. 3 (August 1965), pp. 1142–47, and in a series of five articles compiled under the title "Fighting Space-Age Quackery," *Today's Health,* Vol. 44, No. 12 (December 1966), pp. 50–53. The articles are: William H. Gordon, "Why People Go to Quacks," pp. 50–51; James L. Goddard, "Quackery in the Market Place," pp. 51–52; H. Thomas Ballantine, "Medicine and Chiropractic," p. 52; Mrs. Winthrop Rockefeller, "Mental Health and Counseling," pp. 52–53; and John W. Miner, "The Costs of Quackery," p. 53.

10. The emotional life

Further reading on topics in this chapter calls for an international perspective. Jerome D. Frank discusses the psychiatrist's relationship to international politics in his provocative article "The Psychiatrist and International Affairs," *Journal of Nervous and Mental Disease,* Vol. 114, No. 6 (June 1967), pp. 479–84. T. A. Lambo writes of "Socio-economic Change, Population Explosion and the Changing Phases of Mental Health Programs in Developing Countries," *American Journal of Orthopsychiatry,* Vol. 36, No. 1 (January 1966), pp. 77–89, with an insightful cross-cultural viewpoint, and Bryant Wedge, "Psychiatry and International Affairs," *U.S. Navy Medical News Letter,* Vol. 50, No. 6 (September 22, 1967), pp. 7–12, briefly presents another viewpoint about psychiatry's international responsibilities.

A historical book of a basic nature is Franz G. Alexander and Sheldon T. Selesnick, *The History of Psychiatry* (New York: Harper & Row, 1966). Paul J. Stern's *The Abnormal Person and His World* (New York: Van Nostrand Reinhold, 1964) is a brief text on emotional problems. Anna Freud has delimited the concept of personality more sharply than her famous father in her slender book, *Ego and the Mechanisms of Defense,* tr. by Cecil Baines (New York: International Universities Press, 1946). A recent selection of contributions towards the understanding of both normal and disturbed children is *Annual Progress in Child Psychiatry and Child Development—1968,* ed. by Stella Chess and Alexander Thomas (New York: Brunner/Mazel, 1969). Similarly interesting is an account of emotionally sick patients who have emerged from the hospital: William W. Michaux *et al., The First Year Out* (Baltimore: Johns Hopkins Press, 1969).

More specific topics are pursued by the following selected authors. Their articles exemplify the wide range of subjects now considered in the study of child development and growth in emotional life from infancy through adolescence. Bruno Bettelheim's unforgettable "Joey: A 'Mechanical Boy,'" *Scientific American,* Vol. 200, No. 3 (March 1959), pp. 119–27, depicts the shell of a boy devoid of emotional responsiveness. Erik H. Erikson should never be disregarded, for his theory about the development of personal identity during the psychosexual stages of life is classic; it can be further studied in his *Childhood and Society* (New York: W. W. Norton, 1950). R. S. Illingworth writes interestingly on "Punishment: A Personal View and Historical Perspective," *Clinical Pediatrics,* Vol. 7, No. 10 (October

1968), pp. 577–82. Also recommended is Sylvia Brody, *Patterns of Mothering* (New York: International Universities Press, 1967).

The following articles about the adolescent period and the few years beyond should particularly interest the college student. Two articles on crises are especially recommended: Henry W. Brosin, "Adolescent Crises," *New York State Journal of Medicine*, Vol. 67, No. 14 (July 15, 1967), pp. 2003–11, and Robert M. Counts, "Family Crises and the Impulsive Adolescent," *Archives of General Psychiatry*, Vol. 17, No. 1 (July 1967), pp. 64–71. Seymour L. Halleck's "Psychiatric Treatment of the Alienated College Student," *American Journal of Psychiatry*, Vol. 124, No. 5 (November 1967), pp. 642–50, and Armand M. Nicholi, Jr.'s "Harvard Dropouts: Some Psychiatric Findings," *American Journal of Psychiatry*, Vol. 124, No. 5, (November 1967), pp. 651–58, are other relevant articles. A valuable volume for parents is *How to Raise a Human Being* by Lee Salk and Rita Kramer (New York: Random House, 1969); problems of infancy through adolescence are discussed with wisdom and insight. An entire symposium of the Second Annual New York Congress for Mental Health was devoted to "The Adolescent Crises Today," *New York State Journal of Medicine*, Vol. 67, No. 14 (July 15, 1967), pp. 1979–81. Lewis L. Judd writes of "The Normal Psychological Development of the American Adolescent," *California Medicine*, Vol. 107, No. 6 (December 1967), pp. 465–70; a similar topic is taken up by Tom Hickey and Richard A. Kalish in "Young People's Perception of Adults," *Journal of Gerontology*, Vol. 23, No. 2 (April 1968), pp. 215–19. The latter article reflects upon how the adolescent looks out on his world. The July 1968 issue of *Mental Health* (Vol. 52, No. 3) is entitled "Focus on the Young." It contains almost two dozen articles considering the emotional problems of young people of various ages.

A timeless yet timely topic is investigated in David Abrahamsen, "A Study of Lee Harvey Oswald: Psychological Capability of Murder," *Bulletin of the New York Academy of Medicine*, Vol. 43, No. 10 (October 1967), pp. 861–88. It is likely to be of interest to the student who reads broadly.

Articles on deviant emotional conditions such as suicide, mental illness, and sexual deviation abound. Four articles on "Suicide and Its Prevention" make up an entire section of *Mental Hygiene*, Vol. 53, No. 3 (July 1969), pp. 340–63. The articles are: David Lester, "Suicidal Behavior in Men and Women," Richard Singer and Irving Blumenthal, "Suicide Clues in Psychotic Patients," Robert Jarmusz, "Some Considerations in Establishing a Suicide Prevention Service," and I. William Weiner, "The Effectiveness of a Suicide Prevention Program."

Further recommended readings on suicide include the following:

A. E. Bennett, "Recognizing the Potential Suicide," *Geriatrics*, Vol. 22, No. 5 (May 1967), pp. 175–81.

Graham B. Blaine, Jr., and Lida R. Carmen, "Causal Factors in Suicidal Attempts by Male and Female College Students," *American Journal of Psychiatry*, Vol. 125, No. 6 (December 1968), pp. 834–37.

Herbert Hendin, *Black Suicide* (New York: Basic Books, 1969).

George E. Murphy and Eli Robins, "Social Factors in Suicide," *Journal of the American Medical Association*, Vol. 199, No. 5 (January 30, 1967), pp. 81–86.

Philip Solomon, "The Burden of Responsibility in Suicide and Homicide," *Journal of the American Medical Association*, Vol. 199, No. 5 (January 30, 1967), pp. 99–102.

"Suicide Attempts Increase Minute by Minute: Prevention Centers Total Sixty-three," an editorial in the *Journal of the American Medical Association*, Vol. 204, No. 2 (April 8, 1968), pp. 24–25.

Discussions on sexual deviance can be pursued in these selections:

Alfred Auerback, "Understanding Sexual Deviation," *Postgraduate Medicine:* Part I in Vol. 42, No. 8 (February 1968), pp. 125–29; Part II in Vol. 42, No. 9 (March 1968), pp. 169–73.

Daniel Cappon, "Understanding Homosexuality," *Postgraduate Medicine*, Vol. 42, No. 4 (October 1967), pp. A-131–36.

Harvey E. Kaye *et al.*, "Homosexuality in Women," *Archives of General Psychiatry*, Vol. 17, No. 5 (November 1967), pp. 626–34.

H. M. Ruitenbeek, ed., *The Problem of Homosexuality in Modern Society* (New York: E. P. Dutton, 1963, paperback).

William Simon and John Gagnon, "Sexual Deviance in Contemporary America," *Annals of the American Academy of Political and Social Science*, Edward Sangarin, ed., Vol. 376, 1968, and William Simon and John Gagnon, eds., *Sexual Deviance, A Reader* (New York: Harper & Row, 1967, paperback).

Ralph Slovenko, ed., *Sexual Behavior and the Law*, (Springfield, Ill.: Charles C Thomas, 1965).

Typical of the available bibliographies is that on the "Battered Child Syndrome," consisting of 78 citations in the New Bibliographic Series No. 15–65 (Washington, D.C.: National Library of Medicine, Mid-1963–July 1965).

11.   Anxieties in the 1970s

One topic for further reading arising from this chapter is that of authority and control. A fascinating study is reported by Donald J. Marcuse in "The 'Army' Incident: The Psychology of Uniforms and Their Abolition on an Adolescent Ward," *Psychiatry: A Journal for the Study of Interpersonal Processes*, Vol. 30, No. 4 (November 1967), pp. 350–75. Also relevant is an article by Stanley Milgram, "Some Conditions of Obedience and Disobedience to Authority," *International Journal of Psychiatry*, Vol. 6, No. 4 (October 1968), pp. 259–76. A comparison of animal and human control is developed in Joseph P. Coogan's article, "The Remote Control of Animal Behavior," *SK&F Psychiatric Reporter*, No. 39, (July–August 1968), pp. 21–23. Five companion articles collectively entitled "The Child" in *Saturday Review* (December 7, 1968) examine various aspects of a child's concerns. The articles are: N. J. Berrill, "His Ancient Inheritance," pp. 71–73; John Lear, "His Momentary Ancestor," pp. 73–75; Carlo Valenti, "His Right To Be Normal," pp. 75–77; Robert E. Hall, "His Birth Without Permission," pp. 78–79; and Jerome Kagan, "His Struggle for Identity," pp. 80–82, 87–88.

On the subject of parents, read David Belais Friedman, "Parent Development," *California Medicine,* Vol. 86, No. 1 (January 1957), pp. 25–28. Haim G. Ginott's two small books *Between Parent and Child* (New York: Macmillan, 1965, also in paperback, Avon) and *Between Parent and Teenager* (New York: Macmillan, 1969) are insightful, humane treatises.

Student protest also brings its anxieties to bear upon the citizens of the 1970s—if not upon students, at least upon those in authority. Kenneth Keniston has written two revealing books in this area: *Uncommitted: Alienated Youth in American Society* (New York: Harcourt, Brace & World, 1965, also in paperback) and *Young Radicals: Notes on Committed Youth* (New York: Harcourt, Brace & World, 1968, also in paperback). Erich Fromm's fine *Revolution of Hope* (New York: Harper & Row, 1968, also in paperback, Bantam) is also recommended. Anthropologist Margaret Mead has written provocatively about the generation gap in *Culture and Commitment* (Garden City, N.Y.: Doubleday, 1970). Also of interest is a collection ed. by G. K. Smith, *Stress and Campus Response: Current Issues in Higher Education* (San Francisco: Jossey-Bass, 1968). Some analyses may be found in three articles by Seymour Halleck: "The Roots of Student Despair," *Think,* Vol. 33, No. 2 (March–April 1957), pp. 22–23; "Why Students Protest: A Psychiatrist's View," *Think,* Vol. 33, No. 6 (November–December 1967), pp. 2–7; and "Why They'd Rather Do Their Own Thing," *Think,* Vol. 34, No. 5 (September–October 1968), pp. 2–7. Also recommended is Eugene Rabinowitch, "Student Rebellion: The Aimless Revolution?" *Bulletin of the Atomic Scientists,* Vol. 24, No. 7 (September 1968), pp. 7–10. Another provocative writer about youth is Robert E. Kavanaugh; see, for instance, his "The Grim Generation," *Psychology Today,* Vol. 2, No. 5 (October 1968), pp. 50–55.

The definition and search for love is a topic of major interest. A valuable book is Morton M. Hunt, *The Natural History of Love* (New York: Alfred A. Knopf, 1959). Also recommended is *Animal Social Psychology: A Reader of Experimental Studies* (New York: John Wiley & Sons, 1969), ed. by R. B. Zajonc. Two selections that are profound and provocative are Erich Fromm, *The Art of Loving* (New York: Harper & Row, 1951, also in paperback) and Harry F. Harlow's classic "The Nature of Love," *American Psychologist,* Vol. 13, No. 12 (December 1958), pp. 673–85. Erich Fromm's distinctions among the kinds of loving are renowned and Harry F. Harlow's study of mother love in monkeys provided landmark findings for the study of humans. Lawrence Casler provides a valuable listing in "Maternal Deprivation: A Critical Review of the Literature," *Monographs of the Society for Research in Child Development,* Vol. 26, No. 2 (1961), p. 64. A recent book by the distinguished psychotherapist Rollo May, *Love and Will* (New York: W. W. Norton, 1969), analyzes love and the role of will in its realization. Apathy, to May, is withdrawal of love and will; his sophisticated discussion is appropriate to these times.

Another concern for some in the 1970s is that generated by illegitimate pregnancy. Three articles are recommended: Jean Pakter and Frieda Nelson, "The Unmarried Mother and Her Child, the Problems and the Challenges" in National Council on Illegitimacy, *Illegitimacy: Data and Findings for Prevention, Treatment and Policy Formulation* (October 1965), pp. 31–50; Susan Strom, "The Schools and the Pregnant Teen-Ager," *Saturday Review* (September 16, 1967), pp. 80–81, 97–98; and Seymour Shubin, "The 'Forgotten' Men—A Program for Unmarried Fathers," *SK&F Psychiatric Reporter,* No. 37 (March–April 1968), pp. 8–9.

12. Drug dependence: escape into captivity

Those interested in investigating further the subject of drugs and other toxifying substances will find reports of current studies helpful. For example, the Public Health Service (U.S. Department of Health, Education, and Welfare) has issued *The Health Consequences of Smoking,* 1969 Supplement to the 1967 Public Health Service Review (Washington, D.C.: U.S. Government Printing Office, July 1, 1969) and *Alcohol and Alcoholism,* Public Health Service Publication No. 1640 (Washington, D.C.: U.S. Government Printing Office, 1967). Another source of information is the Cooperative Commission on the Study of Alcoholism, which has published Thomas F. A. Plaut, *Alcohol Problems—A Report to the Nation* (New York: Oxford University Press, 1967).

Thousands of articles on the subject of alcohol are available. Writings addressed to alcohol as a general and historical topic include J. C. Furnas, *The Life and Times of the Late Demon Rum* (New York: G. P. Putnam's Sons, 1965), and Donald Horton, "The Function of Alcohol in Primitive Societies," in *Alcohol, Science and Society* (New Haven, Conn.: Quarterly Journal of Studies on Alcohol, 1945, paperback). Other general discussions are found in Morris E. Chaefetz, *Liquor, the Servant of Man* (Boston: Little, Brown, 1965); Berton Roueche, *The Neutral Spirit, A Portrait of Alcohol* (New York: Harper & Row, 1960); and Norman Taylor, *Flight from Reality* (New York: Duell, Sloan & Pearce, 1949). Also recommended are Jorge Valles, *How to Live with an Alcoholic* (New York: Simon and Schuster, 1967), and Lincoln Williams, *Tomorrow Will Be Sober* (New York: Harper & Row, 1960). A book containing fuller data is David J. Pittman, ed., *Alcoholism in America* (New York: McGraw-Hill, 1966). An important article by J. A. Waller, "Alcoholism and Traffic Deaths," *New England Journal of Medicine,* Vol. 275, No. 10 (September 1966), pp. 532–36, reports on a relationship that is becoming more evident as methods of investigation become refined.

On the general topic of tobacco, readings such as the following are recommended: Alton Blakeslee, *It's Not Too Late to Stop Smoking Cigarettes,* Public Affairs Pamphlet No. 386 (New York: Public Affairs Committee, 1966); Eugene H. Guthrie, "What's Happened Since the Surgeon General's Report on Smoking and Health?" *American Journal of Public Health,* Vol. 56, No. 12 (December 1966), pp. 1–6; and Bernard Mausner and Ellen Platt, *Behavioral Aspects of Smoking: A Conference Report,* Health Education Monographs, Supplement No. 2 (Albany, N.Y.: Fort Orange Press, 1966).

In C. M. Fletcher *et al., Common Sense About Smoking* (Baltimore: Penguin, 1963, paperback), some behavioral aspects of smoking are described. Three authors who write on smoking among the young are: Arthur H. Cain, *Young People and Smoking* (New York: John Day, 1964); Dorothy Dunn, "Cigarettes and the College Freshman," *Journal of the American Medical Association,* Vol. 199, No. 1 (January 2, 1967), pp. 77–80; and Charles L. Leedham, "Pre-Teen Smokers," *Clinical Pediatrics,* Vol. 6, No. 3 (March 1967), pp. 135–36.

Harold S. Diehl's recent book, *Tobacco and Your Health: The Smoking Controversy* (New York: McGraw-Hill, 1969), reports factually about the positive relationship between smoking and disease. Two editorials in *Clinical Pediatrics,* "The Effects of Tobacco Smoking in Children," in Vol. 40, No. 3 (September 1967), p. 362, and "Smoking and Pregnancy," in Vol. 7, No. 10 (October 1968), p. 623, state the beliefs of most pediatricians.

Finally, the reader may wish to peruse E. Corti, *A History of Smoking,* tr. by Paul England (London: George G. Harrap, 1931), and an article on the advertising of cigarettes: Frederic C. Decker, "The Economic Effect of Reduced Cigarette Consumption on Advertising," *American Journal of Public Health,* Vol. 56, No. 12 (December 1966, supplement), pp. 29–32.

Drugs and other mood-modifying substances are considered in total in several books. Donald B. Louria's *The Drug Scene* (New York: McGraw-Hill, 1968) is a discussion with a historical and international flavor. Sidney Cohen's book, *The Drug Dilemma* (New York: McGraw-Hill, 1969), is a straightforward objective compendium of information. A worthwhile volume on the drug crisis and youth is Joel Fort, *The Pleasure Seekers* (Indianapolis: Bobbs-Merrill, 1969). An interesting appraisal of sedatives, tranquilizers, and stimulants is available in an article by Hugh J. Parry, "Use of Psychotropic Drugs by U.S. Adults," *Public Health Reports,* Vol. 83, No. 10 (October 1968), pp. 799–810. Kenneth Keniston, in his article "Heads and Seekers," *American Scholar,* Vol. 38, No. 1 (Winter 1968–69), pp. 97–112, discusses the problem of drugs on the campus.

The following list of articles attempts to provide interesting reading about a number of mood modifiers:

Amphetamines: John C. Kramer, V. S. Fischman, and Don C. Littlefield, "Amphetamine Abuse," *Journal of the American Medical Association,* Vol. 201, No. 5 (July 31, 1967), pp. 89–93.

LSD: Neil L. Chayet, "Law, Medicine and LSD," *New England Journal of Medicine,* Vol. 277, No. 5 (August 3, 1967), pp. 253–54, and Reginald G. Smart and Karen Bateman, "Unfavorable Reactions to LSD," *Canadian Medical Association Journal,* Vol. 97, No. 20 (November 11, 1967), pp. 1214–21.

Marihuana: Lester Grinspoon, "Marihuana," *Scientific American,* Vol. 221, No. 6 (December 1969), pp. 17–25; David Solomon, ed., *The Marijuana Papers* (Indianapolis, Ind.: Bobbs-Merrill, 1966); and Leonard M. Zunin, "Marijuana: The Drug and the Problem," *Military Medicine,* Vol. 134, No 2 (February 1969), pp. 104–10.

Morning-glory seeds: Sidney Cohen, "Suicide Following Morning-Glory Seed Ingestion," *American Journal of Psychiatry,* Vol. 120, No. 4 (April 1964), pp. 1024–25; and P. J. Fink, M. J. Goldman, and I. Lyons, "Morning-Glory Seed Psychoses," *Archives of General Psychiatry,* Vol. 15, No. 2 (August 1966), pp. 209–13.

Narcotics: W. Z. Guggenheim, "Heroin: History and Pharmacology," *International Journal of Addictions,* Vol. 2, No. 2 (Fall 1967), pp. 328–30, and Milton Helpern and Yong-Myun Rho, "Deaths from Narcotism in New York City," *International Journal of Addictions,* Vol. 2, No. 1 (Spring 1967), pp. 53–84.

Plastic Cement: Edward Preble and Gabriel V. Laury, "Plastic Cement: The Ten Cent Hallucinogen," *International Journal of Addictions,* Vol. 2, No. 2 (Fall 1967), pp. 271–81.

13.   Human overproduction and reproduction

This chapter covers three major topics that some readers may wish to investigate more critically: world resource scarcity and population growth, population density and space planning, and the reproductive system of man.

Current information on population studies is obtainable from the Population Reference Bureau at a minimal cost. The Bureau issues two releases: *Press Release* and *Population Profile.* Published in Washington, D.C., the releases contain the latest figures from governmental agencies as well as findings from independent studies and international sources on population density and control.

Two recent issues of *Bioscience* are devoted to the subject of population adjustment to world resources. In Vol. 18, No. 7 (July 1968) two articles are particularly recommended: LaMont C. Cole, "Can the World Be Saved?" pp. 679–84, and E. James Archer, "Can We Prepare for Famine?" pp. 685–90. Volume 19, No. 1 (January 1969) contains three excellent articles delineating concerns about food production and population control: William D. McElroy, "Biomedical Aspects of Population Control," pp. 19–23; H. F. Robinson, "Dimensions of the World Food Crisis," pp. 24–29; and H. David Thurston, "Tropical Agriculture—A Key to the World Food Crises," pp. 29–34. *Bioscience* is a somewhat technical journal, but those with a minimum amount of scientific training will benefit from the extremely thoughtful manner of preparation of the topics and the challenging writing style of the authors.

An excellent reference for the major issues of population problems is a compendium of articles by respected authors, Stuart Mudd, ed., *The Population Crisis and the Use of World Resources* (The Hague: W. Junk, 1964). The charts and tables are easily read and the discussions are fully developed. Still another volume of similar interest is Charles Morrow Wilson, *The Fight Against Hunger* (New York: Funk & Wagnalls, 1969). For those who seek a lively biography of a pioneer in the birth control movement, Emily Taft Douglas has written *Margaret Sanger: Pioneer of the Future* (New York: Holt, Rinehart and Winston, 1970). A book of international and historical scope, Georg Bergstrom, *Too Many* (New York: Macmillan, 1969), describes the scarcity of world resources.

The January 1970 issue of *Natural History* (Vol. 79, No. 1) contains a special supplement on population problems entitled "The State of the Species: 1970," ed. by Alan P. Ternes, who has also provided excellent introductions. Half a dozen worthwhile articles are included: C. Loring Brace, "The Origin of Man," pp. 46–49; Irene B. Taeuber, "The Chinese Peoples," pp. 52–56; Henri Leridon, "Fertility in Martinique," pp. 57–59; Kendall W. King, "Malnutrition in the Caribbean," pp. 64–67; Gordon Harrison, "The Mess of Modern Man," pp. 68–69; and John P. Wiley, Jr., "Space: A Barrier to the Species," pp. 70–73.

A publication concerned more with population control is a monograph, *The Sixth International Conference on*

Planned Parenthood (The Hague: International Planned Parent Federation, 1959). One article of this collection, Juitso Kitaoka, "How Japan Halved Her Birth Rate in Ten Years," pp. 27–36, describes Japan's solution to overreproduction. Another compilation, ed. by Roy O. Greep, *Human Fertility and Population Problems* (Cambridge, Mass.: Schenkman, 1963), also emphasizes population control.

The technical aspects of reproduction can be obtained from a wide variety of texts among which the following are standard: R. G. Harrison, *A Textbook of Human Embryology*, 2nd ed. (Philadelphia: F. A. Davis, 1964), and A. S. Parkes, *Marshall's Physiology of Reproduction*, 3 vols., 3rd ed. (Boston: Little, Brown, 1965). The endocrinology and physiology of the reproductive process is rarely presented in a simple fashion when authors strive for accuracy. Accordingly, these books are not easy reading. An interesting approach to the reproductive and birth processes is found in C. A. Smith, "The First Breath," *Scientific American*, Vol. 209, No. 4 (October 1963), pp. 27–35.

14. Some premarital considerations and advisements

Historical works on courtship and marriage include Willystine Goodsell, *A History of Marriage and the Family*, rev. ed. (New York: Macmillan, 1934); George Elliott Howard, *A History of Matrimonial Institutions*, 2 vols. (Chicago: University of Chicago Press, 1904); E. S. Turner, *A History of Courting* (London: Michael Joseph, 1954); and Edward Westermarck, *The History of Human Marriage*, 2 vols., 5th ed. (New York: Allerton, 1921). These offer the needed perspective in viewing the dynamic changes in modern courtship and marriage practices; Turner's small and entertaining volume can be read with profit in a few hours. The student can turn, thereafter, to more contemporary writings such as Robert O. Blood, *Marriage*, 3rd ed. (New York: Free Press, 1969); James A. Peterson, *Education for Marriage*, 2nd ed. (New York: Charles Scribner's Sons, 1964); and Austin L. Porterfield, *Marriage and Family Living as Self-Other Fulfillment* (Philadelphia: F. A. Davis, 1962). These provide some analyses of more recent trends and views of premarital and marital life. Henry A. Bowman's *Marriage for Moderns*, 5th ed. (New York: McGraw-Hill, 1965) is also well worth exploring, as are C. Byer *et al.*, *Dating, Marriage, and Human Reproduction* (New York: Free Press, 1969), and Evelyn M. Duvall and J. D. Johnson, *Art of Dating*, rev. ed. (New York: Association Press, 1967, also in paperback). Margaret Bastock's *Courtship: An Ethological Study* (Chicago: Aldine, 1967) is also of considerable value for the serious student.

Some specific information about the choice of marital partners is provided in a compilation ed. by Robert F. Winch, Robert McGinnis, and Herbert R. Barringer, *Selected Studies in Marriage and the Family* (New York: Holt, Rinehart and Winston, 1968, paperback). Dated yet informative articles by Harold T. Christenson and Hannah H. Meissner ("Premarital Pregnancy as a Factor in Divorce") and Judson T. Landis ("Marriages of Mixed and Non-Mixed Religious Faith") are included in that volume. Other articles that discuss marital choices made across racial and religious lines include David M. Heer, "Intermarriage and Racial Amalgamation in the United States," *Eugenics Quarterly*,

Vol. 14, No. 2 (Spring 1967), pp. 112–20; Todd H. Pavela, "An Exploratory Study of Negro-White Intermarriage in Indiana," *Journal of Marriage and the Family*, Vol. 26, No. 5 (May 1964), pp. 209–11; and Marshall Sklare, "Intermarriage & the Jewish Future," *Commentary*, Vol. 37, No. 4 (April 1964), pp. 46–52. A delightful book by Alan C. Valentine, ed., *Fathers to Sons: Advice Without Consent* (Oklahoma City: University of Oklahoma Press, 1963) is a light but wise commentary about some of the concerns of youth.

A book that has received much recent attention is Vance Packard, *The Sexual Wilderness* (New York: David McKay, 1967). It contains interesting data on premarital sex activity but has serious shortcomings. Data collection methods are not without loopholes. Moreover, the significance of the data is inadequately explained. The book, particularly the section on premarital sex activity, should be read with these weaknesses in mind. The results of the Packard study, as well as those of a few other workers, are presented in the present volume. However, one would hope that a more scientific approach will be achieved by researchers in this important area of human behavior. John H. Gagnon and William Simon briefly mention one of their disagreements with the Packard work in a recent article, "Prospect for Change in American Sexual Patterns," *Medical Aspects of Human Sexuality*, Vol. 4, No. 1 (January 1970), pp. 100–17. These highly regarded writers state, "On the level of prevalence, it does not appear that there is any body of research evidence leading to a belief that the figures generated by Kinsey *et al.* for the period 1925–1945 from an admittedly limited sample have radically changed . . . What Packard's data do indicate is that for the college-educated the arena for premarital coitus has moved from the post-college to the college years." Still another article relating to the area of premarital sex is Beverley T. Mead, "The Case for Chastity," *Medical Aspects of Human Sexuality*, Vol. 4, No. 1 (January 1970), pp. 8–15. Also recommended is Mary Harrington Hall, "A Conversation with Masters & Johnson," *Psychology Today*, Vol. 3, No. 2 (July 1968), pp. 50–58. In this interesting interview William H. Masters points out that occasionally a woman who takes the pill for "18 months to three years . . . finds herself losing effective sexual function." Some physicians feel that this infrequent complication of the pill may be due to many other associated factors. Robert Bell's *Premarital Sex in a Changing Society* (Englewood Cliffs, N.J.: Prentice-Hall, 1966) is also of some limited interest. An article by Seymour Halleck, "Sex and Mental Health on the Campus," *Journal of the American Medical Association*, Vol. 200, No. 8 (May 22, 1967), pp. 684–90, also contains interesting ideas.

15. Marriage: "the craft so long to lerne"

Readers who wish to investigate the subject of human sexual response further should consult the dated but invaluable volumes by Alfred C. Kinsey *et al.*, *Sexual Behavior in the Human Male* (Philadelphia: W. B. Saunders, 1948) and *Sexual Behavior in the Human Female* (Philadelphia: W. B. Saunders, 1953). Kinsey's is the classic study of human sexual behavior during the immediate post Second World War era. William H. Masters and Virginia E. Johnson's *Human Sexual Response* (Boston: Little, Brown, 1966) is an important report of their research findings. It is the most

616   BIBLIOGRAPHY

valuable book in this area. Articles drawing heavily upon the Masters and Johnson work include Mary Jane Sherfey, "The Evolution and Nature of Female Sexuality in Relation to Psychoanalytic Theory," *Journal of the American Psychoanalytic Association,* Vol. 14, No. 1 (January 1966), pp. 28–128, and Harvey D. Strassman, "Sex and the Work of Masters and Johnson," *GP,* Vol. 38, No. 4 (October 1968), pp. 109–14. Sherfey's highly technical paper merits the widespread professional discussion it has created. It is recommended for the advanced student. A valuable and much less technical approach to sexuality is Willard Dalrymple, *Sex Is for Real: Human Sexuality and Sexual Responsibility* (New York: McGraw-Hill, 1969, also in paperback). Still another excellently written approach is Joseph B. Trainer, *Physiologic Foundations for Marriage Counseling* (St. Louis: C. V. Mosby, 1965). Other helpful books in this area are James A. Peterson, *Married Love in the Middle Years* (New York: Association Press, 1968), and Jerome and Julia Rainer, *Sexual Pleasure in Marriage,* rev. ed. (New York: Simon and Schuster, 1969, also in paperback).

The following works, though not strictly in the tradition of reported research, nevertheless shed light upon human sexual responses: Warren J. Barker, "Female Sexuality," *Journal of the American Psychoanalytic Association,* Vol. 16, No. 1 (January 1968), pp. 123–45; Desmond Morris, *The Naked Ape* (New York: McGraw-Hill, 1969, also in paperback); and Leon Salzman, "Psychology of the Female," *Archives of General Psychiatry,* Vol. 17, No. 2 (August 1967), pp. 195–203. An interesting view, which has a philosophical bent, is Rollo May, *Love and Will* (New York: W. W. Norton, 1969).

The books on marriage mentioned in the bibliography for Chapter 14 are, of course, also useful with respect to this chapter. Added to these are Robert R. Bell, *Marriage and Family Interaction,* rev. ed. (Homewood, Ill.: Dorsey Press, 1967); Lester A. Kirkendall, *Reading and Study Guide for Students in Marriage and Family Relations* 4th ed. (Dubuque, Iowa: William C. Brown, 1968, paperback); William J. Lederer and Don D. Jackson, *Mirages of Marriage* (New York: W. W. Norton, 1968); and Marvin Sussman, *Sourcebook in Marriage and the Family,* 3rd ed. (Boston: Houghton Mifflin, 1968, paperback).

16.   On continuing the human beginning

Students who may wish to pursue the topics of heredity and evolution, genetic disorders, pregnancy, abortion, and contraception will find the works listed here useful. Two books by Theodosius Dobzhansky, *Mankind Evolving: The Evolution of the Human Species* (New Haven, Conn.: Yale University Press, 1962) and *Heredity and the Nature of Man* (New York: Harcourt, Brace & World, 1964) provide excellent writing and highly informative content on the subject of heredity and evolution. H. L. Carson takes a humanistic approach to the subject of the biological process of evolution in *Heredity and Human Life* (New York: Columbia University Press, 1963). For a poetic vision of man and his place in the universe, one may wish to peruse Pierre Teilhard de Chardin's *The Phenomenon of Man* (New York: Harper & Row, 1959).

Genetic structure and change is discussed in numerous publications. A lucid little book, especially well-composed for the uninitiated reader, is Charlotte Auerbach, *Genetics in the Atomic Age,* 2nd ed. (New York: Oxford University Press, 1965). The prolific and popular writer, Isaac Asimov, has written a general reader, *The Genetic Code* (New York: New American Library, 1962, paperback). This may be supplemented with two much more complex articles from *Scientific American* by two of the most distinguished scientists of this generation: F. H. C. Crick, "The Genetic Code," in Vol. 207, No. 4 (October 1962), pp. 66–74, and Marshall W. Nirenberg, "The Genetic Code," in Vol. 208, No. 3 (March 1963), pp. 80–95.

Genetic disorders are of growing concern as these problems proliferate and affect an ever greater number of people. A good reference is a compendium of articles written by experts in the field and ed. by Morris Fishbein, *Birth Defects* (Philadelphia: J. B. Lippincott, 1963). V. Apgar and G. Stickle's "Birth Defects: Their Significance as a Public Health Problem," *Journal of the American Medical Association,* Vol. 204, No. 5 (April 29, 1968), pp. 371–74, is also recommended. Some selected genetic disorders are discussed in the following articles: "Haemophilia, a Royal Complaint," *World Health* (June 1968), pp. 34–35; Ashley Montagu, "Chromosomes and Crime," *Psychology Today,* Vol. 2, No. 5 (October 1968), pp. 43–49; and Audrey Redding and Kurt Hirshhorn, "Guide to Human Chromosome Defects" *Birth Defects, Original Article Series,* Vol. 4, No. 4 (September 1968), pp. 1–16.

A basic, clearly written reference on pregnancy and the birth process is M. Edward Davis and Reva Rubin, *De Lee's Obstetrics for Nurses,* 18th ed. (Philadelphia: W. B. Saunders, 1966). For a discussion of natural childbirth see Deborah Tanzer, "Natural Childbirth: Pain or Peak Experience?" *Psychology Today,* Vol. 2, No. 5 (October 1968), pp. 16–21, 69. In addition, Hyman Spotnitz and Lucy Freeman's *How To Be Happy Though Pregnant* (New York: Coward-McCann, 1969) can be recommended. It is an easily read and practical consideration of some of the emotional problems that may occur during pregnancy.

Numerous articles on abortion present the position of the medical profession and the views of eminent scientists on the subject. A significant summary of the problem is the article by Mildred B. Beck *et al.,* "Abortion: A National Public and Mental Health Problem—Past, Present, and Proposed Research," *American Journal of Public Health,* Vol. 59, No. 12 (December 1969), pp. 2131–43. This article also contains 43 excellent references providing a rich source for continued student investigation. Two statements by leading medical groups are "Abortion and the Doctor," *Annals of Internal Medicine,* Vol. 67, No. 5 (November 1967), pp. 1111–13, and "AMA Policy on Therapeutic Abortion," *Journal of the American Medical Association,* Vol. 201, No. 7 (August 14, 1967), p. 544. The Nobel Prize winner Joshua Lederburg offers his unique perspective in "A Geneticist Looks at Contraception and Abortion," *Annals of Internal Medicine,* Vol. 67, No. 3, Part II, Supplement 7 (September 1967), pp. 25–27. Also recommended is Christopher Tietze and Sarah Lewit, "Abortion," *Scientific American,* Vol. 220, No. 1 (January 1969), pp. 21–27. R. Bruce Sloane's "The Unwanted Pregnancy," *New England Journal of Medicine,*

Vol. 280, No. 22 (May 29, 1969), pp. 1206–13, discusses some of the central issues around which the controversy about abortion rages.

A historical review of contraception is a solid base for the continued accumulation of knowledge about the subject. The standard reference is Norman E. Himes's fascinating *Medical History of Contraception* (Baltimore: Williams & Wilkins, 1936). More recent sources on this particular subject include Arturo Esquival and Leonard E. Laufe, "Contraception Control by a Single Monthly Injection," *Obstetrics and Gynecology*, Vol. 31, No. 5 (May 1968), pp. 634–36; "The Long-Acting Contraceptives: Quarterly Injections Pass Three-Year Trials" in the "Medical News" section of the *Journal of the American Medical Association*, Vol. 204, No. 11 (June 10, 1968), pp. 35–36; and Christopher Tietze, *A Summary of Contraceptive Methods* (Chicago: G. D. Searle, December 15, 1966).

17. The last chapter: health for the freeman

The reader who wishes to anticipate trends of the next quarter-century will find that a number of fine articles have been written on the subject of health in the future. Informative articles such as the following provoke reflection about emerging changes in health care systems: Charles A. Berry, "Space Medicine in Perspective," *Journal of the American Medical Association*, Vol. 201, No. 4 (July 24, 1967), pp. 232–41; A. Marcus, "The Computer Comes to the Patient's Bedside," *World Health* (August 1968), pp. 8–15; and a report in *Science News*, "Engineering the Body," Vol. 94, No. 20 (November 16, 1968), p. 493. An interesting nontechnical account of the effects, both physiological and psychological, of prolonged space flight is provided by the Russians Yuri Gagarin and Vladimir Azrael in their book *Survival in Space* (New York: Praeger, 1969). For still another interesting sidelight, one can turn to Alexander Alland, Jr., "War and Disease: An Anthropological Perspective," *Bulletin of the Atomic Scientists*, Vol. 24 No. 6 (June 1968), pp. 28–31.

Some unresolved problems of public health economics are discussed in William H. Forbes, "Longevity and Medical Costs," *New England Journal of Medicine*, Vol. 277, No. 2 (July 13, 1967), pp. 71–78, and Greer Williams, "Needed: A New Strategy for Health Promotion," *New England Journal of Medicine*, Vol. 279, No. 19 (November 7, 1968), pp. 1031–35. They emphasize the disparities between medical advances and feasible implementation. Eli Ginsberg and Miriam Ostow have written a good review of the changing structure of health services in this country entitled *Men, Money and Medicine* (New York: Columbia University Press, 1970). Some important issues worthy of further investigation are discussed by Nevin S. Scrimshaw, "The Death Rate of One-Year-Old Children in Underdeveloped Countries," *Archives of Environmental Health*, Vol. 17, No. 5 (November 1968), pp. 691–92. Every year, Myron E. Wegman writes an "Annual Summary of Vital Statistics," the latest in *Pediatrics*, Vol. 44, No. 6 (December 1969), pp. 1031–34. In his reviews numbers are used to interpret human needs. John Bryant discusses the health problems of Africa, Asia, and Latin America in *Health and the Developing World* (Ithaca, N.Y.: Cornell University Press, 1970).

Literature on aging and longevity is particularly prolific. A summary of the problems of aging is found in Ernest W. Burgess, ed., *Aging in Western Societies* (Chicago: University of Chicago Press, 1960). Nathan W. Shock provides an interesting discussion of how aging occurs due to the progressive loss of body cells in "The Physiology of Aging," *Scientific American*, Vol. 206, No. 1 (January 1962), pp. 100–10. A technical article by Albert M. Kligman, "Early Destructive Effect of Sunlight on Human Skin," *Journal of the American Medical Association*, Vol. 210, No. 13 (December 29, 1969), pp. 2377–82, may be of particular interest to the young person; Kligman, a dermatologist, writes, "Sunlight, not innate aging, is mainly responsible for the worst manifestations of senile skin." A symposium on "Advances in Medical Care of the Elderly" has been published in *New York State Journal of Medicine*, Vol. 67, No. 24 (December 15, 1967), pp. 3205–18. In addition, the following can be recommended: A. J. Comfort, *The Process of Aging* (New York: New American Library, 1964, paperback); Matilda W. Riley and Anne Foner, *Aging and Society*, Vol. I (New York: Russell Sage Foundation, 1968, Vols. II and III in preparation); and Arnold M. Rose and W. A. Peterson, *Older People and Their Social World* (Philadelphia: F. A. Davis, 1965).

Two cross-cultural views of the elderly may be found in Margaret Clark and B. G. Anderson, *Culture and Aging: An Anthropological Study of Older Americans* (Springfield, Ill.: Charles C Thomas, 1967), and Leo W. Simmons' classic *The Role of the Aged in Primitive Society* (New Haven, Conn.: Yale University Press, 1945).

Finally, an overview of international health can be obtained through World Health Organization publications such as *World Health, World Health Statistics Report*, and *WHO Chronicle*. A suggested summary of the WHO activities is "The Second Ten Years of the World Health Organization," *WHO Chronicle*, Vol. 22, No. 7 (July 1968), pp. 267–312.

Bruno Bettelheim, for excerpts from Bruno Bettelheim, "Joey: A 'Mechanical Boy,'" *Scientific American,* Vol. 200, No. 3 (March 1959), pp. 117–27. Copyright © 1959 by Scientific American, Inc. All rights reserved.

California Medicine, for Table 11-1, "Parent and Child Development," from David Belais Friedman, "Parent Development," *California Medicine,* Vol. 86, No. 1 (January 1957), pp. 25–28.

Canadian Medical Association Journal, for Table 12-5, "Causes of Death of Current Male Cigarette Smokers," adapted from E. W. R. Best *et al.,* "Summary of a Canadian Study of Smoking and Health," *Canadian Medical Association Journal,* Vol. 96 (April 15, 1967), p. 1104.

Jonathan Cape, Ltd., for an excerpt from George Seferis, *Collected Poems, 1924–1955,* tr., ed., and intro. by Edmund Keeley and Philip Sherrard, published by Jonathan Cape, Ltd., in the British Commonwealth and Canada.

Criterion Books, for Table 13-3, "Number of Survivors at Various Attained Ages for Eighteenth-Century France, India 1941–50, and Norway 1946–50." Reprinted by permission of the publisher, from Alfred Sauvy, *Fertility and Survival* (New York: Criterion Books, 1961).

M. Edward Davis, for Table 16-6, "Stages of Labor," from M. Edward Davis and Reva Rubin, *De Lee's Obstetrics for Nurses,* 18th ed. (1966), published by W. B. Saunders Company.

Doubleday & Company, Inc., for a poem from *An Introduction to Haiku,* by Harold G. Henderson. Copyright © 1958 by Harold G. Henderson. Reprinted by permission of Doubleday & Company, Inc.

Environment Magazine (formerly *Scientist and Citizen),* for data used in Table 4-1, "Radioisotopes of Major Biological Importance Occurring in Fallout," from Dan I. Bolef, "Bomb Tests," *Scientist and Citizen,* Vol. 6, Nos. 9–10 (September–October 1964), p. 8.

W. H. Freeman and Company, for excerpts from Bruno Bettelheim, "Joey: A 'Mechanical Boy,'" *Scientific American,* Vol. 200, No. 3 (March 1959), pp. 117–27. Copyright © 1959 by Scientific American, Inc. All rights reserved. For data used in Table 4-1, "Radioisotopes of Major Biological Importance Occurring in Fallout," from J. R. Arnold and E. A. Martell, "The Circulation of Isotopes," *Scientific American,* Vol. 201, No. 3 (September 1959), p. 90. Copyright © 1959 by Scientific American, Inc. All rights reserved.

David Belais Friedman, for Table 11-1, "Parent and Child Development," from David Belais Friedman, "Parent Development," *California Medicine,* Vol. 86, No. 1 (January 1957), pp. 25–28.

Paul W. Gikas, for Table 4-2, "How Seat Belts Might Have Saved Drivers' Lives," adapted from Donald F. Huelke and Paul W. Gikas, "Causes of Death in Automobile Accidents," *Journal of the American Medical Association,* Vol. 203, No. 13 (March 25, 1968), p. 1106.

Harcourt, Brace & World, Inc., for Table 7-2, "Some Typical Functions of the Endocrine Glands," from Ernest R. Hilgard and Richard C. Atkinson, *Introduction to Psychology,* 4th ed., copyright © 1953, 1957, 1962, 1967 by Harcourt, Brace & World, Inc., and reproduced with their permission.

Harper & Row, Publishers, Inc., for Table 12-2, "Phases and Symptoms of Alcoholism," from "Chart of Phases and Symptoms" from Lincoln Williams, *Tomorrow Will Be Sober.* Copyright © 1960 by Lincoln Williams. Reprinted by permission of Harper & Row, Publishers, Inc.

Gerald A. Heidbreder, for Table 6-3, "Natural History of Acquired Syphilis"; Table 6-4, "Natural History of Acquired Gonorrhea"; and Table 17-2, "Organization of the County of Los Angeles Health Department," courtesy of Gerald A. Heidbreder, Health Officer, County of Los Angeles Health Department.

Holt, Rinehart and Winston, Inc., for data used in Table 9-1, "A Dozen Leading Nutrients," and Table 9-2, "Caloric Values for Representative Foods, Classified by Food Groups," adapted and reprinted from Ethel Austin Martin, *Nutrition in Action,* 2nd ed. Copyright © 1963, 1965 by Holt, Rinehart and Winston, Inc. Used by permission of Holt, Rinehart and Winston, Inc.

Donald F. Huelke, for Table 4-2, "How Seat Belts Might Have Saved Drivers' Lives," adapted from Donald F. Huelke and Paul W. Gikas, "Causes of Death in Automobile Accidents," *Journal of the American Medical Association,* Vol. 203, No. 13 (March 25, 1968), p. 1106.

Indiana University Press, for Table 13-1, "Estimate of Births in Three Periods of Human History," and for Table 13-2, "Estimated World Population: A.D. 1000–A.D. 2000," from Annabelle Desmond, "How Many People Have Ever Lived on Earth?" from Stuart Mudd, ed., *The Population Crisis and the Use of World Resources* (The Hague, 1964).

Journal of the American Dietetic Association, for Table 9-4, "Energy Equivalents of Food Calories Expressed in Minutes of Activity," from F. Konishi, "Food Energy Equivalents of Various Activities," *Journal of the American Dietetic Association,* Vol. 46 (1965), p. 186.

Journal of the American Medical Association, for Table 4-2, "How Seat Belts Might Have Saved Drivers' Lives," adapted from Donald F. Huelke and Paul W. Gikas, "Causes of Death in Automobile Accidents," *Journal of the American Medical Association,* Vol. 203, No. 13 (March 25, 1968), p. 1106; and for Table 12-4, "Marihuana Psychoses Among U.S. Soldiers in Vietnam, 1967–68: Twelve Cases," and excerpts adapted from John A. Talbott and James W. Teague, "Marihuana Psychosis," *Journal of the American Medical Association,* Vol. 210, No. 2 (October 13, 1969), pp. 299–302.

The Julian Press, Inc., Publishers, for Table 14-1, "Impact of Premarital Sexual Experience on Two Hundred Young Men," adapted from Lester A. Kirkendall, *Premarital Intercourse and Interpersonal Relationships* (1961).

Alfred A. Knopf, Inc., for excerpts from Erik H. Erikson, "Growth and Crises of the Healthy Personality," in Clyde Kluckhohn, Henry A. Murray, and David Schneider, eds., *Personality in Nature, Society and Culture.* Copyright 1948, 1953 by Alfred A. Knopf, Inc. Reprinted by permission. For "On Marriage" and an excerpt from "On Children," reprinted from Kahlil Gibran, *The Prophet,* with permission of the publisher, Alfred A. Knopf, Inc. Copyright 1923 by Kahlil Gibran; renewal copyright 1951 by Administrators C.T.A. of Kahlil Gibran Estate, and Mary G. Gibran.

F. Konishi, for Table 9-4, "Energy Equivalents of Food Calories Expressed in Minutes of Activity," from F. Konishi, "Food Energy Equivalents of Various Activities," *Journal of the American Dietetic Association,* Vol. 46 (1965), p. 186.

J. B. Lippincott Company, for Table 9-3, "Caloric Values for Common Snacks," adapted from Helen S. Mitchell *et al., Cooper's Nutrition in Health and Disease,* 15th ed. (1968); for Table 9-6, "A Typical Female College Student's Activities for One Day," adapted from Helen S. Mitchell *et al., Cooper's Nutrition in Health and Disease,* 15th ed. (1968); for a poem by an Oklahoma high school boy, quoted in Evelyn Duvall, *Family Development,* 2nd ed. (1962); and for Table 12-3, "Comparative Strengths of LSD and Other Hallucinogens (Approximate)," from Sidney Cohen, "Pot, Acid and Speed," *Medical Science,* Vol. 19, No. 2 (February 1968), p. 31.

Little, Brown and Company, for quotes used in Table 11-1, "Parent and Child Development": From "Tarkington, Thou Should'st Be Living in This Hour," from Ogden Nash, *Verses from 1929 On,* copyright 1947, by Ogden Nash; originally appeared in *The New Yorker.* From "Pediatric Reflection," copyright 1931 by Ogden Nash. From Ogden Nash, "The Kitten," copyright 1940 by The Curtis Publishing Company. From "A Child's Guide to Parents," copyright 1936 by Ogden Nash. From "The Parent," copyright 1933 by Ogden Nash. All from Ogden Nash, *Family Reunion.* For an excerpt from "Allergy Met a Bear," from Ogden Nash, *I'm a Stranger Here Myself,* copyright 1938 by Ogden Nash. Acknowledgment also for excerpts from William H. Masters and Virginia E. Johnson, *Human Sexual Response* (1966). All by permission of Little, Brown and Company.

619

County of Los Angeles Health Department, for Table 6-3, "Natural History of Acquired Syphilis," for Table 6-4, "Natural History of Acquired Gonorrhea," and for Table 17-2, "Organization of the County of Los Angeles Health Department," courtesy of the Records and Statistics Division, County of Los Angeles Health Department, May 1969.

Los Angeles County Medical Association, for excerpts from "℞ for Heavy Smog Attacks," from *The Bulletin*, Los Angeles County Medical Association (October 3, 1968), p. 11.

The Macmillan Company, for Table 9-5, "Energy Expenditures for Various Everyday Activities," adapted from C. M. Taylor, Grace MacLeod, and M. D. S. Rose, *Foundations of Nutrition*, 5th ed. Reprinted with permission of The Macmillan Company. © by The Macmillan Company, 1956. For excerpts from W. B. Yeats, "A Prayer for My Daughter." Reprinted with permission of The Macmillan Company from W. B. Yeats, *Collected Poems*. Copyright 1924 by The Macmillan Company, renewed in 1952 by Bertha Georgie Yeats.

Metropolitan Life Insurance Company, for Table 9-7, "Desirable Weights in Pounds for People Twenty-five or Over," for Table 9-8, "Overweight and Excess Mortality," and for Table 9-9, "Overweight and Excess Mortality from Some Major Diseases," from the Metropolitan Life Insurance Company. Derived primarily from data of the Build and Blood Pressure Study, Society of Actuaries, 1959.

National Dairy Council, for data used in Table 9-1, "A Dozen Leading Nutrients," adapted from Ruth M. Leverton, *A Girl and Her Figure* (National Dairy Council, 1955).

The National Foundation–March of Dimes, for Table 16-5, "The More Common Birth Defects," adapted from a booklet (PR-45-5) published by The National Foundation–March of Dimes.

The New York Times Company, for quotes from *The New York Times*. © 1966 by The New York Times Company. Reprinted by permission.

Nutrition Today, for Table 16-4, "Childbearing Children in the United States, 1965," from Lucille B. Hurley, "The Consequences of Fetal Impoverishment," *Nutrition Today*, Vol. 3, No. 4 (December 1968), p. 9.

Princeton University Press, for an excerpt from George Seferis, *Collected Poems, 1924–1955*, tr., ed., and intro. by Edmund Keeley and Philip Sherrard. Copyright © 1967 by Princeton University Press; supplemented ed., 1969.

Saturday Review, Inc., for excerpt from John Lear, "Spinning the Thread of Life," *Saturday Review* (April 5, 1969), pp. 63–64. Copyright 1969 Saturday Review, Inc.

W. B. Saunders Company, for Table 16-6, "Stages of Labor," from M. Edward Davis and Reva Rubin, *De Lee's Obstetrics for Nurses*, 18th ed. (1966).

Charles Scribner's Sons, for Table 14-1, "Impact of Premarital Sexual Experience on Two Hundred Young Men," which, as Table 16, is reprinted with the permission of Charles Scribner's Sons from *Education for Marriage*, page 166, by James A. Peterson. Copyright © 1956 Charles Scribner's Sons. Copyright © 1964 James A. Peterson.

G. D. Searle & Co., for Table 16-7, "A Summary of Contraceptive Methods," adapted from "A Summary of Contraceptive Methods," G. D. Searle & Co.

Smith, Kline, and French Laboratories, for data used in Table 9-3, "Caloric Values for Common Snacks."

John A. Talbott, for Table 12-4, "Marihuana Psychoses Among U.S. Soldiers in Vietnam, 1967–68: Twelve Cases," and excerpts adapted from John A. Talbott and James W. Teague, "Marihuana Psychosis," *Journal of the American Medical Association*, Vol. 210, No. 2 (October 13, 1969), pp. 299–302.

A. P. Watt & Son, for Table 12-2, "Phases and Symptoms of Alcoholism," from Lincoln Williams, *Tomorrow Will Be Sober*, published now by Evans Brothers in the British Commonwealth and Canada. Reprinted by permission of the Author's Estate. For the poem "At last the happy truth is out . . ." by Sir Alan Herbert, quoted in W. S. C. Copeman, *Arthritis and Rheumatism*. Reprinted by permission of Sir Alan Herbert. For excerpts from "A Prayer for My Daughter," from W. B. Yeats, *Collected Poems*. Reprinted by permission of Mr. Michael B. Yeats and The Macmillan Company of Canada.

John Wiley & Sons, Inc., for Table 16-3, "Mean Birth Weights According to Socio-Economic Status," from WHO, *Nutrition in Pregnancy and Lactation*, cited in Miriam E. Lowenberg et al., *Food and Man* (1968).

World Health Organization, for Table 16-3, "Mean Birth Weights According to Socio-Economic Status," from World Health Organization, *Nutrition in Pregnancy and Lactation*, Tech. Rept. Series No. 302 (Geneva, Switz., 1965), p. 14.

The World Publishing Company, for a poem by Marie Ford, "The Junkies." Reprinted by permission of The World Publishing Company from Herbert Kohl, *36 Children*. Copyright © 1967 by Herbert Kohl.

ILLUSTRATIONS

Chapter 1: pp. 2–3, Gerry Cranham/Rapho Guillumette; 1, C. R. Carpenter, Pennsylvania State University; 2, *The New York Times*; 3, courtesy Edouard Kellenberger; 4, Arents Collection, The New York Public Library, Astor, Lenox and Tilden Foundations; 5, courtesy Helmut A. Gordon, M.D., from *Triangle*, the Sandoz Journal of Medical Science, Vol. 7, No. 3 (1965), p. 115; 6, *New York Daily News*; 7, Radio Times Hulton Picture Library; 8, Mansell Collection; 9, Courtesy of The American Museum of Natural History; 10, courtesy John F. Bertles, M.D.

Chapter 2: pp. 30–31, courtesy WHO; 1, courtesy USDA; 2, p. 36, Wayne Miller/Magnum (top left), courtesy WHO (top right), Roger-Viollet (bottom), p. 37, Bettmann Archive (top left), courtesy Yale–New Haven Hospital (top right), courtesy Australian News and Information Bureau (bottom); 3, Mansell Collection; 4, Picture Collection, NYPL.

Chapter 3: pp. 54–55, Aero Service, Division of Litton Industries; 1, Stephenson Blake; 2, Bettmann Archive; 3, courtesy USDA; 4, Ken Heyman; 5, Mansell Collection.

Chapter 4: pp. 80–81, Wide World; 1, courtesy FAO; 2, courtesy Michigan Department of Natural Resources; 4, courtesy Eastman Kodak Company, from *Medical Radiography and Photography*, published by Radiography Markets Division; 7, *The New York Times*; 8, courtesy David M. Lipscomb, Ph.D.; 9, courtesy Liberty Mutual Insurance Companies; 10, courtesy Corning Glass Works; 11, Pictorial Parade.

Chapter 5: pp. 122–23, "The King," "The Physician," and "The Noblewoman," courtesy The National Gallery of Art, Washington, D.C., Rosenwald Collection, "The Cardinal" and "The Plowman," The Metropolitan Museum of Art, Rogers Fund, 1919; 1, courtesy WHO; 2, Mansell Collection; 3, Spencer Collection, The New York Public Library, Astor, Lenox and Tilden Foundations; 4 and 5, Mansell Collection; 6, Giraudon; 7, courtesy County of Los Angeles Health Department; 8, courtesy New York Academy of Medicine; 9 and 10, Mansell Collection.

Chapter 6: pp. 152–53, Dr. R. W. Horne; 1, courtesy New York Academy of Medicine; 2, Lester V. Bergman & Assoc., Inc. (top), courtesy The Upjohn Company (center), courtesy Lewis M. Drusin, M.D., and George B. Chapman, Ph.D. (bottom); 3, courtesy WHO; 4, courtesy New York Academy of Medicine; 5, Bettmann Archive; 6, courtesy Ny Carlsberg Glyptothek, Copenhagen; 8, Picture Collection, NYPL; 9, Dr. R. W. Horne; 10, Dr. R. W. Horne and Dr. Jack Nagington; 11, King Features Syndicate; 12, courtesy Division of Virology, National Institute for Medical Research, London.

Chapter 7: pp. 196–97, Wide World; 1, Ewing Galloway; 2, courtesy NIH; 3, *1970 Cancer Facts and Figures*, with permission of the American Cancer Society; 4, courtesy NIH; 5, with permission of the Epidemiology and Statistics Department, American Cancer Society, October 1969; 6, Picture Collection, NYPL; 8, courtesy Austin Johnston, M.D.; 10, UPI (left); 12, José M. R. Delgado, M.D., from "Evolution of Physical Control of the Brain," James Arthur Lecture on the Evolution of the Human Brain, The American Museum of Natural History, New York, 1965; 13, courtesy Eli S. Goldensohn, M.D.; 14, from Ernest R. Hilgard and Richard C. Atkinson, *Introduction to Psychology*, 4th ed., copyright, 1953, 1957, 1962, 1967, by Harcourt, Brace & World, Inc. and reproduced with their permission; 15, Wide World; 17, courtesy Eckhard H. Hess, University of Chicago; 18, courtesy National Society for the Prevention of Blindness; 22, Syndication International/Gilloon.

Chapter 8: pp. 242–43, courtesy WHO; 1, Thames and Hudson, Ltd.; 3, adapted from James E. Crouch, *Functional Human Anatomy* (Philadelphia, 1965), with permission of Lea & Febiger; 5, Eugene L. Gottfried, M.D.; 6, Keith R. Porter, M.D., and Clifton Van Zandt Hawn, M.D.; 7, Mansell Collection; 8, adapted from James E. Crouch, *Functional Human Anatomy* (Philadelphia, 1965), with permission of Lea & Febiger; 9, courtesy Carl A. Smith, M.D.; 10, from H. S. Mayerson, "The Lymphatic System." Copyright © 1963 by Scientific American, Inc. All rights reserved; 12, courtesy American Heart Association; 13, courtesy Jack C. Geer, M.D.; 14, courtesy C. Walton Lillehei, M.D., Ph.D.; 15, adapted from Theodore W. Torrey, *Morphogenesis of the Vertebrates,* 2nd ed. (New York, 1967), with permission of John Wiley & Sons, Inc.; 16, courtesy W. S. Hammond, M.D.; 17, Spencer Collection, The New York Public Library, Astor, Lenox and Tilden Foundations.

Chapter 9: pp. 274–75, courtesy WHO; 1, Mansell Collection; 2, courtesy Cambridge Scientific Industries, Inc., exclusive manufacturers of the Lange Skinfold Caliper; 3, courtesy WHO; 4, Metropolitan Museum of Art, Whittelsey Fund, 1959; 5, photographs courtesy American Dental Association; 7, adapted from James E. Crouch, *Functional Human Anatomy* (Philadelphia, 1965), with permission of Lea & Febiger.

Chapter 10: pp. 318–19, Ken Heyman; 1, courtesy Collection Palais de la Découverte; 2, Bruno Bettelheim, Ph.D.; 3, W. Eugene Smith; 4, Lennart Nilsson; 5, Eve Arnold/Magnum; 6, Julio Mitchel; 7, Sybil Shackman/Monkmeyer; 8, Bill Bridges/Globe Photos.

Chapter 11: pp. 350–51, courtesy WHO; 1, p. 364, courtesy WHO (top), Ken Heyman (bottom), p. 365, Regional Primate Research Center, University of Wisconsin; 2, Leon Levinstein; 3, June Finfer.

Chapter 12: pp. 384–85, Steve Schapiro/Consolidated Diamond Minds; 1 and 2, Arents Collection, The New York Public Library, Astor, Lenox and Tilden Foundations; 3, Metropolitan Museum of Art, Egyptian Expedition; 4, Newberry Library, Chicago; 5, Dick Davis/DPI; 6, Sansoni; 7, courtesy William F. Geber, Ph.D.; 8, Bud Lee; 9, p. 425, from Julius Comroe, "The Lung." Copyright © 1966, by Scientific American, Inc. All rights reserved (top), courtesy Eastman Kodak Company, from *Medical Radiography and Photography,* published by Radiography Markets Division (bottom); 10, courtesy WHO; 11, courtesy Oscar Auerbach, M.D., and L. J. Walker; 12, from *Smoking in Relation to Death Rates of One Million Men and Women, 1966,* with permission of E. Cuyler Hammond, Sc.D.

Chapter 13: pp. 432–433, Julio Mitchel; 1, Göran Hansson/Naturfotograferna, p. 446, Ben Ross; 5, adapted from Robert Latou Dickinson, *Atlas of Human Sex Anatomy,* 2nd ed., copyright 1949, with permission of Williams & Wilkins Co., Baltimore, Md. 21202, U.S.A.; 6, Cecil B. Jacobson, M.D. (bottom).

Chapter 14: pp. 492–93, Ken Heyman; 1, courtesy New York Academy of Medicine; 2, Jean Prevost; 3, Pantheon Books, permission SPADEM 1969 by French Reproduction Rights, Inc.; 4, © *Punch,* London; 5, courtesy National Gallery of Art, Washington, D.C., Rosenwald Collection; 6, from Judson T. Landis, "Marriages of Mixed and Non-Mixed Religious Faith," *American Sociological Review,* Vol. 14, No. 3 (June 1949), pp. 401–07, with permission of Judson T. Landis and the *American Sociological Review,* adapted from Robert K. Kelley, *Courtship, Marriage, and the Family,* copyright © 1969 by Harcourt, Brace & World, Inc. and reproduced with their permission.

Chapter 15: pp. 492–93, Ken Heyman; 1, Mansell Collection; 2, Charles Harbutt/Magnum; 3, Katrina Thomas; 4, courtesy Philadelphia Museum of Art, The Louise and Walter Arensberg Collection.

Chapter 16: pp. 518–19, courtesy O. L. Miller, Jr., and Barbara R. Beatty, Biology Division, Oak Ridge National Laboratory; 1, courtesy Albert E. Vatter, M.D.; 2, courtesy Dorothy Warburton, Ph.D., and W. Roy Breg, M.D. (left), courtesy The Upjohn Company (right); 3, courtesy Jon Beckwith, M.D., and Lorne MacHattie, M.D.; 6, courtesy Dorothy Warburton, Ph.D., and W. Roy Breg, M.D.; 7, courtesy Albert E. Vatter, M.D.; 8, from Masayasu Nomura, "Ribosomes." Copyright © 1969, by Scientific American, Inc. All rights reserved; 12, courtesy O. J. Miller, M.D.; 13, courtesy David H. Baker, M.D.; 14, courtesy Eva McGilvray, M.D.; 15, courtesy WHO; 16, reproduced by gracious permission of Her Majesty Queen Elizabeth II; 17, from B. M. Patten, *Human Embryology,* 3rd ed., copyright © 1968 by McGraw-Hill, Inc. Used with permission of McGraw-Hill Book Company (top left and bottom); 18–22, Cecil B. Jacobson, M.D.; 23, photographs courtesy Museum of Science and Industry, Chicago.

Chapter 17: pp. 578–79, courtesy NASA; 1, courtesy Harry A. Wilmer, M.D., Ph.D.; 2, courtesy Michael E. DeBakey, M.D.; 3, Arthur Kornberg, M.D.; 5, Henri Cartier-Bresson/Magnum; 6, Larry Burrows, *Life* Magazine, © Time, Inc.; 7, courtesy WHO; 8, Raymond F. Chen, M.D., Ph.D./NIH (top), Ralph Bredland/NIH (bottom); 9, Bob Brooks.

Index

(Page numbers in *italics* refer to illustrations;
body charts refer to the color insert;
n refers to footnotes.)

Cancer (*cont.*)
  of stomach, 207 (table), *211*
  survival rates in, for selected sites,
    211
  treatment, 94, 205
  twins, incidence in, 209
  urinary, *206,* 207 (table), *211,* 426
  of uterus, *206,* 207 (table), 208, *208,*
    211, 460, 463
  viral causes, 188, 200, 202–05, *204*
  warning signals, 207 (table), 210
Candida albicans, 25
Candidiasis, 25
Canine teeth, 299
Cannabis, *see* Hashish; Marihuana
Capillaries, *247,* 248, *248,* 252, 253, *253,*
    254, 255, 266, 423, *424,* body
    chart 9
  diseases, 256 (table)
  glomerular, *270, 270,* 271, *271*
  in lung, *424*
  in small intestine, *313*
Caplan, Nathan S., quoted, 39–40
Carbohydrates, 279, 286 (table), 311,
    313, 546
  calories, 284
  food sources, 286 (table)
Carbon 12, atom of, *90*
Carbon dioxide
  atmospheric, rise in, 77
  and circulation of blood, 252, 253,
    254, 423
  used by green plants, 279
Carbon monoxide, 72, 73, 79
Carcinogens, chemical, 201
Carcinoma, 200, 583; *see also* Cancer
Cardia, 309
Cardiac sphincter, 309
Cardiovascular apparatus, 244, 257,
    268
Carlyle, Thomas, quoted, 71
Carrier
  of hemophilia trait, 250, *251*
  of microbes, 155, 181, 182, 182n
Cartilage, 423, body charts 5, 6
  and arthritis, *215*
Castration anxiety, 369
Cataract, 233
Catatonic, *335*
Cato the Elder, 469
Catullus, Gaius Valerius, quoted, 363
Cavities, in teeth, 303, 304, 305, 306
Cecum, *308,* 312, 312n
Cell culturing, 184
Cell differentiation, 526
Cells, 518, 520, *521*
  blood, *see* Blood cells
  cytoplasm, 185, 520, 523, 527, 528,
    530, 532n, 533, 541, 583
  ecosystem, 199, 523, 526
  germ (gametes), 524, 536, 537

multiplication, *see* Meiosis; Mitosis
nerve, *see* Neurons
nuclei, *521,* 522, 523, 526, 527, 528,
    530, 541
organelles, 520, *521,* 523
plasma, 158, 163
sex, *see* Gametes
somatic, 524, 525
structure, *521*
Cellulose, 279
Cementum, *302,* 303
Central nervous system, 219, 221–23,
    225, 227, 237, 404, 407, 414, body
    chart 8
Cereals, 286 (table), 288 (table), 290
    (table)
Cerebellum, 222, body charts 7, 8, 15
Cerebral palsy, 228
Cerebral thrombosis, 256 (table), 576
Cerebrospinal fluid, 223
Cerebrovascular disease, 256 (table),
    257, 257n
Cerebrum, 222, 257, body charts 7,
    8, 15
Cervantes, Miguel de, quoted, 303
Cervical cap, 574 (table)
Cervix, 453, *454, 459,* 460, 461, 561
  cancer, 208, *208,* 208n, 453
  in labor, 565, 566 (table), *566–67,* 568
  and venereal disease, 175, 176
Cesarean section, 565
Chambon, Dr., and vaccination, *160*
Chancroid, 172
Character disorders, 333, 334, 339–40
Charas, 414
Charlemagne, 125
Charles I, of England, 244
Charles IV, Emperor, 129
Charles VIII, of France, 170
Charles IX, of France, 276
Chastity, and health, 479
Chaucer, Geoffrey, quoted, 390, 491,
    493
Chekhov, Anton, 44
Chesterton, G. K., 293–94
Chevreul, Michel, 258
Chickenpox, 170n, 192, 296
Child
  adoption, 572
  anxiety, 351, 352, 361–70
  hazards, 117–21
  preschool, *see* Preschool child
  school-age, industry versus inferi-
    ority in (Erikson), 329, *329*
  as toddler, 325, 357, 358 (table), 369
Childbearing children, in U.S., 548
    (table)
Children's Crusade (1237), 130
China, 42–43, 58, 127, 157, 240, 276,
    390, 447
Chlorination of water, 53, 61, 63

Chlorine, 282
Chlorophyll, 279
Chlorpromazine, 346
Cholera, 57, 61, 143, 150
Cholesterol, 258, 259, 259n, 264, 265,
    279n, 311, 312
Chopin, Frédéric, 45, *45*
Chordae tendineae, *246*
Chorion, 558, 559, *560*
Choroid, 231, *231,* 232
Christianity, early, 469, 470
Chromium, 282
Chromosomes, 522, *522,* 524, *524,* 525,
    525, 526, 527, 533, 534, *536,* 541,
    546
  chart, 525, *525, 536*
  and competition in athletics, 538–39
  and crime, 538
  deletion, 535
  disorders of number, during
    meiosis or mitosis, 535–40
  and infectious hepatitis, 545
  karyotype, 525, *525, 526*
  and LSD, 410, 411, 412
  and meiosis, *see* Meiosis
  and mitotic division, *522,* 525, *526*
  radiation damage, *546*
  translocation, 535
  X, *see* X-chromosomes
  XXY, 538, 555
  XYY, 534, 538, 538n
  Y, 524, 525, 537, 538, 541
  see also Genes; DNA; Heredity
Chronic diseases, 196–273 *passim,* 590
Ch'ung Ch'en, 390
Cigarette smoke
  carbon monoxide in, 73
  during smog conditions, 78
Cigarette smoking, *see* Smoking
Cilia, 425, 426, 427, 428
Ciliary body, *231,* 232
Circadian biological cycles, 10
Circulatory diseases, 242–72 *passim*
Circulatory system, 244, 248, 252–54,
    247, 248, 255, 257, 258, body charts
    9–10
Circumcision, 372n, 453
Cirrhosis, 292 (table), 311n, 402, 542
    (table)
"Civil Disobedience" (Thoreau), 447
Clarke, George L., 26; quoted, 13, 15
Claustrophobia, 337
Clean Air Act (1963), 79
Cleft lip (harelip), 550 (table), 553
Cleft palate, 549, 550 (table)
Clement VI, Pope, 127, 129
Cleopatra, 282, *282,* 384
Cleveland, Grover, 145
Climacteric, 463
Climate, as factor in ecosystem, 22
Clinic, psychiatric, 344

Clinical psychologists, 344
Clitoris, *454,* 464, 503, 504, 511, 512, 513, 514
Clotting of blood, 250, 282, body chart 2
Clubfoot, 550 (table)
Clyne, John, quoted, 127-28
Coagulation of blood, 250, 282, body chart 2
CNI (Greater St. Louis Citizens' Committee for Nuclear Information), 97
Coal
  and rise in atmospheric carbon dioxide, 76-77
  and smog, 56, 71
Cobalt, 282
Cocaine, 386, 387, 388 (table), 389
Cocci, 154, *154*
Cochlea, *99,* 100, 101, 236
  of guinea pig, 102, *104*
Cochlear duct, 100, 101
Codeine, 391
Codon, 530, *531,* 532
Coitus, 504, 514; see also Sex
Coitus interruptus, 573, 574 (table)
Colchicum, 214
Cold, common, 41, 190-91, 280
Cold sore, 154, 183, 188, 192
Colitis, 542 (table)
  ulcerative, 314n
Collagen, 307
Collagenase, 307
Colon, 308, *308,* 312, 314, *454*
  cancer, *206, 207* (table), 210, *211*
Color blindness, 235
Colostrum, 464, 564
Combat exhaustion, 338
Combat neuroses, 338
Combau, Tha, 25
Commoner, Barry, quoted, 77
Commonwealth Fund, 604
Communicable disease, 152-95
Community resistance to disease, 49-53
Compulsive, 333
Computer, 580, 581
Conception, see Fertilization
Condom, 573 (table)
Conducting system in heart, 246-47
Conductive deafness, 235
Cones of retina, 232
Confinement, see Birth
Congenital defects, see Birth defects
Congestive heart failure, 261, 262-63
Congreve, William, 496
Conjunctiva, *231,* 234
Conjunctivitis, 234, 416
Constipation, 314
Contact dermatitis, 213
Contraception, 441, 448, 449, 572

ancient writings on, 575
education concerning, 576
methods, 460. 573-75 (table), 576-77
oral, 444-45, 460, 573, 575 (table), 576
"Contract, The" (Hogarth), *483*
Conversion hysteria, 337
Convulsion, see Epilepsy
Cooper, Edward, 133
Cooper's ligament, *465*
Copper, 282
  food sources of, 287 (table)
Cornea, 231, *231,* 232
Coronary arteries, 248, 257, 258, 260, 268, 269, 430, body chart 10
  lipids in, *260*
Coronary circulation, 248
Coronary occlusion, 260
Coronary profile, 263-64
Coronary thrombosis, 260, 262, 576
Corpus luteum, 451, *456,* 458, 459, *459,* 460
Corpuscles, see Red blood cells, White blood cells
Cortex, adrenal, 237 (table), 238, 549
Cortex, cerebral, 222, 223, 236, 349, 399, 449, 507
Cortez, Hernando, 24
Corti, organ of, 100, 101, *104*
Cortisone, 238, 271, 272
Cosmic clock, outer, 10, 11
Cosmic radiation, 10, 91
Courtship, 471, *472,* 482-83, 499
  modern, 471-73
  nonhuman, 467-68, *468*
  primitive, 470-71
Cowper's glands, *450,* 451, 452, 453
Cowpox virus, 159, *160,* 161
Coyotes, and biological imbalance, 26
Cranberries, and ATZ, 82
Crane, Stephen, 376
Cranial nerves, 221, 223
Cranium, 221, body charts 1, 2, 8
Creosote, as carcinogen, 201
Cretinism, 238, 544
Crib death, 191
Criminal behavior, 333
  and genetics, 538, *539*
Crocodiles, found in sewage systems, 62n
Cro-Magnon man, 54
Crown of tooth, *302,* 303
C-type RNA virus, 205n
Culture
  and acceptance of death, 38
  and health, 30-46, *31, 32, 36-37,* 40, *45*
  and human ecology, 17-19
  as learned behavior, 32, 34-35
  of poverty (Lewis), 48, 49
Curie, Marie, 92, 317
Curie, Pierre, 92

Cuspids, *302*
Cyanosis, 261
Cyclazocine, 394
Cystic fibrosis, 238-39, 551 (table)
Cytomegalic inclusion disease, 193
Cytopathogenic effect, 184n
Cytoplasm, 185, 520, 523, 527, 528, 530, 532n, 533, 541, 583; see also Cells

Dacron graft, 582, *582*
Dairy foods, 286-90 (tables)
"Dance of Death, The" (Holbein), *122-23*
Dancing mania, 129-30
Daphnis & Chloe (Longus), 468
"Daphnis and Chloe" (Maillol), *468*
Darwin, Charles, 16, 321
Dating, see Courtship
Da Vinci, Leonardo, *557,* body chart
Davis, Maxine, quoted, 507, 508
DDT, 20, *21,* 22, 26, 53, 85, 86-88, 443
  banned by Nixon administration, 88
  excretion, 87
  in fatty tissue, 86
  insects resistant to, 87
  and louse-borne typhus, 84, 85
  and malaria mosquito, 81, 84-85
  persistence, 86, 87
  and reproduction, effect on, 87, *87*
  river blindness eliminated by, 84, 85
  and yellow-fever mosquito, 84
Deafness, 103, 105, 106, 235, 236
  conductive, 235
  nerve, 236
Death
  acceptance, 38
  awe, 46
  of child, pain caused by, 47
  excess of male over female, 540 (table), 540-41
  in U.S., due to selected causes, 542 (table)
Death rates
  of cigarette smokers, *429*
  decline in, for selected diseases, *588*
  infant, in U.S., 587, 591, 591n, 596, 596n
  maternal, *588*
  world, 442 (table)
Decibels
  defined, 101
  harm from high levels, 102, *104*
  scale, *102*
  see also Noise pollution
Deciduous teeth, *302,* 303
Defoe, Daniel, 134-35
Deglutition, 307
Deletion, chromosomal, 535
Delirium tremens, 402
Delivery of baby, see Birth; Labor

Immunization, *see* Immunity; Vaccine
Immunological memory, 158
Implantation of zygote, 455n, 456, 458, 460, 526, 558, 558n
Impotency, 511, 515–16
Impulse, nerve, 218, *218,* 219, *219,* 225
Incest, taboo against, 516
Incisors, 299, *302*
Incubator, *37, 601*
Incus, 99, *99,* 101
India, 27, 42, 127, 141, 143, 277, 420, 441, 447, 543
Indians, American, 61, 407, 414
   in culture of poverty, 49
   decimated by smallpox, 24
Infancy, 318–20, 323, 357, 358 (table), 362, 382, *588; see also* Baby
Infant mortality rates
   U.S., 587, *588,* 591, 591n, 596, 596n
   world, 442 (table)
Infanticide, 572, 575
Infection
   bacterial, 154
   deaths due to, in U.S., 542 (table)
   defined, 153
   etiological agents, 154–56
   gastrointestinal, 197
   heart injured by, 261
   during pregnancy, 545
   resistance to, *see* Resistance to infection
   subclinical, 164
   transmission, 155
   viral, 154, 185, 187, 188
   and vitamin C, 280
Influenza, 25, 150, 183, 190, 196, 569, 589, 590, 590n
   and antigenic shift, 166
   deaths due to, in U.S., 542 (table)
   Hong Kong, 25, 166, 190
   immunization, 162 (table), 165–66
   and meningococcic meningitis, 182
   virus, 25, 165, 166, 183, *184,* 190
Inoculation, *see* Vaccine
Insecticides, *see* Pesticides
Insects, 15, 31–32, *32,* 83, *84,* 88, 89
   disease carried by, 155
   governed by instinct, 20
   nonchemical controls, 88–89
   see also Pesticides
Instinct, 20, 466–68
Institute for Sex Research, 341
Insulin, 40, 239, 240, 241, 310, 311, 347, 546
Intercourse, sexual, *see* Sex (sexuality)
Interferon, 188–89, *188, 189,* 191
International Directory of Genetic Services, 555
International Health Division, of Public Health Service, 150
Intersexuality, 538, 538n

Intervillous spaces, 558, *560*
Intestinal glands, 313, *313*
Intestine
   large, *308,* 312, 314, body charts 13, 14, 15
   small, 297–98, 309, 310, 312–14, *313,* 398, body charts 13, 14
Intoxication, *see* Alcoholism
Intrauterine devices, 575 (table)
Intrinsic factor, 309
Inversion, temperature, 71
Iodine, 93 (table), 282, 282n
   food sources, 287 (table)
   for pregnant woman, 544
Iodized salt, 84
Ionizing radiation, 90
   damage from, 91–93
   sources, 91
   uses, 94–95
   see also Radiation
Ions, 91
Ireland, 22, *22,* 23, 144, 277
Iris of eye, *231, 232, 235*
Iron, 95, 282, 283
   deficiency, 249, 283
   food sources, 287 (table)
   for pregnant woman, 283, 543, 544
Ischemia
   cardiac, 256 (table), 257, 260
   cerebral, 257
   renal, 257
Islets of Langerhans, 239, 310, 311, 546
Isoniazid, 178, 179, 587
Isotopes, 90; *see also* Radioisotopes
Israel, 361, 437
Issa, quoted, 83
Issac, Alick, 189
IUdR, 190
Ivan IV, of Russia, 500

Jacobi Hospital, adolescent ward in, 374, 374n, 378
James I, of England, 301n; quoted, 421
Japan, 58n, 76, 432–33, 447, 448, 592
Jaundice, 194, 311n, 312, 547
Jefferson, Thomas, 276
Jejunum, *308,* 312
Jenner, Edward, 151, 159, 161, 244, 259; quoted, 243
Jews, 486
   ancient, 42, 170, 397, 461, 469, 575
   persecution, and Black Death, 130
Joan of Arc, 144–45, 147
Joey ("the mechanical boy"), 323–24, *324,* 325–26, 328, 329n
Johnson, Lyndon B., 107
Johnson, Samuel, 482
Johnson, Virginia E., 503, 505, 514, 515; quoted, 509–10, 511, 512

Joints, 213–16, *215, 216,* body charts 1, 2, 5
Journal of the Plague Year (Defoe), 134, 135
Judeo-Christian culture, 469, 470, 553
Julian, Emperor, quoted, 371
Justinian, Emperor, 125, 126, 134
Juvenal, quoted, 155

Karyotype, 525, *525,* 536
Kavanaugh, Robert E., quoted, 477
Keats, John, quoted, 44
Kellogg Foundation, W. K., 604
Kemble, James, quoted, 148, 466
Kendeigh, Charles S., 5
Kennedy, Rose (Mrs. Joseph P.), 604
Ketone bodies, 240
Khat, 389
Kidneys, 253, *253,* 254, 269–71, *270,* 283, 404, 580, body chart 15
   artificial, 272, 306n, 583
   cancer, 426
   diseases, 271–72, 273, 542 (table), 569, *588*
   ischemic, 257
   in pregnancy, 564
   transplant, 272, 583
Kinsey, Alfred C., 341, 466, 475, 476, 506, 514; quoted, 340, 480
Kirkendall, Lester A., 478, 479
"Kiss, The" (Brancusi), *502*
Kitasato, Shibasaburo, 124
Klinefelter's syndrome, *536, 537,* 538
Klobukowska, Ewa, 539
Koch, Robert, 152, 179, 440
Korean War, 22, 495
   and anxieties of U.S. prisoners, 352
   time lapse between injury and surgical care, 116
Korsakoff's psychosis, 402

La Barre, Weston, quoted, 470–71
La Rochefoucauld, Duke de, 262, 262n
La Salle, Pouletier de, 258
Labia majora, *454,* 464, 503, 504
Labia minora, *454,* 464, 503, 504, 505, 512, 513, 514
Labor
   dry, 565
   pain, 568
   stages, 565, 566 (table), *566–67*
Lacrimal apparatus, *235*
Lactation, 464
   caloric demands for, 284
   "witch's milk," 563
Lacteal, *313*
Lactiferous duct, 464, *465*
Lactiferous sinus, 464, *465*

Lagrange, Joseph L., 283
Lamb, Charles, 8; quoted, 9, 431
Lamb, Mary, 8, 9, 11
Lambs, fetal, in synthetic amniotic
    fluid, *601*
Land, limited arable, 436–37, 443
Lanugo, 561, 562
Lao Tzu, quoted, 265
Large intestine, *308*, 312, 314, body
    charts 13, 14, 15
Larynx, 307, *308*, 423, body charts 11, 12
    cancer, 207 (table), 426, 431
Laser beam, 95
    for eye surgery, 53
Latency period (Freud), 329
Lavoisier, Antoine L., 283, 284
L-dopa, 230, 230n
Lead poisoning, 404
Lear, John, quoted, 306n, 528
Lee, Philip R., quoted, 48
Lee, Robert E., 145
Leeuwenhoek, Anton van, quoted, 152,
    440
Lemmings, *434*, 435
Lenin, Nikolai, 242, 244, 258, 259
Lens of eye, *231*, 232, 233
Leonardo da Vinci, *557*, body chart
Leper, in medieval Europe, *40*, 40n
Leprosy, 153, 544n, 596
Lesbians, 342, 343
Leukemia, 200, 201, 204–05, *204*, *206*,
    207 (table), 250, 306
Leukocytes, *see* White blood cells
Leukocytosis, 250
Lewis, Oscar, 48, 49
Librium, 395
Ligaments, *231*, 460, body charts 1, 2,
    3–4, 5
Limbaugh, Conrad, quoted, 16
Limbs, artificial and replanted, 225,
    226, 581
Lindenmann, Jean, 189
Lipase, 309, 310, 311
Lipids, in arteries, *260*
Lister, Joseph, 440
Lithium carbonate, 347
Liver, 253, *253*, 254, 258, 269, *308*, 310,
    311, 313, 398, 399, 404, body charts
    13, 14, 15
    and bile, 254, 258, 311, 312, 314
    cell, *521*
    circulation, *247*
    cirrhosis, 292 (table), 311n, 402, 542
    (table)
Lobotomy, prefrontal, 347
Locusts, 83, *84*
Lockjaw, *see* Tetanus
London
    Great Fire, 137
    Great Plague (1665), 131, 132, 134–37,
    135, 143

smog disaster (1952), 74, 75
London-type smog, 71–72, *73*, 77
Loneliness, 380
Longevity, 441, 441 (table), 587, 587n,
    589, 590, 591, 592, 594
Longfellow, Henry Wadsworth, 118;
    quoted, 68
Longus, quoted, 468
Los Angeles
    gonorrhea case rates, 173, 174, 175
    (table)
    plague (1924), 139–42, *141*
Los Angeles County Health Depart-
    ment, organization of, 602 (table),
    603
Los Angeles County Medical Associa-
    tion, 78
Los Angeles-type smog, 71, 72–73, 75,
    78, 79
Louse
    body, 20, 22, 26
    and DDT, *21*
    typhus transmitted by, 144
Love
    anxiety versus, 382–83
    as art of giving, 383
    discipline required by, 381
    in marriage, 482, 499, 502
LSD, 388, 389, 405, 407–12, 413 (table)
    and chromosomes, 410, 411, 412
    nonpsychic effects, 410–12, *411*
    psychic effects, 408–10
    tolerance, 408
Lucan, quoted, 168
Lucretius, quoted, 56, 227, 492–93
Lumbago, 216
Lunar months, 556, 561–63
Lung cancer, 200n, 207 (table), 427
    (table), 590
    atmospheric factors, 76
    death rate from, 426
    incidence, *206*
    prevention, 207 (table)
    and radiation, exposure to, 18, 208
    and smoking, 200, 208, 428–29, 431
    survival rates, *211*
    in uranium miner, 18, 201, 208
    warning signals, 207 (table)
Lungs, 245, *247*, 254, 269, *308*, 398, 399,
    404, 423, *424*, *425*, body charts 11,
    12, 13, 15
    bronchogram, *425*
    cancer, *see* Lung cancer
Luteinizing hormone (LH), *456*, 457,
    458, 459, 460
Lydall, Sarah, 133
Lymph, *253*, 255, 313, *313*
Lymphatics, 158, 199, 200, 244, 250, *253*,
    255, *255*, 313, *313*
    tumor, 210
Lymphangitis, 255n

Lymphangiograms, *255*
Lymphatic ducts, 244, 313, *313*
Lymphatic system, 244, 254–55, *255*,
    313, *313*
Lymphocytes, 194, 255, 410, 410n
Lymphogranuloma venereum, 172
Lymphoma, *206*, 207 (table)
Lynch, Henry T., 555
Lysosomes, *521*, 523

Mabaan tribe, keen hearing of, 105
Macaque monkey, 5, *5*
MacArthur, William, quoted, 136
McCormick, Michael, 368
McElroy, William D., quoted, 448
Macfadden, Bernarr, 315
Macular area of retina, *231*, 232
Magic, belief in, 38, 40
Magnesium, 282
Maillol, Aristide, *468*
Malaria, 150, 443, 469, 598
    cause, 154
    resistance to, and sickle-cell trait, 29
    transmission, 81, 84–85, 155
    see also Mosquito, malaria
Male reproductive system, *450*, 451–53
Malinowski, Bronislaw, quoted, 38
Malleus, 99, *99*, 101
Malnutrition, *274–75*, 296, 297, 406, 569
    in alcoholism, 401 (table), 402
    and mental retardation, 541
    and poor resistance, 156
    and tuberculosis, 179
    see also Vitamins, deficiency
Malocclusion, 306
Malthus, Robert Thomas, 435–36
Maltose, 299
Mammary glands, *see* Breasts
Mandrake, 384
Manganese, 282, 544
Manic-depressive psychoses, 333, 334,
    336
Mansfield, Katherine, quoted, 44
Mantoux test for tuberculosis, 167,
    177, 178
Marat, Jean Paul, 145
Marboran, 190
Marcuse, Donald J., quoted, 375
Marihuana, 388 (table), 389, 405, 413
    (table), 414–20
    effects, 414–19
    and law, 419–20
    and sex, 416
    Vietnamese, 416–18, 418 (table), 419
Markle Foundation, 604
Marriage, 27, 347, 481–91, 493, 494
    age as factor, 490–91
    and anxieties in sexuality, 508–16
    passim
    campus, 496–99

Sebum, 451
Seconal, 395
Sedatives, 395–96
Seizure, see Epilepsy
Selenium, 282
Self-love, 382
Semashko, Nikolai Alexandrovich, 242
Semen, 435, 452, 453
Semicircular canals, 99, 100, 100n
Semicircular ducts, 100, 100n
Seminal vesicles, 450, 451, 505
Seminiferous tubules, 451
Semmelweis, Ignaz, 155, 440
Seneca, Lucius Annaeus, quoted, 71
Senescence (aging), 591–95
Senility, 334, 542 (table)
Septic tank, 67, 67n
Septum, atrial, 245, 247
Serendipity, 586
Serum, 250, 252, 252 (table)
Seventh-Day Adventists, 604
Sewage disposal, 59, 62, 63
Sex (sexuality), 369–70, 383, 481
    in aged people, 514–15
    and alcohol, 400
    anxieties, 508–16 passim
    chromosomal, 537–39
    determination, 524, 525
    effect in circulatory disease, 268–69,
        269 (table)
    in female, 504–05, 506, 507, 508, 509,
        510, 510n
    and frequency of intercourse, 507
    guilt associated with, 510, 510n, 511
    illness patterns influenced by,
        540–41
    intercourse, 503ff.
    in male, 505–06, 507, 508, 509, 510,
        510n
    and marihuana, 416
    in marriage, 502–16
    misconceptions regarding, 509–15
    normality, question of, 508
    nuclear, 539
    oral-genital, 508
    and orgasm, see Orgasm
    phases (Masters and Johnson), 503,
        504–05
    premarital, see Premarital sex
    tumescence, 504, 505
    variety, 508
    see also Reproduction
Sex-flush, 504, 505
Sex-linked illness, 235; see also
    Hemophilia
Shakespeare, John, 131
Shakespeare, William, quoted, 105, 117,
    122, 131, 132, 170, 213, 227, 235,
    248, 273, 278, 300, 320, 384, 400,
    473, 474, 592
Shame, 325, 379, 511

Shaw, George Bernard, 293, 315
Shearer, Marshall, quoted, 341
Shelley, Percy Bysshe, quoted, 71
Shigella, 181
Shigellosis, 181
Shingles, 170n
Shock therapy, 347
Shope, Richard E., 189, 202
Sickle-cell anemia, 29, 29, 541, 552
    (table)
Sigalert, 78
Sigerist, Henry E., quoted, 149
Sight, see Vision
Sikkim ecosystem, and DDT, 81
Sinoatrial node, 246, 247
Skene's ducts, 464
Skiing, precautions taken for, 120–21
Skin
    and allergies, 213
    cancer, 200, 201, 201n, 206, 207
        (table), 208, 208n, 211
    congenital defects, 550 (table)
    diseases, 41, 213, 451n
    ecology of, 36, 37
    receptors, 219, 219
Skin-diving, 120
Skinfold calipers, 285, 285
"Skin-in" and "skin-out" biology
    (Bates), 13
Skydiving, 120, 121
Small intestine, 297–98, 308, 309, 310
    312–14, 398, body charts 13, 14
Smallpox, 150, 157, 190, 598
    American Indians decimated by, 24
    cause, 157
    reported cases in U.S., 163 (table)
    and Turkish ingrafting, 157, 158, 161
    vaccination, 53, 151, 159, 160, 161,
        162 (table)
Smegma, 208
Smell, sense of, 298, 299
Smith, John, 421
Smith, Sydney, quoted, 212
Smog, 54–55, 59n, 70, 73, 201
    disasters caused by, 74
    London-type, 71–72, 73, 77.
    Los Angeles-type, 71, 72–73, 75, 78,
        79
    medieval, 56–57
    protective measures during, 78
    and sickness, 75–77
    tolerance levels for, 12
    see also Air pollution
Smog alert, 72, 72n
Smoking, 419
    and adolescents, 421–22
    and advertising, 422–23
    and atherosclerosis, 430
    and bronchitis, 428
    death rates for, 426, 427 (table), 428,
        429 (table), 430

economic aspects, 422–23
emotional roots, 422
health consequences, 426, 427 (table),
    427–31
and heart disease, 264, 427 (table),
    430
history, 421
and hypertension, 267
and lip cancer, 428, 431
and lung cancer, 200, 208, 428–29,
    431
and peptic ulcer, 310
during pregnancy, 430–31, 553
social aspects, 423
and tooth loss, 430
Smoking and Health, 426
Snail, 466, 466
Snake venom, as toxin antigen, 168
"Snorting," 404
Snuff, 386, 386
Socrates, 374, 592, 594
Sodium, 282
Soil, 57–58
Solid-waste disposal, 68–70, 69
Solid Waste Disposal Act (1966), 70
Somatotherapy, 344
Sonic boom, 107
Sophocles, 369, 594; quoted, 198
Sound waves, 98
    measurement, 101
    speed, 100
    see also Ear; Hearing
Space exploration, 585
Speck, Richard, 538
Spectro-Chrome, 316
"Speed freak," 405, 406
Spermatozoa, 369, 435, 451, 453, 453,
    457, 458, 459, 502, 507, 524, 524, 525,
    525, 526, 536, 537, 538, 556, 572
    route, 452
Sphincters, 309, 309, 450, 454
Spina bifida, 552 (table)
Spinal cord, 199, 199n, 219, 219, 220,
    221, 223, 224, 225, 229, body charts
    7, 8
    tumor, 227
Spinal nerves, 221, 223, 227
Spinal tap, 223
Spinoza, Baruch, 320–21, 328; quoted,
    508
Spirilla, 154, 154
Spleen, 158, 210, 255, 308, body chart 9
Spock, Benjamin, 358 (table)
Sponge and foam, as contraceptive,
    576 (table)
Stalin, Josef, 242
Stapes, 99, 99, 101
Staphylococci, 180 (table), 181, 191
Staphylococcus aureus, 19, 20, 26
Starches, 279, 286 (table)
Stefansson, Vilhjalmar, 276

Traumatic neuroses, 333, 338
Trench mouth, 306
Treponema pallidum, 154, *154,* 171, 172 (table)
Trichinosis, 42, 276n
Tricuspid valve, 245, *246,* 254
Triglycerides, 265
Triiodothyronine, 282n
Triple X syndrome, *536*
Trisomy, 536, 540
Trophoblast, 558, *560*
Trust, basic, *318–19,* 322, 332, 357, 358 (table), 362
Trypsin, 310
Tuberculin, 177, 179
Tuberculosis, 23, 24, 25, 177–79, 196, 197, 541, 589, 596, 598, 604
   BCG vaccine for, 167, 167n, 179
   cause, 154, 177
   deaths due to, in U.S., 178, 178 (table), 542 (table), *588*
   isoniazid as preventive, 178, 179, 587
   Mantoux test for, 167, 177, 178
   primary infection, 177
   reinfection, 177
   streptomycin for, 179, 587
   symptoms, 177
   transmission, 155, 178
   world-wide cases, 179
Tumescence in sexual response, 504
Tumor
   benign, 199, *199,* 204
   brain, 95, 225, 226, 232, 334, 346, 534
   malignant, *see* Cancer
   "solid," 200
   spinal cord, 227
Tundra, 437
Turbinates, body charts 11, 12
Turner's syndrome, *536, 537, 537*
Twain, Mark, quoted, 378
Twins, cancer incidence in, 209
Tympanic membrane (eardrum), 99, *99,* 100, 101, 236
Tympanum, 98, 98n
Typhoid, 20n, 58n, 61, 66, 147, 150, 180, 590, 596
   immunization, 168
   transmission, 155
Typhus, 20, 23, 84, 85, 143, 144, 147, 150, 154
   causative microorganism, 144

Ulcer, peptic, *see* Peptic ulcer
Ulcerative colitis, 314n
Ultracentrifuge, 523
Ultraviolet rays, 91, 91n
Umbilical cord, 559, *560,* 561, 562
Umbilical vessels, *560*
Underweight, 295–96
United Nations, 420, 597

United States
   health work by agencies of, 599
   population statistics, 444–45, *445,* 486
U.S. Department of Health, Education, and Welfare, 599, *600*
Universal donor, 252
Universal recipient, 252
Unwed mother, 380, 381, 382
Uranium, 90–91
Uranium miner, lung cancer in, 18, 201, 208
Uremia, 272
Ureter, *270,* body chart 15
Urethra, *450,* 452, 453, *454,* 464, body chart 15
Urethritis, nonspecific, 176n
Uric acid, 214
Urinary bladder, *see* Bladder
Urinary system, *see* Bladder; Kidneys
Urine, 254, 273, *273,* 283, 452
Uterus, 199, 449, 453, *454,* 455, 456, 458, *459,* 460, 461, 504, 526, 556, 558, *560*
   cancer, *206, 207* (table), 208, *208, 211,* 460, 463
   cross section, *560*
   in labor, 565, *566–67*
   lining, 455, *456,* 458, 459, *459,* 460, 461, 526, 558, 559, *560*
   and menstruation, 460–62
Utricle, 100n
Uvula, 307

Vaccine, 163, 598
   adenovirus, 191, 191n
   bacterial, 167–68
   BCG, 167, 167n, 179
   diphtheria, 162 (table), 169
   DTP, 169
   German measles, 162 (table), 164–65, 167, 192, 236, 545
   influenza, 162 (table), 165–66
   of living attenuated bacteria, 167
   measles, 48, 50, 53, 162 (table), 164, 170, 191, 192, 545
   mumps, 162 (table), 164, 167, 170, 191, 193
   of nonliving bacteria, 168
   pertussis, 162 (table), 168, 169
   poliomyelitis, 162 (table), 164, 167, 170, 604
   rabies, 51, 52, 52n, 53, 161
   rubella, 162 (table), 164–65, 167, 192, 236, 545
   smallpox, 53, 151, 159, *160,* 161, 162 (table)
   tetanus, 162 (table), 169
   tuberculosis, 167, 167n, 179
   typhoid, 168
   viral, 164–67

Vaccinia virus, 161, 162 (table), 167
Vagina, 453, *454,* 457, 458, *459,* 460, 461, 463, 464, 504, 505, 512, 513, 514
   in labor, 565
Vaginal contraceptives, 573 (table), 576, 577
Vaginal thrush, 176n
Vagus nerve, 223, body chart 7
Valley fever, 154, 191
Valves, of heart, *see* Heart valves
Vas deferens, *450,* 451, 453, 505
Vegetables, 286–88 (tables)
Veins, *247,* 248, 253, *313,* body charts 9, 10
Vena cava, 245, *246,* 253, body charts 9, 10
Venereal diseases, 25, 170–77
   historical notes, 170–71
   infants infected by, 176
   penicillin for, 173
   public protection against, 176
   in young people, 174–75
   see also Gonorrhea; Syphilis
Venom, snake, as toxin antigen, 168
Ventricles of heart, 245, *246, 247, 247,* 254, 260, 424, body chart 10
Venules, 248, *248,* 253, *253,* 254, *313*
Venus, 438
Vergil, 129, 390
Vermiform appendix, *308,* 312, 312n, body chart 14
Vernix caseosa, 562, *563*
Vespasian, Emperor, 46
Vesuvius, eruptions of (A.D. 79), 56, 60
Victoria, Queen, 250, *251,* 293, 568
Videotape, in psychotherapy, *580*
Vietnam War
   effect of defoliation, 596n
   gamma globulin used for U.S. troops, 194
   time lapse between injury and surgical care, 116
   and use of marihuana by U.S. troops, 416–18, 418 (table), 419
Villi, chorionic, 559, *560*
Villi, intestinal, 254, 312–13, *313,* body chart 14
Vincent's angina, 306
Virchow, Rudolf, 258
Virulence of microorganisms, defined, 153
Virus, 6, *15,* 25, 41, 89, *152, 153,* 154, 183, *184,* 186
   bacteria invaded by, 15, *15, 153,* 185
   and cancer, 188, 200, 202–05, *204*
   and common cold, 190
   DNA, 183, 185, 187, 188, 202, 203, 204
   drugs versus, 190
   growing, in culture of cells, 183, 184